Mosby's
FUNDAMENTALS OF MEDICAL ASSISTING
ADMINISTRATIVE AND CLINICAL THEORY AND TECHNIQUE

Mosby's
FUNDAMENTALS
OF
MEDICAL ASSISTING
ADMINISTRATIVE AND CLINICAL THEORY AND TECHNIQUE

Sharron M. Zakus, RN, BA, MS, CMA
Educator, Health Science Department
City College of San Francisco
San Francisco, California

De A. Eggers, BS, MBA
President, De A. Eggers & Associates
Health Care Consultants
San Rafael, California

Margaret A. Shea, RN, BA, MBA
San Francisco, California

SECOND EDITION

with 551 illustrations

The C.V. Mosby Company
ST. LOUIS · BALTIMORE · PHILADELPHIA · TORONTO 1990

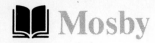 Mosby

Editor: Richard A. Weimer
Assistant Editor: Adrianne H. Cochran
Production Editor: Cynthia A. Miller
Production: Cracom Corporation
Book Design: Rey Umali

Printed in the United States of America

The C.V. Mosby Company
11830 Westline Industrial Drive, St. Louis, Missouri 63146

Library of Congress Cataloging-in-Publication Data

Zakus, Sharron M., 1942-
    Mosby's fundamentals of medical assisting: administrative and
clinical theory and technique / Sharron M. Zakus, De A. Eggers,
Margaret A. Shea.—2nd ed.
      p.   cm.
    Shea's name appeared first on previous ed.
    Includes bibliographical references.
    ISBN 0-8016-4280-9
    1. Medical assistants. I. Eggers, De A. II. Shea, Margaret A.
III. Title. IV. Title: Fundamentals of medical assisting.
    [DNLM: 1. Physicians' Assistants. W 21.5 Z21m]
    R728.8.Z343 1990
    610.73'7—dc20
    DNLM/DLC
    for Library of Congress

89-14010
CIP

C/VH/VH 9 8 7 6 5 4 3 2

To

"The Important Ones"

They Know Who They Are

Preface

THIS BOOK is the realization of a collaborative effort to provide the foundation for all administrative and clinical courses needed to prepare the professional medical assistant for a variety of employment opportunities. This book reflects contemporary concerns in medical assisting and focuses on the practical aspects of the profession while providing the theory needed for successful functioning in this challenging field.

Emphasis has been placed on quality patient care as the medical assistant's primary goal based on the development of a positive attitude toward individual responsibilities and a commitment to the other members of the health care team.

In each section of this book, the chapters are organized in an order of increasing complexity, helping the student develop the foundation of knowledge and skill required to perform the more complex and advanced procedures presented in subsequent chapters.

In addition to the logical organization of the material, the most current theoretical information available is presented with an emphasis on practical application. To assist the student in applying theory to actual patient care situations we have included numerous and varied photographs to illustrate correct technique and the facilities and equipment used to accomplish medical procedures. Each subject area is presented as a complete unit, including chapter objectives, extensive vocabulary with pronunciation keys and definitions, detailed step-by-step clinical procedures with rationales, review questions, and valuable suggested readings. Unique chapters have been included to provide students with practical aids for seeking employment, an understanding of specialization in health care and the need for teamwork, and an overview of holistic health to emphasize the role of the medical assistant in educating patients about the importance of preventive health care.

This book is designed to provide the foundation for all general, administrative, and clinical courses needed to prepare the medical assistant for employment in varied medical settings.

The general and administrative sections of this book have been redeveloped and expanded by De A. Eggers as a result of her extensive knowledge of the administrative side of the medical practice. She has long recognized the need for the medical assistant to be thoroughly trained to execute the administrative portions of the practice. Since it is rare that a physician receives any type of business training during the whole process of education, this burden frequently falls on the medical assistant. Thus De shares her extensive knowledge and practical applications with others in a combined administrative and clinical theory and skills textbook for medical assistants.

The clinical section of this book and the appendixes were developed as a result of extensive involvement with inpatient and outpatient care and medical assisting education and from a detailed textbook on clinical skills and theory by Sharron M. Zakus. To meet the needs of programs of study that require a combined clinical and administrative textbook, *selected* information from her clinical textbook has been incorporated into this new text. For a more comprehensive and complete textbook on clinical skills and theory, we refer you to *Clinical Skills and Assisting Techniques for the Medical Assistant*, second edition, by Sharron M. Zakus (St. Louis, 1988, The CV Mosby Co).

Part One of this book, "Fundamentals of Health Care," sets the stage by providing an overview of medical assisting, externing and job hunting, medical science and specialization, medical ethics and law, and a holistic approach to patient care. Part Two, "Administrative Theory and Techniques," provides much of the foundation needed for effective management, application of practical skills, and updating insurance requirements for the business side of the medical office or agency. Much of these two sections has been completely updated and expanded to meet the ever-growing needs of the trained medical assistant. The functioning of a medical practice, no matter what its entity, has become extremely complex over the last four years. To meet this need a tremendous amount of new information has been added to several chapters, and a new chapter on computers is included.

Part Three, "Clinical Theory and Techniques," has also been updated and expanded and presents the fundamental theories and related skills needed for clinical expertise and assisting. A special section on Universal Blood and Body Substance Precautions is included.

Appendixes have been written for convenient reference. The topics include common medical terminology combining word parts, common medical abbreviations, special vocabulary with definitions and pronunciation keys used to record information obtained from the review of systems and physical examination, sample medical reports, two-letter state abbreviations, and English and medical words frequently misspelled.

Overall, it is our intent and goal to provide a comprehensive and current textbook for training new medical assistant students as well as a reference and review source for individuals actively employed in the health care field or in need of a refresher course if anticipating a return to work.

The core curriculum for the medical assistant, as defined by the Curriculum Review Board of the American Association of Medical Assistants, Inc., has been our guide throughout the writing of this text.

Keeping in mind the diverse background and preparation levels of our readers, we have attempted the following:

- To write a readable and interesting textbook that will stimulate learning and motivate each reader;

- To lay a solid foundation of fact and principle in the field;

- To provide orientation for the student and active or inactive assistant by presenting a coherent, consistent, and meaningful analysis of the major issues encountered;

- To present the best ideas and most current information on the subject in such a way as to form a sound basis for teaching procedures; and

- To challenge the student to develop a permanent interest in the medical field and a desire for continued growth and knowledge.

It is our hope that you will find this book a welcome change and that it will be a textbook to benefit all educators, medical assistant students, practicing medical assistants, and those wishing to reenter this challenging field in allied health careers.

We wish to express our most sincere thanks to many friends, family, colleagues, and other specialists in the medical and health care fields for their support, encouragement, inspiration, and assistance given while this book was being written.

Our appreciation is also extended to the authors and publishers who have given their kind permission to use some of the illustrations from their books and to all firms and their representatives who cooperated with us in supplying illustrations and descriptive literature of their products. Their names are given appropriate credit throughout the book.

Special appreciation and recognition are due our outstanding publishing team for their expertise, patience, support, and guidance.

Finally, we wish to acknowledge all our past and present students, whom we have had the pleasure of knowing and working with in the classroom, and also to thank each other for the support, critiques, and reviews of our individual materials for this textbook.

Sharron M. Zakus
De A. Eggers

Contents

APPENDIXES

Mosby's
FUNDAMENTALS OF MEDICAL ASSISTING
ADMINISTRATIVE AND CLINICAL THEORY AND TECHNIQUE

Part One

Fundamentals of Health Care

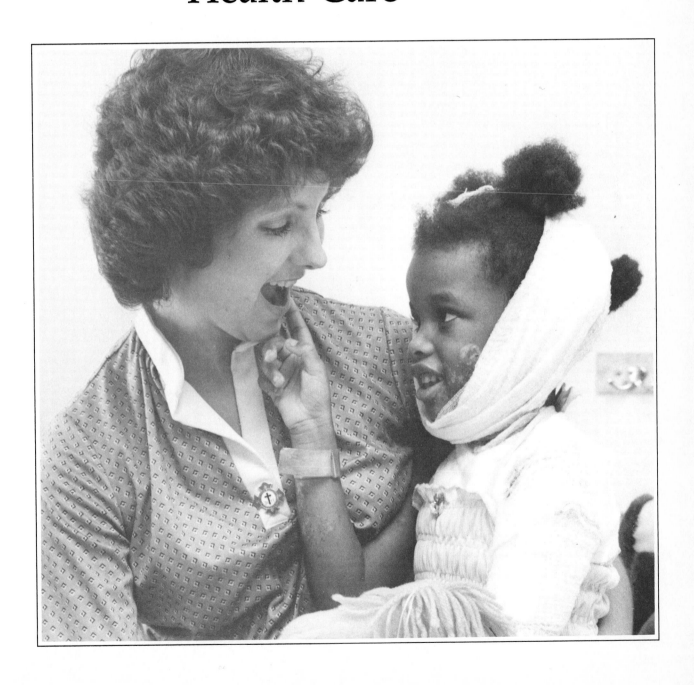

Chapter 1

The Professional Medical Assistant

- Development of professional medical assisting
- Qualifications of a medical assistant
- Areas of responsibility
- Rewards of a health care career

Objectives

On completion of Chapter 1 the medical assistant student should be able to:

1 Define the terms listed in the vocabulary.

2 Discuss the concept of health care teams.

3 State the sources of training available for medical assistants and the advantages and disadvantages of each.

4 List the purposes and functions of the American Association of Medical Assistants.

5 List 11 personal attributes that a medical assistant should possess.

6 List the basic skills needed in medical assisting and the integration process for the student.

7 Discuss the possible members of the health care team.

8 Describe the outpatient and inpatient facilities available for possible employment.

9 List and discuss the eight areas of responsibility that apply to medical assisting.

10 Discuss the rewards of a career as a professional medical assistant.

Vocabulary

confidential Private, secret.

consumer An individual who utilizes the services of a health care provider or practitioner.

health care facility The site at which health care is provided.

health care service The performance of a function related to health care.

health maintenance organization A health care organization that, for a fixed periodic premium, provides the subscriber with health care with an emphasis on preventive services.

health provider One who supplies or furnishes health care services.

independent physician association A health care organization that has a select group of health care providers to provide health care services to the public on a fee-for-service basis. The payments come from the IPA, which usually withholds a percentage for what is called a risk factor and which is later paid to the physician if the association makes a profit.

interpersonal relationships Interactions between individuals recognizing the need for communication and understanding.

job description A statement of the duties, skills, and responsibilities of a position.

patient education The provision of informa-

tion and support to a patient about an illness or condition or about methods of
maintaining general well-being.
practitioner Physician, nurse, or other individual licensed to dispense health care in a
variety of settings.

primary care The evaluation, advice, and
treatment of patients by physicians.
provider Generic term used to describe a
health care facility at all levels of care.
tangible Definite, real.

The need for health care is universal, and the
health sciences have a direct or indirect influence
on the life of every individual. Medical developments and events are being reported on television
and in newspapers, and consumers of health care
are becoming more interested in maintaining their
well-being and receiving the best medical care.

In the recent past medical care was relatively
simple. The few people who held paraprofessional
jobs associated with health care had little, if any,
training. As medical science advanced, new knowledge, extensive equipment, and complex treatment
techniques developed. In addition, the means of
providing care for increasing numbers of patients
changed from basic one-physician offices to sophisticated medical practices, clinics, and hospitals.

Health care providers, particularly physicians,
have come to rely on a variety of personnel in the
delivery of medical services. Medical assistants
have emerged as unique among allied health professionals. This is because of the broad scope of
training that prepares medical assistants for administrative or clinical positions. Professional medical
assisting is a career, not just a job, and the professional medical assistant is a valued member of the
various health care teams formed to provide necessary health care.

DEVELOPMENT OF PROFESSIONAL MEDICAL ASSISTING
Transition

The concept of training personnel specifically for
work in the physician's office was initiated by Dr.
M. Mandl, a biologist and former teacher in the
New York City Public Schools. Dr. Mandl established the first school for medical assistants in
1934. Today there are many private schools and
public community colleges throughout the country
with programs for training medical assistants for
diverse positions and career opportunities.

In its brief history, the medical assisting profession has undergone a remarkable transition. From
a humble beginning as the physician's general
helper, the medical assistant has evolved to be a
special member of the health care team. The medical assistant of today has a variety of options in

choosing where to work and, if it is desired to specialize, what area of specialization to consider.

Methods of Training

A career as a medical assistant can be attained
through one of the following:
* On-the-job training;
* Training at proprietary (private) schools; or
* Training at junior or community colleges.

At one time, on-the-job training was the most
common way of learning the duties and skills
needed in a medical office. After an individual acquired a position, he or she would learn how to assist the physician and perform other duties as the
occasion arose. Today, on-the-job training is rarely
the only preparation needed to work as a medical
assistant. More common today is attendance at either a proprietary school or a community college.
Once a program of training is completed and the
graduate obtains a position, he or she receives limited on-the-job training. At this time the new employee is introduced to the specific needs and requirements of the medical practice at which he or
she will work. There are advantages and disadvantages to each method of training, as described in
Table 1.1. All prospective medical assistants
should be aware of the advantages and disadvantages of each training method so that they are capable of responsibly making a decision that will affect their future professional career.

The Medical Assistant's Professional Organization

In 1959, about 25 years after the founding of the
first school for medical assistants, the American
Association of Medical Assistants (AAMA) established national headquarters in Chicago, Illinois.
Since its founding, the AAMA has grown to a
present membership of thousands of dedicated
medical assistants. As a nationwide organization,
the AAMA has the advantage of monitoring the
needs and status of medical assistants throughout
the country. In an effort to serve its membership
the AAMA participates in the accreditation of
training programs and supports continuing educa-

Table 1.1
Advantages and disadvantages of training methods

	Advantages	Disadvantages

On the job	1. Personalized training
	2. Income while learning
	3. Job security
	4. Depend on employer
		1. Training unique to facility/
		   environment
		2. Skills may not be transferable
		3. Salary may be lower
		4. Limited medical and related
		   knowledge

Proprietary school	1. Short-term courses
	2. Job placement services
	3. If accredited, graduates eligible
	   for certification examinations
	4. Higher potential earning power
	   than untrained personnel
		1. High cost of course
		2. Inflexible, predetermined course
		   of study
		3. Concentrated, short-term studies

Junior/community college	1. Broad scope of college-level vo-
	   cational and elective courses
	2. Low or no fees
	3. Graduates earn associate degree
	4. Many courses transferable to
	   4-year colleges for students inter-
	   ested in bachelor's degree
	5. Higher potential earning power
	   than untrained personnel
	6. If accredited, graduates eligible
	   for certification examinations
		1. Length of curriculum; either 1 or
		   2 years
		2. Loss of income-earning time
		3. Predetermined course of study

tion. It has also developed a mechanism for certifying the professional medical assistant. State and local divisions of the AAMA serve as links between the medical assistant and the national organization by distributing information about decisions made at the national level and providing information to the AAMA on local and regional needs.

Training programs for medical assistants are accredited and periodically reevaluated by a joint team from the AAMA and the American Medical Association (AMA). After a careful examination of all aspects of a program seeking accreditation, the accreditation team makes a recommendation to the Independent Committee on Allied Health Education and Accreditation of the AMA. A favorable recommendation will result in the accreditation of the proprietary-school or community-college program.

In 1962, in an effort to standardize the quality of medical assistants' knowledge, the AAMA developed a national examination for certifying graduates of accredited training programs or individuals with documented work experience. These examinations are given semiannually (in January and June) in over 100 cities throughout the United States. A medical assistant need not be a member of the AAMA to be eligible for the examinations. A state or local branch of the AAMA will be able to assist a candidate for examination by providing application forms and information about the examination site. Successful completion of the basic examination will result in the award of the title, certified medical assistant (CMA). After the basic CMA examination has been passed, specialty-area examinations are available. These examinations and subsequent credentials include the following:

- Administrative (CMA-A);
- Clinical (CMA-C);
- Combined administrative and clinical (CMA-AC); and
- Pediatric (CMA-P).

A priority of the AAMA is continuing education for medical assistants. This is accomplished through professional publications, annual meetings, and accredited continuing education courses.

The Professional Medical Assistant is a bimonthly journal that publishes articles on clinical advances, opinions, and experiences. These articles provide medical assistants with information on developments in their profession and other medical and allied health fields. In addition, an annual AAMA convention held in different cities throughout the country offers medical assistants the opportunity to participate in workshops, share ideas with colleagues, and attend lectures and view exhibits planned to disseminate the most current information about the medical and allied health professions. Continuing education courses developed at local and state levels give the medical assistant another source for acquiring knowledge about new administrative and clinical techniques. Any qualified person, organization, or educational facility that develops a course may submit the curriculum to the AAMA for approval so that medical assistants can receive recognized continuing education units when they attend and meet the standards of the course. Continuing education is not currently required of medical assistants as it is for physicians and registered nurses, but it may be required in the future. In either case, medical assistants will find that participating in continuing education courses is a source of continued advanced learning, increased self-confidence and self-esteem, and increased value as an employee.

QUALIFICATIONS OF A MEDICAL ASSISTANT
General Qualifications

A successful medical assistant must possess the educational background and personal attributes necessary for working with people. Try to remember a time when you required the services of a physician in private practice or care in another health care facility. Whether you were having a routine examination or you were ill and seeking aid, you may recall that you perceived yourself as the most important person in the process. Regardless of his reason for being in a medical setting, the consumer-patient's attention is directed toward his own personal well-being. Patients who are well are seeking reassurance that they will continue to be well, and patients who are ill are concerned about the outcome of their illness and anxious to be well. In both cases, the emotional state of the patient is altered, and the patient needs special emotional support as well as physical care.

Personal Attributes

The health care consumer expects the attention of individuals who are prepared to meet his special needs. People who wish to become members of the health care team will need to evaluate their attributes and determine whether they possess qualities compatible with those recognized as important for success in these professions. The required personal attributes include the following:
- Ability to communicate clearly with others;
- Common sense;
- Diplomacy;
- Honesty;
- Interest in helping others;
- Integrity;
- Dependability;
- Empathy;
- Tolerance;
- Sense of humor;
- Consideration;
- Attentiveness to personal appearance;
- Calm manner; and
- Courtesy.

Basic and Technical Skills

Personal attributes of the medical assistant are qualities that must be developed over time through family and interpersonal relationships, experience, and education. The technical skills required of the assistant can be acquired through a sequence of courses designed to meet the needs of the student and the medical community. The required professional cognitive and performance knowledges and skills are presented in this book. Previously acquired basic skills that will enhance the medical assistant student's success include the following:
- Mathematics;
- Grammar;
- Written communication;
- Spoken communication;
- As well as a knowledge of human behavior.

Integration of Qualifications

After acquiring the necessary theoretical foundation, the medical assistant student will be eased into the work environment through a student work experience program. This program allows the student to observe and participate as a member of an actual health care team. This concept is discussed further in Chapter 2.

A team is a group of individuals, each with a different function, who coordinate their efforts to accomplish a specific goal. The team concept of health care has evolved to cope with the complex environment of health promotion, maintenance, treatment, and rehabilitation. A health care team is made up of a variety of health care providers

Table 1.2
Health care team members

Personnel	Duties
Electrocardiogram (ECG) technician	Obtains electrocardiographic tracings from patients and prepares tracings for interpretation by physician
Electroencephalogram (EEG) technician	Obtains electroencephalographic tracings from patients and prepares tracings for interpretation by physician
Licensed practical nurse (LPN) Licensed vocational nurse (LVN)	Clinical practitioners who work under supervision of physician
Medical technologist	Obtains, prepares, and examines samples of body tissues and fluids to assist in determination of presence of disease processes
Medical records technician (MRT)	Extracts data, organizes records, and maintains medical records and health statistics for a facility under direction of registered records administrator (RRA)
Medical transcriptionist	Prepares reports, records, and correspondence from physician's dictation
Nuclear medicine technologist	Under direction of physician-specialist, obtains diagnostic data or treats disease processes with radioactive nuclides
Occupational therapist (OT)	Under direction of physician-specialist, designs and executes a program to retrain patients for new or expanded job descriptions
Orthotist	Under direction of physician-specialist, designs braces or equipment to assist patients in regaining as close as possible previous levels of personal or job functioning after a debilitating injury.
Physician	Directs and monitors health care services
Physician's assistant (PA)	Certified to conduct specified diagnostic evaluations and/or treatment plans under supervision and assumed responsibility of physician in certain specialty areas
Psychiatric technician (PT)	Under direction of psychiatrist, works one-on-one to bring patients back to previous level of social functioning.
Registered dietician (RD)	Plans therapeutic nutrition programs, instructs patients in plan, and develops sample menus as guides
Registered nurse (RN)	Administers treatment under direction of physician and plans and organizes nursing procedures for health maintenance, rehabilitation, and prevention of complications
Registered physical therapist (RPT)	Under direction of physician-specialist, designs and executes therapy designed to rehabilitate patients to previous functional levels.
Respiratory therapist	Obtains diagnostic information on patient's respiratory functions and prepares data for interpretation by physician; treats patients with respiratory conditions under physician's orders
Work hardening therapist (WHT)	Under direction of physician-specialist, works with patients in their actual work situation to retrain them to previous levels of functioning after a disabling injury.
X-ray technician	Obtains x-rays from patients and prepares x-ray film for interpretation by the physician.

(Table 1.2) whose primary concern is the health and welfare of each individual patient. The medical assistant is an essential member of the team.

AREAS OF RESPONSIBILITY
General

Health care services are provided in three basic types of facilities that provide either outpatient or inpatient services. Outpatient services are available for patients who are ambulatory and able to go to a physician's office, a clinic, or a health care center for required medical services or for patients who are cared for at home.

Inpatient care is provided in hospitals, nursing homes, or hospices in which patients reside temporarily or permanently. All necessary medical services are provided through these facilities. The pro-

Table 1.3
Possible job opportunities

Type of facility	Description of facility services	Medical assistant's role
Outpatient		
Testing centers	Collect specimens or record data and evaluate and report results to physician	Administrative
Rehabilitation centers	Assist patient return to optimum functioning	Administrative or clinical
General practice or specialist-physician's office	Private health care	Administrative or clinical
General clinic	Primary care	Administrative or clinical
Speciality clinic	Care required for specific condition, e.g., surgery, gynecology, cardiology, dermatology	Administrative or clinical
Health maintenance organizations (HMOs)	Total care; emphasis on preventive medicine	Administrative or clinical
Hospital-based care plans	Outpatient services with easily available ancillary services; similar to HMOs	Administrative or clinical
Accredited Surgical Center (ASC)	Freestanding short term surgical cases with associated records and staff	Administrative and clinical
Inpatient		
Treatment rooms	Perform minor procedures and diagnostic examinations	Administrative or clinical
Surgery	Surgical cases (major and minor) with associated records and staff assignments	Administrative
Patient care units	Provide all basic inpatient services	Administrative (ward clerk, unit secretary)
Admissions department	Initiates record	Administrative

fessional medical assistant can select a position from among a vast array of opportunities in outpatient and inpatient facilities; some of these job options are presented in Table 1.3.

Employee Interaction

Medical assistants are most often employed in outpatient health care facilities, particularly by physicians in private medical practice. A medical assistant working in this area may work with administrative personnel such as bookkeepers, insurance clerks, receptionists, and clinical personnel such as electrocardiogram technicians, laboratory technicians, nurses, and physician's assistants. The health care team in a medical office varies with the number of physicians, number of patients cared for, and specialty of the practice.

The office medical assistant frequently has to communicate with health care team members employed in various other outpatient settings. These team members can be considered extensions of the medical office staff, since the services they provide must be coordinated with the services provided in the physician's office. Outpatient services, also called ancillary services, with which medical assistants may communicate include medical testing facilities (laboratory, radiology), rehabilitative services (physical therapy, occupational therapy), and support services (home health aid, transportation). The office medical assistant's relationship with ancillary service personnel begins when office patients are referred for necessary ancillary medical services.

A medical assistant employed in an outpatient setting can expect some patients to require hospitalization. The medical assistant will communicate with hospital admitting clerks, giving information regarding patient insurance plans, unit secretaries, and nurses when arranging for the patient's hospital admission, during the course of the patient's stay, and when the patient is about to be discharged.

Other options for medical assistants who wish to work in outpatient care facilities include positions in one of the ancillary care settings, in general or specialty clinics or agencies, in health maintenance organizations (HMOs), or in hospital-based care plans. Another possibility for the medical assistant is employment in inpatient facilities such as hospital treatment rooms, hospital surgical suites, hospital admissions departments, emergency room (ER), walk-in clinics, urgent care centers, accredited surgical centers, trauma centers, and burn units.

These examples demonstrate some of the employment opportunities available to medical assistants. The roles that the medical assistant can assume are increasing as the options in health care expand. In addition, there is an increasing awareness of the role and function of the medical assistant. Physicians, nurses, therapists, and technicians recognize a well-trained medical assistant as a vital part of the health care team.

Basic Preparation

Part One of this book will provide the medical assistant with a broad foundation of information that will be necessary regardless of the employment opportunity selected. Discussion of the beginnings of medical science, medical law, and medical ethics and how they influence the practice of medical care will provide the basic information necessary to understand why and how the procedures described throughout this book developed. The methods of obtaining a desired job will assist students during the remaining course of study by preparing them to evaluate their attributes and skills. Finally, an overview of holistic health care, which emphasizes health maintenance and maximizing each individual's potential, will allow students to approach their varied studies from an integrated perspective.

Administrative Assisting

Administrative assisting is viewed as the business portion of the medical assisting profession. The administrative assistant works in the part of a facility that is commonly referred to as the "front office" and handles the business portion of the practice. The size and patient volume of a practice or agency will determine the number of assistants necessary to perform the administrative duties. The solo administrative assistant's job will include all of the responsibilities discussed in Part Two of this book. In an office or other health care agency that employs more than one administrative assistant, the responsibilities will be divided among these individuals. The administrative assistant sets the tone for an efficiently run facility and creates the public's initial impression of the personnel and the facility.

Clinical Assisting

The clinical assistant working in the examination or treatment area (the "back office") must provide an environment that is safe, private, and comfortable for the patient. Depending on the number of assistants working in the clinical area, responsibilities will include all or designated portions of the knowledge, skills, and techniques presented in Part Three of this book. The clinical assistant will prepare the patient for routine and special examinations, assist the physician, and collect clinical data when appropriate. In addition, the clinical assistant can sustain the patient's confidence and provide a communication link between the patient, the physician, and the other staff members.

A medical assistant may choose to work in a facility that will allow him or her to function in both the administrative and clinical areas or may select one specialty area.

Patient Education

As a member of the health care team, the medical assistant has the opportunity to perform a vital service for all patients who enter the health care facility. This service is patient-consumer education. The benefit that the patient derives from this education is well worth the time spent on providing it and will reflect favorably on the good will of the provider. An informed patient is generally more relaxed and cooperative than an uninformed one when receiving care in any medical situation. In the role of medical educator, the medical assistant can also provide valuable information to the patient about medical care facilities and providers with which the patient may come in contact, such as laboratories, therapeutic agencies, and hospitals.

Patient education within the facility

In the course of your work as a medical assistant, regardless of your position, you will have numerous opportunities to perform this vital service of patient education. Again, try to put yourself in the position of the patient. The anxiety and stress of being in a medical setting can easily be appreciated when the patient does not understand why a procedure is necessary or how it will be accomplished.

As a source of information for patients, the medical assistant can anticipate patients' needs for certain information and provide it without being asked. A receptive environment will provide the patient with a comfortable atmosphere in which to ask questions (for example, "Why do I have to get in this position for the examination?" "What is the doctor going to do?" "How do I get my insurance company to pay for this?"). Medical assistants must work with the rest of the health care team to create an atmosphere that will inspire the patient's confidence and trust.

Within the work setting, the medical assistant can anticipate the patient's need for basic information regarding administrative and clinical procedures. The *administrative assistant* can volunteer information regarding appointment schedules, billing, insurance services, telephone hours, the physician's office hours, and how to reach the physician before or after office hours. The medical assistant should also emphasize the office policy on confidentiality. All of these measures will help establish rapport between office personnel and patients and give them added confidence to ask questions.

Patients often feel inhibited (because of shyness or awe) about questioning the physician directly. The medical assistant can acknowledge this common situation and let the patient know that he or she is available to transmit the patient's questions to the physician. The medical assistant may suggest that patients write down their questions before the appointment and show the list to the physician or verbally ask their questions one by one to the physician. The role of the medical assistant as the patient intermediary will help establish rapport between the patient, the physicians, the medical assistant, and other personnel in the health care agency. The *clinical assistant* can continue the patient education process by perceiving the patient's lack of understanding of the various examination and treatment procedures. Explaining a process before it begins will alleviate anxiety and again provide an atmosphere receptive to patient questions.

Patient education for referred patients

Providing information about services and facilities outside of the immediate work area may also become the medical assistant's responsibility. You may be called on to provide information about support services available in the community, such as transportation and visiting-nurse services. It may also be necessary to assist the patient in obtaining financial assistance for medical services through appropriate insurance coverage or through public medical assistance provided for those unable to pay for care.

The more common situation in which the medical assistant may have to provide educational services occurs when a patient requires hospitalization or is referred to another health care facility for medical tests or consultation. The medical assistant can do a great deal to alleviate the patient's fears by telling the patient what to expect in the new setting. This readily available information will reassure the patient that such referrals are routine, because you are demonstrating that you have made such referrals before.

Medical information and new treatment methods are favorite topics with the popular media (television, radio, magazines, newspapers). Patients may ask questions about the medical news they have heard on television or radio or bring articles with them when visiting the physician. Although patients may be hesitant to approach the physician, they may attempt to involve the medical assistant in a discussion on the validity of the information or the effectiveness of the treatment. Again, the medical assistant can help patients by alerting the physician of their concerns or by encouraging patients to speak directly to the physician.

Interpersonal Relationships

Interpersonal relationships are diverse in all medical settings. The foundation for any positive interpersonal relationship in the medical setting is communication, both oral (see Chapter 9) and written (see Chapter 11).

Patients in a medical setting are subject to stress that may alter their behavior. They may be apprehensive, distrustful, or belligerent because of their fear or their denial of possible outcomes. The responsibility for establishing an effective medical assistant–patient relationship rests with the medical assistant. This relationship often serves as the foundation for the patient's relationships with the physician and other staff members. The effective medical assistant must be skilled, tactful, and empathetic in handling patients and must have a genuine interest in the individual person.

Interpersonal relations within the office or agency will be evident to patients and must be positive and consistent. All staff members will have a different relationship with the physician-employer, varying with each personality and area of responsibility. The medical assistant must be able to communicate effectively and work together to meet the primary goal of patient care. The physician and the medical assistant must work together in a relationship based on consideration, trust, and professionalism. Individual relationships become a part of all staff relations in the office or agency. Positive relations in any work setting require compromise, support, and cooperation. Each staff member must contribute to the team effort. The team spirit will inspire confidence and trust in the patient.

Public Relations

The medical assistant is the public representative of the physician or health care agency. In this role the medical assistant can expect to have contact with outside physicians, staff members of other offices or facilities, salespersons, supply company representatives, and service representatives. Courtesy, patience, and effective communication skills will help you present a positive public image of the physician's office or the agency and its staff. These skills will also establish you as an asset to your employer.

REWARDS OF A HEALTH CARE CAREER

The tangible rewards associated with any career are measured by job security and salary. Job security includes availability of positions and acceptable performance of designated responsibilities. Job security also relates to an established working environment. Once a medical assistant is established as part of a health care team, the option to remain in the same position or be promoted to a level of increased responsibility exists. While salaries vary in different areas of the country and in urban or rural locations, the trend is toward improved wages and benefits.

Although job security and adequate salary are necessary to provide for basic needs, most people also seek other rewards from their work. The higher needs of self-esteem and personal satisfaction can be met in a health care career because it provides opportunities for the following:
- Satisfaction through helping others;
- Personal growth and development;
- Pride through participation on a professional health care team and performance of professional skills; as well as
- Continuing education.

Conclusion

Individuals choosing a career in medical assisting will find themselves in a challenging profession that provides numerous opportunities to demonstrate acquired skills. In return the professional medical assistant will receive personal satisfaction and enhanced self-esteem for a job done well. Becoming part of a health care team is a rewarding experience. As a member of that team, the medical assistant can anticipate an ever-increasing level of responsibility as medical science and the medical professions continue to advance.

Review Questions

1. Why is health care considered a team effort?
2. Describe the method of training you are using to become a medical assistant. Compare and contrast your method with the other methods available.
3. What is the purpose of the American Association of Medical Assistants (AAMA)?
4. How can personal attributes affect your work as a medical assistant?
5. How will you integrate your personal, basic, and theoretical preparation as a medical assistant?
6. List and describe the duties of the possible members of a health care team.
7. Compare and contrast outpatient and inpatient services.
8. What responsibilities can you expect to assume throughout your career with regard to co-workers, patients, and public relations contacts?
9. What personal rewards do you expect to acquire from a career in health care?

SUGGESTED READING

American Medical Association: Winning ways with patients, Chicago, 1979, The Association.

Chapter 2

Extern Experience and Obtaining a Job

- The extern experience
- The job search

Objectives

On completion of Chapter 2 the medical assistant student should be able to:

1 Define the terms listed in the vocabulary

2 Determine the purpose of an externship program and describe where an externship might be conducted.

3 List the three advantages of an externship program to the school.

4 State the three theoretical and the two personal advantages of an externship program.

5 List the three possible personal opportunities of an externship program.

6 Establish his or her own externship program if necessary.

7 Define the relationship between an externship program and a course seminar.

8 Determine a method of assessing personal attributes.

9 State the primary purpose of the resume and cover letter.

10 Develop one basic and one alternative resume.

11 List the fundamental considerations in resume preparation.

12 List and describe the factors evaluated during the first-impression phase.

13 List the points evaluated in a formal application.

14 Describe the steps in preparing for an interview.

15 State the two purposes of a written follow-up to an interview.

16 List the five steps in the goal-setting process.

Vocabulary

attitude A way of thinking or feeling; also, a bodily position assumed to show feelings or mood of an individual.

attribute A personal trait or characteristic.

externship A limited experience in an environment in which students can apply learned theory under supervision.

goal The point or purpose determined to be a desirable end result.

integrity The condition of being competent, upright, honest, and sincere.

interpersonal relationship A connection or dealings between individuals, as in business interactions.

long-term Far reaching or extended into the future.

mannerism A habitual action, gesture, or style of speech unique to or identified with an individual.

objective An aim or end toward which any action is directed.

personal assessment The act of objectively determining the value of an individual's qualities or attributes.

perspective The ability to view incidents in correct relation to each other; the proper relationship of things to one another.

reference An individual to be consulted for information regarding another person.

resume A synopsis or summary of an individual's education, work experience, or skills prepared as an aid in obtaining a job.

seminar An unstructured meeting of individuals of similar education or training for the purpose of exchanging ideas and theories.

short-term Limited, lasting for a brief period of time.

theoretical Pertaining to abstract principles; based on ideas rather than practical experience.

As a medical assistant student you are preparing for an important position in the health care field. In this chapter the concept of an externship program and the process of obtaining a permanent position are introduced. One of the goals that you have set for yourself is to become an effective and efficient medical assistant. The administrative and clinical training available through an externship program will help you attain this goal, and the guidelines presented here for obtaining a job will help you acquire the position as a medical assistant that you want. The externship experience and obtaining a job are presented together in this chapter because they are closely linked in two ways.

First, the externship program occurs simultaneously with or soon after a theoretical foundation has been developed in the classroom. The externship program will provide you with information on and reinforcement of your skills. Second, the externship experience will expose you to potential employers and provide you with references for job hunting. This information is presented early in this book because it should be kept in mind throughout your future studies; each subject you study will eventually be put into practice.

The externship program provides you with an opportunity to make a smooth transition from student to paid employee and can be viewed as a period of personal adjustment. You will be involved in new interpersonal relationships and will begin to integrate the theories and skills you have been studying. With the support of instructors who are prepared to offer guidance through the externship program, you will have the opportunity to test yourself in a receptive environment.

The externship period can be used to evaluate your skills and preferences objectively in preparation for paid employment. The opportunity to experience administrative and clinical responsibilities under "real-world" conditions will allow you to develop, with your instructor's assistance, a method of evaluating your potential. The externship period will allow you to recognize your preference, select the areas of primary interest to you,

and examine the areas in which you create the most positive effect. You will also be able to determine areas that you may need to develop further or that you may wish to consider studying in future continuing education courses.

THE EXTERN EXPERIENCE

Many schools with programs for medical assistants provide a course entitled Externship or Work Experience. If the program is accredited by the American Association of Medical Assistants (AAMA), an externship is mandatory. In this course the student participates in a practical application of the theories learned in the classroom. The term *externship* is derived from the word *external,* because the externship experience occurs away from the self-contained environment of the classroom. The externship experience is offered in cooperative medical offices or hospitals in the community for a predetermined period of time. The course may extend from several weeks to several months. It involves working in one facility or rotating to several settings 1 or 2 days each week, 3 to 8 hours each day. During an externship program the experience is guided by an instructor who arranges for appropriate work settings for the student, monitors the student's adjustment and progress as an extern, and provides feedback for the student to make necessary adjustments.

Advantages to the School

While the primary purpose of an externship program is to benefit the student, it also provides secondary benefits to the school. By working cooperatively with community facilities, the school and the medical assistant program benefit by having the use of a variety of settings and equipment that are not available at the school. The externship program also provides a public relations link with the community. The presence of students, in community settings, reminds the public that the school and the medical assistant program are available for future students and that program graduates are available for employment. In addition, the externship period gives the medical assistant program director the opportunity to monitor community needs. This is accomplished because the externship instructors have ongoing contacts with the facilities, employers, and employees in the community. Students will also provide feedback on the observations they have made in the facility at which they serve their externships. The evaluation of community needs allows the individuals responsible for the medical assistant program to make appropriate decisions when adjusting the curriculum to meet student and community needs.

Advantages to the Student

The most important concerns in an externship program are the student and the advantages to the student of working in an actual medical setting. The basic advantages of an externship program are presented here as a guide to what should be sought from the experience. Keep them in mind as you proceed through the externship process. These advantages relate to your educational endeavors and to your personal growth.

Theoretical advantages

First, an externship program provides you with the opportunity to gain experience that will help you when you are ready to seek permanent employment. Second, you can begin to integrate the information learned separately in various clinical and administrative courses by applying this information in a practical setting. Third, the real-world setting of the externship provides you with the opportunity to observe and participate in the dynamics of the various interpersonal relationships that occur in a medical facility (medical assistant–medical assistant, physician–medical assistant, physician–patient, medical assistant–patient).

Personal advantages

The personal advantages of the externship program include the opportunity for you to develop a base of information to help determine which type of work, clinical or administrative, interests you most. You may also take advantage of this opportunity to recognize your strengths and weaknesses and develop or correct these personal characteristics as necessary.

Opportunities

When a health care facility or medical office accepts a student-extern they are accepting an im-

plied responsibility. This responsibility includes having staff members willing to supervise the student's activities, seeing that the student participates in a wide variety of experiences, and allowing the student to assume increasing responsibility. The willingness of the facility's health care team to work with the externship program provides the student with several opportunities. The opportunity with the greatest immediate impact is the opportunity for the medical assistant student to develop skills and test theories that were learned in the classroom in a supportive environment. This is especially important before the student ventures into a job setting of greater personal and medical responsibility. The supervising personnel in the health care facility will assist the student with decisions and help him or her recognize when increased responsibilities may be undertaken. The student must recognize that the office supervisor is a substitute for the school instructor and that the other personnel provide an example of teamwork in action.

A more long-term opportunity that you should keep in mind is that by working in one or more facilities during an externship, you can acquire references for future job hunting. You should approach the externship with a positive attitude and accept any guidance or responsibility offered as a learning experience. Your attitude and willingness to learn will create a positive impression of you among your externship supervisors, and this will develop potential reference sources. As your externship experience in a facility nears an end, speak frankly with your work supervisors regarding your interest in a reference. If you have established rapport with your supervisors this will be a simple exchange that will result in a favorable reference. You may request a general reference addressed to "To whom it may concern" that you can take with you when you have completed your student work experience. The other option is to let your supervisors know you would like to give their names as references, thereby notifying them that they may be contacted in the future by prospective employers. The first option is the most considerate choice, since your externship supervisors will need to write only one letter, which you can photocopy when references are requested. Your prospective employer can follow up with a phone call if confirmation is necessary.

A final opportunity that may develop from your externship is an offer of a permanent position at the office or facility. If the interest is mutual your potential employer may be willing to keep the position open for you until you have completed your training program, or you may be able to arrange a part-time work schedule in the interim.

Programs Without an Externship

If your school does not include an externship program you still have two options. First, you can volunteer your services in a willing medical office, hospital, or agency. Second, you can secure a part-time job in an entry-level position in a health care facility. You can use this opportunity to observe the functions of the various personnel. You may also be able to participate in activities of increasing challenge as you demonstrate your willingness and capability to assume more responsibility. A cooperative instructor in your program may be able to assist you in locating a volunteer or paid position and provide follow-up guidance when you wish to evaluate your work experience.

The Self-Supporting Student

If it is necessary for you to work during your course of study, you should be aware that your medical assistant program probably has a rule against working for pay in the same facility in which you do your externship. If there is no specific rule about this situation in your program you should establish your own guideline. The logic behind this rule is the difficulty in separating the paid and nonpaid (externship) times when they occur in the same setting. Isolating the externship experience allows the student, the instructor, and the externship supervisor to remain objective in evaluating the progress and development needs.

Expanding the Externship Experience

The externship process may or may not be associated with a seminar in the classroom. If a seminar is included, it will offer an opportunity, usually on a weekly basis, for the externship instructor and all of the students in the program to meet. The instructor provides minimal structure to the meeting and guidance or advice when necessary. The primary purpose of the seminar is to provide students with the opportunity to share experiences and observations with one another. This serves as a mechanism to reduce stress and broaden exposure, since each student is unique and is working in a different environment.

If your student work experience is not organized through your school or is not associated with a seminar, you may wish to establish an informal seminar with other students in similar situations.

The result will be supportive and positive. You may also be able to enlist the help of an instructor to act as an informal advisor for your group.

Whether you participate in a formal externship program organized by your school or develop one of your own, you will find externship an important and rewarding experience. What you get out of the process depends on you. Keep in mind the influence the externship experience can have on your development and future employment.

THE JOB SEARCH

As mentioned earlier in this chapter, you are actually beginning the process of obtaining a job by beginning your current program of study. The methods used in a job search are presented in this chapter so that you may begin a personal assessment and develop the tools and skills that will assist you when you begin to look for a permanent position. As you proceed through the training period, your personal assessment will change, your skills will improve, and your tools and skills will be revised. The employment process involves two perspectives: that of the potential employee, which is presented in this chapter, and that of the employer, which is discussed in Chapter 7. Both perspectives should be reviewed both as you pursue your educational preparation and when you are ready to seek paid employment.

Personal Assessment

Positive attributes important for the medical assistant were presented in Chapter 1 on p. 6. You should evaluate these and other positive attributes that you identify in yourself and in other professionals during your training period. You must be honest in assessing your attributes now and in reassessing them periodically throughout the training process and your subsequent career. Instructors and externship supervisors will be able to offer observations that can be integrated into your personal evaluation; keep in mind that these observations are intended to help you and should be accepted in the positive spirit in which they are offered.

The skills you develop in administrative and clinical areas of study should also be evaluated and periodically reassessed as you become more proficient. Accept every opportunity to practice skills in the classroom and in your externship facility. Each time you perform a skill, you improve your performance. The guidance and suggestions for improvement from instructors or externship supervisors also apply as they did in your evaluation of attributes.

To assist you in establishing a format for attribute and skill analysis, you may wish to consult a reference book prepared specifically for this process. *What Color Is Your Parachute?* by Richard Nelson Bolles* provides an excellent collection of data on skills analysis and job-hunting techniques, as well as an appendix that lists hundreds of resource books categorized into areas of primary concern, such as guides for college students, women, and minorities as well as books on career planning, volunteer opportunities, and internships. Also explore bookstores in and around your school for guides to help in the evaluation process. Whatever source of assistance you choose, keep in mind that the objective evaluation of your skills and attributes is the first step in obtaining the job you want.

Sources of Employment

There are many potential sources of employment available when you are ready to enter the job market. The health care field should be viewed as a business, and the process of obtaining a job in health care requires the same approach as obtaining a job in general business. The first thing to keep in mind is that job hunting *is* a job and should be approached in an organized fashion using all available tools and interested individuals. You should explore all possible sources of employment. The recruiting sources that the future employer will use are listed in Table 7.2 (p. 80). These sources should also be reviewed and used by *you.* The section in Chapter 7 on recruitment and selection will alert you to what a potential employer will be evaluating when selecting an employee. Your understanding of the employer's perspective will be an asset throughout your job search. The added advantage available in an externship program will round out the available sources that can be investigated for potential employment. As previously noted, your externship supervisor may be prepared to offer a permanent position after your course of study. Another opportunity that may arise during externship is that employees in your externship facility will know of possible jobs and thus be a good source of employment referral.

Tools of Job Hunting
The resume

A resume is a common tool used in seeking employment and can be an asset to you in your job search. It should be thought of as a method of introduction, an advertisement of your skills and potential value to an employer and a facility, and a demonstration of your written communication skills. Until recently resumes tended to follow one format—the chronological resume, which is a historical account of your education and work experience, beginning with the most recent (see opposite page). This format may not be the most advantageous as you begin a career as a medical assistant. If you are preparing for your first full-time work experience, you will only be able to record your externship in the work history section, in which employers expect to see data on paid work experience. If you are preparing for a change of career to medical assisting, you will only be able to record employment information unrelated to your new career aspirations.

Alternative resume styles. In looking for your first position as a medical assistant, you may wish to explore some of the new, alternative-style resumes. *The Perfect Resume* by Tom Jackson* is an excellent resource for learning to develop a resume that will best serve your needs. Organized in a workbook format, this reference includes step-by-step guidance in selecting and developing the resume, special notes for students and individuals re-entering the job market, sample resumes of all styles, and tips for handling your job search. One alternative, if you are seeking your first position, may be a skills-oriented resume (see opposite page).

Fundamentals of the resume. Regardless of the style of resume you choose there are certain basic considerations that apply to all resumes. Resumes should be clear and concise (one page maximum), typed without error, and on a high-grade bond paper. Resumes are traditionally typed on white paper, but other soft, pleasant shades such as bone, beige, or light grey may be used. Dark or bright shades of paper should be avoided. Once you have a well-planned, well-prepared resume, you can have an instructor review it for information, style, and general appearance. It is difficult to see minor flaws in a project that you have worked on so closely. To reproduce the resume, locate a copy service with a high-grade copier and have the ser-

*Revised ed, 1987, Ten Speed Press.

*1981, Doubleday & Co, Inc.

Chronological Resume

John C. Adams

123 Main Street
San Francisco, CA 94118

Objective

To become a member of a health care team as an administrative assistant in a challenging medical practice.

Education

1989   City College of San Francisco. A.S. degree, Certified Medical Assisting Program. Broad theoretical foundation and externship experience in clinical and administrative positions.

1987   City High School, San Francisco, Calif. Diploma. Successful completion of all required courses and elective course in business skills.

Experience

1989   Sara M. Smith, M.D., San Francisco, Calif. Clinical externship. Experience in assisting with examinations, preparing instruments, stocking supplies.

1988   John Jones, M.D., San Francisco, Calif. Administrative externship. Experience in reception, billing services, banking, and bookkeeping.

Honors

C.M.A. Certified by American Association of Medical Assistants.

References

On request.

Skills Resume

Jane M. Jones

345 Central Avenue
St. Louis, MO 63141

Objective

To attain a challenging position in a dynamic health care facility that would recognize the benefits of including a Certified Medical Assistant on the health care team.

Skills

Administrative   Theoretical and practical knowledge of the vital operations needed to maintain the administrative functions of a medical facility, including telephoning techniques, pegboard and computer billing systems, insurance billing, account collection techniques, bank deposits and statement balancing, and inventory management.
Clinical   Knowledge and skill in the preparation for and care of the patient, including infection control, positioning for and assisting with physical examinations, taking vital signs and health histories, collecting and handling laboratory specimens, preparing and administering medications, and responding to common emergencies.

References

On request.

vice copy directly onto your own paper. The copied resumes are very similar to the original, and this saves you from repetitive typing. If the resume is produced on a word processor, tell the operator to produce multiple copies.

The information provided in resumes today has changed from that provided in the past because of legal restrictions and the need to save space for more vital information. To avoid discrimination, the law states that you need not specify such data as age, marital status, dependents, or physical measurements (height and weight). You should not include this information on a resume. To save space you should also exclude the names and contact information of references from your resume. This information will be included on your employment application. Please include those letters of reference that you have available.

Preparing a resume takes time; therefore, be prepared to rewrite your resume several times to polish the finished product. It will also need to be revised over time as your experience expands and skills develop. Professional resume services are available in many cities to assist in putting together an impressive resume.

The cover letter

When you send a resume to a potential employer it must be accompanied by a cover letter. Like the resume, the cover letter should be clear and concise and attract the employer's attention. Extreme care must be taken to assure that the potential employer's name, title, and address are accurate, with special attention to spelling. Jackson's *The Perfect Resume* includes a section on cover letters, the information to include in them, and writing techniques that put you in a positive position (see below).

The letter and accompanying resume will not secure you a job, but they should accomplish their primary purpose of securing an interview. Remember that the entire process of obtaining a job is salesmanship. You must convince prospective employers that you are exactly the individual they need. You have accomplished the first step if you are invited to interview for a position.

Cover Letter

John C. Adams

123 Main Street
San Francisco, CA 94118

June 22, 1989

Sara M. Smith, M.D.
1482 Tenth Avenue, Suite 2
San Francisco, CA 94123

RE: Medical assistant position

Dear Dr. Smith:

I noted with interest your advertisement in the June 21, 1989 Mercury News. The enclosed resume highlights my skills, which were developed through participation in the Medical Assisting Program at San Francisco City College and affirmed by my certification as a medical assistant through the American Association of Medical Assistants.

Based on the stated requirements of the position, I believe that I will be able to assist you successfully with your patients' needs and contribute to the efforts of your present medical staff.

I look forward to the opportunity of meeting you and discussing my qualifications, which will be an asset to your practice. I am available to work immediately and can interview at your convenience.

Very truly yours,

John C. Adams, C.M.A.
Enclosure

The interview

First impressions. Once you have obtained an interview appointment you should plan carefully for the interview process. The first thing to remember is that your evaluation will begin the moment you arrive in the office and before you have the opportunity to speak. Be prepared for unusual questions, i.e., "What have you done with your life that you are proud of?" Interviewers are becoming more aggressive, try to respond with more than just a "yes" or "no" answer. The factors that will be evaluated at this point include the following:

- Punctuality;
- General appearance;
- Dress;
- Mannerisms;
- Courtesy; and
- Attitude.

Plan to arrive approximately 10 to 15 minutes before the time of your interview appointment. This will give you an opportunity to fill out an application, compose yourself, and observe the general activity within the office or facility. You should carefully plan the time necessary to travel to the interview. However, should you encounter some unusual interference, such as automobile failure or a breakdown in the transportation system, locate a phone as soon as possible and call the interviewer's office. Briefly explain the situation, apologize for the difficulty, and request another appointment.

Your general appearance should be professional. Your hairstyle should be neat and conservative, wear minimal jewelry, and any fragrance should be subtle. If applying for a position in an allergy office, environmental office, or holistic office, do not wear any body scents. Women should apply makeup conservatively. Men with beards or moustaches should have them carefully trimmed. Clothing should be conservative, appropriate day wear, comfortable, and well fitted. Colors should be subtle: blue, grey, or brown. Attention should be focused on the person, not on the clothing. Men should wear a suit or slacks and a complementary jacket, a dress shirt, and a tie. Men's dress shoes should be a black or brown as appropriate. Women should wear a dress or suit with a skirt. Although pantsuits may be conservative and stylish, dresses are considered to make a better initial appearance. Women's stockings should be free of flaws, and shoes should be conservative. Avoid bright colors, heels that are too high, or sandal styles. Avoid long acrylic or lacquered nails.

In preparation for the interview you will want to evaluate yourself for the presence of distracting mannerisms. Seek the constructive criticism of observant friends or helpful instructors. Such mannerisms include excessive hand movements such as moving your hands to your face or hair, failure to make eye contact with the interviewer, frequently shifting position in the chair, chewing gum, or using redundancies of speech such as "fillers" ("ahh" "you know" "like").

Above all be courteous and maintain a positive attitude. Your attitude is demonstrated by all of the factors that make up the potential employer's first impression of you. Your dress, general appearance, mannerisms, tone of voice, self-confidence, and courtesy demonstrate your willingness to develop a positive interpersonal relationship with the employer. Maintaining a positive attitude will require work on your part, particularly if you must participate in many interviews before you are offered a position that you want to accept. Repeatedly answering similar questions from multiple interviewers can influence your attitude without your awareness. Being conscious of the possibility of a bored attitude or tone of voice should prevent the problem. Approach each interview as you will approach each patient in the future; each is unique and offers a special challenge. Your attitude will influence the outcome.

The application. Filling out a preprinted application form may or may not be required at the time of the interview. It is to your advantage if you allow the time to fill out the form as completely as possible (even if you provide a resume). Smaller, private medical practices with one or two physician-employers may eliminate this step of the process. In this case your resume will serve as the application. If the potential employer has not received a resume from you before the interview, bring one with you. It will serve as a reminder of your skills and qualifications when the final selection is being made.

Application forms are most often required in such settings as hospitals, clinics, and large group-medical practices. Be certain to answer questions briefly and clearly and in clean, neat printing. The employer will evaluate the appearance of the application as a sample of your work. Answer all appropriate questions. By law you are not required to answer questions regarding your marital status, dependents, religious preference, ethnic origin, and so on. You can leave these blank; no comment is necessary at this time. Even though you are not required to answer a number of questions, it is to your credit and advantage to do so, particularly marital status and number of dependents. Be prepared to supply the names, addresses, and phone numbers of references at this time. You will, of course, have obtained advance permission from your reference sources and have chosen individuals who recognize your positive attributes and skills. Three references are considered the minimum. At this time you may also supply photocopies of the reference letters you may have obtained on completion of your externship.

The interview process. If you have little or no experience in seeking paid employment, anticipating an interview may be intimidating. It does not have to be! You can prepare well in advance of the actual interview. Request time in your externship seminar or form a group of supportive friends to practice interviews. Take turns being the interviewer and the applicant; tape-record the practice if possible. Have the interviewer and any observers report their observations. Retain the positive actions and make any appropriate adjustments to present yourself in a better light. The tape recorder will help you objectively evaluate your speech patterns and give you a permanent record to compare with future tapes.

Your instructor, students with interview experience, and reference books will supply you with questions that may be asked during an actual interview. Some will be very specific, such as the following:

- "What is your typing speed?"
- "Have you prepared blood and urine samples for transport to the laboratory?"
- "What options do you have if a patient does not accept the first appointment time you offer?"
- "Which billing services have you had experience with?"

Other questions may be classified as *open-ended* questions. These might include the following:

- "Tell me a little about yourself."
- "What do you consider your strengths and weaknesses?"
- "In what ways can you contribute to this practice?"
- "What are your career goals?"

Such open-ended questions are intended to provide the interviewer with material by which to evaluate your oral communication skills and your opinion of yourself. Both specific and open-ended questions should be answered clearly and honestly. Take time to think before answering, and answer only the specific question asked. Refrain from giving lengthy answers or volunteering information that is not requested. The interviewer may inquire about the questions you chose not to answer on the ap-

plication. If you still feel that the questions are not appropriate you should not feel pressured into answering. However, you should be careful not to reply in a hostile or defensive manner. An appropriate response might be "I did not feel that the information was important to my professional career."

Toward the end of the interview the interviewer may ask whether you have any questions. If the opportunity to ask questions is not offered, you should request it. Asking pertinent questions demonstrates interest in the position and provides the opportunity to contribute information about yourself that did not surface in answer to the interviewer's questions. You may wish to inquire:

- "Do you encourage your employees to take continuing education courses?"
- "Why did the previous employee leave the position I am applying for?"
- "Do your staff members cross-train so that there is a backup for each position?"

You should *not* begin this phase of the interview by asking about holidays, vacations, or sick leave. This would imply that your primary concern is the time you can spend being paid for time off work.

If salary has not been discussed it should be before the interview closes. A statement on a job description or in an advertisement of "salary negotiable" is inappropriate. It should alert to the possibility of a low salary offer. Before reporting for an interview you should investigate the salary ranges in the area. If the potential employer states a salary that is low, politely say so. If you are asked to state the minimum salary you would accept, do not respond with a dollar amount. Instead, state that you are not interested in minimums but in a challenging career opportunity with appropriate compensation. If you know the salary ranges for the area, you may wish to name a slightly higher range. For example, if the starting salaries average $900 to $1,100 a month, you might state that you consider $950 to $1,150 an appropriate range. This way a counteroffer will still fall within the appropriate range.

As the interview is about to close you should recognize the interviewer's cue. Stand, thank the interviewer for his or her courtesy and time, and shake hands. Ask when you might hear about the final decision if the interviewer does not volunteer the information.

Interview follow-up. The evening of the interview you should write a brief, formal note to the interviewer saying thank you for his or her time and courtesy. This serves two purposes: (1) it demonstrates your conscientiousness, and (2) it will put

Figure 2.1
Example of a follow-up letter.

Sam D. Smith, M.D.
888 Nowhere Street, #201
Anywhere, USA 90000

Dear Dr. Smith / Name of Interviewer:

Thank you for the opportunity to interview for the Administrative Medical Assistant position today. I am truly interested in the position. It not only sounds challenging and rewarding, but will provide the opportunity for utilizing the skills I have developed through educational preparation and practical experience.

I enjoyed meeting you and your staff. There seems to be a strong sense of camaraderie between you and the staff and the patients.

Thank you for considering my application, and I look forward to hearing from you in the near future.

Sincerely,

Person's Name

your name in the interviewer's mind again (Figure 2.1).

You can usually expect to hear the outcome of the application and interview within 7 to 10 days. If the job is offered to you, take time to carefully evaluate the offer and compare the position with others that you are considering. Should you be notified that another applicant was offered the position, take the initiative to ask why in a positive manner. Make it clear that you are seeking constructive assistance for your continued job search and that you will appreciate any suggestions. Many times you will discover that the reason is that the other applicant had more experience, not that the employer had a negative reaction to you. Your openness may stimulate the interviewer to become a source of leads to other positions. Do not be dismayed if the interviewer did not call. Take the initiative, call and ask if the position has been filled. Unfortunately, many interviewers do not take the time to respond to each applicant. Consider the interviewer's point of view; that is, they have advertised a position and suddenly have more than 100 applicants (in large cities). The response time would be incredible. Call and ask. Put yourself in the forefront again.

Conclusion

Your externship experience and preparation for a role on a health care team are, in a sense, a job in themselves. Devote careful attention to the process and keep in mind that it is the first step to your future career. You need to develop skill in interpersonal relationships, pay serious attention to your studies in the administrative and clinical areas, and identify and enhance your talents.

It is in your best interests to develop a close working relationship with your instructors. They can provide you with objective evaluation of your development, can provide references, and are a potential source of job referrals.

Now is also the time to set goals and objectives for your future. Some will be short-term goals, such as completing the medical assistant program and passing the certifying examination, and some will be long-term goals, such as becoming an office manager within 5 years. Overall, these goals should be realistic and developed using an effective method. The goal-setting process includes the following:

- Set positive priorities—determine a goal;
- Determine resources;
- Develop plans and analyze barriers to goals;
- Implement the plan; and
- Evaluate the plan periodically, adjusting and improving it when necessary.

Overall, you need to develop and maintain a positive attitude toward every experience and opportunity you encounter. An optimistic approach will make you an asset in any career setting.

Review Questions

1. Where could you work to fulfill your externship requirements?
2. How is an externship helpful to you in your theoretical courses? How is it helpful to you personally?
3. How could an externship program help you get a job?
4. List your best attributes. How will each one help you in your career?
5. What three basic considerations will you keep in mind when planning a resume?
6. Develop a basic resume based on your education and experience; develop an alternative resume.
7. Write a cover letter to a potential employer.
8. What do you expect a resume and cover letter to accomplish?
9. Prepare five questions that you would ask a potential employee if you were the interviewer.
10. Pair off with a classmate and practice an interview as the employer. Then switch roles and repeat the interview.
11. Write an appropriate follow-up letter to a person with whom you interviewed.

SUGGESTED READINGS

Bolles RN: What color is your parachute? rev ed, Berkeley, Calif, 1987, Ten Speed Press.

Jackson T: The perfect resume, Garden City, NY, 1981, Anchor Press Doubleday.

Chapter 3

Medical Science and Specialization

- Primitive medicine
- Concepts among the ancients
- Dark and Middle Ages
- Effects of the Renaissance (1350-1650)
- Post-Renaissance contributions
- Development of surgery
- Advancement of nursing
- Twentieth century achievements
- Modern medical practices
- The transition of medical practice styles
- Medical associations

Objectives

On completion of Chapter 3 the medical assistant student should be able to:

1 Define the terms listed in the vocabulary.

2 Describe the role of superstition in primitive medicine.

3 Name four common drugs and their primitive sources.

4 Discuss the contributions of the ancient Greeks and Romans to medicine.

5 Discuss four developments of the Renaissance period that influence modern medicine.

6 Name six scientists of the post-Renaissance period and discuss their contributions to medicine.

7 Discuss the two major contributions that allowed the advancement of surgery.

8 Name the three women responsible for modern nursing techniques and discuss their influence on medical care.

9 Describe basic medical education and the two methods of obtaining a medical license.

10 Discuss the development of medical specialization and the requirements of specialty education.

11 List the five primary care specialties, the twenty-two consultative specialties, and the ten surgical specialties.

12 Discuss the concept of continuing medical education.

13 Discuss the three organizational forms a medical practice can take.

14 Discuss the four possible methods of practice from which a physician can choose.

15 List the medical associations to which a physician might belong.

Vocabulary

bacteriology The science or study of one-celled microscopic organisms.

disposition The act of managing or distributing; placement or arrangment.

disseminate To spread, circulate, or disperse.

immunology The science or study of the protective mechanism of the body against disease; the mechanism may be natural or acquired.

internship Period of practical study, usually 1 year, immediately after medical school; the physician is called an *intern* during this time, a term not to be confused with *internist*.

internist A common term for the physician who practices internal medicine; a specialist who has completed an internship and a residency in internal medicine after completing medical school.

microbiology The science or study of microscopic plants and animals.

operative Pertaining to surgical procedures.

primitive Belonging to the earliest ages in time.

proprietor An owner; the one who has legal title to property.

residency A 3- to 5-year period of study after internship during which the physician prepares for the practice of a specialized field in medicine.

Today's health care consumer is accustomed to great numbers of services for all types of health care. Consumers have high and sometimes unreasonable expectations of the health care provider. Patients are accustomed to a vast array of diagnostic and treatment modes and preventive and curative medications and a readily available variety of health care providers. Many patients cannot remember a time when antibiotics did not exist, even though penicillin was not refined or produced in quantity until the demands generated by World War II stimulated research and mass production. Surgery is common, relatively safe, and pain free today, yet a little over 100 years ago it was a dangerous, painful experience because of the lack of knowledge about bacterial infection and anesthesia.

PRIMITIVE MEDICINE

Imagine yourself in primitive times without electricity, exposed to the elements, with few tools, and with a full-time job just obtaining food and avoiding predators. In the earliest days of civilization, mystery, magic, and medicine were synonymous. Without sufficient knowledge to explain cause-and-effect relationships, primitive peoples attributed many phenomena they could not explain to supernatural powers. Superstition played a dominant role in the healing arts, and witch doctors were believed to have special powers to drive away evil spirits. The effective tribal doctor was able to rid patients of the spirits responsible for their symptoms. In performing this function the primitive physician inadvertently discovered and used drugs that are the bases for some of our modern medicines. Since it was accidently discovered that

chewing the leaves of the foxglove plant could slow and strengthen the heartbeat, we now have digitalis. The bark of the cinchona tree was found to control fever and muscle spasms. Quinine is now derived from that same source. Juice from the belladonna plant (deadly nightshade) was found to relieve abdominal pain and intestinal cramps. Our modern drug, atropine, is one of the several medicines made from that plant. Some varieties of the poppy plant produce opium, now used as the medication morphine to relieve severe pain. As the centuries passed and tribal organizations developed, the medicine man grew in importance as both priest and physician, maintaining a link between the spiritual world and the role of healer. Even before people discovered how to control and use fire, the tribal physician recognized the relaxing or stimulating qualities of some plant roots used for nourishment. By isolating or combining these substances, the witch doctor had a means to control people, and he often used this power to assume a position of tribal leadership.

CONCEPTS AMONG THE ANCIENTS

The earliest civilization of which we have any extensive knowledge is that of the Egyptians. The medicine of the Egyptians was made up of a combination of superstition, religion, and some practical considerations. The gods were invoked to heal, but the early Egyptian physicians also administered medicines to the sick and used splints to heal fractures. Egyptian physicians were adept in the diagnosis and treatment of numerous diseases, and even performed surgery as sophisticated as trephination to relieve intracranial pressure.

The first step toward scientific inquiry and a

Figure 3.1
Nuns and monks caring for the sick in a hospice.
From Donahue MP: Nursing, the finest art—an illustrated history, St Louis, 1985, The CV Mosby Co.

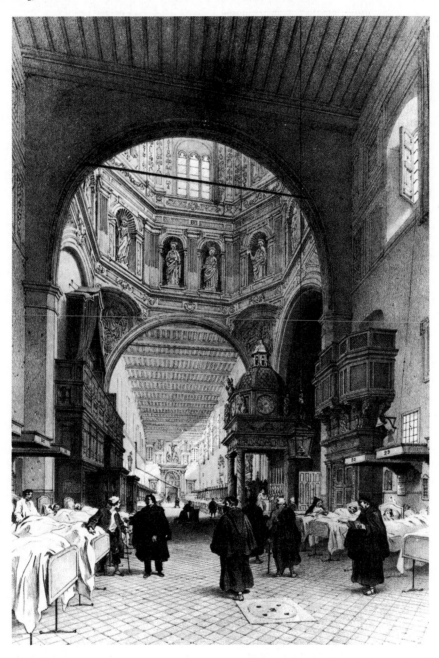

break with the pure superstition and mysticism of the primitives was made by the ancient Greeks. They attempted to study nature objectively by considering the human body and its disease without resorting to the supernatural explanations. The Greeks became the first people to enunciate the value and enumerate the principles of scientific medicine, including the importance of research. They removed mystery from medicine, making medicine a practice of common sense, observation, and logical reasoning.

Hippocrates, often referred to as the father of medicine, lived during the golden age of Greek culture (circa 400 BC) and developed great skill in diagnosis. He enhanced the scientific approach by carefully noting and recording signs and symptoms associated with various diseases. Hippocrates is also credited with establishing a standard of ethics, known as the Oath of Hippocrates, which serves as the foundation for today's principles of medical ethics (Chapter 4).

Religious custom prevented the Greeks from gathering information on anatomy and physiology through dissection of the body after death. Instead, Greek physicians derived their knowledge from bedside observation of patients, noting the signs and symptoms and eventual outcome of the patient's condition. They tried to correlate the information they observed with the experiences of their previous patients.

The Romans became the cultural and scientific descendants of the Greeks, inheriting their knowledge and developing it further. The Greeks are credited with establishing the importance of personal hygiene, and the Romans enlarged the concept to establish principles of public health. From the medical standpoint, the greatest contribution of the Roman era was sanitation. Recognizing the need for a system of sanitary engineering even without having knowledge of microorganisms, the Romans drained swamps, built aqueducts to carry fresh water to their cities, and constructed a system of sewers to carry off wastewater.

Surgery was apparently a well-accepted practice in the Roman Empire, as substantiated by an archeological find of over 200 surgical instruments in the ruins near Pompeii. Postmortem dissection of the human body, however, was still considered a sacrilegious act and was forbidden. The advancement of anatomy and physiology during this period is credited to Galen, a Greek physician who worked and taught in Rome. His experiments led to an excellent overview of anatomy as it was understood at the time. His experiments in physiology were considered brilliant.

DARK AND MIDDLE AGES

After the fall of the Roman Empire, the progress of medical science came essentially to a halt. During the 400 years of the Dark Ages (about 400 to 800 AD) and the 600 years of the Middle Ages (about 800 to 1400 AD) medicine was practiced only in the great monasteries and convents (Figure 3.1). These practices consisted chiefly of custodial care and the use of herbal medication. The monks' greatest contribution to the science of medicine was the collection and translation of the works of Greek and Roman physicians. This breakdown of public health

practices resulted in the tragic spread of communicable diseases, especially the bubonic plague, which killed an estimated 20 million people in Europe.

EFFECTS OF THE RENAISSANCE (1350-1650)

The Renaissance, the period from the fourteenth to the seventeenth century, is considered an era of great cultural and scientific activity. Four developments during this time influenced the future of medical science. First, universities and associated medical schools were founded, providing an environment in which research and instruction in the medical arts could take place in a more systematic manner. Second, a transition occurred in human understanding from unquestioning acceptance to challenge of existing beliefs and exploration of new horizons. Third, the printing press was invented, promoting the rapid dissemination of information, including advances made in medical science. Fourth, the stigma attached to the dissection of the dead was overcome by the realization that knowledge of anatomy and physiology would be advanced only through organized scientific examination. The combined effect of these four factors influenced the future of the art and science of medicine.

POST-RENAISSANCE CONTRIBUTIONS

The path begun in the Renaissance period was zealously followed during the next two centuries. This period was characterized by a tremendous increase in the accumulation of technical facts. Once physicians understood the structure of the human body, they were able to turn their attention to the functioning of its systems. Knowledge of physiology remained in the embryonic stages until the 1600s, when William Harvey, an English physician, accurately described the manner in which blood circulates through the body. Experimenting with animals, he actually witnessed and felt a heart beating. Harvey's great contribution to medical knowledge helped to substantiate the interdependence between the structure of the body and its internal workings.

The discovery of the microscope provided scientists with the tool necessary to examine life forms not visible to the naked eye. In the mid-1600s, Anton van Leeuwenhoek, a Dutch lens maker and scientist, produced the earliest forerunner of today's microscope. He was able to identify bacteria and recognize variations among microorganisms, confirming the presence of numerous forms of micro-

Figure 3.2
Florence Nightingale.
From Donahue MP: Nursing, the finest art—an illustrated history, St Louis, 1985, The CV Mosby Co.

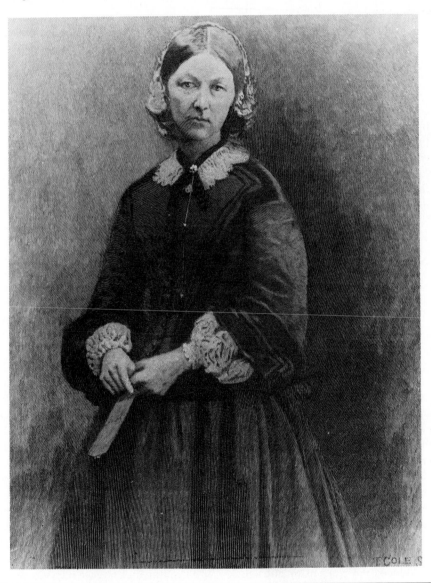

scopic life. However, the role of bacteria in the cause of disease was not recognized until 150 years later.

Although Leeuwenhoek and several other seventeenth century pioneers in the use of the microscope described various forms of microscopic life, the real significance and origin of these bodies was not actually understood until they were investigated by Louis Pasteur. Pasteur was a French bacteriologist and chemist whose work paralleled that of a German physician, Robert Koch. The research of both men showed that bacteria exist everywhere and that sterilization kills bacteria.

Pasteur studied the process of fermentation, assisting the French wine industry, but he is most commonly associated with the process of heating food to prevent the growth of bacteria. This process, called pasteurization, is still used today.

Koch is generally credited with discovering the tubercle bacillus. Although he was unable to determine a cure for the disease it causes, tuberculosis, he developed laboratory aids such as culture plates and dried, fixed, and stained slides of bacteria for microscopic examination.

Edward Jenner (1749-1823) of England made one of the greatest contributions toward the prevention of disease when he discovered a method of vaccination against smallpox. Jenner's discovery led to the science of immunology and eventually to public health preventive medicine.

Medicine progressed quite rapidly during the nineteenth century. Great discoveries in chemistry and physics were applied to research in physiological problems. The medical advances of the nineteenth century, particularly those arising from the demonstration of the bacterial cause of infection, made medicine a social necessity and a guiding force in modern civilization.

Continuing the work of the pioneers in microbiology, Paul Ehrlich (1854-1915) is credited with facilitating the identification and classification of various organisms. His techniques of staining bacteria and cells provided the means for differential analysis.

DEVELOPMENT OF SURGERY

Although surgery had been performed since ancient times, it was not until the late eighteenth century that surgery was elevated to the status of a medical science. Often referred to as the father of modern surgery, John Hunter (1728-1793) developed surgical techniques that were founded on knowledge of anatomy and physiology and the diagnosis of a pathological condition. The English School of Surgery, founded by Hunter, is still in existence.

Recognizing the need for surgery and developing effective surgical techniques solved half of the problems associated with surgery. The remaining problems involved the pain of surgery and the subsequent infection of wounds.

Joseph Lister (1827-1912), using the new knowledge of bacteria and determining the relationship between bacteria and infection of operative wounds, introduced the concept of antisepsis. Lister searched for a substance that, if applied to wounds, would kill the bacteria present and prevent the entrance of other bacteria from the outside, without causing injury to the tissue. His experiments with carbolic acid proved his theories on the bacterial cause of infection. He eventually expanded the use of carbolic acid to a spray for the operating room before surgery, a bath for the surgical instruments, and a washing solution for the surgeon's hands. Lister's development of surgical asepsis proved to be one of the greatest contributions to modern surgery.

Until the early 1840s the necessity for speed to reduce the pain and shock of operations preceded the development of the accuracy and precision by which we characterize modern surgery. In the United States, Dr. Crawford Long, a physician, and Dr. William Morton, a dentist, helped to make anesthesia safe for surgery. Working independently, each man began to use ether as a general anesthetic. The use of anesthetics has made possible the performance of many operations that were previously avoided and thereby has provided the means to cure many diseases.

The alleviation of pain and the reduction of wound infections enabled surgical technique to progress rapidly. With the concern for speed eliminated by general anesthesia, surgical operations could last longer, and the surgeon could devote time to precision and care.

ADVANCEMENT OF NURSING

The nineteenth century also saw the beginning of the recognition of nurses as qualified health care providers. Pioneers of nursing are credited with a perseverance and courage necessary to establish nursing as a profession. Florence Nightingale (1820-1910) (Figure 3.2) received what was considered formal training at the first hospital-based school for nurses in Kaiserswerth, Germany. Recognizing that educated nurses had more to offer patients than hygiene and hand-holding, Nightingale mobilized people in support of her cause. Her efforts during the Crimean War (1850-1853) did a great deal to alleviate the suffering of the ill and wounded and to establish credibility for her theories of training. After many disappointments and a long struggle, Nightingale succeeded in getting public support for her efforts to improve the care of the sick. The principles she established have served as a fundamental guide for nursing progress, and the school she established at St. Thomas Hospital in London has served as the model for subsequent nursing schools.

Clara Barton (1821-1912) was an American nursing pioneer in the American Civil War. The difficulties of tracing the whereabouts of injured or dead soldiers led to Barton's role in the formation of the Federal Bureau of Records. The problems of supply procurement in battle or disaster situations and her exposure to the Red Cross organization in Europe resulted in Barton's establishment of the American Red Cross in 1881. She served as the president of the organization until 1904, 8 years before her death at the age of 91.

The third outstanding contributor to the advancement of nursing was Lillian Wald (1867-

1940), a graduate of the New York Hospital Training School. She is credited with placing public health nursing on a firm and rational foundation. She championed the idea that the health needs of patients were closely related to their social needs. She was instrumental in founding the Henry Street Settlement House in New York City (1893), which is now famous as the seed of public health nursing.

The development of nursing as an adjunct to physicians' health care practices laid the foundation for future complementary professions. The role of formally trained medical assistants in health care will broaden over time just as the nursing and medical professions have advanced.

TWENTIETH CENTURY ACHIEVEMENTS

The strides of medicine since 1900 have been truly magnificent. X-rays, discovered by the German physicist Wilhelm Roentgen, were refined and provided a means to diagnose injuries and disease processes and to provide a method for the treatment of some cancers. The French physicists Marie and Pierre Curie discovered radium for the treatment of malignancies. Radiology has since progressed to include the use of radioisotopes and sound-, heat-, computer-assisted imaging (Chapter 27).

Diagnostic and therapeutic procedures are being discovered and refined at an unprecedented rate. Techniques in laboratory analysis (Chapters 25 and 26), electrocardiology (Chapter 28), and physical therapy (Chapter 29) provide invaluable assistance to the physician and the patient.

The development of natural and synthetic medications to treat illness, prevent diseases, replace substances, and control pain has evolved to a fine art. The techniques of administering drugs have been refined for optimum results, and the control of substances has been required for public safety (Chapter 23).

Infection control (Chapter 20), surgical asepsis, and surgical techniques (Chapter 21) have advanced to the point of maximum patient safety. The potential of surgery is only now being realized as a result of collaboration between technologists and medical scientists.

MODERN MEDICAL PRACTICES
An Era of Specialization
Basic medical education

The individual planning to become a physician will study for a minimum of 9 years. The basic preparation for practicing medicine is 4 years of college with a major in premedical studies or a basic science, 4 years of medical school, and 1 year of internship, a period of practical experience. If the physician does not wish to specialize in one area of medicine, he or she may choose a *rotating* internship, which provides experience in multiple specialty areas throughout the 1-year period.

Licensure

In the United States a physician is eligible to practice general medicine in individual states after successful completion of the required medical school curriculum, an internship, and the state's board examination. In lieu of an individual state examination, some states accept successful completion of the National Board Examination for licensure. Generally the examination is taken just before completion of medical school, and the license issued after the internship experience. This license is issued for the lifetime of the practitioner and is renewed periodically with payment of a fee. The physician who chooses to begin private practice at this time is considered a general practitioner.

Development of specialization

Specialization is a relatively recent phenomenon in the history of medicine. The initial impetus to this division of functions occurred during the past 100 years. The industrial and technological revolution, which began in the late nineteenth century, accelerated the advancement of the sciences and the development of precision instruments. However, the greatest single factor in advancing medical specialization was World War II. This unfortunate period saw individuals with unprecedented injuries. Physicians were not sufficiently prepared to use the scientific and technological advancements of the time to treat these patients. The physicians drafted for the war effort had been out of medical school for varying lengths of time, and the new technological discoveries were being applied with such speed as to preclude the possibility of developing skill in all areas. The usual total educational experience of physicians before this period was limited to what is now considered basic medical education.

Specialty education. The U.S. Army Medical Corps responded to the immediate need by organizing brief, intensive courses for its personnel. Subsequently, medical schools and health care facilities developed programs for individuals interested in developing skill and knowledge in specific areas. The advent of postgraduate study made specialization inevitable, and those physicians who seek out advanced study in one of the specialties tend to restrict their practice to the diagnosis and treatment of ailments falling into that class.

The selection of a specialty by a physician is a highly individual matter; the choice is dictated by personal preference, interest, and special ability. Depending on the specialty, the physician who decides to pursue a specialty must plan to spend an additional 3 to 6 years of study after internship. This period of time is known as *residency,* and the student is referred to as a *resident physician.*

Specialty certification. After residency, the physician is prepared to begin practice as a specialist. Each specialty recognized by the American Medical Association has a national board that has been established to set standards and to certify the competency of its members. The physician applying for certification in a specialty must fulfill certain requirements with regard to education, training, and practical experience and is also expected to pass a written or oral examination. On successful compliance with all board requirements, the physician is awarded a certificate of competency in the specialty and becomes known as a diplomate of the speciality. The common designation of the certified specialist is *fellow,* as in Fellow of the American College of Surgeons (FACS).

Specialty categories. Specialists may practice medicine, surgery, or both. Medicine includes treatment by physical or chemical means; surgery includes treatment by manual and operative procedures. Specialty practices may also be classified as primary and consultative care.

Primary care. The physician who practices primary care is one who provides all basic diagnostic, preventive, and treatment services for patients. The specialties commonly designated as primary care include internal medicine, family practice, gynecology, pediatrics, and gerontology as well as the general or family practitioner. Medical assistants who work for a primary care physician will have the opportunity to use almost every facet of their training and preparation. Variety in duties and responsibilities is the rule, not the exception. A brief overview of the primary care specialties will help medical assistants decide which area they would most care to devote their efforts.

Internal medicine is the medical specialty in which the physician evaluates and advises the patient about the functioning of internal organs and treats disorders by physical or chemical means.

Family practice is similar to internal medicine but differs in that the physician cares for *all* members of a family unit. Involving the family allows the physician to observe and interpret the influence of interrelationships in maintaining or restoring the health of individual members.

Gynecology deals basically with the examination or treatment of the female reproductive organs. It is classified as primary care because the gynecologist is often the only physician a woman sees on a routine basis. Therefore the patient often seeks advice on matters other than gynecology, and the physician performs certain screening evaluations on a periodic basis.

Pediatrics involves the evaluation and treatment of infants, children, and adolescents. The pediatrician is prepared to deal with the special needs of his or her patients because of additional training in the growth and development phases of life and the diseases unique to children.

Gerontology involves the evaluation and treatment of the older adult. The gerontologist is prepared to handle the special needs of patients because of additional training in the evaluation and treatment of diseases unique to the older adult and the aging processes.

Consultative specialties. Some consultative specialists are best able to practice in institutional settings, including hospitals, and educational or research facilities. Since medical assistants working in these settings will have direct or indirect contact with these specialists, a brief description of each follows.

Emergency medicine (EM) specialists practice in the emergency rooms of hospitals or in commercial facilities developed to provide intervention in situations involving sudden, serious, and potentially life-threatening illnesses or injuries. Once the crisis period has passed, the EM physician refers the patient to the appropriate specialist(s) for continued care.

Neonatology specialists practice primarily in the hospital setting to evaluate and treat severely ill infants, many of whom are born either premature or with congenital defects and/or drug related illnesses.

Pathology deals with the etiology of disease, and the pathologist assists other physicians to reach a diagnosis by evaluating tissue or fluid acquired from the patient.

Perinatology specialists provide evaluation and advise patients about possible congenital illnesses of the fetus. Laboratory tests used by the pathologist assist in determining cellular changes that affect the structure or function of the body systems.

Nuclear medicine specialists diagnose and in some cases treat disease processes by means of radioactive substances (Chapter 27).

✻ *Clinical pharmacology* involves the treatment of disease with chemical substances. This physician consults on the selection of appropriate medication, the interaction of various drugs, and the diagnosis of adverse results from the use of drugs.

Preventive medicine is a diagnostic or therapeutic specialty. The diagnostic radiologist assists other physicians in determining a patient's structural or functional status through the use of various imaging techniques. Therapeutic radiologists treat certain disease processes with various radioactive substances.

Consultative specialists who establish private offices will provide the most likely opportunities for jobs for medical assistants. Brief descriptions of the specialties most commonly encountered in private practice follow.

Allergy involves the diagnosis and treatment of allergic reactions that may include both internal and/or external illnesses. A new subspecialty of environmental allergy evaluates, advises, and treats the patient with regard to the patient's reaction to environmental allergies that contribute to the patient's illness or inability to function within the environment in which he or she lives.

Cardiology involves the evaluation and treatment of the patient with a heart condition, but may also include internal and/or external illnesses. The cardiologist is prepared to handle the special needs of his or her patients due to additional training in evaluation and treatment of particular cardiology (heart) problems.

Dermatology concerns the proper care of the skin as well as the treatment of disease affecting the skin. The causes of skin difficulties may be from environmental contact or internal sources. Treatment may be medical or surgical.

Endocrinology is the medical specialty that deals with the ductless glands and their disorders. The diseases include overproduction or underproduction of hormones by the various glands.

Gastroenterology involves the diagnosis and medical or surgical treatment of diseases of the digestive system.

The specialist in *infectious diseases* diagnoses and medically treats communicable diseases. The process includes investigation to determine the causative agent, provision of appropriate treatment, and development of a plan to prevent recurrence or spread of the infectious organism.

The relatively new field of *legal medicine* developed as a result of the increasing complexity of the health care field and the increasing number of legal cases involving medical situations. The individual who practices legal medicine may be a physician who serves as an expert witness in specific areas of medicine or may limit his or her practice to the perspective of the defendant or the plaintiff. The legal medical specialist also may be an individual with degrees in both law and medicine who chooses either to practice law, specializing in medical cases, or to practice medicine, specializing in cases involving legal issues.

Neurology involves the diagnosis and treatment of disorders of the central and peripheral nervous systems. These disorders may be caused by injury, disease, or infection. The neurologist is concerned primarily with the diagnosis and treatment of conditions by medical means.

The specialty of *obstetrics*, often practiced in combination with gynecology, relates to the care of women during pregnancy, labor, birth, and the recovery period after birth, usually 6 weeks. Throughout pregnancy, labor, and birth, the obstetrician has a dual responsibility to the mother and the developing fetus or fetuses.

Ophthalmology is the evaluation of the structure and function of the eye and the medical or surgical treatment of any disorders. The ophthalmologist is a physician and is not to be confused with the *optometrist*, who is limited to the evaluation of visual ability and the adaptation of the lens, or the *optician*, who prepares corrective lenses according to the directions of the physician or optometrist.

Otorhinolaryngology is commonly referred to as ENT, because the specialist medically or surgically treats disorders of the ear, nose, and throat.

✝ *Physical medicine and rehabilitation* involves the evaluation of an individual's functional status and the development of a treatment plan designed to return the patient to an optimum level of physical performance. The physiatrist's patients may be referred because of organic disorders such as cerebrovascular accident (CVA), or injuries, such as quadriplegia caused by an auto accident. The physiatrist works with other health care providers such as physical, occupational, and recreational therapists.

Pulmonary is the medical specialty that deals with the lungs and the respiratory system. Many of these disorders may be caused by injury, disease, or infection.

Psychiatry is the branch of medicine that deals with the etiology, diagnosis, treatment, and prevention of mental disorders. The foundation of psychiatry is the one-to-one relationship between the physician and the patient. The treatment of more serious psychiatric disorders has been greatly enhanced in recent times by the development of mood-stabilizing drugs.

Oncology is the medical specialty that primarily treats patients with cancer. These physicians will utilize either radiation therapy (megadoses of radiation) or chemotherapy, intravenously giving drugs that are considered very powerful.

✳ *Surgical specialties.* Surgery, as previously noted, is treatment by manual or operative procedures. Combined advances in anesthesia and drugs, physiology, and technology have enhanced the scope and safety of surgical treatment. These advances have created specialized subcategories of surgery.

Breast surgery involves the evaluation and treatment of the breast, which may involve biopsies for breast cancer, removal of the breast, and reconstruction of the breast.

General surgery involves the treatment of neoplasms and functional disorders of the abdominal organs, breasts, subcutaneous tissue, and extremities.

Colon and rectal surgeons limit their evaluation and treatment to the lower segment of the digestive system.

Cardiovascular surgery is limited to the heart, heart valves, and the vessels that serve the heart muscle.

The musculoskeletal system is the concern of the *orthopedic surgeon*. Orthopedic surgery includes treatment of structural or functional disorders of the muscles, ligaments, tendons, bones, and joints.

Neurosurgery is the invasive treatment of the brain, spinal cord, and peripheral nervous system.

Plastic surgery involves the repair or restoration of tissue for cosmetic or functional purposes. Cosmetic restoration is commonly the first thought that comes to mind when plastic surgery is mentioned, but restoring function, often in cooperation with orthopedic surgeons, and neurosurgeons is an important aspect of plastic surgery. The specialist may consult on cases involving burns, amputations, or birth defects.

The *thoracic surgeon* treats disorders of the structures within the chest, such as the lungs, bronchi, esophagus, and diaphragm.

In *urology* the specialist medically or surgically treats diseases and dysfunctions of the urinary tract and the male reproductive system.

Vascular surgery is the invasive treatment of the veins and arteries throughout the body.

• • •

Medical specialization of physicians has become common, and the specialization of ancillary personnel is following the precedent. Laboratory technicians, medical assistants, nurses, and other health care providers may offer unique services designed to meet special needs. Regardless of the setting or specialty, medical assistants will find a growing need for their services in administrative or clinical areas.

Relicensure and recertification

License renewal. An increasing number of consumer advocates and other interested individuals feel that lifetime licensure of physicians is inappropriate and that physicians should be required to prove periodically that they are keeping abreast of developments in their field. Many physicians are beginning to agree that there is a need for more public accountability by the medical profession. The report of the 1970 Carnegie Commission on Higher Education pointed out that physicians who do not remain *lifelong* students "face partial obsolescence in five to ten years." As yet no state requires periodic examinations before allowing license renewal; however, most states now require a significant number of hours of continuing medical education (CME).

Specialty recertification. The increasing concern with medical proficiency is also influencing the 22 medical specialty boards recognized by the American Medical Association. Although board certification is not legally required to practice a specialty, it is frequently necessary before a hospital will grant a physician staff privileges in the particular specialty. Many proponents of recertification argue that this trend and the considerations noted in the discussion of relicensure will promote higher-quality medical care by forcing all physicians to maintain their skills and keep up with rapidly changing medical knowledge.

Continuing medical education. Continuing medical education is one mechanism for fulfilling the need for physicians to keep up to date in their knowledge of medical trends. Some states now require proof of continuing education for license renewal. In 1971 New Mexico became the first state to implement a license reregistration law. Now physicians in New Mexico will lose their right to practice unless they accumulate 150 hours of CME credits every 3 years. As of August, 1977, medical practice acts in 19 states allow the state board of medical examiners the authority to require evidence of CME as a condition of reregistration of the license to practice medicine.

The trend among state medical associations to require CME as a condition of membership is evident but is progressing at a slow rate. As of 1985, all states require CME credits.

The effort toward making physicians more accountable is expected to spread. CME required for recertification and relicensing will probably be a fact of life in the relatively near future.

THE TRANSITION OF MEDICAL PRACTICE STYLES

Just as science and technology have caused a trend toward specialization in the practice of medicine, medical and legal environments have stimulated a change in the manner in which physicians choose to organize their practices. The most common legal forms for medical practices are sole proprietorship, partnership, professional corporation, or association. The manner in which physicians can provide care include employer-employee, association, group, or institutional relationships.

Organizational Form
✕ Sole proprietorship

The physician in a sole proprietorship has total authority and responsibility for all administrative decisions in the practice. This physician may or may not choose to employ another physician to assist with clinical duties. If there is a physician-employee, he or she is a salaried member of the staff subject to the authority of the physician-owner. Physician-owners in each of the other practice forms identified here may also employ other physicians in their practices. The physician-owner has total right to all assets and is responsible for all expenses.

✕ Partnership

A partnership is a legal agreement and association of two or more physicians who act as co-owners of the business. Each partner is legally responsible for all professional (clinical) and financial actions of all other partners.

✕ Professional corporation

Over the 10-year period between 1961 and 1971, each state passed legislation allowing professionals (individually or in groups) to incorporate. A professional corporation gives the physician-owner(s) and employees many legal and financial benefits. Since 1975 the majority of medical practices in the United States have been incorporated.

Methods of Practice
Employer-employee

The physician who chooses the position of employee in a medical practice is usually a recent graduate of a training program who is interested in evaluating practice forms, various communities and opportunities, and other methods of practice. In this position, the physician-employee is relieved of the responsibility of administrative decisions and financial burdens.

Associate

Associate relationships generally imply a sharing of facilities and possibly staff by two or more physicians. The physicians may have a contract detailing the privileges and responsibilities of each associate, but this must not be confused with the legal entity of a partnership. Associate physicians may not share information about or responsibility for one another's patients and are not *usually* legally responsible for one another's actions. Within the last 2 years, however, legal test cases have developed around "ostensible partnerships," that is, *apparent* or assumed partnerships. In this situation, one physician may become legally responsible for the clinical actions of an associate. A partnership may be *assumed* when patients perceive shared responsibility. This situation may be suggested by such simple actions as sharing the services of personnel or placing both physicians' names together on the office door or stationery without clearly indicating that a partnership does not exist. Physicians who plan to associate need to be aware of this potential problem and select associates with the same care as they would partners.

Group

Following is the definition of group practice according to the Medical Group Management Association and the American Group Practice Association.

Group practice is the provision of health care services by a group of at least three licensed physicians or dentists engaged full-time in a formally organized and legally recognized entity; sharing the group's income and expenses in a systematic manner; and sharing equipment, facilities, common records, and personnel involved in both patient care and business management.

Group practices can include one or several specialties and tend to employ a wide variety of allied health personnel.

Institutional

Physicians may practice in an institution in which patients are in residence or to which individuals come for medical care. Residential health care institutions include hospitals, skilled-nursing facilities, and extended care facilities. Nonresident patients may seek care at public health facilities, clinics, or health maintainance organizations. Institutions that individuals encounter for other than medical purposes may also provide periodic medical care or evaluation. Large industrial and work settings often maintain medical departments, as do educational institutions and boarding facilities. Physicians working in institutions have the added advantage of freedom from the concerns of establishing an office and all that it entails.

MEDICAL ASSOCIATIONS
General Medical Associations
Local medical societies

The physician interested in developing relationships with other physicians in the community usually joins the local medical society or association. The size of the local society is usually determined geographically by county. Member-physicians develop policy, establish committees, perform community services, and select representatives to communicate local needs and views to the state and national associations.

State medical associations

Associations at the state level establish health care policy, monitor state political activity that affects medical care, assist in the censure of negligent physicians, promote continuing medical education, and provide services unique to the area.

National medical association

State and local medical associations send delegates to the national organization, the American Medical Association (AMA). The AMA establishes guidelines for the ethical practice of medicine, monitors and initiates federal political activity with regard to health standards and legislation, and serves as a representative for state and local organizations of physicians.

In most situations the physician who joins the local society automatically becomes a member of the state and national associations. A portion of the dues paid to the local society is designated to the state and national organizations. If state and national membership is optional, physicians will decide at which level they wish to belong. The structure of the AMA is similar to that of the American Association of Medical Assistants (AAMA).

Specialty Associations

Many physicians choose to maintain membership in organizations established to serve their special interests. Some associations relate to the physician's medical specialty, such as the American College of Surgeons, the American Academy of Family Practice, or the American Society of Clinical Pathologists. These organizations provide current medical information and serve as the mechanism by which physicians become certified in their specialty. Physicians may also choose to participate in specialty public service organizations such as the American Heart Association, the American Cancer Society, or the Muscular Dystrophy Association.

Conclusion

The present advances in medical science were not even dreamed of as recently as 100 years ago. Today people are living longer, communicable diseases are being conquered, organs are being transplanted, and joints and limbs are being replaced. Technological and scientific advances can be expected to escalate and accelerate progress in the future. Progress in medical science has generated the specialization of physicians and the limitation of medical practices to illnesses or injuries of one type. Members of allied health professions may also opt to specialize. The medical assistant who develops a diverse foundation of knowledge and theory will be able to make an intelligent decision about future employment options.

Review Questions

1. What is superstition? What role did it play in primitive medicine?
2. Which drugs do we use today that were discovered in primitive times?
3. How did the ancient Greek and Roman physicians contribute to today's medical care?
4. Name and describe four major developments of the Renaissance period that influenced modern medicine.
5. State in your own words the contributions of the following post-Renaissance scientists to modern medicine: William Harvey, Anton van Leeuwenhoek, Louis Pasteur, Robert Koch, Edward Jenner, and Paul Ehrlich.
6. Describe in your own words how modern surgery was made safe.

7. What is the basic education required for an individual to be prepared to practice medicine?
8. How does a physician become a specialist?
9. What is primary care? Which specialists are considered primary care physicians?
10. Briefly describe the relicensure process today and proposed changes.
11. List and describe the possible organizational forms a physician may choose for his or her practice.
12. What are the four methods of practice from which a physician can choose?
13. Name and describe the general and specialty organizations to which a physician might belong.

SUGGESTED READINGS

The Medical Assistant, CCMA, Chicago (monthly publication).

The Professional Medical Assistant (monthly publication).

Chapter 4

Medical Ethics

- Medical ethics
- The AMA Principles of Medical Ethics
- The Judicial Council of the AMA
- The physician and the medical assistant

Vocabulary

bylaw A rule or regulation made by an organization for the purpose of governing the conduct of business.

collaboration The act of another or others, especially in literary or scientific work.

colleague A professional associate.

confidential Secret or private.

consent A state of agreement, or to grant approval.

ethics The science of moral behavior; principles or guides for moral behavior.

fraud A technique of reaching a goal by deceptive or deceitful means.

health maintenance organization (HMO) A means of providing health care with an emphasis on preventive medicine. *All health care is provided for a fixed annual fee.*

independent physician association (IPA) A group of physicians who have enrolled within the IPA to service enrolled patients.

judicial Pertaining to the administration of justice or to the courts of law.

mandatory Related to or as a part of an official command; compulsory.

medicolegal Pertaining to the relationship of medicine and law.

mode The manner or way of accomplishing an activity.

preferred provider organization (PPO) A means of providing health care to a select group of patients by physicians who have agreed to provide services to that select group.

philosophical Pertaining to the principles that explain events, facts, or a specific system of beliefs.

principle A truthful or honest foundation that forms the basis for other truths or laws.

standard An established quality or degree that is accepted as desirable.

statute A law passed by a recognized governing body, such as a state legislature.

Ethics is considered a system of correct conduct for an individual or a group with a single objective. The term *ethics* has its origin in the Greek word *ethos,* meaning custom or habitual mode of conduct, and the Latin word *ethicus,* meaning related to moral character. Ethical systems are primarily concerned with voluntary acts. It is assumed that individuals responsible to a code of ethics possess sufficient knowledge and freedom of choice to participate in the system.

The ethics of a particular profession is the code by which it attempts to regulate the actions of its members and establish general standards. One of the chief purposes of formulating a professional code of ethics is to elevate the standard of competence in a given field by strengthening the relationships among its members, thereby benefiting the entire community.

MEDICAL ETHICS
Historical Development

The earliest known written code of medical ethics dates back to 2500 BC. The document was created by the Babylonians and was known as the Code of Hammurabi. It was extremely detailed and would not have easily adapted to rapid developments in modern medical science and complex cultural patterns.

In the fifth century BC, during which Greece was experiencing a period of intellectual enlightenment, a brief statement of principles that has lasted through history was developed. The Oath of Hippocrates, named for the physician who developed it (Figure 4.1), has survived in a statement of ideals to be followed by medical practitioners. The Oath of Hippocrates protects the rights of the patient and guides the physician by appealing to moral instincts rather than imposing sanctions or penalties. It also functions as a basic frame of reference for much of the law connected with the practice of medicine.

After the Oath of Hippocrates the most outstanding contribution to the development of medical ethics was made by Thomas Percival, a British physician, author, and philosopher. Percival's interest in the advancement of sociology and his association with the Manchester Infirmary led to the development of a code of conduct based on hospital situations. His code was published in 1803.

Development of the AMA Principles of Medical Ethics

The American Medical Association (AMA) held its first official meeting in 1847 in Philadelphia. At that meeting, the two major items on the agenda were the establishment of minimum requirements for the education and training of physicians and the creation of a code of medical ethics. The code adopted at that meeting was clearly based on Percival's code.

While the basic language and concepts of the 1847 code went unchanged over time, some revisions were necessary to reflect the needs of the times. The desire to state the basic concepts in the clearest possible way led to revisions in 1903, 1912, and 1947. At a revision attempt in 1955, the AMA House of Delegates was asked to accept a proposal for a two-part code designed to separate medical ethics from matters of etiquette. The delegates rejected the proposal on the basis that little if any of the language in the 48 existing principles was changed.

In 1957 a drastic revision of the principles was accepted by the AMA House of Delegates after wide publication and much discussion among physicians. Preserving the basic principles while stating them in language better suited to clear explanation and practical codification, the code was reduced to a preamble and 10 short sections.

A 1977 revision was done to respond to contemporary legal standards, and the most recent revision, adopted in 1980, was done at the request of the AMA Judicial Council. This last revision eliminated all reference to gender and addressed con-

Figure 4.1
Hippocrates.
From Donahue MP: Nursing, the finest art—an illustrated history, St Louis, 1985, The CV Mosby Co.

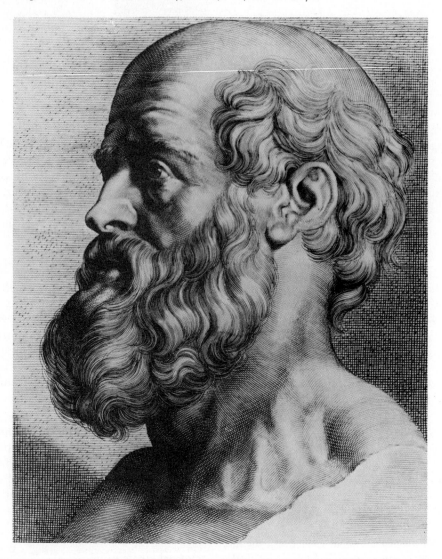

temporary medicolegal guides in a preamble and seven principles (see p. 39).

American Association of Medical Assistants Code of Ethics

Purpose

The American Association of Medical Assistants (AAMA) Code of Ethics serves as a standard of practice for the professional medical assistant. Medical assistants need to be familiar with the five specific guides of conduct in their code, reprinted on p. 39 with the permission of the AAMA. The code is included in the Association bylaws. After a review of the AAMA code, the physician's princi-

ples will be presented and evaluated. Sections of the *AMA Principles of Medical Ethics* appear in italic type. The medical assistant student will note the similarities in the two codes. These parallels demonstrate the close alliance of the two professions (see Table 4.1).

Medical assistants' responsibilities

The general nature of the AAMA code of ethics provides an ethical foundation for the medical assistant. It also provides the latitude necessary to incorporate new information as technological developments occur. The AAMA code of ethics has a philosophical link with the code of the AMA. Professional medical assistants use the AAMA code of

American Medical Association Principles of Medical Ethics

Preamble:

The medical profession has long subscribed to a body of ethical statements developed primarily for the benefit of the patient. As a member of this profession, a physician must recognize responsibility not only to patients, but also to society, to other health professionals, and to self. The following Principles adopted by the American Medical Association are not laws, but standards of conduct which define the essentials of honorable behavior for the physician.

  I. A physician shall be dedicated to providing competent medical service with compassion and respect for human dignity.
 II. A physician shall deal honestly with patients and colleagues, and strive to expose those physicians deficient in character or competence, or who engage in fraud or deception.
III. A physician shall respect the law and also recognize a responsibility to seek changes in those requirements which are contrary to the best interests of the patient.
 IV. A physician shall respect the rights of patients, of colleagues, and of other health professionals, and shall safeguard patient confidences within the constraints of the law.
  V. A physician shall continue to study, apply and advance scientific knowledge, make relevant information available to patients, colleagues, and the public, obtain consultation, and use the talents of other health professionals when indicated.
 VI. A physician shall, in the provision of appropriate patient care, except in emergencies, be free to choose whom to serve, with whom to associate, and the environment in which to provide medical services.
VII. A physician shall recognize a responsibility to participate in activities contributing to an improved community.

Principles of Medical Ethics of the AMA, 1980. Reprinted with permission of the American Medical Association.

AAMA Code

The Code of Ethics of the AAMA shall set forth principles of ethical and moral conduct as they relate to the medical profession and the particular practice of medical assisting.

Members of AAMA dedicated to the conscientious pursuit of their profession, and thus desiring to merit the high regard of the entire medical profession and the respect of the general public which they serve, do pledge themselves to strive always to:
A. render service with full respect for the dignity of humanity;
B. respect confidential information obtained through employment unless legally authorized or required by responsible performance of duty to divulge such information;
C. uphold the honor and high principles of the profession and accept its disciplines;
D. seek to continually improve the knowledge and skills of medical assistants for the benefit of patients and professional colleagues;
E. participate in additional service activities aimed toward improving the health and well being of the community.

ethics in their work, but they must also understand the physician's code. As the physician's representative, the medical assistant must carry out clinical and administrative duties within the guidelines of the AMA Principles of Medical Ethics.

To help the medical assistant student understand the AMA code, each section and its interpretation and application is examined here separately.

THE AMA PRINCIPLES OF MEDICAL ETHICS*
Preamble

The medical profession has long subscribed to a group of ethical statements developed primarily for the benefit of the patient. As a member of this profession, a physician must recognize responsibility not only to patients, but also to society, to other health professionals, and to self. The following Principles adopted by the American Medical Association are not laws, but standards of conduct which define the essentials of honorable behavior for the physician.

---

*Interpretation and application of the *AMA Principles of Medical Ethics* and overviews of *Current Opinions of the Judicial Council* are the author's own and do not represent the official interpretation of the AMA Judicial Council.

Table 4.1

Similar sections in the AAMA Code and the AMA Principles of Medical Ethics

AAMA	AMA
Members of AAMA. . . . do pledge themselves to strive always to:	A physician shall . . .
A. render service with full respect for the dignity of humanity;	I. . . . be dedicated to providing competent medical service with compassion and respect for human dignity.
B. respect confidential information obtained through employment unless legally authorized or required by responsible performance of duty to divulge such information;	IV. . . . safeguard patient confidences within the constraints of the law
C. uphold the honor and high principles of the profession and accept its disciplines;	II. . . . deal honestly with patients and colleagues and strive to expose those physicians deficient in character or competence, or who engage in fraud or deception.
D. seek to continually improve the knowledge and skills of medical assistants for the benefit of patients and professional colleagues;	V. . . . continue to study, apply, and advance scientific knowledge, make relevant information available to patients, colleagues and the public, obtain consultation, and use the talents of other health professionals when indicated.
E. participate in additional service activities aimed toward improving the health and well-being of the community.	VII. . . . recognize a responsibility to participate in activities contributing to an improved community.

Principle I

A physician shall be dedicated to providing competent medical service with compassion and respect for human dignity.

The physician must treat each individual with respect and understanding, without regard to race, creed, sex, or social status. Each patient has the right to expect personal attention and all necessary services that are within the physician's capabilities.

Principle II

A physician shall deal honestly with patients and colleagues, and strive to expose those physicians deficient in character or competence, or who engage in fraud or deception.

The appropriate channel for dealing with ineffectual, incompetent, or impaired physicians is through the official medical associations, beginning at the local level.

Inquiries or complaints about physicians may be made in writing to the professional relations committee of the county medical society. Member-physicians will contact the physician in question and, if appropriate, secure the records of the patient involved. If the complaint appears accurate, the committee will hold a hearing, make a determination

on the case, and report its findings to the physician and the complainant. If it appears that legal matters are involved, the issue will be referred to the state board of medical examiners.

If the professional relations committee determines that the physician is impaired, a different approach is attempted. An impaired physician is one who is incapable of optimally performing professional duties because of substance abuse or mental or physical illness. Impaired physicians are offered professional help in an effort to avoid legal difficulties or association censure. Many state associations have established committees to approach, educate, and obtain help for the impaired physician.

If the state board of medical examiners initiates the investigation of a physician based on a complaint by a physician, patient, or interested individual, the process is similar to that used by the medical society. Facts are gathered, the physician is allowed to submit information, and formal hearings are held. Once a complaint has been filed with the state board the information is considered public, and a copy of the complaint is forwarded to the appropriate medical society. The society may or may not initiate proceedings to censure the physician.

Principle III

A physician shall respect the law and also recognize a responsibility to seek changes in those requirements which are contrary to the best interests of the patient.

There is a distinct relationship between ethical standards and the law. The standards of conduct established to guide the professional physician never demand less than the law or conflict with established laws. In some cases, the Principles of Ethics require more from the physician than do the state statutes. As reinforcement of this relationship, the AMA Principles direct the physician to respect all laws as they stand.

Principle III also indicates to physicians that they have a responsibility to their patients and the profession to work toward the removal of laws that interfere with patients' well-being. Such laws might include those that restrict services for state-supported indigent patients, disclose patients' records inappropriately, or deny sex education to teenagers. Physicians who wish to change the law should work through appropriate channels and support organizations that work toward laws affecting patient issues.

Principle IV

A physician shall respect the rights of patients, colleagues, and other health professionals, and shall safeguard patient confidences within the constraints of the law.

The first part of Principle IV is an addition to the Principles that affirms the physician's responsibility to each individual with whom he or she comes into contact in the fulfillment of professional duties. The physician must always keep in mind the rights of consumers or other providers of health care services. Mutual respect enhances the end result—effective patient care.

The second part of Principle IV addresses the issue of patient confidentiality. Patients have the right to expect protection of the information acquired by the physician, and professionals recognize the need for confidentiality of the oral and written communications of a client. By educating the patient on the policy of confidentiality, health care professionals provide the patient with the freedom to reveal all of the information necessary to arrive at an accurate diagnosis and provide effective treatment. The release of confidential records or information requires the *written* consent of the patient except in limited legal situations. Instances that override the need for written submission involve required reports to state and county agencies,

patient involvement in a criminal act, or a lawsuit instituted by the patient. The legal issues involving confidentiality will be discussed further in Chapter 5.

Principle V

A physician shall continue to study, apply and advance scientific knowledge, make relevant information available to patients, colleagues and the public, obtain consultation and use the talents of other health professionals when indicated.

Although the AMA opposes *mandatory* continuing medical education, this principle clearly indicates that physicians have a responsibility to remain abreast of or enhance developments in their field and to share their skill and knowledge. In addition, physicians are morally bound to request the collaboration of other physicians when collaboration will enhance the patient's welfare or hasten the course of recovery or when the patient requests a second opinion. Physicians should recognize the patient's rights and be sensitive to the fact that patients may not realize their rights or may be too timid to request consultation. If the physician suspects that the patient is feeling insecure, he or she should offer the opportunity for another opinion.

Finally, Principle V encourages physicians to use the specialized skills of other health care professionals when such skills will benefit the patient. This can involve clinical and administrative assistance, and it relates to any individual who can provide necessary health care services.

Principle VI

A physician shall, in the provision of appropriate patient care, except in emergencies, be free to choose whom to serve, with whom to associate, and the environment in which to provide medical services.

Rendering appropriate emergency care depends on the environment in which the emergency occurs and the equipment that is available or can be improvised. In any case physicians are ethically bound to offer whatever assistance they can. Good Samaritan laws in every state protect the physician from legal recourse if the results of aid are less than optimal.

Emergency assistance does not establish a physician-patient relationship. Such a relationship is established when the patient or another physician acting as the patient's agent requests the services of a physician, and the physician agrees to accept the patient. This relationship is implied once an appointment has been made for the patient. Dismissing a patient or discontinuing the physician-patient relationship involves legal restrictions that will be discussed in Chapter 5. Ethically, the physician must provide the patient with adequate written notice of intent to withdraw from the case and allow appropriate time for the patient to secure the services of another physician.

Although physicians may choose with whom they wish to associate, they may not voluntarily associate with individuals who use unscientific methods of treatment. Associating involves sharing responsibility for the treatment of a patient. An association does *not* exist when a patient is referred to another physician for care. In this situation the physician who accepts the referral assumes total responsibility for the patient's care and is therefore not associated with the referral source. Basically the physician may accept a patient referral from any available source.

In choosing the environment in which to provide medical care, the physician may prefer private practice, an institutional setting, or a health maintenance organization (HMO). The physician's ethical responsibility in making this selection is to choose an environment in which nonmedical considerations do not restrict his or her ability to provide optimal care to patients.

Principle VII

A physician shall recognize a responsibility to participate in activities contributing to an improved community.

Physicians acquire knowledge that can be of value not only to individual patients but also to the general public. Physicians may assist the public by serving on medical association committees, which provide for community needs and educate the public regarding scientific developments or potential health hazards. Voluntary participation in charitable and research organization functions also assists the community.

THE JUDICIAL COUNCIL OF THE AMA
Defining the Council

The Judicial Council of the AMA consists of five members nominated by the AMA president and elected by the House of Delegates for a 5-year term. One member's term expires each year, so that a new member is elected at each annual convention. The Judicial Council performs several functions, including the interpretation of the *Prin-*

ciples of Medical Ethics. The Council has absolute authority in judicial matters, and its decisions are final.

The Purpose of the Council Opinions

The *Current Opinions of the Judicial Council* was published in June, 1982. It is an appendage to the latest revision of the *Principles of Medical Ethics* approved at the 1980 annual convention.

The opinions presented by the Judicial Council are guides to responsible professional behavior. The Council insists, however, that its opinions are not the only means to achieve medical morality. For clarity the Council's opinions are grouped into nine major headings, with subheadings, by number and subject matter. The subheadings are numbered as decimal points of the major numbers; thus 1.00 is the number for the heading *Introduction,* and 1.01 is the number for the subheading for *Terminology.*

The numbering for the Council subject headings does not coincide with the numbering of the subject matter covered in the *Principles of Medical Ethics.* The *Current Opinions of the Judicial Council* is also more detailed than the principles, because it must address the increasing number of situations unique to the complex medical environment. Only a brief overview of each major subject will be presented.

Council Subjects
1.00 Introduction

Section 1.00 is titled *Introduction* and deals with the terminology of ethics and the interdependent relationship of law and ethics. In particular this section points out that legal proceedings and medical organization censure are conducted separately. However, evidence of possible criminal action by a physician that is discovered by a medical society must be reported to the proper government authorities.

2.00 Opinions on social policy issues

Section 2.00 is the largest section of the Council Opinions. This indicates the complexity of social, medical, and technological developments. Subjects covered include the following:
- Abortion;
- Artificial insemination by standard and test-tube techniques;
- Clinical investigation for treatment or for the accumulation of scientific knowledge;

- Consideration of the cost of health care;
- Genetic engineering;
- Guidelines for organ transplantation;
- Quality of life;
- Terminal illness; and
- Unnecessary or worthless services.

Each of these subjects is controversial and can be the foundation of misunderstandings on the part of the public. Entering into discussions with patients on these issues may be unwise because of the emotional responses of many individuals to the subject matter. If such questions are pursued by patients they should be referred to the physician.

3.00 Interprofessional relations

The physician has many opportunities to request the services of other health care professionals. These requests may be for diagnostic services or treatment services, and physicians are responsible for selecting practitioners who will provide competent care in accordance with accepted standards.

4.00 Hospital relations

The hospital is a necessary facility for the practice of medicine, and the physician is necessary for the continued functioning of the hospital. Therefore it is important that the relations between physicians and hospitals be positive for the ultimate benefit of the patient. The Judicial Council develops its opinions on physicians fees for hospital care, physician ownership of health facilities, physicians as hospital employees, and the organization of hospital medical staff members to enhance physician education and professional skills.

5.00 Confidentiality, advertising and communications media relations

Section 5.00 of the Council Opinions involves some very complex issues that have changed recently because of technology and federal regulations.

Confidentiality of patient information is discussed in relation to attorney-physician relations, the potential impact of computers, insurance company representatives, and industrial cases.

Advertising and publicity are discussed in relation to the form of the communication (print, radio, or television), the content of the advertising, and the federal standards for commercial advertising.

The final area covered in Section 5.00 involves the release of information to the press. In routine cases information regarding a patient's condition, illness, or disease cannot be released to the press without the consent of the patient or the patient's legal representative. The only situation that does not require the patient's authorization occurs when the information is in the public domain. The category of public domain involves births, deaths, accidents, and police cases. In these cases the physician may reveal the demographic data on the patient such as name, address, age, and sex, the general nature of the accident, the diagnosis and prognosis, and the patient's present condition.

6.00 Fees and charges

The basic theme of Section 6.00 is avoiding the charging or collecting of fees that are illegal or excessive. Fees for medical services must be reasonable as determined by such criteria as the complexity of the service, the customary fee for the locality, the quality of the services provided, and the experience of the physician.

Fee splitting, paying a physician only for the referral of a patient, is *always* unethical. This practice includes payments to the referring physician by other physicians, clinics or laboratories, or drug companies for prescriptions written.

Section 6.00 of the opinions also presents three points regarding charges that involve the medical assistant in the education of patients and the establishment office policy: (1) charging for completion of insurance forms, (2) interest and finance charges on unpaid balances, and (3) billing for outside laboratory services. It is the opinion of the Council that a fee should *not* be charged for routine, simple insurance forms, though a customary fee may be charged for more complex forms. Charging interest and finance charges is ethical if the patient is aware in advance that these fees will be charged. The notice must be *in writing* and may be accomplished by a posted sign, a patient information pamphlet, or a notice on the statement sent to the patient. However, harsh collection practices are not appropriate. Billing for outside laboratory services is done when a laboratory specimen is collected in the physician's office and sent to a clinical laboratory for analysis. The laboratory, in an effort to reduce cost to the patient, prefers not to send statements to individual patients. Instead the laboratory bills the physician for all services performed each month, itemized by patient, and at a reduced rate because of the saved billing charges. The physician's statement to the patient will then state the actual fee charged by the laboratory and a minimal separate charge for the professional skill required in obtaining the specimen. The latter is often called a handling charge. The total charge to patients is less than if they had gone to the laboratory for the services and been billed separately.

One final area in the discussion of fees involves the method of charging for physicians' assistants in surgery. Each physician involved in the surgery should send a separate bill for his or her services. In the rare case in which the primary surgeon bills for all of the physicians' services and distributes the fees, the practice is considered ethical *if* the patient understands the financial arrangement in advance.

7.00 Physician records

Section 7.00 of the Judicial Council Opinions deals with the ownership and transfer of patient records. The progress notes made in a patient's chart and the data gathered are considered the physician's personal property. The information should not be withheld from other physicians, attorneys, or other persons designated by the patient in writing. Record requests accompanied by an appropriate release may not be denied for any reason, including nonpayment of a bill for medical services.

Many states have enacted laws that give patients access to their medical records. However, some of these laws include a restriction on the availability of psychiatric records. If the patient has a legal right to his record, the physician must supply a copy of the file or a narrative summary, depending on local statute. The physician should *never* release the actual chart. A reasonable charge may be made to cover the cost of photocopying the records or supplying a narrative report.

On the retirement or death of a physician the patients must be notified and their records transferred to the physician of their choice on receipt of a written authorization. If the patient does not request a transfer, the records should be retained by an individual legally permitted to act as a custodian of records. If a medical practice is sold, the new physician acquires the furniture, equipment, and *goodwill*. The goodwill of a medical practice involves the opportunity to continue the care of the patients formerly treated by the physician selling the practice. Patients must be notified that the records are to be transferred to a new physician and offered the opportunity to transfer them to a physician of their choice.

8.00 Opinions on practice matters

Practice matters are discussed in 12 subsections that cover a variety of subjects. Some are related to the mode of practice and outline the physician's ethical requirements when working for a clinic or under contractual arrangements. Physicians in these situations must be satisfied that all members of the group also practice ethical medicine.

Fees and income are discussed with regard to source and influence. A patient may be charged for a missed appointment or for one not cancelled with a 24-hour notice if the patient is fully aware that this charge may be made. Physicians are advised, however, to resort to this tactic infrequently and only after careful consideration of the patient's circumstances. The physician's preferences in drug prescription may not be influenced by any financial interest in a pharmaceutical firm, and the patient should have free choice of where to fill the prescription. Patients should not be discouraged from requesting a written prescription, nor should they be encouraged to patronize a specific pharmacy because the physician has a direct intercom line to that pharmacy.

Other practice matters discussed involve the patient's right to informed consent, to pertinent information about the condition under treatment, and to the attention of the physician. Once a physician-patient relationship is established, the physician may not neglect the patient and must give adequate notice in the event of withdrawal from a case.

The final area discussed under practice matters involves substitution of a surgeon without the patient's knowledge or consent. In popular literature and medical jargon, this is known as "ghost surgery." In all respects, substituting a surgeon without the patient's knowledge violates the patient's right to free choice of physician. Should the surgeon become incapacitated for any reason, the patient must be informed and allowed to decide whether or not to accept the substitute. An emergency situation may preclude the consent of a patient, and the selection of the surgeon may rest with the health care facility if there is no available next of kin.

9.00 Professional rights and responsibilities

The last section of the Council's Opinions deals with the civil rights of physicians and their right to membership in professional associations without regard to race, religion, ethnic origin, or sex. Physicians can expect discipline according to association rules, review by their peers, and the right to due process.

Patients can also exercise their right to free choice of physician or health care plan. They can expect ethical conduct from their physician of choice, whether the physician practices in a private setting, a clinic, an HMO, a group practice, or a closed panel, which is a relatively new method of practice involving a group of physicians who serve a selected group of patients who agree to a health care plan with a limited number of physicians from which to choose.

Obtaining a copy of the Opinions

A detailed copy of the 1982 *Current Opinions of the Judicial Council of the American Medical Association* may be obtained by writing to:

Order Department OP-122
American Medical Association
PO Box 10946
Chicago, IL 60610

When requesting a copy, note that you are a medical assistant student.

THE PHYSICIAN AND THE MEDICAL ASSISTANT

As shown in Table 4.1, the five sections of the medical assistant's Code of Ethics are clearly aligned in concept with the physician's Principles. Three of the AMA principles deal with matters that can only be controlled by the physician. Responsibility for respect of legal boundaries and for working toward changes of inappropriate statutes rests solely with physicians (Principle III). In addition, only physicians can determine who they will serve, in which environment they will practice, (Principle VI) and which activities they can perform to improve their community (Principle VII), just as Section E of the AAMA code, the equivalent of AMA Principle VII, is under the control of the medical assistant.

Aside from the three sections of the Principles that are strictly under the physician's control, the medical assistant is expected to conduct business and perform clinical skills according to the standards set for and expected of physicians. A working knowledge of the AMA Principles will provide the guidelines necessary for the medical assistant to avoid an inadvertent error or a breach of ethics. Understanding the AMA Principles also means understanding the medical assistant's Code of Ethics. The medical assistant is responsible for both.

Conclusion

As a professional medical assistant you will have a responsibility to the patient, the profession, and the community. If you follow the physician's Principles and the medical assistant's Code of Ethics, you will be performing according to the highest possible standards.

It is rare but possible that a physician or facility will conduct business outside of the guidelines established by the professional principles of ethics. If you believe that the codes of ethics are not being upheld in the place in which you are working, you should attempt to evaluate the situation objectively. Perhaps you are not aware of all the factors involved or have misunderstood an event. In that case, seek the guidance of a more experienced individual or discuss the situation with the physician. In either case, you should not presume to mention unethical behavior. Instead, state that you do not understand a certain situation and would appreciate help in understanding the basic reasons for it. If the question is still not resolved to your satisfaction, seek the advice of knowledgeable professionals without revealing confidential information. If you determine that unethical practices are taking place, you must decide whether to stay in the practice or seek other employment. If you choose to stay in the hope of changing the situation, remember that others may be equally aware of the unethical conduct. This awareness may reflect on you negatively when you seek employment in another office or agency. If you choose to leave the situation, be discreet in explaining the reason why to your present and future employers.

Review Questions

1. What two conditions are necessary for an individual to be capable of participating in a system governed by a code of ethics?
2. When was the first code of ethics adopted by the AMA? Why has it been revised?
3. How did the 1957 revision greatly differ from previous revisions?
4. How many principles are there in the AMA Principles of Medical Ethics? How many in the AAMA Code of Ethics? State in your own

words the sections that are similar in both statements on ethical behavior and briefly interpret each.

5. State the three principles of the AMA code that are under the sole control of the physician.
6. Discuss the purpose of the Judicial Council of the AMA.
7. Briefly discuss the Judicial Council Opinions on

social policy issues, interprofessional relations, confidentiality, fees and charges, and physicians' records.

8. Describe the responsibilities of the medical assistant in relation to medical ethics.
9. Describe your options if you believe that the Principles of Medical Ethics are not being respected in your place of employment.

SUGGESTED READINGS

American Medical Association: Current opinions of the Judicial Council, Chicago, 1982, The Association.
American Medical Association: Medicolegal forms with legal analyses, Chicago, 1981, The Association.
Lewis MA and Wardon CD: Law and ethics in the medical office, Philadelphia, 1983, FA Davis.

Chapter 5

Medical Practice and the Law

- Definition of legal medicine
- Relationship of law and ethics
- Purpose of medical practice acts
- Medical licensure
- Role of the medical assistant
- Duty to patients

- Professional liability
- Handling liability claims
- Good Samaritan acts
- Controlled substances
- Uniform Anatomical Gift Act
- Reporting responsibilities

Objectives

On completion of Chapter 5 the medical assistant student should be able to:

1 Define the terms listed in the vocabulary.

2 Discuss medical practice acts, their purpose, and their relationship to licensure.

3 State the difference between permissive and informed consent; discuss who can give consent for treatment.

4 Define professional medical liability.

5 List and discuss the three common causes of professional liability suits.

6 List the four elements of negligence.

7 Describe the physician's legal responsibility for others.

8 Discuss the three options for handling professional liability claims.

9 Discuss Good Samaritan acts and their limitations.

10 State briefly the 10 elements of the Uniform Anatomical Gift Act.

11 Discuss briefly the reporting responsibilities for births, deaths, communicable diseases, medical examiner cases, and child abuse cases.

12 Discuss the two circumstances under which permissive reports are allowed.

Vocabulary

binding arbitration A method of settling a dispute in which the facts are heard by a neutral third party and the decision of the arbiter is final; neither party may subsequently pursue the issue in court.

burden of proof The responsibility of verifying beyond a doubt the facts in an issue; usually the responsibility of the plaintiff.

civil law The area of the legal system that decides issues and protects the rights of individuals in relation to the actions of other individuals.

contributory negligence An act or omission by a defendant that can be directly linked to the cause of injury.

criminal law The area of the legal system that decides issues in relation to the actions of individuals against the state and society in general.

defamation An injury to an individual's

47

public image or reputation through deliberate false, misleading, or malicious statements.

defendant An individual accused of wrongful action in a civil or criminal matter.

emancipated minor An individual at least 16 years of age who lives independent of the financial support of a parent or legal guardian.

felony A criminal offense of a serious nature that is usually punishable by imprisonment.

judicial Pertaining to the administration of the law.

jurisprudence The philosophy on which the legal system is based.

libel Written or printed defamation of the reputation of an individual that results in public ridicule, degradation, or disgrace.

malfeasance An action that is in every respect considered wrong or unlawful.

non compos mentis A general term relating to the alteration of the mental status of an individual.

offeree An individual who invites an offer, such as a physician who, by establishing a medical practice in a community, invites potential patients to offer themselves for care.

offeror The individual who makes an offer, such as the potential patient who approaches a physician for care.

plaintiff The individual who initiates a legal action against another person; the person who instigates a lawsuit or files a complaint.

quackery The inappropriate practice of medicine by an individual with neither the appropriate knowledge of nor skill in the field.

res ipsa loquitor Literally "the thing speaks for itself," in other words, the action is obvious or self-explanatory.

res judicata A matter settled according to the process established by law.

rule of discovery The point in time at which a patient realizes or should have realized that he has been injured; the starting point of the statute of limitations.

slander Spoken defamation that results in injury to the reputation of another individual.

statute of limitations A period of time established by law during which an individual may file a civil lawsuit. The period, often 1 year, begins at the time an injury occurs or at the time an individual discovers the injury.

subject (in experimental studies) A person who agrees to participate in a program involving an experiment for treating or gathering information about a disease or illness.

subpoena A legal order (writ) to appear at a given time and place to present evidence in a civil or criminal matter. Records, correspondence, and documents may also be required by subpoena.

tort A civil injury or wrongdoing.

DEFINITION OF LEGAL MEDICINE

Legal medicine is determined by the laws of the state in which the physician practices or has a license to practice medicine. The licensing board in each state receives its authority from the statute or law known as the medical practice act and polices the activity of the physicians practicing in the state. The medical practice act of each state defines the limitations of medical practice, prescribes the penalties for practicing without a valid license, and specifies the conditions that would warrant the revocation of a physician's license. Some of the more common reasons for the revocation of a medical license include the following:
- Drug addiction or substance abuse (drugs, alcohol);
- Conviction of a felony;
- Mental illness;
- Crime involving moral turpitude;

- Prescribing drugs without examining the patient or performing a good-faith examination of the patient;
- Prescribing drugs for known addicts;
- Insurance claim fraud; and
- Gross negligence in the care of patients.

RELATIONSHIP OF LAW AND ETHICS

Legal medicine and the ethics of the medical profession are philosophically linked. Medical laws and ethics complement one another and serve as guides to reach the same goal: to make the best possible health care available to consumers. Although physicians are responsible to different authorities for legal matters and ethical concerns, both are easily accomplished by one course of action. The principles of medical ethics support legal requirements and are never less demanding of the physician's behavior. Medical ethics frequently requires more of the physician than does the law.

PURPOSE OF MEDICAL PRACTICE ACTS

The consumer is the reason for medical practice acts. The sole purpose of laws that regulate methods of providing health care is to protect the rights and the health of patients. Before the existence of medical practice acts, quackery was not uncommon, medical care was inconsistent, and patient welfare was jeopardized. By 1900 medical science was developing at a rapid pace, which increased the risk of patients' exposure to inadequate care. By the same time each state realized the need to pass laws to protect consumers and to develop standards by which the public could be assured of appropriate care. Statutes regarding medical practice are introduced in state legislatures as needed in response to social changes and scientific developments.

MEDICAL LICENSURE

All 50 states and the District of Columbia have licensing statutes, and it is illegal to practice medicine without a license anywhere in the United States. In most states the physician may acquire a license by *written examination, endorsement,* or *reciprocity.* Each state medical board provides a written examination for physicians and sets the required level of proficiency necessary to receive a license to practice. In an effort to develop national standards for the practice of medicine a National Board Examination was developed and is taken by most medical students before graduation. Many states accept a passing national board score in lieu of the state examination and are said to issue licenses by *endorsement.* The third method of obtaining a license to practice medicine is by reciprocity. If a physician wishes to change residence from one state to another, the medical licensing board of the new state may grant the physician a license on the basis of his or her qualification for a license in the original state. This usually occurs when both states have similar requirements for licensure. The requirements for license renewal vary from state to state. The current situation and some of the anticipated changes were discussed in Chapter 2. Regardless of how a license to practice medicine is acquired, the physician is responsible for fulfilling the responsibilities outlined by the state and for practicing medicine within the guidelines of the state's medical practice act.

ROLE OF THE MEDICAL ASSISTANT

The medical assistant is the legal representative agent of the physician and can be held individually responsible or involve the physician in a legal dispute. Therefore it is vital for the medical assistant to conduct business within the legal guidelines established to regulate the physician's responsibilities (Table 5.1) and protect the patient's rights. The common areas of responsibility for the physician and the medical assistant will be discussed in this chapter.

DUTY TO PATIENTS
Establishing a Physician-Patient Relationship

Patient care is a mutual agreement made after sufficient consideration, to do or not to do certain things. This becomes a contract which may be either expressed or implied. An *expressed* contract is developed in distinct oral or written language. An *implied* contract is one not necessarily produced by or documented in an explicit agreement between the involved parties. However, an implied contract is recognized by law and based on the conduct of the parties involved. The established relationship between a physician and a patient is considered an implied contract.

Patient expectations

Physicians and medical assistants must remember that patients are not aware of all of the legal fine points of medical care and frequently are very distracted by the anticipation of medical care. It is not uncommon for patients to become restless when diagnostic and treatment plans take longer than expected or to make demands that are impossible to fulfill.

Careful and consistent patient education and the establishment of an open communication system are important. Patients who understand why certain procedures are necessary or know what to expect during treatment programs are usually more cooperative and realistic in their expectations.

Consent
General considerations

Each individual who receives medical care and treatment has the legal right to participate in decisions that affect his well-being. In fact, the final decision regarding care rests solely with the patient or the patient's legal guardian, whether or not the physician feels the decision is in the patient's best interest. The physician must respect the patient's

Table 5.1
Responsibility to the patient

Requires physicians to:	Does not require physicians to:
1. Use due care, skill, and diligence in treating patients. 2. Keep informed of the best methods of diagnosis and treatment. 3. Perform to the best of their ability whether or not the fee is paid. 4. Exercise the best professional judgment in all cases. 5. Consider the established customary treatment for similar cases as determined by the profession. 6. Abstain from experimental treatment except with the complete understanding and approval of the patient. 7. Provide proper instructions to the person caring for a patient during the physician's absence. 8. Furnish proper and complete instructions to each patient. 9. Take every precaution to prevent the spread of contagious diseases. 10. Advise patients against needless or unwise treatments or operations.	1. Accept employment from anyone who solicits their services. 2. Restore the patient to the same condition as before treatment was initiated. 3. Possess the *highest* skill or the *maximum* education available. 4. Effect a recovery with every patient. 5. Be familiar with every possible reaction of patients to *all* anesthetics or drugs. 6. Be skilled as specialists if they are general practitioners. 7. Make correct diagnosis in every case. 8. Be free from errors of judgment in every case, particularly difficult cases. 9. Display infallibility of judgment. 10. Continue services after they have been discharged by a patient or the patient's legal representative, even if harm should be anticipated for the patient. 11. Guarantee the successful result of any treatment or operation.

right to decide and his decision and provide appropriate care based on the limitations of the patient's consent. There are two types of consent for treatment: permissive consent and informed consent. Informed consent is the type most commonly and extensively discussed; permissive consent is considered implied when informed consent is obtained. Any consent may be implied, that is understood or assumed, or expressed either orally or in writing. A consent may be withdrawn by the patient at any time.

Permissive consent

In the course of examination and treatment, the physician must touch the patient. Permissive consent authorizes the necessary body contact and is usually an implied consent. Touching an individual without consent can result in a charge of assault and battery against the physician. In legal terminology *assault* is the threat of unauthorized contact and *battery* is the actual unauthorized contact. Even if the services provided have positive results, the patient may sue the physician for damages, pain, and suffering.

If a question or objection should arise during the course of examination, the physician should suspend the examination and answer the patient's questions or offer further explanation. The examination should resume only with the patient's permission. When a female patient is to be examined by a male physician a female assistant should be present. A patient might misunderstand a method of examination, and the presence of a female assistant will be reassuring. This person's presence will also guard against inappropriate charges of unauthorized body contact.

Informed consent

Purpose. Informed consent is a means of involving patients in decisions regarding their medical care and of legally protecting the physician. To make a knowledgeable decision, a patient *must* understand what is planned, who will provide care or perform a procedure, the expected outcome of the treatment, the risks involved, and alternative care or treatment possibilities.

Situations requiring informed consent. Consent problems are more common in situations involving surgery than diagnostic procedures or medical care, but informed consent should be acquired for any situation that involves risk. When procedures are conducted in an office, informed consent is often oral. In this case the physician must be careful to note in the patient's record that the necessary information was supplied to the patient and that the patient agreed with the treatment plan.

Providing the necessary information. Written informed consent requires the patient's signature on a preprinted form with the details of the specific procedure included. The patient's signature is witnessed by an employee who supervises the acquisition of the written permission. The patient is expected to carefully read the consent form before signing, but this step is often ignored because of anxiety, trust, or disinterest. The person signing the form as a witness, often the medical assistant, must be aware that this means that he or she acknowledges the patient read the form before signing. If there is any doubt, the witness should review each section of the form with the patient before either of them signs the form.

Avoiding omissions. Many techniques may be employed to assure that all aspects of the consent are adequately covered. For frequently performed procedures physicians may develop their own information sheet, purchase one prepared by a commercial medical education organization, or use videotapes. Any educational material from an outside source must be *carefully* reviewed by the physician for accuracy before it is made available to patients. However, such printed material must *never* replace oral communication between the patient and the medical care provider.

A prepared checklist of the elements of an informed consent may help assure that all important information is passed on to the patient. The minimum information to be discussed for an informed consent to exist includes the following:

1. The date;
2. The specific planned procedure;
3. Any potential risks;
4. The anticipated benefit or result;
5. Any alternative treatments or procedures;
6. Any exclusions (reasons the patient provides that alter the options available, such as allergies to substances or respiratory conditions that will influence the choice of anesthesia);
7. Assurance that the patient's questions are always welcome;
8. The patient's right to withdraw consent at any time;
9. Any unusual circumstances;
10. The signature of the patient or the patient's legal guardian or representative; and
11. The signature of the witness to the consent procedure.

Who can give consent. It is vital that consent for treatment be obtained from the appropriate individual. As in contracts, the individual providing consent must be of legal age and capable of providing permission. In most instances a minor (under the age of 18) may not legally contract for medical care. A legal guardian must be advised of all of the information involved in an informed consent. A legal guardian has the power to grant permission. Exceptions to this rule that allow minors to provide their own consent occur in the following circumstances:

1. The minor is serving on active duty in the armed services;
2. The minor is emancipated (self-supporting and at least 16 years old);
3. A communicable disease is involved, including sexually transmitted disease;
4. An unwed pregnancy;
5. Illness related to substance (drug) abuse; or
6. Advice regarding birth control and abortion.

Mental capacity is an important criterion for a valid consent. Mental illness, diminished capacity, or mental retardation interfere with the possibility of an individual contracting for care or granting informed consent for treatment. Individuals who are temporarily incapacitated because of medication or shock or who are in a reduced state of consciousness are also incapable of granting informed consent. A legal guardian must be appointed to act on the patient's behalf.

Emergency care and consent

In the case of a life-threatening emergency, the survival of the patient is the *only* consideration. Regardless of the age, capacity, or consideration of the patient, it is understood that treatment cannot be delayed. The physician's judgment prevails in an emergency, and consent is not required.

Abandonment and Dismissal

An established physician-patient relationship requires the physician to provide services when needed and to attend to the obvious needs of the patient. Abandonment is the failure to meet the requirements of the physician-patient relationship. However, the relationship may be discontinued by the mutual agreement of the patient and the physician, or the patient may dismiss the physician either orally or in writing. Should the physician wish to dismiss the patient, certain details must be considered to avoid a legal charge of abandonment.

Avoiding abandonment charges

A physician may wish to terminate a relationship because the patient refuses to follow advice or cooperate in the agreed treatment program or continually fails to keep appointments. It is also necessary to terminate the physician-patient relationship when the physician retires, relocates the practice to another community, or has to discontinue practice for any reason. The patient may charge abandonment unless the physician does the following:

1. Provides adequate notification of the intention to terminate care;
2. Remains available to the patient during the notification period;
3. Provides competent substitute care when continuing care is necessary; and
4. Cooperates with the new physician by supplying the information necessary to provide appropriate care.

The physician and medical assistant must be aware that abandonment can also be charged in less obvious situations. A physician may be sued if a telephone message requesting help is not relayed, if hospitalized patients are not visited daily by the physician or a competent substitute, if "on-call" coverage is not provided during the physician's absence, or if the physician does not provide the patient with a means of contacting him or her 24 hours a day.

Procedure for patient dismissal

When the dismissal of a patient is necesary for any reason, a predetermined procedure should be followed to avoid missing an important step. A sample procedure follows.

Once an effective procedure has been developed, it should be integrated into the office procedure manual and used as needed. A sample letter that might be used in completing the procedure is shown on p. 53.

Standards of Care

Patients expect a certain standard of care, a level of quality that includes professional skill and diligence. In a legal sense the standard of care is determined by the care that would be provided by an average practitioner under the same or similar conditions. In each circumstance physicians are expected to do the following:

- Apply their best judgment in diagnosis and treatment;
- Refer a patient to a specialist or request consultation when necessary; and
- Advise patients of their physical condition, limitations, or need for continued care.

If a physician becomes involved in a legal dispute over a standard of care, the law presumes that the defendant physician provided appropriate care. The responsibility for proving that the physician did not meet the standard of care rests with the plaintiff. If other physicians are used as witnesses in this type of case they must be of similar training and experience and practice under similar conditions.

Procedure for Dismissing a Patient

Procedure	*Rationale*
1. Determine that a dismissal notice is necessary.	The change is unavoidable, or a change of physician will be in the patient's best interest.
2. Determine the appropriate notification period—usually a minimum of 14 days.	Different environments will require varying periods to acquire another physician's services (easier in urban areas).
3. Prepare the dismissal letter. Include date, reason for dismissal, period for change, available interim assistance, transfer of records, and physician's signature.	
4. Retain a copy of the letter in the patient's medical record.	This documents the contents of the letter.
5. Address the envelope specifically to the patient or guardian.	The letter should be considered confidential.
6. Send the letter by certified mail, requesting a return receipt.	The receipt must be signed by addressee, proving that the letter was received.
7. Retain the signed receipt in the patient's chart, attached to the letter copy.	This documents that the letter was received by the patient.

Experimental Procedures

The first consideration in experimental procedures involves medical ethics. This consideration has evolved since the trials at Nuremberg that followed World War II. These trials dealt with physicians who performed experimental procedures on involuntary human subjects. When the trials were over, the World Medical Association developed the Declaration of Helsinki, which was subsequently endorsed by the American Medical Association. With some modification, the Declaration remains as the foundation for the modern medical ethics regarding experimentation on human beings.

Scientific experimentation is classified as either primarily for treatment or for the gathering of scientific knowledge. In general the latter category does *not* provide medical benefits to the individual participating in the study. It is designed to help a segment of the population eventually. Experimentation with treatment, on the other hand, is used in anticipation of helping an individual recover from or survive an illness. In both situations it is the responsibility of the physicians working with the experimental process to assure the safety, health, and welfare of the patient or subject. It is also vital that the patient give informed consent especially in regard to risks, expected outcome, and alternative treatment.

The Food and Drug Administration (FDA) has established rules to regulate informed consent if drugs are involved in the experiment. Drug experiments are classified as Phase I, Phase II, or Phase III experiments. *Written* informed consent is required for Phase I or II experiments. A Phase III experiment is the final step before a drug is released to the market, and the physician has the option of obtaining either oral or written consent. However, the responsibility to inform the patient of all relevant information still applies.

PROFESSIONAL LIABILITY
General Law

The law of each state involves two types of actions and responsibilities that are classified as criminal law and civil law. In very limited terms, criminal law deals with actions against the state and in theory against *all citizens;* civil law involves the actions of individuals against individuals. Civil lawsuits are covered by the segment of the law known as *tort* and include professional liability determinations.

Sample Dismissal Letter

Physician's Name
Street address
City, state, zip code

September 23, 1989

Ms. Jane Doe
123 Main Street
Anywhere, USA 12345

Dear Ms. Doe,

As we discussed at your last appointment on September _____, 1989, I feel it is very important for you to have further diagnostic studies and possible surgery because of your abnormal Pap smear, dated September _____, 1989.

Since you have refused appointments for follow-up care offered by my staff on four separate occasions, it is necessary for me to withdraw as your physician effective October 15, 1989. You require continued medical care and I urge you to select another physician before that date. On receipt of your written request I will supply your new physician with all information necessary to continue your care.

If you should require medical care before October 15, 1989, I will be available to you.

Very truly yours,

Physician's name, MD

Defining Professional Liability

Professional liability claims must have two components to be valid:

1. The physician fails in his or her duty to a patient as required by the medical practice acts.
2. The failure in duty results in a discernible injury to the patient.

The common term for professional liability is *malpractice,* a word that medical professionals shun because of its negative implications. The use of the word should always be avoided in the course of performing professional duties.

Liability Insurance

Insurance policies are available specifically to protect the physician's assets in the event that liability claim is made by or settled in favor of a patient. The number of lawsuits filed against physicians has increased steadily since the early 1960s. Increased technology, the complexity of available medical services, and the raised expectations of patients contribute to the rise in the number of claims. As claims and the dollar amounts of settlements increased, the cost of liability insurance increased, until it reached unprecedented proportions in the early 1970s. During 1974 and 1975 some insurance premiums were raised 300% to 400%, and this created what was considered a crisis for physicians. The cost of professional liability is determined by the potential risk of the medical speciality. The medical practices considered the lowest risks include internal medicine, psychiatry, and general practice; the highest-risk specialties include neurosurgery, anesthesiology, and obstetrics.

As with any insurance policy, the purchaser may set the limits of the coverage and the basic functions of the policy. The limits of a professional liability policy are usually stated in two separate dollar amounts, such as $1-$3 million coverage. The lower figure relates to the maximum amount of money available to settle any single incident, and the higher figure represents the maximum amount of money for all incidents that occur within the policy period. A policy period is usually 1 year, therefore policies must be renewed on an annual basis.

Professional liability insurance may be purchased to cover the physician for an incident, regardless of when the claim is made, as long as the policy was in effect when the incident took place. This is called an occurrence policy. The other type of policy, called a claims made policy, will protect the physician *only* if the policy is in effect when the incident occurs *and* when the claim is made. Physicians with this type of policy must purchase what is called a "tail" to provide coverage after they retire.

Common Causes of Lawsuits

The most frequent grounds cited in professional liability suits are negligence, lack of informed consent, abandonment, and missed diagnoses. Professional insurance analysts and medicolegal experts believe that the primary reason a patient will file a professional liability suit against a physician, regardless of the grounds, is a break-down in the physician-patient relationship because of a lack of communication. It has also been determined that a majority of the suits filed are unfounded, but before this is determined the physician and the insurance company attorneys will invest a great deal of time and money on the complaint.

Being aware of this gives physicians the ability to control a major factor in lawsuits. By developing and maintaining rapport with patients throughout all aspects of care, physicians can prevent most unfounded lawsuits. This is not to say that communication can take the place of competent, diligent patient care; all these factors are necessary for the best possible practice of medicine. Overall the important considerations remains the welfare of the patient.

Negligence and Liability

Negligence in the performance of duty constitutes malpractice in any profession. Attorneys, accountants, and clergy are as capable of malpractice as medical professionals. Negligence of professional duty may be the result of an action or an omission. In other words, a physician is negligent if he or she performs a service that is not in accordance with the expected standards of care or fails to perform a service that is necessary for the well-being of a patient. When a patient is injured (physically or mentally) because of the physician's negligence the patient may sue for financial compensation. A physician's liability (responsibility) is determined to exist if four distinct elements are present.

AMA criteria of negligence

The American Medical Association's 1963 Committee on Medicolegal Problems produced a report discussing the elements necessary for negligence to exist. These elements have become known as the "four Ds." They are as follows:

- Duty;
- Derelict;

• Direct cause; and
• Damages.

The plaintiff in a negligence suit against a physician must be able to support the claim with evidence of *each* of these elements.

Mutual agreement establishes a contract for medical care between the physician and the patient. Once a physician accepts the responsibility for a patient's care, he or she has a *duty* to provide medical services according to the standards of care.

The *derelict* physician fails in the performance of duty to the patient by either falling short of the expected standards of care or abandoning the patient.

The principle of *direct cause* means that the explicit act or omission by the physician is directly linked to the injury suffered by the patient. The plaintiff must prove that the physician's actions and no other possible cause resulted in an injury.

Damages are the result of actions by a physician that could have been predicted or anticipated. The measure of damages in a professional liability case are classified as compensatory. *General compensation* is a dollar amount for injury, pain, suffering, potential loss of earning, and so forth, that do not have to be confirmed. *Special compensation* might involve actual added costs of medical care, hospital services, rehabilitation, and so on, that must be documented.

California Medical Association "ABCDs" of negligence

The California Medical Association Committee on Professional Liability restated the necessary elements for negligence to exist in slightly different and perhaps simplified language. This version may help the medical assistant remember the relationship of the various factors to one another. As stated in the CMA 1971 report, negligence in medical practice involves the following:

A—Acceptance of a person as a patient;
B—Breach of the physician's duty of skill or care;
C—Causal connection between the breach by the physician and the damage to the patient; and
D—Damage of foreseeable nature.

The criteria for negligence is demonstrated in the following example:

A board-certified orthopedic surgeon is asked by a pediatrician to treat a 10-year-old boy for a simple displaced fracture of the ulna and radius just above wrist level. The orthopedist examines the child, reviews the x-ray films, and determines the necessary treatment. After discussing the treatment plan and need for anesthesia with the parents and obtaining the parents' written consent, treatment begins. The child is given a general anesthetic, the fracture is reduced, and the proper position of the bones is confirmed by x-ray film. As the physician begins to apply the cast a message is delivered that the office medical assistant received an important call that should be returned as soon as possible. In haste, the physician applies the cast too loosely and without sufficient layers of plaster to provide adequate support. Four weeks later a follow-up x-ray film reveals that the bones have changed position and are no longer in alignment. Surgery is necessary to attempt correction of the alignment. After complete healing it is determined that the child will never have complete range of motion with the arm.

If the parents sue the pediatrician on the child's behalf the defendant (the pediatrician) should be cleared. The pediatrician fulfilled his or her duty by recognizing the need for a specialist and referring the patient to a qualified orthopedist. If the parents sue the orthopedist the judgment should be in favor of the plaintiffs (the parents). Negligence could be demonstrated in each area:

• Duty—the orthopedist did not provide appropriate care for the patient according to acceptable standards of care;
• Derelict—the physician was derelict in not applying a proper cast;
• Direct cause—direct cause can be demonstrated between the weak cast and the subsequent bone displacement; and
• Damages—the case involves permanent disability.

In a true legal sense this example is extremely simple and the outcome very obvious. Actual medicolegal cases are usually very complex and require a great deal of research to determine if the four necessary elements are present.

Statute of Limitations

Each state determines a statute of limitations, the period of time in which a civil lawsuit may be *filed*. Filing a claim with the court establishes the lawsuit process; the process does not have to be completed within the statute of limitations. It is possible that determination may not be made on a claim for several years after the suit is filed. Regardless of the time limit, the typical statute of limitations is worded in such a manner that the claimant may file a claim within a certain period from the time an injury occurs or from the time it is *discovered* that an injury has occurred.

For example, a state may have a statute of limitations of 1 year. A patient has an annual examina-

Table 5.2
Physician's responsibility for other personnel

Associates	Physician's responsibility
Employees	Under the legal doctrine of respondeat superior, physicians are responsible for *any* act or omission by their employee in the course of treatment or care.
Borrowed employees (hospital, clinic)	Depends on the physician's control over the selection and direction of the facility's employee, varies by state.
Fellow employees (several physicians employed by a facility)	Each physician is responsible for own actions but *not* for the acts of others not under direct supervision or control.
Substitute physician	No responsibility if the original physician takes reasonable care in selecting the substitute.
Referral physicians	Referred physicians are responsible for their own acts or omissions while treating the patient. The referring physician is *not* responsible if care was taken in selecting the referred physician.
Partners	Each partner is responsible for his or her own actions and the actions or omissions of all legal partners whether or not a partner participated in the care of a patient.
Members of professional corporations	Action may be taken against the responsible physician, direct employee supervisors, and the limited assets of the corporation. Physicians not involved in an incident cannot be held responsible for the actions of other corporate members.
Hospital employees	Physicians are not responsible for employees under the direction and control of the facility. The hospital is legally responsible.

tion, including a Pap smear by her gynecologist. A week later the smear is reported by the pathologist as "negative, Class I," and the gynecologist notifies the patient that everything is fine. Six months later the patient schedules an appointment with the gynecologist because of intermittent vaginal bleeding. A repeat Pap smear reveals a carcinoma insitu (Class IV), and a recheck of the original smear reveals that the slide had been misread. It should have been reported as a Class III with further study recommended by the pathologist. Although the error occurred 6 months earlier, the patient has 1 year from the date of the *second* Pap smear to file a claim against the pathologist.

Liability for Others

It is well established that physicians are responsible for their own actions and for the well-being of their patients. In the course of protecting patients, physicians are responsible for and potentially liable for the actions of certain associates and employees.

The other personnel that physicians are possibly responsible for are discussed in Table 5.2.

The Medical Assistant's Role

In every situation the physician-employer is responsible for the actions and omissions of each employee. Therefore, a basic understanding of the essential legal principles governing the performance of professional duties and limitations under the law will be of great assistance in avoiding legal action.

It is imperative that physicians be assured that the medical assistants they employ are adequately trained to perform the tasks delegated to them. Medical assistants must also be aware of the legal limits of their role in a practice. The medicolegal risk to the physician can be minimized when assistants have some guidelines about their duties, responsibilities, and limitations. A policy and procedure manual can serve this purpose (see Chapter 7).

The medical assistant functions as the representative or agent of the physician and must constantly be aware that patients perceive him or her as the spokesperson for the physician. Any comment or directive from the medical assistant can be construed as a message relayed from the physician. As a result the patient can rightfully assume that a legal contract is in effect. Even an innocent remark, intended to demonstrate support for a positive outcome, can be misunderstood as a promise for a cure.

In general, adhering to the guidelines of the physician's and medical assistant's code of medical ethics, the general statutes covered in this chapter, and the policy of the practice will protect the medical assistant, the physician, and the patient in medicolegal matters.

HANDLING LIABILITY CLAIMS
The Best Option: Prevention
Communication

As stated in the section on the causes of lawsuits, a lack of rapport or a breakdown in communication is the primary factor in most professional liability claims. It therefore follows that communication is the most important element in *preventing* liability claims. Communication may be spoken or unspoken, and both types are involved in a medical relationship.

Spoken communication is rightfully given a great deal of consideration. The medical assistant can inadvertently involve the physician in an unwanted contract, promise impossible results, or give treatment advice and thereby become liable for practicing medicine without a license. The physician may omit information necessary for the patient to provide informed consent, inappropriately guarantee results, or withhold information of the true condition from the patient. A third possible error in spoken communication may be the result of conversations among members of the health care team. Patients are anxious about their status and keenly aware of the activities and interactions within the facility. When personnel speak carelessly it is possible for patients to overhear information out of context, learn information about their condition before it is presented properly, or incorrectly apply information about another patient to their own case. Even if such conversations are not misinterpreted by patients or applied to their own cases, the patients may rightfully question the degree of confidentiality practiced by the facility's personnel.

Unspoken (nonverbal) communication is an element in patient relations and the responsibility of all members of the health care team. Patients are as attuned to nonverbal communication as they are to verbal communication. Medical assistants may inadvertently imply a problem with, for example, a frown while taking a blood pressure reading or disgust at the sight of a wound or by avoiding eye contact when a patient expresses concern for his prognosis. If the physician ignores a patient's questions or answers brusquely, the patient may interpret this action as a lack of concern for or attention to his needs.

In any situation involving communication about or with patients the medical care team should keep in mind that effective, appropriate communication is the foundation of liability claims prevention.

Records and documentation

The medical record is the most important tangible element in legal medicine. The patient's record provides documentation (proof) of the care provided, including when and how it was provided and the consideration of options. The record provides the information necessary to determine if medical services were given in accordance with the standards of care recognized by law, and it should include the patient's acceptance or refusal of medical advice. The record should clearly indicate the patient's failure to comply with treatment plans or keep necessary appointments for follow-up care and the physician's attempts to inform the patient of the necessity of care.

The physician and any other personnel responsible for making contributions to the patient's record should be careful to avoid unprofessional comments. Such comments include the following:
- Slang or colloquial terms;
- Criticisms of patient's life-style, previous physicians, or medical care; or
- Terms such as *error, mistake,* and *inadvertently.*

Although the medical record is considered the property of the physician because he or she acquired, compiled, and interpreted the information, other persons have legal access to the record. Patients or their attorneys may acquire copies of the record for review. If a lawsuit is filed, the patient's records become available to the legal representatives of the plaintiff and defendant and to the court. The records are also available to federal or state agencies responsible for payment of the medical care or private (health, life, or disability) insurance companies with the written consent of the patient.

It is in the patient's and the physician's best interests if the records are accurate, complete, and legible. If these three criteria are met the physician can be assured of having an important tool in the prevention of or defense against professional liability claims.

Arbitration

A method of settling a dispute between two individuals or two groups of individuals without resorting to a civil lawsuit is *arbitration*, a common technique in labor issues. Arbitration of medical disputes increased in popularity as an alternative to lawsuits during the professional liability insurance crisis of the mid-70s. An agreement of arbitration is a contract for care between the physician and the patient. A court is involved only in determining the legality of the contract, not the issue or the settlement.

How does arbitration work?

Many states have statutes that allow arbitration. Your state medical association can advise you about the availability of arbitration and information about it. Where arbitration is available, it is viewed as an alternative to large liability insurance premiums. The physician may build a fund for the possibility of having to pay a settlement. Another option is for a group of physicians to form an arbitration association and pool their funds for possible settlements. In either situation physicians invest much less than they would if they were paying insurance premiums, because they avoid the expense of attorneys and the court costs associated with lawsuits. A popular term for doing without professional liability insurance is *going bare*.

The physician's and medical assistant's roles

In a practice that uses arbitration, each patient should be given an information sheet and an arbitration agreement to read at the time of registration. The medical assistant should tell patients that the agreement is office policy and that the physician will discuss the agreement, discuss any questions, and sign the agreement with the patient before the examination.

It is important that the medical assistant and the physician do not attempt to legally interpret the agreement to the patient. Specific words such as *tort* or *personal representative* may be defined, but the patient should be advised to seek interpretation from his attorney.

A typical agreement

In many respects an arbitration agreement is similar to an informed consent for medical care. The arbitration agreement clearly lists the method of settlement if a dispute arises over the fulfillment of medical care duties or the quality of care. The agreement signed by the physician and the patient usually covers the following:

- Possible issues of dispute;
- The voluntary nature of the arbitration contract;
- The patient's relinquishment of the right to sue in a court of law;
- The binding nature of the agreement;
- The method of settlement;
- The patient's right to revoke the agreement;
- A statement that the agreement is not mandatory for treatment; and
- A statement of understanding of the agreement.

Who arbitrates a settlement?

A dispute covered by an arbitration agreement is settled by a neutral individual or a panel of three neutral individuals acceptable to both the physician and the patient. Arbiters are individuals who are knowledgeable in the field in which a decision is required. The professional medical associations or the American Arbitration Association can provide a list of acceptable arbiters. The latter organization assures the qualifications of the arbiters it recommends, and one of the requirements necessary to be considered as an arbiter by the organization is 100 separate endorsements of neutrality.

The results of arbitration

The binding nature of an arbitration agreement means that the physician and the patient *must* abide by the decision of the arbiter. Patients who agree to arbitration may not pursue the dispute in a court of law if they do not agree with the settlement established by the arbiter. Should either party believe that the arbiter was not knowledgeable or neutral, an appeal may be made to the arbitration association.

Court Cases

Physicians not using arbitration must settle disputes through the civil court system or with an out-of-court settlement. In either situation professional liability attorneys are necessary. If the physician has professional liability coverage the insurance company will provide attorneys. Otherwise the physician must provide his or her own legal counsel.

When a liability claim is made a legal case and pursued through the courts, it is likely to be several years before a decision is reached. During these years the physician will lose practice time to legal conferences, depositions, and court appearances, and the office schedule will be disrupted. In some cases, because of the nature of a claim or the anticipated time involved, a physician may be advised to settle out of court. This type of settlement involves negotiations by the attorneys of the defense and plaintiff until a mutually acceptable settlement is determined. While an out-of-court settlement may be appealing, physicians should resist this option, and they will need the support of their staff during the legal process. Although some claims settled in court favor the plaintiff, and settlements for these are steadily rising in dollar amount, the majority of claims are in favor of the defendant (the physician).

GOOD SAMARITAN ACTS

As the number of lawsuits filed increased, physicians realized that they must practice defensive medicine. In other words, they had to use any means available to avoid a lawsuit being filed against them. Physicians even became reluctant to give voluntary care to unknown injured persons at the scene of an accident or sudden illness. In 1959 California became the first state to recognize this trend and to pass a law protecting physicians and encouraging them to offer aid when needed. Since that time most states have passed similar statutes, which are known as Good Samaritan acts.

Good Samaritan acts encourage voluntary help by protecting physicians from legal liability under civil law. These statutes generally make the physician immune from any suit arising out of emergency care, provided that the care is given with reasonable care under the circumstances and in good faith. In some states the Good Samaritan act extends to registered nurses but not to medical assistants. Medical assistants who wish to offer help at the scene of an accident should be trained in first aid, ideally through a certified program, and offer help as a private citizen.

In general, Good Samaritan laws do *not* protect the physician in professional settings such as medical offices, clinics, and hospitals. They also do not provide immunity if a fee is charged or collected for the service. A physician who provides emergency care as a Good Samaritan should relinquish the patient to emergency medical personnel or an attending physician as soon as possible.

CONTROLLED SUBSTANCES

A physician who administers, prescribes, or dispenses any drugs listed under the Controlled Substances Act has certain legal restrictions and responsibilities. These restrictions and responsibilities and the role of the medical assistant when drugs are involved are discussed in Chapter 23.

In general, medical assistants in facilities that dispense controlled substances must be aware of the following:
- The drugs considered controlled;
- The records required by law;
- Inventory control;
- Order forms;
- Security for drugs and prescription forms; and
- Reporting responsibilities.

It is *most* important for the medical assistant to be aware that only a physician may prescribe drugs and that only a physician or a licensed pharmacist may dispense drugs. Most states have statutes regarding the administration of medication to a patient. When a medical assistant administers medication, it is assumed that this is done under the direct supervision of the physician. The physician bears the responsibility for the act and the outcome.

UNIFORM ANATOMICAL GIFT ACT
Reason for the Act

Technological advances now permit the transplantation of many organs. Many states have passed laws allowing individuals to declare their wishes with regard to the disposition of their bodies or specific organs after their death. Since state laws varied and some states had no organ-donor laws, individuals who wished to donate their organs or body could only be assured that their wishes would be carried out in the state in which they legally declared their intentions. To correct this and encourage a valuable service to society, the National Conference of Commissioners on Uniform State Laws approved the Uniform Anatomical Gift Act in 1968. This act serves as the model for state statutes.

Elements of the Act

The basic elements of the Uniform Anatomical Gift Act include the following:
- The donor must be at least 18 years of age;

- The wish to donate should be in writing;
- The donor may stipulate specific organs for transplantation, the entire body for research or transplantation, or any acceptable organs or tissues;
- The donor's valid statement takes precedence over anyone else's wishes, except when the law requires an autopsy;
- An individual's survivors may act on his behalf;
- If aware of the donor's wishes, the attending physician may dispose of the body under the act;
- The physician accepting the donor's organs in good faith is protected from lawsuits;
- Death of the donor may not be determined by any physician involved in the transplantation;
- The donor may revoke the gift, or the gift may be refused; and
- No financial arrangements can be made for donated organs.

In many states the department that issues driver's licenses provides Uniform Donor Cards that may be attached to the license. Law enforcement and emergency medical personnel automatically check the license in the event of an accident. In addition to completing the necessary written documents, potential donors should make their wishes known to their physicians, family, and friends.

REPORTING RESPONSIBILITIES

In the course of doing business medical practices must fulfill certain reporting responsibilities to various legal agencies. Again, state laws vary, but some general issues can be discussed here.

County Statistics

Physicians are required to complete and file information on births and deaths that occur within a county. Birth certificates must be filed within 5 days after the birth and include information about the child and both parents. Death certificates must be signed by the physician attending the patient at the time of death and include the patient's statistics and the place and cause of death.

Public Health

Health departments require that physicians report certain contagious diseases discovered during the course of attending a patient. These diseases include cholera, plague, smallpox, meningitis, scarlet fever, measles, mumps, tuberculosis, and sexually transmitted diseases. Because these diseases have a potential effect on the general public, the patient's consent is not necessary to release information. The physician and the health department do, however, respect the confidentiality of the patient.

When sexually transmitted disease or tuberculosis is involved, the physician must advise the patient of the need for treatment and of the patient's responsibility to prevent the spread of the disease. Physicians and health department authorities often work together to assure that the advice is carried out.

Medical Examiner Cases

The medical examiner or the individual serving as coroner must be notified of a death in certain circumstances. Depending on the county, these circumstances include the following:
- Uncertain cause of death;
- No medical care in a given period of time;
- Death within a certain time after hospital admission or major surgery;
- Death as a result of violence or during the commission of a crime; and
- Child abuse cases.

In the past the person reporting a suspected case of child abuse or neglect was subject to a possible lawsuit for libel and slander. In 1967 California passed a statute protecting individuals who honestly and without malice report a possible case, and other states have adopted similar laws. Many states have since gone one step further and now *require* physicians, nurses, teachers, and other responsible adults to report suspected cases. Suspected cases may be reported to the police or to the department of public welfare.

Permissive Reports

Physicians may supply information without liability or the patient's consent under statutes that allow permissive reports. The two circumstances that allow permissive reports are the following:
1. When information is requested by medical organizations, health agencies, or facilities conducting studies to control or cure disease.
2. When information is requested by a facility or institution currently treating a patient who was formerly under the care of the physician providing the information.

The agency that gathers information by permissive report has the responsibility of maintaining confidentiality and protecting the patient's privacy.

Conclusion

Legal medicine is a complex field that requires specialized training and experience. The overview presented in this chapter is intended as a guide for medical assistants in the course of their professional career and is not an absolute statement for legal interpretations. In a doubtful situation medical assistants should seek clarification of a situation from a physician-employer or another knowledgeable source. In every case, confidential patient information must be absolutely protected.

Review Questions

1. Name the statute that controls the method of providing care for patients.
2. List six reasons a physician might lose his or her license to practice.
3. Why is it important to obtain informed consent before treating a patient?
4. What is professional liability?
5. What situations might cause a patient to charge a physician with abandonment?
6. Compose a letter of dismissal to a patient.
7. Name and describe the four Ds *or* the ABCDs of negligence.
8. Decide whether or not physicians are responsible for the following individuals. If they are responsible, explain why.
   a. Employees
   b. Borrowed employees
   c. Fellow employees
   d. Substitute physicians
   e. Referral physicians
   f. Partners
   g. Comembers of a professional corporation
9. State in your own words the eight elements of a typical arbitration agreement. How is an arbitration dispute settled?
10. When will a Good Samaritan act protect a physician from a liability suit? When will it not protect the physician?
11. How can an individual indicate the wish to donate organs for transplantation?
12. What is the responsibility of medical personnel in a suspected case of child abuse?

SUGGESTED READINGS

Hirsch CS, Morris RC, and Moritz AR: Handbook of legal medicine, ed 5, St Louis, 1979, The CV Mosby Co.

Private Practice, Physician's Management and Marketing (published monthly by Health Care, Atlanta).

Stetler J and Moritz AR: Doctor and patient and the law, ed 4, St Louis, 1962, The CV Mosby Co.

Chapter 6

Holistic Approach to Patient Care

- Role of the medical assistant in holistic health
- Approaching well-being
- Physical fitness
- Life cycles

Objectives

On completion of Chapter 6 the medical assistant student should be able to:

1 Define the terms listed in the vocabulary.

2 Discuss the holistic approach to health care and the role of the medical assistant as a member of the holistic health care team.

3 Describe the problem analysis approach to evaluation of behavior that influences well-being.

4 Define mental health and list the human problems that can influence it.

5 Discuss the role of stress in daily life, common responses to stress, and methods of coping with stress.

6 Discuss the influence of diet, exercise, rest, and substance use on physical fitness.

7 Discuss human sexuality and life cycles, including childbirth, parenting, aging, and death and dying.

Vocabulary

aerobics Exercise, such as bicycling or jogging, that stimulates the heart and lungs by increasing the intake of oxygen.

beliefs Convictions that certain things are true or factual.

holistic Pertaining to the concept that the integrated whole is greater than the sum of the individual parts; in health care, referring to the concept that the whole person, not separate parts, is the focus of care.

psychoactive A chemical or drug that has an altering effect on the mind.

self-esteem Respect for or belief in oneself.

sociocultural Pertaining to the environmental and developmental elements of an individual's life.

threshold The physiological or psychological point at which a stimulus begins to produce a response.

values The goals, standards, or principles held as important to an individual or group

The term *holistic* is frequently seen in reference to health care in both professional and popular current literature and is discussed by many individuals. Basically it refers to the whole or total person in contrast to individual parts of the whole. Health is defined as the state of physical, mental, and social well-being of an individual and not merely the absence of disease. Holistic health represents a concept or philosophy based on this simple definition. It assumes that the body, mind, emotions, spirit, and social aspects of the person are integrated.

Factors that influence our well-being include the following:

- Environment—fetal, physical, sociocultural;
- Life-style—knowledge, attitude, behavior, experiences;
- Value systems; and
- Medical care services and systems—prevention, treatment, maintenance, rehabilitation.

Influencing our level of wellness and all of the factors just listed are our natural resources, cultural systems, ecological balance, and human satisfaction.* According to Malcolm C. Todd, former president of the American Medical Association, holistic health is†:

A state in which an individual is integrated in all his/her levels of being: body, mind, and spirit. It has been suggested that all modalities of treatment may be used in holistic healing; that is, surgery, medicine, chemotherapy, radiation, nutrition, rehabilitation, yes, hypnosis, acupuncture, psychics, and, of course, religion . . . to teach an individual to assume responsibility for him/herself and to heal him/herself by modifying any unhealthy attitude, values, or life-styles.

Holistic health care is an aspect of today's emerging wellness movement, which emphasizes increasing the quality of our lives and the lives of others, preventing illness, and promoting a lifestyle that will enhance wellness. This concept, which is becoming essential for the future, places major emphasis on the individual to make informed decisions and to take responsibility for his own level of health and wellness.

Holistic health is a dynamic process that stresses a balanced relationship among all of these factors. In the holistic health care process individuals are encouraged and assisted to assume responsibility for their levels of wellness. Patient education, aimed at behavior change, is an important aspect of this process. It allows the individual to develop attitudes that may and should result in positive health behavior and life-styles and a subsequent high level of wellness. H.L. Dunn defines high-level wellness for the individual as "an integrated method of functioning which is oriented toward maximizing the potential which the individual is

capable of within the environment where he/she is functioning."*

Key dimensions for wellness and the growing significance of holism are exemplified as individuals become more self-aware, take more responsibility for themselves, and become more interested in physical fitness, improved nutrition, stress management, meditation, natural childbirth, and sensitivity to their environment and personal needs. Holistic health care providers deal with all of this in addition to the traditional medical and surgical care.

The holistic and wellness concepts have led to the development of various wellness inventories. The purpose of these inventories is to help individuals assess the various aspects of their lives that may need improvement and also to spotlight lifestyles that promote wellness. This guides them toward decisions that will improve their levels of health and wellness. Since patient education is a vital part of this process, the wellness inventories must be discussed with patients so that positive behavior can be reinforced and plans can be made for any areas in which changes are required.

ROLE OF THE MEDICAL ASSISTANT IN HOLISTIC HEALTH
Understanding the Concept

As a medical assistant you will have the opportunity to assist patients in the development of effective health behavior. To do this it is important that you develop an understanding of the basic concepts of the integrated components of wellness. Since entire courses are taught on the subject of holistic health, a detailed description is beyond the scope of this book. However, an overview is provided in this chapter to introduce you to the areas that must be considered in the integration of holistic health care.

Resource Person

You will contribute to the general well-being of the patients you work with by being prepared to be a resource person. Acquaint yourself with the educational and self-help programs available in your community. A patient-teaching program, coordinated and approved by the physician, can be used to make patients understand their role in the process. Patients must be made part of the team for any program to be effective and for behavior changes to take place, and you can be a source of

---

*See Blum HL: Planning for health, New York, 1974, Human Sciences Press.
†Combs BJ, Hales DR, and Williams BK: An invitation to health: your personal responsibility, ed 2, Menlo Park, Calif, 1983.

---

*Dunn HL: What high-level wellness means, Health values 1(1):9, 1977.

information and encouragement to them. Overall, the most important contribution you can make to a program of holistic health care is to instill in patients the understanding that they are responsible for the foundations of their own well-being and should take an active part in decisions that affect their care. In other words, you should assist patients to become discriminating health care consumers.

Attitude

Change of any kind can be a source of confusion and stress; it can be even more so when it involves such intangible elements as beliefs, values, and behavior. You will need to help patients develop and maintain a positive attitude throughout the process. Reassuring patients of your understanding and ongoing support will reduce their anxiety and resistance.

APPROACHING WELL-BEING
Health Behavior: Problem Analysis

Once you have instilled in patients a sense of responsibility for their own well-being, including informed participation in responsible decision-making, you can begin development of an effective wellness program. Planning is the important first step. It will include consideration of each patient's current situation and needs, an appropriate time frame for the development of the plan, and stages at which changes can be expected.

The next step is the identification of problem behavior. Various health or risk inventories are available from health departments, educational institutions, and special-interest groups such as the American Cancer Society, the American Heart Association, and the American Lung Association. Assist patients with filling out the forms, help the physician interpret the information, and educate patients regarding the necessary changes and means to attain a more positive life-style.

Behavior change can be difficult and stressful for patients. One of the most helpful roles you can play in this phase of the process is that of a supportive ally. Patients will need help sustaining their commitment to a program of change, and your ongoing encouragement can make a difference in attitude and outcome.

Mental Health

There are numerous possible definitions of mental health that are based on a variety of models devel-

oped by various scientists and physicians over time. For the purpose of this book, mental health is considered the effective interplay between individuals and their environment. Mentally healthy individuals might be seen as possessing the qualities noted by Abraham Maslow, which include the following:
- Ability to accept their environment as it is;
- Ability to accept themselves;
- A continuing freshness of appreciation for activities in their environment;
- Being self-directed;
- Trusting their senses and feelings; and
- Being democratic in their attitudes.

Human problems

The spectrum of human behavior ranges from "normal" to insane. Behavior that is classified as "normal" encompasses a portion of the continuum, not a single point on the scale. Within the normal range, everyone experiences certain human problems, including the following:
- Manipulation;
- Rejection and alienation;
- Anxiety;
- Depression;
- Stress; and
- Conflict.

The issue is not that individuals experience these problems from time to time but the manner in which they deal with them. You will be able to assist patients to keep these problems in perspective and help them realize that the important factor is that problems are recognized and solutions are sought.

Promoting mental health

One of the key things you can do for patients in promoting mental health is to create an environment and attitude that encourage them to communicate their concerns and needs. It is appropriate for you to listen to patients, encourage them to discuss the issues with the physician, or act as the liaison between patients and physician. It is not appropriate for you to make a determination regarding patients' needs or to make suggestions regarding possible therapy.

Identifying mental health as a real part of patients' overall well-being, educating them about the interrelationship of emotional needs and physical response, and being responsive to, but nonjudgmental of, patients' needs will be of great service to the patients and to your health care team. In addition, effectively fulfilling this function and the other services you perform will enhance your self-esteem and add an element of fulfillment to your career.

Methods of therapy

Although you will not recommend therapy or directly refer patients to therapists, it is helpful for you to recognize the various treatment methods available. It is gradually becoming more generally accepted that individuals should not be stigmatized for seeking assistance with personal and interpersonal problems. However, you will recognize a reluctance on the part of some individuals to acknowledge the need or accept the physician's recommendation for therapy. The fact that you recognize a method of treatment and are able to acknowledge that to a patient in a nonjudgmental manner will communicate acceptability to the patient. Your "matter-of-fact" attitude will be perceived as supportive. Regardless of the method of therapy suggested to or chosen by a patient, your role should be one of encouragement and support. A brief overview of treatment methods follows.

Biological therapy. Biological therapy methods may involve prescribed drugs or electroconvulsive shock therapy or a combination of the two. These methods are often used in combination with other treatment plans. Drug therapy, often involving tranquilizers or mood elevators, is needed to alleviate symptoms of depression or hyperactivity. This is done to bring patients to a level of functioning that will allow problem-solving discussions to take place. Shock therapy is usually reserved for more serious forms of depression, often beginning in middle age, that fail to respond to drug therapy. This method is reserved in most cases until other methods have been exhausted.

Psychoanalysis. Psychoanalytical therapy involves a retrospective review of the elements that have contributed to the present state of the patient's mind and the influence these contributions have made to the patient's current attitudes and actions. It is based on the principles that responses are based on cumulative previous events, and that understanding and acknowledging those events will result in acceptance or modification of current and future responses. Psychoanalysis typically occurs over an extended period of time, usually several years.

Psychotherapy. *Psychotherapy* is a generic term that includes several forms of treatment, all of which are based on communication or talking about the problem areas. The therapist may take an active or passive role in the process. The active therapist will guide the discussions and offer advice; the passive therapist will allow patients to control the topics discussed and to arrive at their own conclusions and solutions with minimal guidance.

Group therapy. A therapy method that brings together several individuals with similar problems is referred to as group therapy. The sessions are guided by a therapist, but the benefit to participants results from interaction among the group members. The advantages to patients include recognizing that others experience similar problems and that there are several perspectives from which to view the problems and more than one solution. Some self-help groups, such as Alcoholics Anonymous and Weight Watchers, base themselves on a group-therapy model and attribute their success in part to the supportive atmosphere generated by the participants.

Stress Management

Today's social, cultural, and economic environment includes stressors that require recognition and attention. Since humans are adaptive, it is possible to integrate stress into our daily lives without realizing the impact it has on our physical, mental, spiritual, and social well-being. Therefore it is important to develop mechanisms to recognize and cope with the stressors that cannot be changed and to reduce stress whenever possible.

The first step in stress management is the evaluation of personality and ability to cope with stress. Each individual has a different threshold of stress and exhibits a different response when that threshold is crossed. Some people attack verbally and in anger when under stress, while others retain a calm exterior but react to the stress in another way, such as developing stomach ulcers. As a medical assistant you should always be aware that stress is likely to play some role in the actions or reactions of patients. Simply being in a medical environment generates some stress, and this will enhance a patient's acceptance or rejection of diagnostic or therapeutic plans. Understanding stress and adapting your approach to patients to include the stress factor will increase your effectiveness as a health care provider.

Evolution and stress

Changes, expected and unexpected, are a common source of stress in our everyday lives. Response to change is termed *evolution,* and humans are capable of responding both biologically and culturally.

Biological evolution is a process so slow that it is measured in massive spans of time, and until recent times cultural evolution was also considered a relatively slow process. However, the industrialization that has taken place through the nineteenth and twentieth centuries has created essentially new societies that change several times within single generations. Family units, employment, mobility, methods of travel, and production of items to fulfill our basic and higher needs have all contributed to a dramatically changing cultural environment. The fact that change contributes to stress reinforces the theory that each individual is influenced in some manner by attempts to adapt to environmental changes.

Responding to stress

Individuals may respond to stress psychologically, physiologically, or in a combination of the two ways. Psychological responses may include a reduction in self-esteem, feelings of guilt or remorse, depression, or a lack of enthusiasm for life. Stress and the physiological reactions to it are only recently being recognized as having a legitimate cause-and-effect relationship. Some disease processes that are now associated with stress include ulcers, hypertension, heart disease, and colitis.

Some factors that are recognized as psychosocial contributors to stress include the following:
- Social change (changing jobs, marrying, divorcing, moving to another geographical location);
- Urban living; and
- Occupation and work environment.

Coping with stress

Recognition of stress and its influence on mental and physical health is the first step to putting it into perspective and controlling its influence. Each individual must first identify his threshold of stress, determine the sources of stress, and develop a plan to reduce stress. Since it is impossible to eliminate all stress from our lives, it is necessary to cope with stress as it exists. Some general techniques that are suggested include the following:
- Rest and relaxation;
- Proper nutrition;
- Humor;
- Supportive relationships; and
- Exercise.

Testing the various stress-reduction options will allow individuals to determine which technique or combination of techniques works best. There is no universal formula for stress reduction.

PHYSICAL FITNESS

Physical well-being involves the balance of nutritional substances taken into the body as well as exercise, rest, and control or avoidance of potentially harmful substances, including tobacco, alcohol, and other drugs. Your understanding of these elements of fitness is important to your ability to assist patients to maintain their health.

Dietary Considerations
Nutrition

The basics of nutritional science provide the information necessary to evaluate the needs for human life support, to determine the foods that will fulfill those needs, and to explain the processes involved in assimilating food for growth and tissue replacement. There are certain essential substances that the body must have to maintain structure and function. These substances are:
- Proteins;
- Carbohydrates;
- Fats;
- Vitamins; and
- Minerals.

They must be supplied from an external source on a daily basis. Once food is ingested it is metabolized, that is, altered or modified to a form that can be used at the cellular level. Many nutrients in varying combinations are necessary for all of the processes that allow individuals to continue to function.

Appropriate diet

Nutritional science has been able to determine minimum needs for survival and appropriate intake levels to maintain optimum body weight but has not yet been able to explain how eating certain foods affects individuals differently. Based on currently available knowledge, including an understanding of essential nutrients, patients should be encouraged to select a balanced diet from the foods of the four basic food groups. The basic foods are categorized as follows:
- Milk or milk products;
- Meat;
- Fruits and vegetables; and
- Breads and cereals.

Depending on age and activity, you can adjust the amounts of food selected from each category and still fulfill the basic needs (Figure 6.1). Individuals who have special dietary restrictions for personal, religious, or health reasons need to be counseled regarding alternative sources of any nutrients they

Figure 6.1
Four basic food groups.
From Sorrentino S: Mosby's textbook for nursing assistants, St Louis, 1984, The CV Mosby Co.

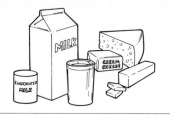

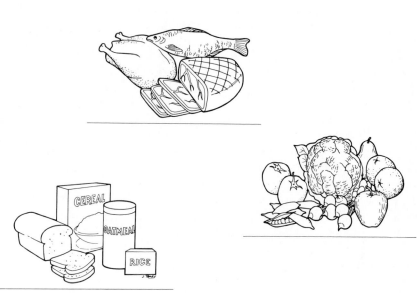

may be missing. If vitamin, mineral, or nutrient supplements are recommended, patients will need instructions to avoid consuming more than the recommended doses. Some nutrients can be toxic when taken in quantities greater than necessary to meet daily requirements.

Diet and weight control

Ideal weight. Current social attitudes include a strong emphasis on diet and weight control. At one time charts produced by life insurance companies were the main source of information on appropriate ranges of weight for height and bone structure. Now a vast array of professional and popular literature presents charts and formulas to determine ideal weight, and this may add to the confusion of both lay and professional people. Patients should be encouraged to discuss their concerns with their physician, using him or her as the single source to work with to determine their ideal weight.

Obesity. *Obesity* is the term that identifies the physical condition of excessive weight caused by accumulation of a disproportionate amount of fat tissue. Individuals are considered obese if they are 20% or more over the average ideal weight for

their height and body structure. Numerous theories and studies have been developed in an attempt to determine the causes of obesity. Certain factors have been identified as contributory, including the following:

- Genetic factors;
- Developmental factors;
- Metabolic factors;
- Physical activity;
- Social factors; and
- Emotional factors.

Each obese person needs to be evaluated individually so that a determination can be made of the factor or factors contributing to his obesity. Identification of these factors will assist in the treatment plan devised for the person.

Controlling weight. Weight is maintained or altered depending on the balance of caloric intake and energy expended. The value of food is measured in calories, which is a measure of energy. If the calories you take in during the course of a day equal the calories you use in your activities, your weight should remain constant. If your intake exceeds your output, you will gain weight; if output exceeds intake, you will lose weight. Therefore a

Figure 6.2
Exercise as part of group outing.
From Godow A: Human sexuality, St Louis, 1982, The CV Mosby Co.

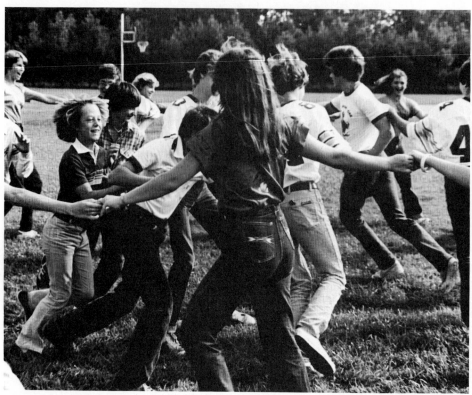

very elementary approach to weight control or reduction is to adjust either intake or activity appropriately.

Exercise

In the 1960s President John F. Kennedy drew national attention to the general lack of physical fitness of U.S. citizens, particularly among young people, and began a program to improve the situation. It is now understood that routine exercise plays an important role in our general well-being and provides definite benefits in the treatment or prevention of some specific disease processes.

Exercise can influence both physical and mental health (Figure 6.2). Aggressive exercise, including aerobics, affects the heart and vascular system and also has positive effects on glands, enzyme use, blood volume, body weight, blood pressure, and ability to cope with stress.

Initiating an exercise program should include planning and input by the physician. A physical examination, including an electrocardiogram, may be indicated depending on the patient's age and previous exercise experience. During the planning phase, the medical assistant can help patients by pointing out the value of various activities that use the most muscle groups and involve aerobics for the cardiovascular system. Patients should be encouraged to select activities that they like and can accomplish without such hindrances as lack of time, travel to initiate activities, and dependence on others. Removing as many obstacles as possible will increase commitment to the program.

An exercise plan should be implemented in stages, especially for previously sedentary individuals. Time spent exercising should be increased gradually, usually at weekly intervals, until the maximum level of benefit has been reached. Once individuals have arrived at this point, a maintenance plan can be implemented for continued benefit and well-being.

Rest

Rest, particularly sleep, is an element of well-being that is often neglected, particularly by young adults. Although individuals vary in the amount of rest they require for feeling their best, the need for adequate rest and sleep is universal. It is important to point out to patients that rest influences both physical and psychological responses and is as vital to well-being as food, air, and shelter. In addition, the rested individual is more capable of dealing with the stressors that influence him on a daily basis. Rest is required every day.

Substance Use and Abuse

Substances that can have detrimental effects on health include tobacco, alcohol, and other drugs (prescription and nonprescription).

Tobacco

The effects of smoking are widely publicized, and warnings on each package of cigarettes are mandated by the federal government. It has been conclusively proven that smoking causes numerous diseases of the respiratory and cardiovascular systems and new evidence is being generated on the effects of secondary smoke, that is, smoke which individuals who do not smoke are exposed to at home, at work, or in other settings. Since smoking seems to involve psychological as well as a physiological dependence, patients who are encouraged to or wish to quit smoking will need a great deal of support. The American Lung Association and the American Heart Association can provide you with literature for patients, and you can provide them with positive reinforcement of their efforts to eliminate the use of tobacco.

Alcohol

Alcohol is of great concern to health care providers, because it is a legally available, socially acceptable, and potentially lethal substance. Ingested alcohol is absorbed from the stomach and intestines into the circulatory system, where it is transported to the liver for metabolizing. It is subsequently distributed throughout the tissues of the body.

Alcohol is a drug and should be dealt with as such. Physiologically it acts as a depressant to the brain and central nervous system, the musculoskeletal system, and the cardiovascular system. Alcohol interferes with the control of inhibitions, enhances assertiveness, and reduces coordination and reflex response time. The relationship of psychological factors and alcohol can be perceived in two ways. Some observers feel that a person with a particular psychological profile is more susceptible to alcohol abuse, while others feel that the dependence alters the individual psychologically. Either way, it is important to remember that there is a psychological

component to alcohol abuse that must be considered when evaluating the problem.

Alcohol and alcohol abuse have social ramifications that include the involvement of alcohol in family problems, violent crimes, automobile accidents and deaths, and illnesses resulting in time lost from work. The needs of the alcoholic have been identified, and a vast array of approaches to treatment have been developed. Authorities agree, however, that the first step to effective treatment for alcohol abuse involves the desire to change and the commitment of the abuser to a treatment program. You may wish to acquire literature from local treatment plans to be prepared for questions from patients.

Drugs

The term *drugs* is a broad one that includes many substances in a variety of categories. Working in the medical profession initially limits thinking to prescription drugs, but over-the-counter (OTC) and "street" drugs must also be considered.

Legal drugs, either prescription or OTC, should be respected, taken only when needed, and taken as directed. "Street" drugs should be avoided because of their inherent consequences and their potential for contamination by unknown substances. This basic philosophy can be your guide when discussing drugs with patients. Of particular concern to health care providers are the psychoactive drugs. This group includes drugs that modify moods or influence psychological responses. They are receiving attention because of their increased use as a means of coping with stress. Patients request prescriptions for tranquilizers, sedatives, or antidepressants and need to be educated regarding potential dependence. They also need to know that these drugs treat only their symptoms, while the causes of their problems still need to be identified and resolved. Your contact with users of street drugs may be limited, but you should be prepared for the possibility.

The availability of OTC drugs can encourage individuals to self-diagnose and self-medicate. Responsible health care providers will make the effort to educate consumers about the potential hazards of this practice and encourage them to be discriminating consumers. Many people need to learn to change their attitudes toward OTC drugs and to be less responsive to mass advertising that encourages consumption. One additional area in which you can assist the consumer involves the packaging safety of readily available items. Unfortunate incidents in recent years have led to many safety considerations in packaging, and consumers need to be taught to look for signs of tampering and potential contamination when purchasing OTC drugs.

LIFE CYCLES
Sexuality

The cycles of life that individuals have completed and will encounter are linked together through human sexuality (Figure 6.3). Regardless of the area of health care in which you choose to participate, you can anticipate encountering some aspect of sexuality and patient concerns about it. Because of the potential need for patient education and reassurance, you should be prepared to recognize patients' needs for information and to offer appropriate information. Some of the areas that can be confusing for patients include misinformation about or misinterpretation of the following:
- Physical sexual response;
- Emotional sexual response;
- Evaluation of sexual needs;
- Responsibility to sexual partner; and
- Birth control methods.

It is advantageous for all members of a health care team to work together in developing a patient education plan that includes human sexuality. It is most important that patients receive accurate and consistent information, regardless of the stage of life in which the educational process is initiated. All members of the health care team need to be prepared with educational materials, agency references, or support group information regarding sexual education that is safe sex, moderate sex, unsafe sex, with controls and methods of same.

Childbirth

The stages of life are begun during pregnancy and are evidenced at childbirth. The process of childbirth receives a great deal of attention from professional and public perspectives through the entire gamut of the media. During pregnancy it is ideal to involve both parents in the planning and decision processes, and you can anticipate many questions regarding new techniques for childbirth. Traditionally, a child is delivered in a hospital delivery room

Figure 6.3
Human sexuality includes sharing, affection, and understanding between partners.
From Godow A: Human sexuality, St Louis, 1982, The CV Mosby Co.

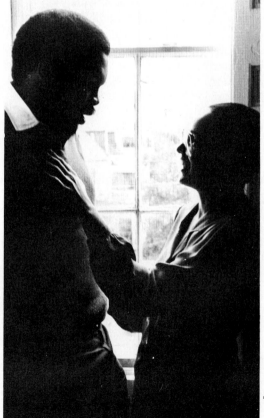

or surgery suite if cesarean section is required. For an uncomplicated vaginal delivery, however, some parents are considering alternatives to the perceived impersonal atmosphere of the hospital. Some midwives and obstetricians will assist parents with a home delivery, although most discourage this alternative because of the lack of equipment in the event of an emergency with the mother or child. Many hospitals, in an effort to respond to parents' needs, have developed birthing rooms within the hospital. These can fulfill the parents' wishes while sustaining the safety factor. Birthing rooms are furnished to appear as similar to a bedroom in the home as possible, and barring complications, the entire birth process can take place in this environment (Figure 6.4). If complications should arise, the mother and child are within the medical facility and can have the immediate attention of necessary medical personnel with the equipment needed to cope with the problem. If you are involved in the area of obstetrical care, familiarize yourself with the facilities and resources that are available to patients.

Parenting

The stage of life in which individuals deal with the responsibilities of being a parent can be equally rewarding and stressful. Members of the health care team must understand the needs of parents during this time. Parents are responsible for providing for the physical and emotional needs of their children and must do so in an increasingly stressful environment. You can assist them as they attempt to reach the ultimate goal of parenting, the independence of the child, by being supportive and informed and by providing them with a comfortable atmosphere in which to express their needs. You may also assist them by being aware of which local colleges or agencies provide courses for new parents or parents who seem to be struggling with the role of parenting. These courses are normally provided in most well populated areas.

Aging

Aging is an inevitable process that takes place as individuals pass through the various stages of life. It can be approached from the perspective of physiology, psychology, or sociology or from the overall study of gerontology, the science of aging. The goals of health care providers should be support and education to assist individuals as they go through the aging process, particularly the latter stages. Health care providers can help individuals maintain dignified, high-quality lives.

People tend to cope better with change when they understand why certain events are taking

Figure 6.4
Entire family together following the birth of new member in alternative birth center.
Photograph courtesy of Mount Zion Hospital and Medical Center, San Francisco, Calif.

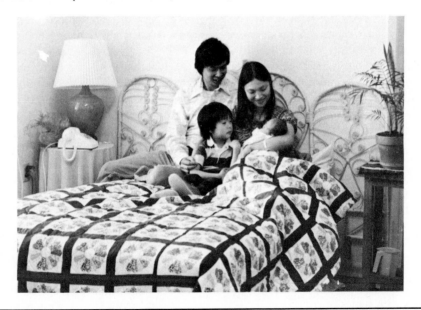

Figure 6.5
Physical activity and related socializing assists individuals to adjust to aging process.
From Ebersole P: Toward healthy aging, St Louis, 1981, The CV Mosby Co.

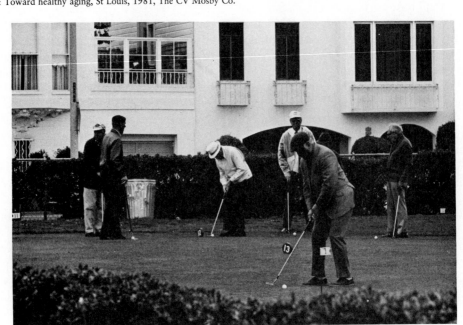

place. By understanding the physiological and psychological effects of aging and being able to explain them to patients, you will be performing a valuable service. You may also want to determine what programs and services are available for "senior citizens" in your community that can help them cope with personal and environmental changes.

Gerontologists have determined that the aging process and response to change can produce serious consequences for the elderly if allowed to go undetected. It is the opinion of most experts on aging that the best approach to the situation involves preventive measures, including the following:
- Maintaining proper nutrition;
- Stimulating the mind;
- Staying physically active; and
- Interacting with people of all ages.

Being able to counsel patients on these matters and offer resources to help accomplish them can result in some very positive physiological and psychological results (Figure 6.5).

Death and Dying

The definition of death varies greatly from the religious to the medical perspectives. Overall, death is change and the cessation of the life of an organism as we know or recognize it. For medical purposes, death is related to the cessation of function of one or more vital organs, particularly the brain or the heart.

The process of dying, whether it takes moments or months, is difficult psychologically for the patient and for those close to the patient, particularly since our society supports an attitude of denial where death is concerned. Fortunately, popular and professional literature has begun addressing the issue of death and dying in recent years. Bringing the issue to the foreground should serve as a means of eliminating the fear and superstition surrounding the death process and should make death easier to cope with when it occurs.

One concept being reported on involves the right of individuals to make and declare decisions regarding their wish to die peacefully and with dignity in the event of a terminal illness or injury. A "living will" may be written requesting that physicians, family members, and friends provide for the patient's comfort and not use any extraordinary means of life support. This arrangement, although not legally binding, allows the initiator to feel that he will have some control over the decision that affects his life and relieves his survivors of potentially guilt-producing decisions.

Figure 6.6
Hospice outpatient with support team including nurses, social workers, physical therapist, nutritionist, home health aide, and volunteer.
Courtesy Hospice of San Francisco, Calif.

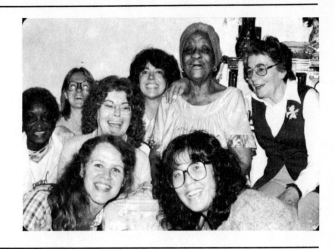

Figure 6.7
Hospice philosophy.

Hospice Philosophy

Hospice affirms life.
Hospice exists to provide support and care for persons in the last phases of incurable disease so that they may live as fully and comfortably as possible.

Hospice exists in the belief that through appropriate care and the promotion of a caring community patients and families will be free to attain a degree of mental and spiritual preparation for death that is satisfying to them.

Hospice movement

Another development in the area of death and dying is the hospice movement. Named for the medieval hospices or waystations that provided comforts for travelers, a modern hospice provides inpatient or outpatient services designed to meet the holistic needs of the dying person and his loved ones (Figures 6.6 and 6.7).

The hospice movement and current literature also address the need for survivors to go through a process of mourning for the dead person. In your work you can expect to encounter dying patients and their families and should be prepared to assist them. Understanding the needs of survivors and encouraging them to express themselves will be a great service that will help them cope with the loss they have suffered.

Conclusion

This limited overview of holistic attitudes for health care is designed to make you aware of the concept and to stimulate your interest in further exploring the theory as you proceed to study the administrative and clinical areas of your chosen profession. Your attitude and behavior toward patients will influence the results of your work, and an ongoing consideration of the individuality of your future patients will help you succeed in the health care field.

Review Questions

1. How would you describe holistic health to a patient who heard the term on a radio talk show?
2. What three areas of responsibility do you have as a medical assistant in a holistic health environment?
3. List and describe the three components of problem analysis.
4. List the six qualities of mentally healthy individuals as determined by Maslow.
5. List the six human problems that everyone can be expected to encounter in varying degrees.
6. List and describe four common methods of psychotherapy.
7. Describe the role of stress in daily life and list five general techniques for coping with it.
8. List and describe the four major influences on physical fitness.
9. Describe two alternatives to traditional childbirth techniques.
10. Describe the role of the medical assistant in working with patients who are experiencing problems with parenting, aging, and dying.

SUGGESTED READINGS

Briggs JL and Calloway DH: Bogent's nutrition and physical fitness, ed 10, Philadelphia, 1979, WB Saunders Co.

Combs BJ, Hales DR, and Williams BK: Invitation to health: your personal responsibility, ed 2, Menlo Park, Calif, The Benjamin Cummings Publishing Co.

Farquhar JW: The American way of life need not be hazardous to your health, New York, 1979, WW Norton & Co, Inc.

Goldfried MR and Merbaum M, editors: Behavior change through self-control, New York, 1973, Holt, Rinehart & Winston.

Part Two

Administrative Theory and Technique

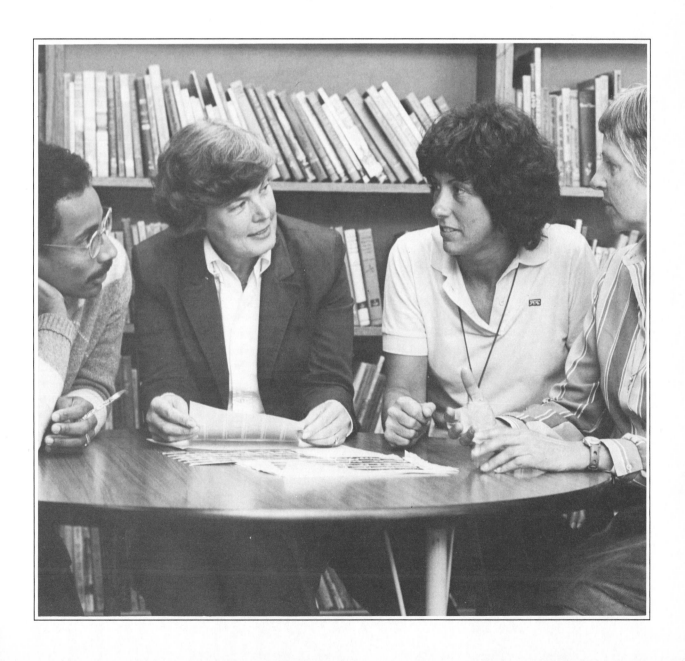

Chapter 7

Administrative Systems Management

- Administrative systems management

Objectives

On completion of Chapter 7 the medical assistant student should be able to:

1 Define the terms listed in the vocabulary.

2 Discuss the concept of administrative systems and the primary purpose of systems management.

3 List the six types of administrative systems.

4 List the six basic qualities that are necessary for an office manager.

5 Discuss the duties and responsibilities of the office manager.

6 List and discuss the seven possible recruiting sources for new employees.

7 Discuss the steps to be followed when selecting a new employee.

8 Discuss the three elements of the employment process.

9 Discuss the two elements of employee compensation and the associated record responsibilities.

10 List and discuss the eight general topics that should be covered in a procedure manual.

11 Describe a facility procedure manual.

12 Define communication systems, scheduling systems, records management, financial management, and facility and equipment management.

Vocabulary

administrative system An organized approach to the elements that make up the business portion of a medical practice, based on the goals and objectives of the physician-owner.

agency A facility developed and organized for the purpose of providing health care. An agency may be public, such as a county health department, or private, such as a health maintenance organization.

consumer An individual who takes advantage of the services of a facility. In a medical facility the consumer is also referred to as a patient.

cost containment An effort to provide high-quality services by the most economical method.

dynamic process The progressive, adaptive quality of an administrative system, allowing for changes in the internal and external environment of a medical practice.

facility The site at which medical care is provided.

integrated Various components of an organization joined or brought together to function cooperatively and produce a positive effect.

level of care A determination of the degree of care required to assist the patient's return to optimum well-being. An acute-care hospital is the highest level of care

77

because it can provide all necessary specialized personnel and equipment. The cost of care is proportional to the level of care; an acute-care hospital is the most expensive care.

management The process of directing or controlling the functions of an organization.

manual A book developed as a reference source of the policies or procedures used in an office or agency.

outpatient setting A level of care provided to individuals capable of residing at home and able to report to a facility for a specific examination or treatment; the most cost-efficient level of care.

patient recall A method of notifying individuals that a return visit is necessary for examination or treatment.

policy An established course of conduct based on the goals and objectives of an organization or medical practice.

private sector Any service, including health care, provided by funds from nongovernment sources.

procedure A detailed course of action; a step-by-step method of accomplishing an activity.

provider An individual who supplies a service for others. Health care providers include physicians, technicians, medical assistants, and nurses.

provider services Professional functions performed by individuals for the well-being of others.

public sector Any service provided or supported by a government agency.

system A combination of parts that function together in an orderly manner to accomplish a predetermined task.

Medical assistants of today find an increasing demand for their skills. The growing complexity of medical services and the trend toward specialization require greater numbers of well-trained medical assistants. In addition, both public (government) and private (insurance companies) agencies responsible for paying for medical services are encouraging and in some cases demanding an emphasis on care in outpatient settings. This shift will likewise create positions for medical assistants and expand their roles through increased contact with the patient-consumer. The purposes of this shift toward treatment in outpatient settings are to ensure consumer use of the appropriate level of care and to encourage cost containment. Since patients may not understand the restriction to outpatient services, the medical assistant as educator will, whenever possible, be responsible for explaining these requirements and reassuring the patient that the staff will coordinate other necessary outpatient services to minimize inconvenience.

As payers place more emphasis on outpatient care and the complexity of provider services increases, the need for careful organization emerges. The professional medical assistant is the key to an effective, efficiently managed medical practice. The physician and the facility staff are concerned chiefly with the care and treatment of patients, but there are many other details that must be attended to in maintaining a successful practice.

Administrative systems management is based on the planning and organization of the various components that make up the administrative (business) portion of a medical practice. The primary purpose of systems management is to achieve patient care and comfort by maintaining an efficient and effective medical practice.

ADMINISTRATIVE SYSTEMS MANAGEMENT

In the management of administrative systems, the medical assistant must be aware of the following principles:

- Each system is used in every medical practice or agency in varying degrees of complexity;
- The various systems are integrated and function simultaneously; and
- The efficiency of each system depends on and affects all of the other systems.

After each system has been planned, developed, and instituted, the medical assistant observes, monitors, and evaluates the process for efficiency and effectiveness. As long as a system supports the goals of a medical practice, it may continue unchanged; when a system is not functioning optimally it must be revised.

To prepare for work in a medical office, the medical assistant student will need to develop an understanding of the elements of the following administrative systems:

- Personnel management;
- Communication systems (oral and written);
- Scheduling systems;
- Records management;
- Financial management; and
- Facility and equipment management.

Personnel management will be discussed in this chapter. The remaining five systems will be introduced in this chapter and expanded on in subsequent chapters.

Personnel Management
Solo assistant office

All systems are equally important, and the employee is the foundation on which all systems are based. In a limited medical practice employing a single medical assistant, the physician-owner takes the role of manager. The physician is the decision maker. The medical assistant is responsible for carrying out directives and maintaining all systems necessary for the efficient operation of the facility. The medical assistant in this position must be an especially organized and self-directed individual.

Multiple-employee office

Selecting the office manager. As a practice grows, increased clinical responsibilities require more personnel, and the management time available to the physician is reduced. To allow the physician the freedom to concentrate on the primary goal of providing patient care, an office manager is needed. The office manager in turn coordinates the staff duties necessary to promote total patient care.

After the need for an office manager has been established and a job description has been written, the employer has two options for filling the position; to select one of the current employees or to hire a new employee. Each option has advantages and disadvantages that must be recognized and evaluated (see Table 7.1). Each office or agency is different, and the office manager should be selected to fulfill the responsibilities unique to the setting.

Qualifications of the manager. Each office or agency will require different qualifications for the office manager. However, there are some general qualities that are basic requirements for any manager. These qualities include the following:
- Objectivity;
- Organizational skills;
- Creativity;
- Effective communication skills (written and oral); and
- Diplomacy.

Duties of the manager. The office manager is responsible to both the physician and the other staff members, and he or she serves as the informational link between the two. The information that must flow in both directions between the physician-employer and the staff relates to the six administrative systems listed on p. 78.

Just as the office staff is the foundation of the medical practice, the office manager sets the tone for the effective and efficient management of the remaining five systems. The manager will either work with the physician-owner or be delegated total responsibility for the various functions of personnel management.

Recruiting and selecting employees

Recruiting sources. When a medical practice or agency needs to replace personnel or add personnel to the existing staff, the process should be ap-

Table 7.1
Selection options for office managers

	Advantages	Disadvantages
Current employee	1. Acquainted with staff	1. May create friction with nonselected employees
	2. Knowledge of existing systems	2. Will have preexisting opinions
	3. Established trust and rapport with employer	3. Inexperienced as manager
	4. Known skills and loyalty	4. Disruption of routine during transition
New employee	1. Offers a fresh perspective	1. Orientation time
	2. Offers objectivity	2. May not be accepted by current employees
	3. Able to select individual with proven managerial experience	3. Will probably command a higher salary
	4. No established interoffice relationships	4. Unknown loyalty

Table 7.2
Employee recruiting resources

Resource	Advantages	Disadvantages
Newspapers		
Office phone given	1. Reach vast audience 2. Least expensive 3. Quickest results	1. Heavy influx of calls 2. Disrupts routine
Newspaper box number	1. Initial screening simplified 2. Demands sample of writing skills	1. No personal contact 2. Discourages applicants
Private employment agency	1. Prescreening done by a professional 2. Specialized medical agencies available	1. Expensive 2. Fee paid by employer
Professional association placement service	1. Applicants generally rated good to excellent 2. Fees less than private employment agencies	1. Screening for specific skills may be weak
State employment offices	1. Good for paraprofessional employees 2. No fees	1. Inadequate screening
Local formal training programs	1. Candidate graduate of accredited program 2. No fees	1. Availability based on program completion dates
Friends or relatives of current employees	1. Quick, convenient contact 2. New employee begins with a positive attitude toward practice	1. Feeling of favoritism among other employees 2. Ill will if referral is not selected
Walk in/write in	1. Approach demonstrates the applicant has initiative and is self-directed	1. May arrive at a time when no positions are available

proached in a logical manner. The first concern is how to recruit enough applicants to make an intelligent choice. There are many possible recruiting sources, and the person responsible for hiring new employees may want to use one or more of them. The common recruiting sources and the advantages and disadvantages of each are noted in Table 7.2. One source of potential employees that is relatively common and was eliminated from Table 7.2 is called *pirating*. This resource involves seeking out and hiring qualified employees away from other medical offices or facilities in the community. Pirating was not included in Table 7.2 because it is not openly acknowledged and is not considered professional. It does, however, exist. The personnel manager must be aware of this practice to prevent the loss of valuable employees to others who use this method.

Selection process. Once you have recruited candidates for the available position you will begin the selection process. The tendency at this point may be to rush the selection in an effort to fill the va-

cant position quickly. This should be avoided, regardless of the urgency. Hasty selection may result in hiring an individual who is not qualified for the position or does not work well with the other employees. The appropriate selection process is an orderly one that should follow these steps:

- Accept employment applications;
- Conduct interviews;
- Contact references;
- Rank applicants; and
- Select the most qualified applicant.

The application form can be designed specifically for your facility or you may use one that has been tested and proved appropriate by others. The latter form may be the best to avoid legal problems that may arise from requesting inappropriate information, such as age, marital status, or ethnic origin. The application should include an authorization to contact the applicant's current employer.

Once the applications have been completed, each potential employee is scheduled for an interview. The office manager may have the authority to make the final hiring decision or may only do the screening interview, scheduling appropriate applicants for a second interview with the physician-employer. If the employer conducts the second interview, the office manager usually works cooperatively with the physician throughout the remainder of the selection process. Regardless of who conducts the interviews, the following basic rules apply:

- All interviews should be conducted by the same person. This allows the interviewer to make appropriate, first-hand comparisons of the various applicants;
- Following a brief, precise description of the specific job by the interviewer, the applicant should do most of the talking. This provides a means to evaluate the applicant's oral communication skill;
- The interviewer should use the written application as the foundation for questions asked during the interview;
- An application file should be kept with notes on each applicant recorded immediately after the interview; and
- The interviewer should avoid making any verbal commitment or offering an opinion of the applicant's possibility of obtaining the position.

After the interviews the three or four most acceptable candidates for the position should be selected. These applicants will then be considered until the final selection is made.

The third step in the selection process is checking references. The person responsible for hiring the new employee may wish to trust his or her own intuition about the applicant. However, while impressions are important, they should *never* replace direct contact with former employers, personal references, or both.

References may be checked formally by writing to the reference source to request a written reply, either on a preprinted form or by letter. While this method will provide a permanent record, it has limitations. These limitations can be overcome by checking references by telephone when possible. By speaking directly with the reference sources, you have the advantage of hearing the respondents' vocal inflections and detecting their reactions to questions or omissions in answers to questions. The respondents may also be more candid during a conversation than they might be in a written response for a permanent record. It should be noted, however, that there is an increasing reluctance by employers to provide telephone references, as legally they must have the written con-

sent of the applicant to provide such information.

The final step in the selection process involves choosing the three best candidates and ranking them as first, second, and third choices. The position is then offered to the first-choice applicant. If he or she declines, the job is then offered to the second-choice applicant.

Employment process

The employment offer.   A position should be offered in writing; however, the offer may be made orally with a follow-up written confirmation. At the time the offer of employment is made, the minimum information that should be supplied to the job candidate includes the following:

- Starting salary for the position;
- Salary payments schedule;
- Benefits;
- Job description or list of major duties and responsibilities;
- Employment status;
- Work hours;
- Dress code; and
- Office policies and procedures.

When the job offer has been accepted, it is the responsibility of the office manager to notify the candidates who were not accepted; this should be done in writing.

Employment status.   Employment status relates to a condition of the employee's position. The employee will be categorized as one of the following types:

- Temporary;
- Part-time;
- Probationary; or
- Permanent.

The temporary employee works in the facility for a short time to provide interim services. A temporary employee may be necessary to substitute for permanent staff members who are absent for reasons such as vacations, illness, or jury duty. The temporary employee is usually paid on an hourly basis and is not eligible for benefits.

Part-time employees usually work half-time or less on a predetermined schedule and at a fixed, prorated salary. Generally, benefits such as health insurance are not available to part-time employees.

When an employee is hired with the intention of making him or her a permanent member of the health care team, a trial period of employment is usually established. This period ranges from 30 to 90 days, and the employee is usually not eligible for benefits such as sick leave, vacation, or insurance during this time. The length of the probationary period must be clearly established. At the end of the probationary period the employer and employee will meet to determine whether the employee will remain as a permanent staff member. The option to terminate without prejudice may be made at this time by either the employer or employee.

Permanent employees have established positions and functions in the medical facility. They receive full salaries and are eligible for all benefits.

Terminations. Ending an employer-employee relationship is called a termination. A termination may be classified as voluntary or involuntary.

Voluntary terminations are initiated by the employee who might wish to leave a position to return to school, work in a different type of facility, or move to another area. The possibility also exists that an employee may wish to terminate because of interpersonal difficulties within the facility or because of inability to adapt to particular methods of operation. The voluntary termination process should include the following:

- A letter of resignation from the employee, giving appropriate notice (2 weeks to 1 month).
- An exit interview. This will give the employer the opportunity to determine the possible reasons for the resignation. There may be internal problems of which the employer is unaware and about which the existing employee can elaborate. However, the employee should be careful to relay only significant information accurately and diplomatically; petty information will diminish credibility.
- A current forwarding address for the employee so that documents such as W-2 forms and retirement fund information can be sent.

Involuntary terminations are initiated by the employer or office manager and are usually unpleasant experiences. They must be conducted in the most professional and diplomatic manner possible.

Layoffs occur in such circumstances as a reduction in work load, the relocation of a practice or facility in another area, or the retirement of the physician-owner. Although a layoff may be more easily understood by the employee, it is still an unsettling experience.

Firing of an employee usually follows an accepted protocol that includes the following steps:

- Verbally warning the employee of unacceptable performance;
- Warning the employee in writing if the behavior continues; and
- Terminating the employment, verbally and in writing, if the employee's performance fails to meet established standards.

Usually the person responsible for hiring must also conduct the dismissal process.

The employee who has been terminated should be given notice as predetermined by office policy. Since it may be uncomfortable for all concerned to have the dismissed employee work through the notice period, the employer should pay up-to-date all salary, vacation benefits, sick leave benefits, and/or retirement benefits (if possible) through the notice period and ask the employee to leave immediately. Experience has determined that dismissals should be given privately, preferably at the end of a workday, and on a Friday if possible.

The only situation that precludes the warning process and notice period occurs when the employee is found guilty of a gross breach of ethics, such as betraying a patient's confidentiality or if a legal issue such as embezzlement is involved.

In any involuntary termination, it is absolutely necessary for the employer—office manager to have clear, well-documented records detailing the warning process and the circumstances that led to the termination.

Employee compensation

Salaries. Employee compensation includes salary and selected benefits. Salaries vary depending on the part of the country, the setting (urban or rural), the medical assistant's experience and length of service, and the duties of the position. The trend is toward improved salaries for medical assistants. This trend may be influenced by recognition of the profession, improved training programs, standardized certification examinations, and professional associations.

Salary advances should be scheduled and based on the cost of living as well as considerations of merit. Cost of living increases are based on a set percentage for all employees; merit raises are based on individual performance evaluations. Raises usually occur after the probationary period, at which time the employee becomes a permanent member of the staff. They continue according to the established schedule. Annual salary increases may occur on a fixed date for all employees, on the employee's birthday, after a job performance evaluation, or on the anniversary of the employee's attainment of permanent status.

Benefits. Benefits will vary depending on the employment site and whether a practice is incorporated. However, most employees can anticipate such basic benefits as the following:

- Health insurance;
- Sick leave;

- Vacations and holidays; and
- Retirement plan.

As previously noted, information on salary and benefits should be discussed with the employee at the time the job offer is made.

Records and forms. Personnel files should be complete and well organized. Each employee's file includes the employee's job application, job description, references, salary and performance reviews, and necessary records and forms. The office manager keeps attendance records, W-4 forms, payroll deduction information, and enrollment forms, such as benefit insurance applications.

The information in each employee's personnel file and the tax reports generated from the employee's payroll records must be treated as *strictly confidential*. The personnel file is a matter between the employer or his or her authorized representative and the employee.

Orientation and training

The orientation of a new employee involves introducing the new employee to co-workers, the work environment, and the guidelines that establish the foundation for operations and relationships within the facility.

Since much of the preparation of medical assistants today takes place in formal training programs as described in Chapter 1, on-the-job training requirements have been greatly reduced but *not* eliminated. Formal training provides the theoretical foundation, and the externship or previous experience enhances that knowledge, but each employer or agency involves unique individuals who use particular variations on procedures. The new employee needs a training period to learn and adapt to these variations. This period coincides with the probationary period.

Upon accepting a position, the new employee should not be surprised that the predecessor of the position being filled is not available to train the new employee. Although it is not a desirable situation, many times the position cannot be filled in time to provide adequate orientation and training. Thus the new employee will need to ask the office manager or employer any questions regarding the position. It is not uncommon that the new employee will be placed in a position of self-training or on-the-job training. This is particularly true in the positions of receptionist and insurance billers.

Foundation of a training program. The orientation and training plan is based on the information outlined in the office or agency policy and procedure manuals. All practices, regardless of size, should develop and maintain these manuals. They are necessary as a foundation for all services. The office manager will work with the employer to develop the policy manual and with the health care team to develop the procedure manual. Once the manuals have been developed, follow-up duties include monitoring and evaluating the effectiveness and efficiency of each system and maintaining or revising the procedure manual as needed.

Ongoing training and development. A continuing-training technique that contributes to maintaining the cooperative spirit among the employees and between the employees and employers is the office staff meeting. Staff meetings are preplanned semi-formal gatherings attended by the employer and employees at which issues relevant to staff relations and office management are discussed. Some decisions are by their nature reserved for the employer, and others are decided by the majority.

Staff meetings serve several purposes. They provide a means to discuss issues openly and thereby promote communication among the staff. They also help avoid interoffice gossip and allow issues to be discussed in a logical manner for all to hear at one time. This is preferable to allowing information to be repeated several times and possibly distorted in the retelling. Staff meetings also provide an atmosphere different from the daily work routine and include an element of socialization. This may have a bonding effect by which all involved can see themselves as part of the team.

Staff meetings should be described in the policy manual under the work relations heading. This description should include scheduling and planning information. The box on p. 84 details one possible policy on staff meetings.

Policy manual

A policy is a general statement that serves as a guideline for operating a business and that governs the employee-employer relationship. Policies are based on the goals and objectives of the facility. A policy manual is a binder, preferably a loose-leaf one, in which statements of policy can be organized and stored. The policy manual in a medical practice serves as a reference source for all employees. It is used to orient and train new employees, and it enables the staff to make changes with minimal disruption of routine. Some of the topics that should be discussed in a policy manual are presented in Tables 7.3 and 7.4. Sound management principles indicate that an office policy manual should be well thought out and well designed. Once in use it must also be periodically reviewed and updated.

Table 7.3
Policy manual topic areas

Employment	Attendance and timekeeping	Salary	Employee benefits
Confidential information	Absences	Payroll	Health insurance
Employee status	Work breaks	Employee progress review	Pension plan
Employment procedure	Time off (medical/dental appointments)	Overtime	Vacations
Probationary period	Word schedules	Salary advances	Holidays
Recruiting and selection	Timekeeping		Life insurance
Retirement			Sick leave
Terminations			
Unemployment insurance			
Job description and duties			

Sample Page from Policy Manual (Work Relations)

Staff Meetings

Day Third Wednesday of each month
Time 12:00 noon to 2:00 PM
Place Office, with lunch delivered, or local restaurant
Attendance All staff members, office manager, employer
Recording secretary Administrative assistant
Agenda
Old Business: Typed and copied minutes of the last meeting are distributed by the third Monday of the month and reviewed at the opening of the meeting.
Progress Report: Remedial actions decided on at the previous meeting are reviewed.
New Business: (1) Subjects of interest to physician/ owner, (2) subjects suggested by office manager, and/or (3) subjects suggested by staff members.

Agenda items must be submitted for consideration in writing by 12:00 noon on the Wednesday before the meeting. Subjects for the meeting will be selected by the office manager based on the information submitted and the discussion time available. The planned agenda will be distributed to all attendees with the minutes of the previous meeting. Subjects not selected for discussion may be resubmitted for consideration. Subjects to be considered are introduced in order and discussed, and suggestions for any remedial action necessary are considered. The decision on a course of remedial action will be made by a consensus, by the office manager, or by the employer, depending on the necessary authority position.

Procedure manual

The procedure manual provides a more detailed aid in personnel and systems management. The manual should be a loose-leaf binder with a separate sheet devoted to each staff position and procedure. The manual can be divided in several ways, including the following:

- Into clinical and administrative sections;
- By employee position and job description; and
- By job title.

The first method is the most definitive and can be subdivided easily. The *administrative section* can be arranged according to the six administrative systems listed on p. 78. The *clinical section* can be organized according to the areas discussed in Part Three of this book, using the headings that apply to the specific practice.

Once the format for the manual has been selected, each section is reduced to specific procedures. Each procedure becomes a step-by-step outline or a list of tasks. This serves as an educational tool, because it reduces confusion regarding work distribution and provides a guide for new employees, the employee who must fill in for another, and temporary employees who are brought into the facility. As the manual is developed and revised, the various personnel involved should have a chance to offer their ideas about procedures that affect them. Completed procedures should be dated. As procedures are revised the outmoded procedure sheet should be discarded, and the new procedure sheet should be substituted and dated as a revision (Rev. 00/00/00).

Completed procedure manuals are kept by the physician(s) and the office manager and should be

Work relations	Education and training	Health and safety	General
Suggestion program Complaints	Educational leave Tuition payment	Environment Accident reporting	Professional ethics Confidential information
Staff meetings	Professional association dues payment	Building/office security	Dress code
Reporting responsibilities	New-employee orientation	Recreation/exercise facilities	Hygiene and grooming Parking Standards of personal conduct

Table 7.4
Office policies

1. Requirements for payments from patients.
2. Forms of payments accepted.
3. Policy relating to private insurance.
   a. Full fee due?
   b. When?
   c. Accepting assignment?
   d. Bill insurance for patient?
   e. Fee for rebilling insurance?
4. MediCare/Medicaid.
   a. Does the practice participate?
   b. Does the practice accept new patients with this coverage?
      (1) By referral only.
      (2) By emergency only.
      (3) By family member reference only.
5. Practice policy for payment plans.
6. Policy for other fees that may be charged to the patient.
   a. Broken appointment.
   b. Interest/finance charges.
   c. Lab handling fee.
   d. Rebilling charge.

Sample Job Description from Procedure Manual

Job title Medical receptionist
Reports to Office manager
Job description The receptionist is responsible for controlling the telephone system, scheduling appointments, greeting patients, notifying appropriate personnel of a patient's arrival, and processing mail.
Specific tasks
1. Sign in and out with answering service when opening or closing office for day or lunch hour.
2. Answer and direct all incoming calls to appropriate person for processing.
3. Prepare copies of daily appointment schedule for physician and staff members.
4. Schedule office appointments for patients.
5. Schedule appointments in other facilities for patients.
6. Greet patients when they arrive.
7. Notify personnel when patients arrive.
8. Open incoming mail and distribute to appropriate personnel.

accessible to all employees. Copies of individual sections should be given to the employee responsible for the duties as detailed. Sample procedure sheets are shown above and on p. 86. Other administrative and clinical procedures will be presented in subsequent chapters in this text. The rationale for each step of a procedure is included when appropriate. Procedures are easier to learn when an individual understands *why* they are important.

Communication Systems

A communication system is divided into two areas: (1) oral and (2) written. This system should be thought of as the key link between the physician and the patients. Effective communication is also a form of public relations that links the physician with colleagues and office personnel with professionals in other offices and health care agencies. The impression made through communication reflects on all personnel and on the medical practice in general.

Sample Procedure

Answering Service Sign In/Sign Out

Procedure	*Rationale*
Call service on arrival at desk.	Answering service (exchange) is relieved of responsibility of answering telephone. Patients can make direct contact with facility personnel.
Obtain any messages left with service. Receive report from service on physician's whereabouts. Distribute message to appropriate personnel for processing.	Reduces time involved if physician is needed by office personnel.
If offices closes for lunch, notify service of (1) where and how physician can be contacted and (2) time you will reopen the office. Call service on return from lunch. Sign out end of workday, supplying same information as at lunch-hour sign out.	

Oral communication is the spoken transmission of information between individuals. Information can be transmitted to and from an office or agency very rapidly through the use of the telephone. The telephone is one of the most important means of communication. Telephone equipment, supplies, and support services and effective techniques of telephone use will be discussed in Chapter 8.

Written communication will be discussed in Chapter 11. This chapter includes information on communications equipment, techniques of effective writing, forms that reduce the collection of redundant information, and the processing of incoming and outgoing mail.

Scheduling Systems

A method of time management is necessary for the efficient organization of the work involved in a health care facility. Scheduling systems will be discussed in Chapter 9. These systems must be well developed, since they affect all personnel and, most importantly, the patients who will be using the services provided by the health care agency.

Records Management

The topic of records management is discussed in Chapter 10. Patient registration provides the foundation for the patient's medical record. Various approaches to patient registration, the advantages and disadvantages of each method, and the information necessary for registration will be discussed.

Responsibility for the patient's medical record

usually involves many if not all of the office personnel. Techniques in the development, handling, and storage of this document are also presented in Chapter 10.

Reminder systems, which are internal informational processes, are important in the smooth operation of an office or agency. This form of records management, discussed in Chapter 10, will assist in the coordination of patient recalls, supply reordering, business and medical meetings, reporting requirements, and license and insurance policy renewals.

The other adjunct records discussed in Chapter 10 involve medical correspondence unrelated to patients, business correspondence, and the physician's personal records.

Financial Management

The management of financial systems in a facility involves the following three areas of responsibility:
- Billing systems;
- Insurance; and
- The fundamentals of banking and bookkeeping.

The income generated by billing and insurance is accounted for by banking and bookkeeping techniques. This income provides the funds with which the practice or agency conducts business. One employee may be responsible for all financial records management, or the responsibility may be distributed to various staff members with the skill to handle a specific aspect of the function.

Billing systems are discussed in Chapter 12. This

chapter includes the types of billing systems available for medical practices, the personal data necessary to generate bills to patients for services rendered, and the recording of transactions (charges and payments).

Chapter 14 presents information on insurance and medical practices. Health care insurance pays for all or part of the fees billed to patients. The types of insurance coverage, methods of processing patient's claims, possible office policies regarding insurance services, and insurance company restrictions on some services are among the topics discussed in Chapter 14. Other insurance considerations necessary to protect the employee of a medical practice (Worker's Compensation, unemployment, disability), and the practice (public and professional liability, property loss) will also be presented in Chapter 14.

Chapter 14 presents information regarding computerizing the medical office, including application of software and systems information. The third component of financial management involves

banking techniques (check writing, deposit records, statements reconciliation) and bookkeeping processes (payroll preparation, records, ledgers, tax reports). These techniques and processes are discussed in Chapter 15.

Facility and Equipment Management

The final aspect of administrative management is facility and equipment management. This area of responsibility, discussed further in Chapter 16, involves factors necessary for patient comfort and safety. Facility planning involves the management of the public, administrative, and clinical areas of an office or agency. This includes attending to patient traffic flow and providing for the patient's privacy and security. Attention to equipment planning and maintenance involves considerations of capital (major) equipment and disposable (short-life) equipment and electronic aids to the inventory and storage of such equipment.

Conclusion

This chapter has introduced the medical assistant student to the organization of the administrative aspects of a medical practice or agency through a *systems approach*. In viewing the operation of a medical practice as a series of systems, you will be able to study each system independently while developing an understanding of how the systems affect one another. As you proceed through the re-

maining chapters of this book, you will be building a foundation of theory regarding your potential contribution to a health care office or agency. This theory will be integrated into practice as you participate in the extern program or work experience aspect of your training and, eventually, as you become a member of a functional health care team.

Review Questions

1. Describe the role of the medical office manager.
2. What factors influence the increasing demand for professional medical assistants?
3. What is systems management? Name and describe the six administrative systems involved in a medical practice.
4. What considerations must the medical assistant keep in mind in the management of administrative systems?
5. Discuss the advantages and disadvantages of promoting a current employee to the position of office manager. Discuss the advantages

and disadvantages of hiring a new employee for the position of office manager.
6. Name and discuss the four steps of the process used in selecting new employees for a practice.
7. List and discuss the four possible levels of employment status.
8. What steps should the employee follow in a voluntary termination? What steps should the employer follow in an involuntary termination?
9. Describe the purpose of a policy manual. Describe a procedure manual and explain how it is used to train personnel.

SUGGESTED READINGS

American Medical Association: The business side of medical practice, Chicago, 1979, The Association.

Johnson, HW: Selecting, training, and supervising office personnel, Menlo Park, Calif, 1969, Addison-Wesley Pub. Co.

Chapter 8

Oral Communication

- Interpersonal communication
- Telephone communications
- Auxiliary telephone services

Objectives

On completion of Chapter 8 the medical assistant student should be able to:

1 Define the terms listed in the vocabulary.

2 State and discuss the four factors that are basic to effective spoken communication.

3 Discuss effective techniques for in-person communication.

4 Describe the seven steps for dealing with the angry patient.

5 List and discuss the three reasons that the telephone is the most vital tool in a medical practice.

6 Describe how attitude can influence telephone communication.

7 Identify letter sounds that are troublesome in telephone communication and demonstrate the technique for clarifying these sounds.

8 List and describe the six types of telephone equipment used in a medical office.

9 Describe the methods of using the four types of directories available for locating telephone numbers.

10 List and discuss the four elements of general courtesy when handling incoming telephone calls.

11 Describe the two necessary factors in taking accurate messages, including those from troublesome callers.

12 List the five major categories used to classify incoming calls and the types of calls in each category.

13 Discuss the appropriate disposition of incoming calls.

14 Describe the technique and etiquette of placing local, long-distance, and conference calls.

15 List and discuss the five auxillary services that complete the telephone system.

Vocabulary

communication The exchange of thoughts or opinions between persons or business firms; any means of conveying ideas or information in person or by the use of auxiliary equipment.

conference call A prearranged telephone call that allows many people in many different locations to hear and speak to each other at one time.

directory An alphabetical list of names with

addresses and telephone numbers or telephone extension numbers.

disposition The act of arranging or placing or the power of managing and distributing.

enunciate To declare or state; to pronounce clearly when speaking.

etiquette The rules of conduct observed in social or business interactions; polite behavior.

handset The portion of the telephone that is held in one hand and allows the user to hear and speak with others.

hold (on the telephone) The ability to retain possession of a call in an inactive state.

interconnect telephone systems Telephone service available through private compa-

nies as an alternative to services from public utility (Bell) system.

rapport A level of communication based on trust that allows individuals to express their true opinions and feelings.

telephone cradle The part of the telephone on which the handset rests when not in use.

telephone receiver The part of the telephone, located in the handset, that accepts electrical waves and converts them into sound.

telephone recording device An instrument attached to the telephone that mechanically intercepts calls and preserves the caller's message.

Oral communication is one of the vital systems in a medical office or agency. It is important in any business but is even more important in patient care. The medical assistant has a responsibility to patients and physician-owners to develop effective techniques of oral communication. Each member of the health care team also has a responsibility to maintain communication with the other members of the team.

Oral communication is possible through face-to-face encounters and through the use of the telephone and its auxiliary services.

INTERPERSONAL COMMUNICATION
Basic Considerations

Many factors influence oral communication and affect the way information is presented and received. Regardless of the message that is spoken, other messages are delivered through posture, facial expression, tone and volume of voice, and enunciation. Separately and together these factors influence the effectiveness of spoken communication.

Posture

The way you sit or stand will affect communication in two ways. If your posture is poor, with your back bent forward, your shoulders slumped, and your head down, your speech will not be clear. You will also indicate to the other person that you are not interested in him or his message. On the other hand, if your back is straight with your shoulders in the proper position and your head up so that you make eye contact with the other person, your message will receive more attention, and the person will feel that you are genuinely inter-

ested in him. Good posture also communicates that you are alert and confident and care about your work.

Facial expression

Your facial expression can communicate just as much as the spoken word, and patients are particularly sensitive to anything that might give an indication of their status. Eye contact is important in establishing communication and indicating your interest in the patient. You should be conscious of expressions that might indicate concern about or negative attitudes toward the patient. Wrinkling your forehead, drawing in your eyebrows, or clenching your teeth is evident to the patient and may cause worry. In some specialty work you may encounter individuals with disease processes that include unpleasant stages or permanent results. As a medical assistant in this situation you must be especially careful not to indicate revulsion or pity. This begins with maintaining a neutral facial expression. By establishing rapport with patients you let them know that they are important to you as people and that the disease process is only one aspect of the relationship.

Tone of voice

Your tone of voice can completely change the meaning of the spoken message. When speaking with patients you should use a normal conversational tone that is neither too loud nor too soft. You should remember that tension, anger, or disappointment can come through in your voice and affect its volume. Regardless of the true source of these emotions the people hearing them will assume that they are the source. Your tone is influenced by your attitude, your awareness, and your facial expression. Relaxed facial muscles and a smile will soften the tone of your voice and enhance the encounter.

Enunciation

Speaking clearly is very important in making yourself understood. Factors that may interfere with proper enunciation include muscle tension around the mouth, clenched teeth, eating or chewing gum, and unfamiliarity with the correct pronunciation of a word. Pronunciation is improved by the use of a dictionary, asking the advice of co-workers, and careful listening. You should also speak naturally and use words with which you are familiar and comfortable.

Technique: In Person
Eye contact

Making and maintaining eye contact with the person to whom you are speaking cannot be overemphasized. Eye contact affirms to the individual that you are speaking only to him, that what is being said is important, and that you are listening. Avoiding eye contact will indicate the opposite and may also indicate to the patient that you are trying to avoid him or avoid a certain subject.

Attitude

Your attitude toward patients and your work influences your interactions with everyone in the work environment. What you are thinking or feeling can unknowingly influence your attitude; even events that occur away from your job can have an effect. It is important for the welfare of your patients and your relationships with co-workers that your private life not affect your work. A negative attitude is easily detected and will affect the others with whom you have contact. Likewise, a positive attitude can enhance the work environment and improve the quality of all interpersonal relationships.

Atmosphere

The medical assistant is usually the first person to be in contact with patients and other individuals in the course of business. The proper atmosphere is necessary to encourage communication. Greeting patients or other callers in a pleasant, receptive, and professional manner will encourage them to respond in a similar manner. Addressing patients by name will reinforce that you consider them important individuals. Providing privacy is absolutely necessary for patients to confide in you. Do not ask questions while the patient is in the waiting room or in any location in which the conversation can be overheard. Establishing rapport with patients and developing their confidence in the practice and personnel depends on the initial encounter and the atmosphere projected at that time.

Special situations

Hearing-impaired patients. The degree of impairment will affect the actions you take in communicating with the hearing-impaired individual. Persons with total loss of hearing who cannot lipread may be able to communicate by sign language, or communication may take place by exchanging written notes. Individuals capable of lipreading or who have some degree of hearing can communicate orally. To assist the patient you should stand or sit directly in front of him, ideally at eye level. Raising your voice is not advised and in some instances may interfere with the degree of hearing. It is more important that you speak slowly and enunciate clearly with distinct movement of your lips. It is important that you demonstrate patience and willingness to be of help.

Angry patients. There will be occasions on which you are confronted by an angry patient. In most instances the patient will not be angry with you or with the issue being discussed. The anger is often an indication of anxiety about being in a medical setting or a stage of response to a diagnosis or needed treatment.

Dealing with an angry patient will require your understanding and tact. It is important to recognize anger, not ignore it. Ignoring the patient's feelings will only cause them to grow. Instead you should do the following:

- Acknowledge the patient's anger;
- Provide privacy for the patient;
- Allow the patient to express his feelings;
- Listen; you will learn the real reason for the anger;
- Never respond in anger; communication will cease;
- Resolve issues that are under your control; and
- Relate the situation to the physician.

You may also notice times when the patient will speak angrily to you but not to the physician. Again, you should not take this personally. Many people are shy or inhibited in the presence of physicians and suppress their feelings. This is why it is important to report the situation to the physician. The physician can then introduce the subject and discuss it with the patient. Above all, the patient's feelings must not be ignored.

TELEPHONE COMMUNICATIONS
Importance of Telephone Systems

Most management authorities believe that the telephone is the most important tool in a medical practice. Telephones serve the following vital functions:
- A means of rapid communication;
- A vital link with patients; and
- A link with other practices and ancillary services.

The use and management of telephone systems involves each member of the health care team, and the proper use of the telephone system cannot be stressed too much. It is part of every working day, and it must be treated with respect and used in the most efficient and effective manner.

Telephone policy and procedures

Managing the telephone system requires guidance to ensure consistency among the various employees and possible substitute employees. This guidance can be provided by established office policies and procedures, discussed in Chapter 7. Policy will direct the general office attitude and rules about the management of the system. Procedures detail the method of handling specific situations related to telephone use. You will be able to help develop office policy and procedures with the information discussed in this chapter.

General Considerations
Attitude

The factors previously mentioned that influence oral communication—posture, facial expression, tone of voice, and enunciation—are just as important when using the telephone as when speaking face-to-face. Even though you cannot see the person with whom you are speaking on the telephone your attitude and the value you place on the interaction is evident to him.

Enunciation

Because the individuals communicating by telephone cannot see each other, enunciation is particularly important. The previously noted factors that influence enunciation *all* apply when using the telephone. This especially includes eating or chewing gum. In fact, the telephone tends to magnify the sound of chewing, and it is particularly distracting.

Troublesome letter sounds

On occasion it will be necessary to spell names or words over the telephone because they are complex or unusual. Some letters of the alphabet sound similar, especially over the telephone. You need to be aware of these letters and develop a method of distinguishing them from one another. The letters potentially misunderstood are as follows:

b-d	*d-t*
b-p	*f-s*
b-v	*m-n*
c-z	*p-t*

When it is necessary to clarify any of these letters it is a common practice to state the letter and then a word that begins with the letter. Possible words you can use for this purpose are listed at the top of the next page.

B as in boy	*F* as in Frank
P as in Paul	*V* as in Victor
D as in dog	*M* as in Mary
S as in Sam	*Z* as in zebra
C as in cat	*N* as in Nancy
T as in Tom	

BASIC EQUIPMENT
The Telephone

Options for acquiring equipment. The most common source of telephone equipment is, of course, the Bell Telephone System; however, since deregulation, there are many manufacturers of all types of telephone systems. The necessary equipment may be leased or purchased from many of these companies, although the local servicing entity will have to be contracted for hook-up of the equipment to the local system. Thus the equipment fee will be separate from the monthly service charge. Some services, such as long distance calling, may be supplied by private companies. Private telephone companies are commonly referred to as *interconnective systems.*

Types of equipment. The type of equipment chosen for a medical office or agency depends on the needs at the time and in the near future. Telephone specialists are available to assist with the selection of appropriate equipment when setting up or making changes in a practice. Some of the equipment options are discussed here.

Six-button key set. The six-button key set is one of the more common types of equipment used in a medical office. One of the buttons is red and is used to put a call on hold. This means that the call is temporarily detained or set aside while information is retrieved or the call is transferred. The remaining buttons are clear plastic and may be delegated to incoming lines or com lines. The term *incoming lines* does not indicate that the lines are limited to calls received by the office; it indicates the number of lines from the telephone service company available for use to and from the office. A com line is a line used within the office suite. Personnel are able to communicate with each other via the com line and thereby save time and unnecessary movement about the office.

When a line is in use a steady light is visible through the clear button. An incoming call is indicated by an intermittent flashing light, and a call on hold is signaled by a rapidly winking light. The six-button key set may have a rotary dial but more frequently has the popular push-button dial. The latter is more efficient, usually requiring only 3 seconds to dial a seven-digit number.

10-button telephone. Increased telephone activity in a practice may require a set with more lines available. The 10-button telephone provides one hold button and nine additional lines for external or internal communication.

Com Key. An office that covers a large amount of floor space may want to use a Com Key version of the 10-button phone. It provides seven incoming lines plus the capability of multisite intercom conversations at one time, loudspeaker service, and selection of when and where various phones within the facility will ring.

Desk sets. A facility with several physicians, many patients, and a busy telephone system may need to select among the 11- to 30-button telephones available. Some can serve as a desktop switchboard, allow for operator recall without breaking the caller's connection, or establish conferences by simultaneous depression of the necessary buttons.

Touch-A-Matic. The Bell system Touch-A-Matic phone allows storage of 31 frequently called numbers in a memory. The face of the telephone instrument has a column in which each name or place in the memory is written next to a small button. You may place a call to any number in the memory by lifting the receiver and pressing the button for the person or place you want. The number will be dialed automatically. If you need to call back to a number just dialed either directly or by Touch-A-Matic because of a busy signal or some other reason you may use the *last number dialed* button. This button will automatically redial the number last dialed by the caller.

Speakerphone. An attachment to the primary telephone instrument, the speaker-phone allows an individual to speak to and hear the other person without holding the receiver. This leaves the hands free to handle papers or make notes on the conversation. The user of a speakerphone must be careful, however, to assure privacy if confidential information is discussed.

Placement of telephone. Telephones should be placed with consideration of efficient use and appropriate privacy. Planning where the telephone can be the most accessible to personnel is as important as choosing the right type of equipment. However, telephones should not be placed where they are easily available to patients or visitors to the office. Pay telephones are usually available in medical buildings or facilities; people requesting a telephone should be referred to them.

Head set. Many telephone systems will provide a head set. This feature normally either clips over the head, to glasses, or over the ear with a small tube-like device being inserted into the person's ear and a small wire-like device rotatable in front of the person's mouth. This device has a very powerful but tiny microphone in the tip. There will normally be a connecting wire that clips to the person's clothing, thus allowing the person the freedom to move about and use his or her hands to handle papers or make notes on the conversation while communicating over the telephone.

Telephone service companies are charging for the use of *Information* (411) to locate local telephone numbers. In addition, if you must wait for a prerecorded message to play before you can speak to an information operator, valuable time is wasted. Therefore you should develop a personal system to locate quickly the numbers you need to conduct business.

City telephone directories. The local telephone company automatically provides customers with a city directory. Directories for other cities can also be supplied and should be requested for cities in which you conduct business. City telephone books are divided into two major sections that are commonly called the white pages and the yellow pages. The white and yellow pages may be combined in one volume or may be in separate volumes in major metropolitan areas. The white pages contain the following:

- An introductory section describing available telephone services, including emergency police, fire, and ambulance numbers, area codes, long-distance directions, time zones, and instructions on how to handle obscene or harassing calls;
- Emergency first-aid and disaster-survival guides;

- A government section listing the offices of local, state, and federal agencies; and
- Alphabetically listed names, most addresses, and all telephone numbers of individuals not requesting unlisted numbers. Unless the private customer requests that his number be unlisted, it will automatically be printed in the directory.

The yellow pages list the names, addresses, telephone numbers, and advertisements of businesses according to the service or product provided. Physicians are listed alphabetically and also have the option of a second listing according to specialty. Any listing in the yellow pages results in an additional monthly service charge based on the number of lines and the size of the print requested.

Medical society directories. County medical societies publish an annual directory of all members of the organization. Usually a photograph of each physician is included with his or her name, office address and telephone number, medical school, and year of graduation. This is a convenient alphabetical reference source of many local physicians. If there are some offices that you must call frequently you may want to note the name of the assistant responsible for answering the phone under the physician's entry. People appreciate being recognized by name, and the practice establishes a positive tone for the subsequent conversation.

Hospital directories. Local hospitals may print a directory of hospital services and departments, listing the corresponding extensions or the direct-dial numbers. Knowing the extension number you want will reduce the time required with the hospital operator. If direct dialing to service areas is available you can bypass the hospital operator altogether.

Personalized directories. You will also develop your own system for quick access to numbers that you use frequently. A rotary file or a desktop box suitable for holding 3 × 5 index cards is most commonly used for this purpose. Each is supplied with alphabetical dividers. A separate card should be used for each business or person in the file and should include the following information:

- Name, spelled correctly;
- Complete address, including zip code;
- Telephone number with area code when appropriate; and
- Pertinent information such as services, equipment, or supplies provided.

Emergency numbers can be highlighted by using colored cards or a colored tab or by edging the card with colored tape.

A method of cross-indexing your personal directory involves your office procedure manual. In the section on telephone procedure you should prepare lists of the following:

- Physicians, by specialty, to whom your employer commonly refers patients;
- Professional agencies or services such as hospitals, ambulance companies, pharmacies, home health aides, visiting nurses, laboratories, and specialty clinics;
- Business suppliers or services such as medical-surgical suppliers, bankers, stationers, equipment maintenance companies, instrument repair services, and linen suppliers; and
- Employer's personal and private numbers such as family, friends, insurance broker, accountant, and attorney.

Message recording

A procedure should be developed for recording telephone messages or calls received in the office. Messages may be recorded on individual message pads (Figure 8.1) or in call logbooks (Figure 8.2). The latter allows for the original copy of the message to be delivered to the appropriate person and the duplicate copy to remain in the logbook as a permanent record of the call. The method used for recording messages depends on established procedure, which must be followed consistently by all personnel.

Incoming Calls

Incoming calls make up approximately 80% of the daily telephone activity in an office or agency. Up to 50% of this activity may involve patients or potential patients. Because the telephone is considered a valuable public relations tool, it is imperative that you develop effective telephone techniques.

General courtesy

Answer promptly. The telephone should be answered as quickly as possible, preferably on the first or second ring. This gives the caller an impression of efficiency and consideration. Answering quickly does not mean hastily. If you are rushing and sound breathless it is evident to the caller. If you do have to rush to the telephone, pause briefly, take a deep breath, and then pick up the receiver. If you must answer but are unable to complete the conversation, be courteous. You would not appreciate placing a call that was answered "Doctor's

Figure 8.1
Individual telephone message pad (to be kept in duplicate).

TELEPHONE SYMPTOM SLIP

DATE_____19_____

PATIENT'S NAME _____ AGE_____

ADDRESS _____

PHONE NO._____ TIME OF CALL _____

COMPLAINT_____

_____

HOW LONG SICK _____ TEMP._____

WHAT HAS BEEN DONE_____

                                                PROD.
COUGH_____TYPE_____COLOR_____

EARS_____ NOSE_____

VOMITING_____ DIARRHEA_____

PAIN_____ LOCATION_____

GU_____

BOWELS_____

BLEEDING_____

HOW MUCH_____FROM_____HOW LONG_____

DR'S. INSTRUCTIONS_____

_____

FORM NO. 199   HISTACOUNT CORPORATION, MELVILLE, L. I., N. Y. 11746

office, please hold" and finding yourself on hold before you could respond. A more considerate technique would follow these steps:
- Answer the telephone in the usual manner;
- Allow the caller to identify himself;
- Restate the caller's name;
- Ask the caller if he can hold for a moment;
- Wait for the caller's reply; and
- Thank the caller and depress the hold button.

When you return to the call, thank the caller again and proceed with the conversation.

Hold the instrument properly. Remove the telephone receiver gently from the cradle with your nondominant hand around the center of the handset. This leaves your dominant hand (the one with

which you write) free to write notes or take messages. Place the receiver to your ear with the mouthpiece directly in front of and approximately 1 inch away from your lips. This position will transmit your voice the most naturally. The position can be checked by looking in a mirror or by passing the width of two fingers between the mouthpiece and your lips. Your fingers should just barely pass through.

Never prop the handset between your ear and shoulder. This causes the mouthpiece to be pressed against your chin and distorts your voice, interfering with the ability to enunciate. Should you accidentally drop the receiver, retrieve it, apologize to the caller, and continue the conversation.

Figure 8.2
Telephone message log book.

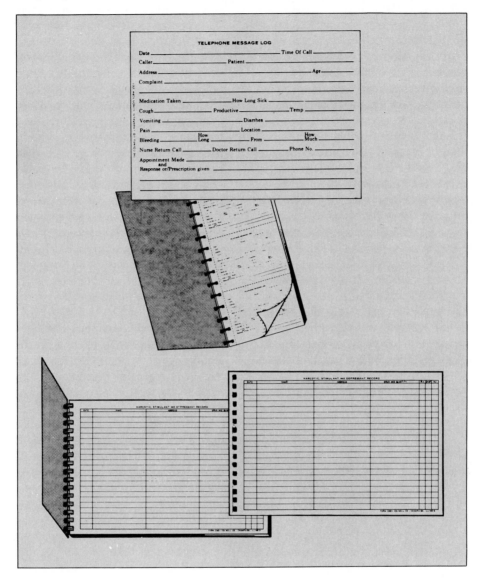

Identify the office and yourself. Office procedure will guide all personnel in the preferred manner of identifying the office and the person answering. Most telephone specialists suggest some variation of "Dr. Smith's office, Ms. Jones speaking." In a multi-physician office each physician's name can be stated, for example, "Drs. Smith, Adams, and Caldwell, Ms. Jones speaking." With more than three physicians you will need to consider answering, "Doctor's office." Some multi-physician offices are incorporated or have adopted a group name. In that case you can answer, for example, "Valley Medical Group, Ms. Jones speaking."

If time permits you may wish to include a greeting such as "Good morning" or "Good afternoon" or ask "May I help you?" after stating your name. The caller will appreciate the pleasant opening.

Some states have regulations regarding the telephone identification of an incorporated medical practice. The physician's attorney will be able to guide you on this matter. Some attorneys have linked the incorporation rules to the need for identifying the office by merely stating the telephone number. This procedure should be avoided if at all possible. It is bewildering to the caller, who usually replies, "Is this Dr. Adam's office?" By the time the identification is made, time has been wasted, and callers infer that they are dealing with an impersonal medical office.

Proper use of hold.   Hold should be used *anytime* you are not speaking with the caller. This includes brief interruptions to retrieve information or a record or to bring another person to the telephone. Placing the receiver on the desk and not depressing the hold button allows the caller to overhear office conversations. Placing a hand over the mouthpiece is an inadequate substitute for hold and may even magnify what is being said.

Hold must also be used when routing a call, that is, directing it to the person for whom it is intended. After the caller is put on hold, you may use the com line to notify the physician or a co-worker of who is waiting on which line.

When you are speaking to one caller and another line rings, you must respond to the new call. An appropriate procedure to follow is listed below.

A caller should not be allowed to wait on hold indefinitely. You should speak with the caller who is on hold at 2-minute intervals to tell him the status of the call. For example, you may have a caller waiting to speak to a physician who is already speaking on another line. When you check back with the caller you might say, "Dr. Smith is still on the other line, would you like to continue to hold, or can the doctor call you back?" This lets the caller know that you have not forgotten him, and your courtesy will demonstrate your understanding of the caller's needs.

Taking messages

Be prepared.   You must always be prepared to take a message as you lift the handset from the telephone cradle. A message pad or note pad should be near the telephone at all times, and you should have a pen or pencil in your hand. A note pad, such as a stenographer's spiral book, may be the appropriate aid for initially answering the telephone, because it can also be used to make notes

to yourself. You may even want to note who is on which telephone line when you are dealing with several calls at once.

Being prepared to note the information received by telephone is the first step in handling messages. To minimize the amount of time spent on each call, develop techniques for controlling calls and procedures on the classification and disposition of calls.

Control the call.   Callers may forget that you must handle a variety of duties and a number of telephone calls each day. In addition, their anxiety may cause them to include a great deal of unnecessary information in their conversation. Toward the goals of acquiring accurate information and saving time, it is important that you control each call.

First, you must acquire the basic information. If the caller has not volunteered a name, you should ask, "Who is calling, please?" If necessary, ask for the correct spelling of the name, which will save time if you need to locate records. You should also obtain the caller's telephone number and the reason for the call.

Retain control of the call by asking distinct questions rather than allowing the caller to give a lengthy account of his reason for calling. You should not be rude or sound rushed, but you can learn to conserve time with each caller. For example, a patient calling for an appointment because of an upper respiratory infection may mention the illness and then attempt to tell you what he thinks happened last week to cause it. At the first opportunity you might interject, "This type of infection is common in this area now. Dr. Smith can see you this afternoon at 2:00 or at 3:30. Which time would you prefer?" With this technique you can intercept a potentially lengthy conversation while demonstrating that you understand the caller's needs and are offering assistance. You can learn additional telephone techniques from articles in *The Professional Medical Assistant* and by observing experienced co-workers.

Procedure	*Rationale*
1. Excuse yourself from the call you are handling.	The caller will appreciate the courtesy, and understanding the reason will generate cooperation.
2. Answer the second call and put the caller on hold as previously suggested.	The caller will be reassured that they have reached the office they want and will be more willing to wait.
3. Return to the first caller, thanking him for waiting and mentioning that the other line is on hold.	Knowing that another caller is waiting may encourage the individual to limit the discussion to business.

There will be occasions on which you receive calls that are considered troublesome. These callers may include the following types:

- The angry caller;
- The repeat caller;
- The appointment juggler;
- The caller seeking aid beyond your duties;
- The caller requesting confidential information; and
- The unidentified caller.

You will need to deal with these callers in a tactful manner but also in a way that indicates you are in control of the situation.

The angry caller. The angry caller should be handled in the manner described in the discussion of the angry patient. It is in your best interest to remain calm, determine the issue, and assure the caller that you are interested in helping. You may be able to reduce the caller's anger by saying, for example, "I understand you are upset, Ms. Jones, but I may be able to help if you will answer a few questions for me." You may then proceed to ask the questions necessary to determine the issue.

The repeat caller. You will occasionally encounter individuals who repeatedly call the office for clarification of the same instructions, for reassurance, or perhaps to discuss information from the public media that concerns them. Many calls may be eliminated by providing patients with printed instructions or diet slips that have been prepared for routine situations in your office. The instructions may be reviewed by patients before they leave the office. This provides them with an opportunity to ask questions. Individuals making repeated calls about items covered in the information sheet may be referred to the guide they were given. This will reduce the time spent on the call and will subtly suggest that the call was unnecessary. Your statement of "I believe that is covered in the instruction sheet you received during your last visit" may be all that is needed. If the caller persists you may need to suggest, "Perhaps you would like to schedule an appointment to discuss your concerns with the doctor." The prospect of spending time and money on another office visit often separates true concerns from insecurity.

The appointment juggler. Patients may occasionally need to change a scheduled appointment. This is certainly understandable, and the change is usually for a valid reason, such as an unplanned business trip, a change in work or school schedule, or car trouble. However, you may encounter the occasional individual who constantly changes appointments, often at the last minute. If you notice this pattern developing, you will need to speak to the patient. At the time an appointment change is requested, you might say, "Mr. Smith, I will try to help you with your requested change, but I think you should know that it helps to have more notice if possible when you cannot keep an appointment. Another patient could be scheduled."

The assistance seeker. Occasionally patients will ask for your help with matters that are beyond the scope of your duties and would require time away from your responsibilities. Many times this involves a request to check with the patient's insurance company about the status of a claim. Patients should be told that the insurance company can provide the information directly to them if they telephone the company. It may be diplomatic to mention that insurance companies prefer to speak to the patient directly because they wish to protect the patient's privacy. Other requests, such as to change appointments with laboratories or other offices, should also be tactfully declined by stating, "I can give you the office's number and you can speak with the appointment secretary directly. That way you can select a time that will best fit your schedule."

Requests for confidential information. There are many situations in which individuals seek information of a confidential nature. Some of these individuals are interested friends, insurance companies, the media if the patient is newsworthy, or employers. You know that the patient's written consent is necessary to release the information and should state this to the caller. If you receive a call from an institution stating that they have admitted your patient and need information from the patient's record you should do the following:

- Request some identifying data on the patient, such as date of birth or social security number.
- Request the caller's name and telephone number, stating that you will call them back immediately. By returning the call you can verify the institution and person to whom you are speaking.

The unidentified caller. You may occasionally receive calls from individuals who refuse to identify themselves or who misrepresent their identity or the nature of their business. Techniques such as this for gaining access to the physician seem to be on the increase among salespersons, particularly those selling financial investments. Some of the statements you may hear in response to your request for information include the following:

- "This is Ms. Jones regarding the doctor's financial statement."

- "This is Mr. Smith regarding the doctor's stock portfolio."
- "This is Simpson from the Human Aid Society to see if the doctor will be matching last year's donation." (When the physician did not make a donation last year.)

Office policy will direct you how to deal with calls of this type. Some possibilities are the following:

- For callers who refuse to identify themselves, advise them that you may not transfer a call without the information you have requested, but they may state their business in a letter to the physician.
- For callers implying that they are the physician's established representative and you know they are not, you might reply, "The doctor's broker handles the portfolio. Thank you for calling. Goodbye."
- If you are in doubt about the validity of the representative, check with the physician.
- For contributions, say, "The doctor reviews contribution requests submitted in writing. If you care to send your literature, the doctor can make a decision. Thank you for calling."

Classification of calls

It is important to establish a policy defining the various classifications of calls. Classifying calls is necessary to determine how and by whom calls will be handled. The common groupings for calls received in a medical office or agency are discussed in the sections that follow.

Emergency calls. Emergency calls require the immediate attention of the physician. Situations that should be considered emergencies include the following:

- Loss of consciousness;
- Heavy bleeding;
- Severe pain;
- Severe vomiting or diarrhea, particularly in children; and
- Fever over 102° F (38.9° C).

If the physician is not in the office he or she should be located immediately. On the average 2% to 5% of calls to an office are true emergencies.

Routine patient calls. The majority of patient-originated calls concern routine matters. Most of them are handled by the medical office personnel. Routine patient calls include the following:

- Requests for appointments;
- Clarification of instructions;
- Inquiries about fees;
- Inquiries about statements;
- Inquiries about laboratory results; and
- Reports on status.

In most offices the first four types of routine calls are handled by the administrative medical assistant; the physician usually prefers to speak to the patient about status reports and laboratory results. It is good to note to the patients that the physician returns nonemergency calls to the patients between 11:30 AM and 1:00 PM, and 4:30 PM and 6:00 PM. This is a valuable service to not only the patient, but to the practice as well to eliminate many additional calls from patients wanting to know when the physician will return calls.

Medical business calls. Medical personnel from other offices or facilities will call the physician's office through the course of the day. Medical business calls can be expected from the following:

- Other physicians;
- Hospitals;
- Pharmacies;
- Laboratories;
- Ancillary services (physical therapy, visiting nurses); and
- Professional associations.

Messages noting the pertinent information will be required from each caller. Preprinted forms are available for recording laboratory data (Figures 8.3 and 8.4). These forms save time because you will not have to write out each element before writing the value found. The laboratory technician will also appreciate this time-saving technique.

The use of a recording device is extremely helpful in offices that receive numerous prescription refill calls. This allows the recorder to log as many as five to six calls regarding prescriptions. Then all charts may be pulled and documented at the same time and sent back for refiling. This type of system usually results in fewer telephone calls on the part of the staff. It is important that information regarding this service should be preprinted in the practice brochure.

Other business calls. Maintaining an office requires contact with a variety of individuals who represent various services, including the following:

- The office accountant;
- The physician's attorney;
- The physician's insurance broker;
- Medical-surgical supply sales representatives; and
- Pharmaceutical company representatives seeking an appointment to talk with the physician.

The physician does not usually interrupt patient care to speak with business callers but returns their calls when possible.

Personal calls. Physicians usually receive some personal calls from family or friends during business hours. Friends tend to call because it is easier to reach the physician at the office, or they may not want to interfere with the physician's limited free time at home. Family members may wish to confirm tentative plans or remind the physician of a personal appointment. On rare occasions you may be asked to perform a service or do an errand for the physician's spouse or children. You must be tactful, but it is best to avoid allowing a habit to develop. You may reply, "I would be happy to help if time is available after completing my office duties," or, "I will check with Dr. Smith to see if our schedule will permit the time you request." Physicians typically prefer to reserve office personnel for business and will support your stand.

You and other members of the staff cannot expect the privilege of receiving or making personal telephone calls at work. Office policy will usually state that staff members should discourage personal calls; if a personal call arrives, employees should advise the caller that they will return the call from home that evening.

Disposition of calls

Once a call has been received and classified, you can determine the disposition or appropriate management of the call. Making the proper choice in handling incoming calls will save time for the caller, the physician, and the office personnel.

Figure 8.3
Preprinted form for recording telephoned laboratory reports.
Courtesy Histacount Corp, Melville NY.

SPECIAL & BLOOD CHEMISTRY ANALYSIS

Date ______________ 19 No.______

Name ______________________________

Glucose___mgms. per 100 cc blood	Basal m. r. ________
Urea ________	Glucose Tolerance ________
N. P. n. ________	________
Creatinine ________	________
Total nitrogen ________	________
Chlorides ________	________
Calcium ________	________
Phosphorous ________	Urine Concentration Tests ________
Cholesterol ________	________
Cholesterol (esters) ________	________
Ph. ________ Test used ________	________
Carbon dioxide ________	Other Tests ________
Combining power ________	________
Serum proteins ________	________
Tests used ________	________
Albumin ________ ratio ________	________
Globulin ________	Conclusions: ________
Iodides:___mgms. per 100 cc blood	________
Alcohol:___mgms. per 100 cc blood	________
Icteric Index: ________	________
Van den Berger: ________	________
Direct: ________	________
Indirect:	

FORM NO. 146 PROFESSIONAL PRINTING CO., INC., MELVILLE, L. I., N. Y.

Continued.

Figure 8.3, **cont'd**
Preprinted form for
recording telephoned
laboratory reports.

BLOOD ANALYSIS

Date_____19   No._____

Name_____

Hemoglobin_____	Leukocytes_____
Hematokrit_____	Small lymphocytes_____
Color Index_____	_____
Bleeding time_____	Large lymphocytes_____
Coag. time_____	Large mononuclears_____
Erythrocytes,	Transitional_____
per c. mm_____	Polynuclear_____
Leukocytes	Neutrophiles_____
per c. mm_____	Eosinophiles_____
Erythrocytes,	Basophiles_____
color_____	Myelocytes_____
Anisocytosis_____	Myeloblasts_____
Poikilocytes_____	Miscellaneous_____
Polychro matophilia_____	_____
Granular	
degeneration_____	Sedimentation Rate_____
Microcytes_____	Method_____
Macrocytes_____	Culture, Parasites, etc._____
Microblasts_____	
Normoblasts_____	
Macroblasts_____	

Remarks:_____
Conclusion:_____

FORM NO. 141-PROFESSIONAL PRINTING CO., INC., NEW HYDE PARK, N. Y.

Referred to the physician. Calls that are typically referred to the physician include the following:
- Emergencies;
- Patient status reports;
- Reports of laboratory results to patients;
- Calls from other physicians;
- Calls from hospitals;
- Calls from professional associations;
- Calls on nonmedical business other than from medical suppliers; and
- Personal calls.

Handled by the medical assistant. The medical assistant will usually be responsible for resolving the needs of the majority of callers contacting the office. These needs include the following:
- Scheduling appointments;
- Clarification of instructions;
- Inquiries about fees and bills;
- Requests from pharmacies;
- Laboratories calling with reports;
- Patient status reports;
- Scheduling meetings with hospital and professional association committees;
- Medical-surgical suppliers; and
- Lab results to patients with physician's OK.

Your policy manual should have a page devoted to a chart to use for quick reference regarding the appropriate disposition of a call. See Table 8.1 for a sample disposition chart.

Outgoing Calls
Use of directories

Directories were discussed earlier in this chapter and should be readily available to personnel need-

Figure 8.4
Preprinted form for
recording telephoned
laboratory reports.
Courtesy Histacount Corp,
Melville, NY.

URINALYSIS

Date_____19   No._____

Name_____

Amount (single)_____   Centrifuged_____
Amount (24 hours)_____   Uncentrifuged_____
Color_____   Microscopic_____
Appearance_____   Casts_____
Reaction_____   Hyaline_____
Specific Gravity_____   Granular_____
Albumin_____   Waxy_____

                                Epithelium_____

Blood_____   _____
Sugar_____   Cylindroids_____
                                White blood cells_____
_____
Urea_____   Red blood cells_____
                                      (per high power field)
Indican_____
Acetone_____   Bacteria_____
Diacetic Acid_____   Crystals_____
Bile_____   Amorphous_____
        Test Used_____Time_____Speed_____
Preservative used_____Method of centrifuging_____
Conclusion_____
_____
_____
_____

FORM NO. 140   SCM HISTACOUNT CORPORATION MELVILLE, NEW YORK 11746

ing to place outgoing calls. The office should acquire or prepare as many directories as necessary to avoid frequently moving them from one site to another. You are likely to require a set of directories at the desks of the office manager, the administrative medical assistant, and the physician.

Directory assistance

Local assistance.   Calling for assistance to locate a number within your area code can be accomplished by dialing 411. As noted, telephone service charges are expected for use of the 411 service, possibly 15¢ for each call over 20 per month. This is another reason for acquiring the directories of nearby cities or counties if they are included in your area code. Dialing 0 for directory assistance instead of 411 will result in an even larger charge, possibly $1 for each request.

Long-distance and international assistance.   Help in locating long-distance numbers may be obtained by dialing the area code of the business or person and then dialing 555-1212. Your telephone directory lists most area codes. International calls may also be dialed directly if you know the local telephone number. To complete an international call you must dial the following, in order:

- 011 (the international access code);
- The country code (available in your directory white pages);
- The city code (from directory white pages);
- The local number; and
- The # button if using a push-button phone.

A sample international direct dial might be:

```
   011      +    61    +   12   +  218-362
(international   (country)   (city)   (local + #
access code)                         number)
```

Table 8.1
Guide for disposition of incoming calls

Disposition	Patient emergency	Patient reporting back on treatment	Patient seeking reinstruction on treatment plan	Other physicians	Hospital, urgent	Hospital, nonurgent	Pharmacies	Laboratories reporting results	Nonmedical business	Personal	Patient: appointment scheduling	Patient: administrative inquiries
Calls requiring physician												
Physician in office												
Interrupt immediately	X			X	X							
Return as soon as possible		X				X						
Return at fixed, routine time (medical assistant to advise caller of approximate time)		X					X		X			
Return when convenient									X	X		
Physician out of office												
Contact physician immediately for handling or instructions	X			X	X							
Hold messages until physician calls for them		X					X	X	X	X		
Calls processed by medical assistant												
Administrative								X			X	X
Clinical			X					X				

You can expect approximately a 45-second wait after dialing before the connection is complete and the telephone rings.

800 Numbers.   Many companies throughout the country provide toll-free (800) numbers so that callers may conduct business or place orders at no charge. If you want to determine whether or not a business provides a toll-free number call 800 information by dialing 800-555-1212.

Emergency assistance.   Some cities have instituted a means of summoning emergency aid by dialing 911. Where the system is in effect you can even dial the number from a pay telephone without inserting a coin. Dialing 911 connects the caller with a public safety answering point, from which the dispatcher can provide the following services:
- Fire rescue;
- Police or highway patrol;
- Ambulance; and
- Paramedics.

This number must only be used in a true emergency. When you use the 911 access number, the number from which you are calling is automatically displayed on the dispatchers message screen, whether or not it is listed. This aids the dispatcher in case you are cut off before completing the call. If you do not wish your number displayed, you must locate and dial the individual number of the service you need.

Planning your calls

Thinking about a telephone call that you need to make and preparing for it will, in the long run, save time for you and for the person answering the call. Planning calls also demonstrates your efficiency. Your preparation in planning a call includes the following:
- Locating the correct telephone number;
- Compiling the information that will be needed during the call; and
- Keeping a note pad and writing instrument on hand for information gathered during the call.

The number and note pad elements of planning have been discussed previously. The information that will be needed will vary depending on the purpose of the call. If it is necessary to set up or change a patient's appointment, you will need the appointment book to know the days and times available. To order supplies, you will need a list of the items needed, including a description of the item, catalog numbers, and the quantity desired. To discuss a patient's account, you will need the billing record and insurance claims filed. Practicing and placing business calls will provide you with the experience of planning for these calls. The preparation will become automatic, will be appreciated by the person receiving the call, and will build confidence in your ability to conduct business.

Types of calls

Local. The majority of calls placed from your office or agency will be local, that is, within your area code. Most local calls are covered by the basic monthly service charge. Some calls within an area code but beyond a predetermined distance are still considered local but will be billed based on the distance, the time spent on the telephone, and the time of day that the call was placed.

Long distance. Long-distance calling is increasing in popularity because it reduces the amount of paperwork necessary to conduct business. The cost of long-distance calls is influenced by the company supplying the service, the method used in placing the call, the distance between the caller and the recipient, the time spent on the call, and the time of day the call takes place.

The company supplying the long-distance call will influence the cost of long-distance calling. In general, the cost of long distance has been greatly reduced in recent years. Interconnect telephone systems, which use microwaves to transmit voices, tend to cost less than the Bell system for long-distance calling. If your office or agency uses long distance often you might want to investigate the options for saving money.

The cost of long distance is also influenced by the method you choose in placing the call. Direct dialing is the least expensive method of placing a call and is termed *station-to-station calling*. To place a station-to-station call you simply dial the area code and the seven-digit number you want. In some areas you must dial 1 before the area code to gain access. Your direct-dial number would be, for example, 1-361-123-4567.

Operator-assisted long-distance calls involve the services of a telephone operator, which increases the cost of the call. The operator is necessary for collect calls, credit card calls, or person-to-person calls. A person-to-person call is used when you want to be assured of reaching a specific person who may or may not be in the office when you call. An operator-assisted call is placed by dialing 0, the area code, and the seven-digit number. The operator will intercept the call, obtain the necessary information from the caller, and then allow the call to proceed.

The time of day must be considered when placing a call. The least expensive times for placing calls do not usually coincide with business hours, but time must be considered for another reason. The world is divided into various time zones. The continental United States is divided into four time zones. From the West Coast to the East Coast these time zones are titled Pacific, Mountain, Central, and Eastern. Each time zone involves a 1-hour difference from the zone on either side of it. For example, when it is 9:00 AM Pacific time, it is 10:00 AM Mountain time. See your telephone directory for the geographical areas included in each time zone. You must consider these time zones when placing calls to reach a business during working hours. A call placed from New York at 10:00 AM Eastern time to an office in San Francisco will be too early, since it will be 7:00 AM Pacific time. A call placed to North Carolina from Colorado at 4:30 PM Mountain time will be too late, since it will be 6:30 PM Eastern time. Your city telephone directory includes a time zone chart to assist you in planning long-distance calls.

Conference calls. Conference calls allow between 3 and 14 different geographic points to be connected at one time. Each person at each different point can speak to and be heard by each other person involved in the call. Conference calls are of great value in sharing information among several physicians or among the physician and members of a patient's family in different geographical areas. Being able to discuss an issue with several people at once saves valuable time.

Conference calls are billed at the person-to-person rate applicable to the two farthest points involved in the call, with each additional line charged at a reduced rate. You can establish a conference call by contacting the local operator and requesting connection to the conference operator. The conference operator will need the name, area code, and number of each person to participate in the call and the time the call will take place. The conference operator will contact the parties in advance and ask each person to hold. Once all connections are made the operator will open the lines to all participants.

Telephone etiquette

When you place a telephone call you should remember that you may be interrupting another person's activities. Your calls should be designed to save time and respect the other person's needs and above all be conducted in a courteous manner.

Business etiquette suggests that it is most appropriate for individuals to place their own calls. Physicians who wish to speak with a colleague, business associate, or medical facility should dial the call, identify themselves, and request the person with whom they want to speak. Because of experience with being placed on lengthy hold, some physicians ask the medical assistant to place their calls for them. This may evolve into a game of protocol, with the medical assistant who receives the call stating, "Put Dr. Smith on the line and I will get Dr. Adams." If you work with physicians who insist that you place their calls, you can reduce the waiting and interoffice manipulation by placing the call when you know your employer is readily available. If the receiving medical assistant demands that the calling physician be put on the line, you may put the call on hold and inform your employer that the call will be put through as soon as he or she is on the line. The colleague's subtle message may be received. If the receiving assistant puts the call directly through, and you are greeted by the party being called, you will be able to say, "Thank you, Dr. Adams, I will put Dr. Smith on immediately."

Dialing errors. If you make a dialing error when placing a call you should always excuse yourself to the person you disturbed. If the call involves an additional charge you should attempt to learn the number you have reached. Many people are understandably uncomfortable about stating their phone number to an unknown caller, and their rights must be respected. In this case, state the number you were calling and ask if it is the number you reached. If it is the number you dialed you will know your file was wrong. If it is not the number you intended to call, call the operator, state the number you were attempting to reach, and request credit for the error. The misdialed call will not be charged on the monthly statement.

AUXILIARY TELEPHONE SERVICES
Answering Services

Physicians or their substitutes must be available to patients 24 hours a day, seven days a week. Since a medical office or agency is open only eight hours a day, some arrangement must be made so that patients can reach the physician after business hours. Ethically and legally, physicians are bound to fulfill their duty to their patients. If patients are unable to reach their physician in a time of need, they may sue the physician for abandonment.

Recording devices

Telephone answering devices are becoming more common in our society. People are used to listening to the recorded message and leaving their name, telephone number, and the reason they want to speak with the physician. There are positive and negative aspects to using recording devices to monitor after-hours telephone calls. These are presented in Table 8.2

Operator-assisted services

Answering services are available with operators who will assist patients in contacting the physician after office hours. The patient can be connected with the answering service in one of two ways. First, the number of the service can be listed in the telephone directory immediately below the private number for the office. The directory entry may read as follows:

Jones, James	
6 Main Street	123-4567
24 hours call	765-4321
or if no answer, call	765-4320

The second option is to arrange with the telephone company and the answering service for an automatic relay of the calls from the office to the service. With this arrangement, the patient is required to place only one call. As the office is closing, the medical assistant calls the answering service and notifies them to begin intercepting the calls. The answering service operators are trained to make decisions regarding the classification and disposition of calls.

There are two types of operator-assisted answering services: general and specialty. General answering services accept clients from a variety of businesses and individuals who require 24-hour telephone coverage, such as attorneys, plumbers, or consultants. Specialty services limit their clients to members of a particular field. Some county medical societies have developed physician-only answering services with operators trained in handling medical situations. If available, specialty answering services are the best choice for a medical practice.

Coordinating after-hours telephone services

The medical assistant is responsible for coordinating the after-hours telephone services. If a record-

Table 8.2
Pros and cons of electronic recording devices

Pros	Cons
Less expensive than operator-assisted services.	Viewed by some as impersonal.
Valuable in areas where answering services are not available.	Requires a back-up number or instructions if call is an emergency.
Medical assistant does not have to call answering service when arriving at or leaving the office.	Systems subject to interruption if there is a failure of electricity or telephone service.
Can be equipped with a remote control device, allowing physician to collect messages from any telephone outside of office.	Systems that page physician via "beeper" in the event of mechanical difficulty are expensive.

ing device is used it must be on and working before the office is closed. The medical assistant should periodically check the recorded message for clarity and quality of sound. If an operator-assisted service is used, the medical assistant will need to notify the service, sometimes referred to as the exchange, when the office closes. When signing out you should be prepared to inform the service how to reach the physician. Telephone numbers should be supplied.

In addition, the efficient medical assistant will periodically check on the manner in which the office telephones are answered when the office is closed. This can be done by calling the office number when the office is closed and evaluating the efficiency and effectiveness of the recording device or answering service. Another method of checking is to ask patients who had to reach the physician after hours if everything was satisfactory.

Pagers

Pagers, commonly called beepers, are small, pocket-sized devices that the physician can carry. If the medical assistant or answering service needs to speak with the physician, an individualized telephone code can be dialed, and the pager will signal the physician. The physician can then call the office to obtain the message or, with some pagers, a button that allows the physician to hear the message without calling in. The one drawback to pagers is that the medical assistant cannot be assured that the message was received.

Pagers are valuable because they save time for the physician and the medical assistant. Pagers eliminate the need for multiple calls to locate physicians who are ahead of or behind the schedule they left with the medical assistant. After office hours the answering service can hold the patient's

call, page the physician, and connect the patient directly with the physician. This is reassuring to the patient and eliminates the need for the physician to place two calls.

Call Forwarding

Telephones may be adapted to forward telephone calls from the physician's offices to any number programmed into the system. This system is an advantage to practices with more than one office and more than one telephone number. Patients calling one office will automatically be transferred to the site at which the physician and staff are at the moment. This reduces confusion for the patient and eliminates the need for redialing.

If call forwarding is used for after-hours calls, physicians may find it a disadvantage, since unwanted callers may easily trace them.

Dictation Services

The need for clear medical records may involve dictating reports for the office files or for the records of hospitalized patients. Private transcription services and hospital medical record departments often provide special telephone dictating equipment. You will be provided with special telephone numbers that the physician can dial for direct, immediate access to the equipment. The dictation is recorded and transcribed by personnel at the facility.

Some physicians prefer to dictate information regarding patients within their office for clear and concise records for the patient's chart. This has a distinct advantage because of today's requirements for clear and legible documentation of medical records. The physician has available numerous types of recording devices; one of the most popular is the voice-activated tape recorder. The data may be typed on plain white sheets or on what is called "sticky sheets" with a self-adhering backing, which after typing may be cut, pulled apart, and placed in the medical record. This data may be transcribed by office staff or sent out to a transcription service.

Telegraph Services

The telephone is used for access to telegraph services. These services include regular and overnight telegrams and Mailgrams. Telegrams are sent through Western Union and Mailgrams through the U.S. Postal Service. If you wish to send a telegraph message, contact the appropriate agency and dictate the message to the operator. The message will be transmitted by telephone or computer to the point of delivery, where it will be printed and delivered to the proper person. Either service can be charged to your telephone number.

Conclusion

Oral communication is one of the most vital systems in a medical facility. Establishing rapport with patients provides the foundation for the subsequent relationship between the patient and the physician. For maintaining communication, the importance of telephone services cannot be overemphasized, and the medical assistant is the key to the efficiency and effectiveness of the system. Keep in mind that the telephone provides the primary link between the patient and necessary medical services. You will need to monitor the operating efficiency of the office telephone equipment, the auxiliary services, and particularly your communication techniques and skills.

All telephone calls must be logged, and the best system to be utilized is a two-part NCR form that allows a copy for the patient's chart and a permanent copy for the office. These logs should be kept a minimum of 7 years, and if treating children, until the child is 21 years old. The importance of documentation cannot be over stressed. At no time should scraps of paper be utilized for patient information or documentation of phone calls. Many pharmaceutical companies provide scratch pads as a method of advertising their product. These pads should not be utilized for message taking; however, if they are, the information should be transferred to the NCR log as quickly as possible.

Review Questions

1. List the four basic factors that influence oral communication and explain how they influence it.
2. Describe how you will apply the standard techniques of effective in-person communication when working with a hearing-impaired patient and with an angry patient.
3. Why is the telephone considered so vital to a medical practice?
4. Which letters of the alphabet are frequently misunderstood on the telephone? What can you do to avoid misunderstandings?
5. List and describe six possible types of medical office telephone equipment.
6. Name four types of directories and what information you can obtain from them.
7. Write a sample dialogue between you and a caller, keeping in mind the four elements of general courtesy. Produce an accurate message from the call.
8. List the five major categories of incoming calls and describe the appropriate disposition of each type.
9. Explain how you would handle the following:
   a. An angry patient
   b. A repeat caller
   c. An appointment juggler
   d. A request for help beyond your capability
   e. A request for confidential information
   f. An unidentified caller
10. What auxiliary services can you expect to encounter in a complete telephone system?

SUGGESTED READINGS

What every telephone user should know, General Telephone System.

Your telephone personality, Bell Telephone System.
Your voice is you, Bell Telephone System.

Chapter 9

Scheduling Systems

- Time management
- Reception responsibilities
- Types of appointment systems
- Necessary equipment
- Scheduling an appointment
- Office scheduling guidelines
- Referral appointments
- Visitors other than patients

Objectives

On completion of Chapter 9 the medical assistant student should be able to:

1 Define the terms listed in the vocabulary.

2 List and discuss the three reasons for time management.

3 Discuss reception responsibilities.

4 List and discuss the four types of appointment systems.

5 Describe the equipment necessary for an appointment system.

6 State the patient information needed to schedule an appointment; state the information given to the patient about the appointment.

7 List and discuss the seven major guidelines for scheduling office appointments.

8 Discuss the medical assistant's role in referring a patient for services in another facility.

9 Discuss the steps that should be taken to protect the physician legally when a patient fails to keep or cancels an appointment.

10 List the information necessary to schedule a patient for the following: an appointment in the physician's office, an appointment with a consulting physician, an appointment for diagnostic studies, and an appointment for admission to the hospital.

11 Describe what to do and say to the visitors who are not patients to the physician's office: other physicians, pharmaceutical representatives, salespersons, family members or friends, and former patients.

Vocabulary

medical emergency A state or condition that if not treated could result in the loss of a patient's life.

no-show A failure to keep an appointment without notification of other person involved.

receptionist The person responsible for initially greeting callers in an office or agency.

scheduling system A preplanned method of dividing available time to provide services efficiently to the greatest possible number of patients.

time management A systematic method of using the time available to the best possible advantage.

Managing the scheduling system, particularly the appointments for patients in your office or agency, is one of the important responsibilities you will have as an administrative medical assistant. Properly managed, the scheduling systems will control the time available in each working day and allow each member of the health care team to plan for patient care. The efficiency of a scheduling system depends on the ability of the person who develops and manages it and the cooperation of the team.

TIME MANAGEMENT
Patient Comfort
Patient needs

A medical office or agency exists to fulfill the needs of patients. Because a patient is often under stress in a medical environment, it is important to develop a scheduling system that reduces confusion and tension. You should keep in mind that the patients also have schedules that they must keep, and an effective scheduling system will provide some flexibility to respond to their needs.

Patients' greatest complaint

The most common complaint of patients surveyed about medical care is the time spent in the office reception area. Most patients make every effort to arrive on time or even early for a scheduled appointment. Unfortunately, some patients have experienced waiting periods as long as an hour before being taken to the treatment area, with another wait before seeing the doctor.

You should not be surprised if the result of this waiting is angry patients, and it is not uncommon for patients to express their anger to the medical assistant rather than the physician. If the delay is unusual, keeping patients informed about the reason for the delay and the anticipated time involved will usually offset the anger. If delays are common you will need to reevaluate the system and observe the staff members' effects on the efficiency of the system.

Acceptable wait

Surveys and the evaluation of patient questionnaires agree that the maximum acceptable wait in an office before seeing the physician is 20 minutes. Most people recognize that the nature of the business requires some flexibility on the part of everyone involved. However, patients who notice a constant pattern of lengthy waits might ignore the appointment time they are given and arrive at their own convenience. They might also begin calling the office in advance to check on the schedule or waiting time, creating more telephone calls for you to answer. The final step a patient might take because of repeated scheduling difficulties is to change physicians.

Stress Reduction

Effective time management reduces stress for patients and for the health care team. Patients always feel more comfortable when they know what to expect and when to expect it, and, as previously stated, the comfortable patient is a cooperative patient. Reduced stress in the medical environment means less time spent dealing with the stressful situation and more time available for patient care. The stress of a disorderly scheduling system also influences the health care team and is disruptive to the working relationships among the staff and between the staff and the physician. Eliminating staff tension will have a good effect on patients and on staff relationships and will enhance a pleasant working environment.

Providing for Emergencies

Scheduling systems must have some element of flexibility, especially in the medical field. Room for adjustment is necessary to provide for emergencies that might occur during the course of any day. Medical emergencies that can be handled in the office will take priority over routine appointments. Emergencies that require the physician's attention at the hospital will also disrupt the schedule. A preplanned procedure will help keep the disruption to a minimum. The options for emergency scheduling will be discussed later in this chapter.

RECEPTION RESPONSIBILITIES
Types of Callers
Patients

Patients are the most important visitors to a medical practice. As an administrative medical assistant your role as receptionist is usually linked with your responsibilities for the appointment system. Having scheduled the appointment, you will also be the first person to greet patients as they arrive. The tone of your greeting will set the tone of the visit. The arrival of patients should take precedence over other visitors to the office.

Other callers

Since a medical office or agency is a place of business, you can anticipate a variety of callers during the day. These could include other physicians, pharmaceutical representatives, medical sales representatives, the physician's family or friends, or former patients. These people should be greeted politely and allowed to see the physician according to office policy, which is discussed later in this chapter.

You might also have salespeople offering a variety of unsolicited products or services. These callers should be discouraged, because they will distract you from your duties and take time away from patient services. You may post a sign that states *No Solicitors,* or you may politely but firmly inform the caller that you are not interested.

First Impressions
The medical assistant

Attitude. All medical assistants should demonstrate pride in themselves and their work. This attitude will be immediately evident to visitors to the office. The medical assistant who serves as the office receptionist establishes the initial impression of the office and of the other personnel that patients anticipate meeting during the visit. Initial impressions, those formed before one individual knows another personally, are also based on general appearance, etiquette, and the appearance of the work environment. The office receptionist should be aware that, as the first person to have contact with the patient, he or she is the one to promote good public relations for the office.

Appearance. The basic elements of an employee's professional appearance are appropriate dress, tasteful makeup and accessories, and proper hygiene.

Office policy will include a dress code statement. Most offices will expect medical assistants to wear uniforms; some may allow the medical assistant to choose between a uniform or street clothes, with or without a laboratory coat.

Uniforms may be the easiest option for you in many respects. Uniforms are appropriately styled, made of easy-care fabric, durable, and attractively designed for variety. Uniforms are planned for professional work, are available in a variety of styles including dresses, pantsuits, and skirt and blouse combinations for women, and slacks with shirt, jacket, or pullover tops for men. The easy-care, durable fabrics used in uniforms allow for daily laundering while retaining a crisp appearance. The use of discreet colors and prints coordinated with or replacing white adds variety to your uniform wardrobe. If street clothes are to be worn at work, they should be tailored in style and subdued in color. A

laboratory coat worn over street clothes will protect them from excessive wear.

Makeup for work should be minimal and conservatively applied. Accessories should be limited to a watch, engagement and/or wedding ring, professional pin, and name tag. If you have pierced ears your earrings should be simple, preferably post-type.

Grooming and hygiene should receive as much attention as your wardrobe and makeup. Personal hygiene, or cleanliness, includes bathing, use of deodorants, hair care, and oral hygiene. Grooming refers to the attention you pay to the condition of your clothing, neatly arranged hair, and subtly manicured nails. In other words, grooming is your overall appearance after preparing for your day.

Etiquette. Courtesy in welcoming people as they arrive at the office is expected of a receptionist. You should greet each person by name and introduce yourself. If the caller is other than a patient, you should determine the reason for the visit. The caller should be invited to take a seat in the reception room and given some indication of the waiting time. The term *reception room* may be preferable to *waiting room,* since the latter term reminds patients of precisely what they are doing— waiting. Popular and educational reading materials can be placed in the reception room. If a person is waiting for longer than 15 minutes to see the physician, you should speak to him and, if possible, give an estimate of the length of wait expected.

The reception area

The administrative assistant's desk will be the caller's focus point on arrival in the office. The desk should be neatly arranged. Unnecessary items should be properly stored and necessary confidential items placed where they are not visible to callers (Figure 9.1). The ideal desk will have a table-level work area for the assistant and a shelf that shields the appointment book, accounting materials, and charts from the caller's view, while providing a countertop area on which patients may register or sign forms (See Figure 9.2).

The reception room

The reception room should be a pleasant, well-lighted area in which patients and visitors can wait comfortably. The seating should be attractively arranged and the type of chairs varied. Some people prefer or require firm, straight-backed chairs while others will want soft, lower seating. The artwork in the reception area will reflect the taste of the physician-owner but should be relatively conservative in color and design. Green plants add a warm

Figure 9.1
Patient's view of
reception desk.

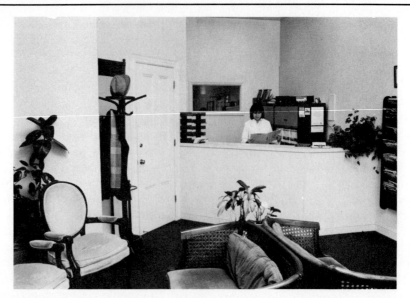

Figure 9.2
Administrative
assistant's desk.

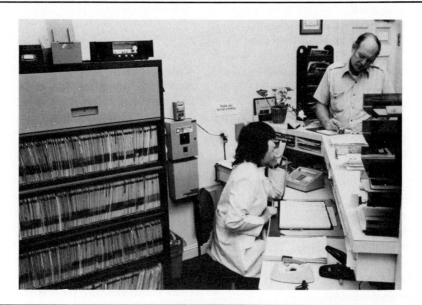

touch to the room and are usually appreciated by patients (see Figure 9.3). Tasteful artwork may be loaned or rented from local galleries or museums.

Monitoring the Reception Area
Patients waiting

It is worth repeating that patients in the reception room should not be ignored. Any waiting period is perceived as longer than it actually is, but a few words from the receptionist will break up the time. You might suggest a magazine you think the patient might enjoy, comment on the outfit the pa-

tient is wearing, or inquire about a hobby you know the patient enjoys. You may tell them the remaining waiting time if you can accurately estimate it. You should not state, "You will be seeing the doctor in just a minute Mrs. Jones" in an attempt to pacify the patient when you know that the wait will actually be 20 minutes or more.

Others waiting

Children. In a pediatric or family practice you can expect and should plan for children in the reception area. Furnishings and diversionary materi-

Figure 9.3
Reception room.

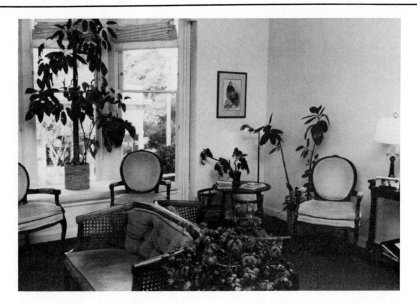

als should be appropriate and safe, especially with small children in mind.

Other practices, however, are usually not prepared for children. On occasion, a parent scheduled to see the physician will either arrive with a child or children or ask at the time an appointment is made if it is all right to bring children. Since a child cannot be with the parent during the visit with the physician, the medical assistant is faced with the responsibility of monitoring the child or children. This will create a hardship, expecially in a solo-employee office. If the child is brought in without your advance knowledge, there is little you can do at the moment but adapt to the situation. As the parent is leaving the office, however, you can politely explain that the office is not sufficiently staffed to accept the responsibility for children, and that the parent should make different arrangements for the next visit. You can offer to arrange an appointment for a time during which the children can be cared for at home. If a request to bring children is made in advance of the appointment, you will have some control over the situation. Again, you should *politely* explain the staff situation and the inadequate facilities. To avoid appearing inflexible you should say, "Yes, you can bring the children, Ms. Adams, as long as you can bring someone with you to watch them while you are with the doctor." The patient usually decides that it is easier to provide a sitter at home than have to provide and transport the sitter to the office.

Relatives or friends of patients. The people who accompany a patient to a physician's appointment may be anxious for the patient or restless with waiting. You can advise them of the approximate time the patient's visit will be completed and perhaps suggest some reading material to pass the time. You should be careful, however, not to answer questions regarding the patient's condition or treatment. This information is confidential. You should respond to these questions by suggesting they discuss it with the patient.

TYPES OF APPOINTMENT SYSTEMS
Individualized Systems

There are two basic types of appointment systems: (1) open office hours and (2) scheduled appointments. Regardless of the system chosen for an office or agency it is necessary that the method be used consistently and meet the needs of the patients, physician, and staff. An individualized system requires evaluation of the type of practice, the preference of the physician-owner, the number of patients seen, and the available facilities. With these considerations in mind you will want to review the standard appointment systems.

Open Office Hours

The least structured and least commonly used method of scheduling patients is the open-hours system. It is equivalent to a drop-in situation. Patients are advised that the office is open during a certain block of time, such as from 12:00 noon to 4:00 PM, and they are told that they may come in anytime between those hours. Patients know in advance that they will have to wait varying lengths of time before seeing the physician. While this method may appear to relieve stress, it prevents planning of the time needed to accomplish the variety of duties associated with a practice. You also encounter the possibility of several patients arriving at the last possible hour, delaying the details that must be attended to at the end of the day. Overall, this is an inefficient method of time management that should be avoided if possible.

Scheduled Appointment Systems
Time-specified

In a time-specified system each patient is given an appointment for a definite time. This method provides time for advance planning to prepare for the patient's needs. The interval between appointments depends on the type of medical practice and the service to be provided during the visit. A complete physical examination may require 1½ hours, while a blood pressure recheck will take only a few minutes. Therefore the medical assistant responsible for scheduling appointments will need to determine the reason for each visit.

Because time-specified systems also provide structure to each day, this method actually allows physicians to see more patients during office hours without the stress of having a backlog of people in the waiting room.

A patient visit most commonly includes a preliminary question-and-answer period, a physical evaluation, and a postexamination discussion period between the physician and the patient. While you never want to interrupt a necessary discussion in progress and understand that some social conversation often occurs before the visit ends, you and the physician will recognize that some patients engage in lengthy, unnecessary conversations. Planning can prevent these conversations from interfering with another patient's time. For example, several minutes before the scheduled end of a visit, you might contact the doctor on the intercom and simply mention the time left until the next appointment. The physician can then gracefully direct the conversation toward closure.

Wave

Some physicians and medical assistants feel that the time-specified system is too structured and prefer a method that provides flexibility. The wave method of scheduling is designed to self-adjust to the unpredictable variances caused by patients. These variances include patients who arrive late,

require more or less time than estimated, fail to keep their appointment, or arrive without an appointment.

The wave system is based on the average time spent with each patient on a routine visit. An hour is divided by the average appointment time to determine the number of patients that can be seen in an hour. Each patient is then told to arrive on the hour. Patients are seen in the order of their arrival. For example, an office staff may determine that an average visit requires 15 minutes; some will be shorter and some longer. Therefore four patients can be seen each hour. Table 9.1 demonstrates the possible outcome of a 1-hour period when four patients are instructed to arrive at 2:00 PM. Many other outcomes are possible, but in general you can expect that patient waiting periods will vary while the office remains relatively on schedule. However, you should know that patients eventually become aware that the 2:00 PM appointment is not exclusively theirs. When patients are waiting in the reception area, they speak to one another, and the topic is often the office. Patients soon learn that others were also scheduled for the same time. Explaining the reason that four people were scheduled for one time is difficult without causing the patients to feel manipulated.

Modified wave

A modified wave system is similar to the wave system in that an hour is the basic block of time. The modification involves prespacing the arrival times of the patients planned for a given hour. Using the previous example, you may schedule two patients for 2:00 PM and two for 2:30 PM, or you might schedule the four patients at 10-minute intervals between 2:00 PM and 2:30 PM, reserving the second half of the hour to complete the visits. The modified wave technique will reduce the possibility of having to answer questions from patients concerned about the scheduling system, but this system may still result in varying waiting periods.

Double booking

Double booking is actually a form of wave scheduling and occurs when two patients, both requiring the physician's attention for the total appointment slot, are scheduled for the same time. Consider an office that schedules patients at 15-minute intervals and also double books. Table 9.2 demonstrates the waiting periods that can occur for patients and the cumulative time the office will be off schedule with double booking. As in the wave systems, patients may compare scheduling and feel manipulated.

Table 9.1
Wave appointment system

Patient	Time of arrival	Time required for visit	Time visit begins	Waiting period (from time of arrival)	Time visit ends
1	2:00	15 min.	2:00	0 min.	2:15
2	2:00	25 min.	2:15	15 min.	2:40
3	2:05	15 min.	2:40	35 min.	2:55
4	2:25	10 min.	2:55	35 min.	3:05

Table 9.2
Effect of double booking

Patient	Appointment time	Time required for visit	Time visit should be finished if on time	Patient's time waiting	Time visit finished	Cumulative time office is "behind schedule"
1	2:00	15	2:15	0 min.	2:15	0 min.
2	2:00	15	2:15	15 min.	2:30	15 min.
3	2:15	20	2:30	15 min.	2:50	20 min.
4	2:15	10	2:30	35 min.	3:00	30 min.
5	2:30	15	2:45	30 min.	3:15	30 min.
6	2:30	10	2:45	45 min.	3:25	40 min.

In general you can see that open office hours, the wave system, the modified wave system, and double booking result in waiting time for patients. More often than not, these methods will put an office behind schedule rather than save time. Time-specified systems are the most efficient if they are respected and provide time for unplanned events.

Grouping Procedures

Booking similar examinations or procedures within specific blocks of time is another method of time management. For example, a pediatrician might decide to reserve three mornings a week and divide them into 1-hour appointment intervals during August to accommodate demands for pre-school physicals. A cardiologist might schedule patients requiring diet counseling in one afternoon so that the nutritionist can assist several individuals in one day. Grouping may be in response to an antici-

pated special situation or may be a routine occurrence. You may need to test a grouping system several different ways until you find an acceptable schedule.

NECESSARY EQUIPMENT
Appointment Book

An appointment book is the foundation of a scheduling system and must be selected to meet the needs of the office and the scheduling system used. Appointment books are available for one physician or several physicians, with one day on each page or a full week on two pages with a column for each day. Each book includes space for scheduling for one calendar year. You may also choose between blank, lined sheets, which allow you to enter the appointment times as you wish, or books with pre-printed time slots, usually at 10- or 15-minute in-

Figure 9.4
Daily log sheet.
Courtesy Colwell Systems,
Inc, Champaign, Ill.

Monday · March 7

HOUR	NAME OF PATIENT	SERVICE RENDERED	CHARGE	CASH	REC'D ON ACCOUNT	√
1	Arnold Wing	on acct.			30 00	√
2	Lester Remick	" "			5 00	√
9:00 3	Mrs. Roger Curry (936 So. Elm)	emergency home visit		10 00		√
9:30 5	Mrs. Mary Feathers	set fracture	50 00			√
10:00 6	Charles Bird	hospital	10 00			√
10:15 7	Mrs. Cecil Dean	"	5 00			√
10:30 8	Betty Witt		5 00			√
11:30 9	John Nyberg	home - Rx	10 00			√
11:45 10	M. C. Kabel	"	7 00			√
1:30 11	Stan Hinton	office cons.		5 00		√
1:50 12	Helen Shelby	" "	5 00		15 00	√
2:00 13	Vern McBride	dressed arm	5 00			√
2:30 14	Russell Steffy	change dressing	5 00			√
2:50 15	Emma Finch	exam	5 00		9 00	√
3:20 16	Gordon Bishop	exam - Rx		6 00		√
3:50 17	Olive Smyth	office cons.	5 00			√
4:00 18	Ella Loftis	treatment		5 00		√
4:10 19	Buella Young	"	4 00			√
4:25 20	Norm Fields	exam - Rx	7 00			√
4:45 21	Marcia Austin	treatment	5 00			√
5:00 22	M. V. Reynolds	"	5 00			√
5:15 23	Fred Mattern	exam - insc.	7 00			√
7:15 24	Mrs. D. Steele	home - Rx	7 00			√

FORM 201   COLWELL CO.; CHAMPAIGN, ILL.

CARRY TOTALS FORWARD TO **BUSINESS SUMMARY**   TOTALS   147 00   26 00   59 00

tervals. Finally, appointment sheets may be in a spiral-bound or loose-leaf book.

Some offices prefer a recording system that is considered a daily log, which serves as a combination appointment book and record of daily fee charges and payments on patient accounts (Figure 9.4). Regardless of the type selected, an efficient appointment book should provide space for at least the following information: date, time, patient's full name, and reason for appointment. If possible, space to note the patient's daytime telephone number near his name will provide a quick reference in case an appointment must be changed.

The appointment book selected should fit comfortably on the medical assistant's desk. It should be readily accessible and not have to be moved constantly to perform other tasks. The book should be maintained in good condition, since it will be retained indefinitely as a back-up legal document.

Pens

Although it has long been taught that a pen is the only appropriate writing instrument, many instructors realize the impracticability of its use. Although a pen provides a permanent record, using it to record information in the appointment book be-

Table 9.3
Appointment book entries

Date	Time	Patient	Additional notations
October 26	2:00 PM	Adams, Sandra	N/S
	3:00 PM	Davis, John	canc. W/C
	4:00 PM	Simpson, Thomas	C 10/28

comes impractical when schedule changes require crossing out a patient's name to insert another. In recent years the appointment book, although written in pencil, has remained a legal document. The appointment book can also be used to verify some information noted in the chart. Should a patient fail to keep an appointment or cancel an appointment with or without rescheduling, this information must be noted. In any of these situations a single line should be drawn through the name and the reason for the cancellation noted. The single line indicates the appointment was not kept, and the name can still be read and verified. You might note *N/S* (no-show) or *F/S* (failed to show) for the patient who does not arrive. *C* or *canc* should be noted after the name of an individual who cancelled an appointment. If an appointment is cancelled you should also note the date of the new appointment if one is made or note *w/c* (will call) if the patient states he will reschedule at another time. (See Table 9.3).

One color of ink, either blue or black, should be selected and used consistently in the appointment book. The neatness and consistency of notations in the book lend credibility to the document.

Some offices select one alternate color to record the name of a patient who is to be seen for the first time. Red is an excellent contrast to the blue or black ink used to record established patients. The alternate color entry will alert the staff at a quick glance as to whether or not new patients are to be seen each day. This will help with time management, since new patients require extra time for registration, chart preparation, and discussion of office policy.

Appointment Cards

The appointment card is an important reminder for patients, since they are likely to have a number of things on their minds by the end of their visit. The appointment cards should be kept in a convenient holder near the appointment book. They will be used each time a patient schedules an appointment while in the office. You may also send an appointment card, along with a patient information pamphlet, to new nonemergency patients who schedule advance appointments or to patients who made advance appointments by telephone but tend to forget them.

The standard appointment card is imprinted with the physician's name, address, and telephone number and a line on which to write the patient's name, usually preceded by the letter *M* (see Figure 9.5). This allows the person filling out the card to follow the *M* with an *r* or *s* to indicate *Mr.* or *Ms.* and then to insert at least the patient's last name. This may take a few extra seconds of your time, but it personalizes the interaction and indicates to the patient that you see him as an individual. Below the line for the name are spaces to enter the day, date, and time of the scheduled appointment. You may choose a card with a preprinted line that states, "If unable to keep appointment, kindly give 24 hours notice." If the office intends to charge for missed appointments, this must be stated either on the appointment card, in the statement of services, or in the patient information pamphlet.

Some appointment cards are designed to serve a second purpose. The back of the card may serve as a business card or provide a map with the location of the office. A dual business/appointment card may serve a purpose in the office but does not look professional when physicians exchange business cards with colleagues. If the office location requires directions they should be provided in the patient information pamphlet. The patient will not require this information before every visit.

SCHEDULING AN APPOINTMENT
Necessary Information from Patient

One of the elements necessary for efficient management of the scheduling system is knowing, in advance if possible, who you will be seeing each day. Advance appointment scheduling is ideal, because

Figure 9.5
Appointment cards.
Courtesy Histacount Corp, Melvill, NY.

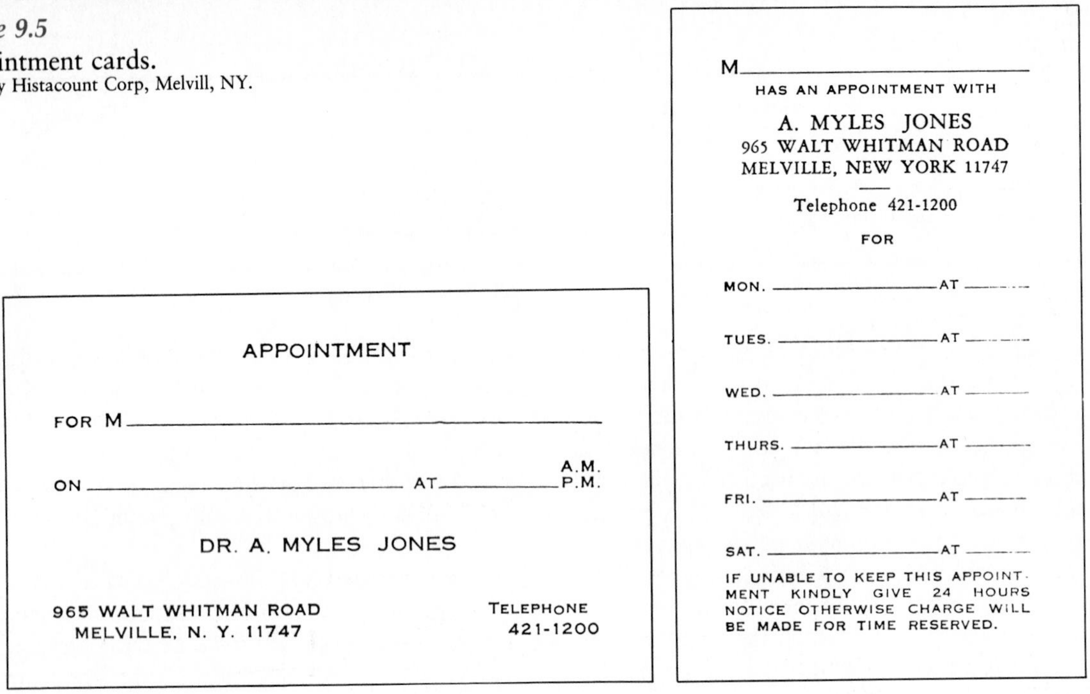

APPOINTMENT

FOR M_____

ON _____ AT_____ A.M.
                                                                P.M.

DR. A. MYLES JONES

965 WALT WHITMAN ROAD   TELEPHONE
MELVILLE, N. Y. 11747   421-1200

M_____

HAS AN APPOINTMENT WITH

A. MYLES JONES
965 WALT WHITMAN ROAD
MELVILLE, NEW YORK 11747
—
Telephone 421-1200

FOR

MON. _____AT _____

TUES. _____AT _____

WED. _____AT _____

THURS. _____AT _____

FRI. _____AT _____

SAT. _____AT _____

IF UNABLE TO KEEP THIS APPOINT-
MENT KINDLY GIVE 24 HOURS
NOTICE OTHERWISE CHARGE WILL
BE MADE FOR TIME RESERVED.

it allows you to save some time each day for unexpected events, such as emergency patients or friends of the physician who drop in. Often, one 15- or 30-minute segment in the morning and one in the afternoon provides enough cushion to end the day on time.

In scheduling advance appointments, the minimum information that you will need is the following:

- Patient's full name, spelled correctly;
- Daytime telephone number;
- Reason for the visit;
- Referral source; and
- Insurance information or ability to pay for new patients.

There are sound reasons for each piece of information gathered when the appointment is made. The correctly spelled name allows you to locate the patient's chart quickly or to label the chart cover, registration form, and account card in advance. Noting the daytime telephone number in the appointment book is for quick reference if you need to change or remind a patient of an appointment. Determining the reason for the visit will allow you to determine the amount of time to reserve for the visit. There will be times when this is a delicate situation that will require perception, tact, and diplomacy. Patients may hesitate to provide the reason because, for example, they are calling from work and lack privacy. If you suspect that this is the sit-

uation, simply ask the patient. You can then suggest that they call you from a private telephone during a break. Patients may also hesitate because they are shy or embarrased about the condition or about speaking to a member of the opposite sex. Your diplomacy and professional manner of speaking will usually relieve the situation. You might say, "Mr. Sims, having a general idea of why you wish to see the doctor will allow me to reserve the correct amount of time for you." With this type of statement you demonstrate consideration of patients and their needs and assure them that you are not pressing for details.

For new patients the referral source should be noted in the appointment book and subsequently on the medical record information sheet and possibly on the financial account card. If the source was a physician, established patient, or professional agency the doctor will want to acknowledge the referral. Also, a referral source may be needed to locate the patient at a future time. Information about insurance or financial responsibility should be acquired without implying that obtaining services is based on finances.

Necessary Information for the Patient

When making an appointment for a patient, either in person or over the telephone, you must be sure the patient has the correct information. State the appointment day, date, and time as you note the patient's name in the appointment book, and state them again before you complete the call. An appropriate closure to the call might be, "Thank you for calling Ms. Adams. I will see you on Friday, March fourth at 3:00 P.M." This demonstrates courtesy, individualized attention, and reconfirms the appointment information.

OFFICE SCHEDULING GUIDELINES

When developing a scheduling system for the office, you will need to consider the needs of the patient, the preferences of the physician, and the personnel, facilities, and equipment available. You will also need to plan for advance scheduling and scheduling exceptions, including emergencies, patients in acute need, and other potential disruptions.

Patient Needs
Work or school schedules

Work or school schedules are important to patients, and they hesitate to disrupt them unnecessarily. Every attempt should be made to accommodate your schedule to the patient's. You might be able to schedule patients with work or school schedules for the first or last appointment of the day so they will be able to limit the time away from their duties.

Travel time

Some patients will be concerned about appointments if they must travel some distance and wish to avoid commuter times. Older patients traveling by public transportation may also wish to avoid being on the bus or train when schoolchildren or business commuters are using the system. You and the patients will be aware of these commuter periods, and you can schedule appointments nearer midday to avoid them.

Child-care needs

The potential problems of having children unsupervised in the reception area have been discussed previously. Therefore you will want to make every effort to accommodate patients who want to work around child-care schedules that they have arranged.

Special needs

Handicapped patients. When scheduling appointments for handicapped patients you must consider their transportation needs and the possible extra time required during the visit to accommodate any mobility difficulties. Handicapped patients may have to adapt their schedules to those of the people who assist them in getting to the physician's office. You should be as flexible as possible in scheduling appointments under the circumstances. You should also include in the planned appointment any extra time you anticipate needing once the patient arrives in the office. It is not necessary to make the patient aware of the extra planning done for his benefit; your actions will be recognized and appreciated.

Communication problems. You will occasionally encounter patients with special communication problems. Hearing impairment was discussed in Chapter 8. Another kind of communication problem may involve non-English speaking patients. If you or your co-workers are not competent in the patient's language, you should request that a translator accompany the patient.

Physician's Preference
Structure

Developing and implementing a scheduling system will depend on the attitude and preference of the physician. Some physicians like a very orderly workday, and others prefer not to be restricted by the clock. These examples represent extreme perspectives, and reality will fall somewhere in between. In most practices absolute structure is impossible because you must allow for emergencies, and complete lack of structure creates long waits and unhappy patients. You should discuss the physician's preferences and evaluate them in relation to the needs of the patients and the staff. The system you devise will have to consider all of these factors to work effectively.

Behavior modification

It may be possible to include a training program for the physician and staff in discussions on the scheduling system at staff meetings. Rather than pointing out the physician's part in disrupting the schedule, the subject can be introduced as an office problem and suggestions for remedies requested. You might state during a staff meeting, "We seem to be getting further and further behind schedule each day. Can we discuss what we can do to remedy the situation either by changing our habits or by altering the system?" Such an introduction to the subject is diplomatic and nonaccusatory and allows each staff member to make suggestions.

Adjusting the schedule

If you identify a specific problem that you are unable to correct with behavior modification, your alternative is to make an adjustment in the system. For example, if patient-care hours begin at 1:00 PM and the physician routinely arrives between 1:15 and 1:25, you could schedule the first patient for 1:30 PM. You may also encounter a patient who is chronically late. The ideal option would be to explain the importance of arriving on time, provided your office functions on schedule, and securing the patient's cooperation. If this approach does not alter the behavior you will simply have to accept it and adjust. Perhaps the late patient can be scheduled next to a patient who typically arrives early. In effect the patients can switch their appointments for you, and your schedule can continue uninterrupted.

Available Personnel

Planning your scheduling system and accepting appointments for office visits requires consideration of the personnel available to provide patient care services.

Routine appointments

Staff members can plan on most patients being scheduled for appointments that are considered routine. Routine visits will vary depending on the type of practice and the specialty of the physicians. In general, routine visits require a limited period of time (15 to 20 minutes), necessitate only basic equipment, and are easily handled by the administrative and clinical staff. The staff can anticipate a predictable transition between routine visits.

Specialized services

Some office or agencies offer specialized services or counseling that requires individuals with training in the specialty. Often the specialty personnel are not full-time members of the staff but come to the office on a limited schedule or on an on-call basis. If they are in the office on a limited schedule, you will need to incorporate some grouping technique in the appointment system so that the specialty therapist and the patients needing the service are in the office at the same time. On-call personnel will come to the office on request to see a specific patient. However, even these visits must be preplanned. The term *on-call* does not imply immediate availability in all situations; it implies "as needed." Some of the specialty personnel you may

be planning for in your office schedule include the following:

- ECG technician;
- EEG technician;
- Nutritionist;
- Occupational therapist;
- Physical therapist; or
- Respiratory therapist.

In managing a scheduling system that involves specialty personnel you will need to keep in mind that you must coordinate time for both the provider and the consumer. The additional temporary staff person will also require your attention to the facilities and equipment necessary to provide the services.

Facilities and Equipment

The nature and number of special examinations or treatments scheduled influences your ability to schedule other visits and is influenced by the availability of facilities and equipment. The types of examinations discussed in Chapters 19 and 28 and the treatments discussed in Chapters 21 and 29 include activities that require special planning. Procedures that need extra time will require shifting patients for routine visits to the remaining examination rooms. You will have to reduce the number of patients seen during the time that includes the special examination.

Equipment is also an important consideration in scheduling special procedures. Equipment can be very expensive. So in some instances, offices have only one piece of a particular item. Such major items might be an echocardiograph machine, cryotherapy equipment, a colposcope, or ultrasound diagnostic equipment. If you only have one of a particular piece of equipment, obviously you cannot schedule two simultaneous appointments for two different people who will need the equipment for diagnostic studies or treatment. You must also remember that some equipment will require special care or sterilization after use. If you have only one of such a piece of equipment you cannot schedule patients needing the equipment one immediately after the other. You must allow a time interval in which to prepare the equipment for the next use. One or more routine appointments can be scheduled during the interim.

Advance Scheduling

Scheduling appointments for a future date depends on the needs of the patient and services to be provided. Advance scheduling refers to an appointment made for any day after the day that you speak to the patient. Advance appointments may be days or weeks ahead.

Types of advance appointments

Preplanned advance appointments can and should be scheduled for routine follow-up visits, physical examinations, and special diagnostic or treatment procedures. The advance planning is to the patient's advantage, because the appropriate amount of time can be reserved to avoid a rushed atmosphere. Occasionally patients will request an appointment on the day they call. You should inquire about the reason for the appointment before making a firm statement about the need for advance planning to fulfill their request. You may be misunderstanding the patient's terminology. Consider the following example. A patient requests a same-day appointment stating that he needs a physical examination. You take the patient literally and explain that physical examination must be scheduled at least 2 weeks in advance. The easily intimidated patient does not disagree but instead accepts your restriction even though he is in need of care on the day of the call. In reality, the patient was trying to request an appointment to have the physician *examine* him for a painful *physical* problem.

Scheduling advance appointments

In person.   At the end of an office visit the physician will advise patients whether they need a follow-up appointment. If a subsequent appointment is necessary it is best to schedule it while the patient is still in the office. The patient will not forget to make the appointment and you can give the patient an appointment reminder card. Also, making the appointment in the office will possibly eliminate a telephone call.

Patients may also telephone for an advance appointment if they want a physical examination, wish to check on a situation that is not urgent, or have been referred by another physician. After the date and time have been agreed on, you may send the patient a written appointment card and, for new patients, a patient information folder (Figure 9.6).

Scheduling by Exception

Scheduling by exception refers to unplanned situations that require an immediate appointment. These situations can include emergency patients, acute-need patients, and physician referrals.

Emergency patients

Criteria of an emergency.   Determining what constitutes an emergency was discussed in Chapter 8 in relation to the classification of incoming telephone calls. Briefly, emergencies are serious situations in which the patient may have a temporary or continued loss of consciousness, heavy bleeding, severe pain, severe vomiting or diarrhea, or fever.

Screening emergency calls.   An experienced medical assistant will be able to determine an emergency call and proceed as necessary. If there is any doubt about the situation the physician, if readily available, should be given the call to make a decision. If the physician is out of the office, he or she should be contacted immediately for instructions. When in doubt it is better to treat the situation as an emergency than to underestimate its severity.

Scheduling emergency patients.   Many emergencies are first evaluated in the medical office or agency. Emergency patients have priority in scheduling and, on arrival at the office, are seen before previously scheduled and waiting patients. The situation may be obvious to the patients who are waiting, but you should briefly explain to them that it is an emergency and that they will be seen as soon as possible.

Acute need patients

Criteria and screening.   Patients in acute need of care should be seen on the same day that they call. Acute conditions include infections, moderately elevated temperature, newly discovered masses, such as a breast lump, or moderate pain of recent onset (for pain terminology see Appendix C, Part 1). Some symptoms, such as slight vaginal bleeding, may seem acute to the patient when actually they are not. However, you cannot disregard the patient's anxiety and need for reassurance.

Scheduling.   Patients in acute need should be given the first possible appointment on the day that they call. If all appointment times are filled you will have to resort to double booking. Patients should be advised of the scheduling situation and made to understand that they may have a limited wait when they arrive. They should be reassured that they will be cared for as soon as possible.

Physician referrals

Physicians frequently refer patients to one another for specialized care or consultation. The referring physician's medical assistant might make the appointment for the patient, or the patient may be given the new physician's name and telephone

Figure 9.6
Patient information folder.
Courtesy Herbert N. Jacobs, MD, San Francisco, Calif.

Patient Information Booklet

WELCOME to our office. Please take a few minutes to read this booklet and acquaint yourself with my policies. We look forward to caring for you and answering any questions you may have.

INTERNAL MEDICINE is that branch of medicine concerned with the diagnosis and treatment of internal organs and functions of the body. My practice is limited to adults and adolescents. I, as an internist, provide consultative services for other doctors in addition to my role as a personal physician. I anticipate a continuing relationship with the majority of my patients to provide advice, therapeutic help, periodic physical exams, and, if necessary, referral to another physician for specialty help.

APPOINTMENTS My receptionist is available Monday thru Friday, from 10:00 a.m. to 6:00 p.m. Routine examinations and annual physicals should be scheduled several weeks in advance, as they may require more time. If a problem arises and you must be seen soon, the receptionist may have you speak with my nurse. She will ask you specific questions about your illness to facilitate scheduling. Urgent appointments usually can be handled the day you call, or we may advise you to go to the emergency room.

I do my best to stay on schedule although emergencies sometimes arise. If we anticipate a delay, we will try to notify you beforehand. Please assist us by being on time for your appointment as this could mean less waiting for you. Occasionally people in the waiting room may be seen out of turn if they are urgent examinations. I ask your patience if you have to wait, and hope my staff will advise you of the waiting time.

YOUR APPOINTMENT If we have mailed you a questionnaire, please complete it and bring it with you at the time of your appointment.

Please be sure to bring with you any medications you are taking. If you have been under the care of another doctor, I may ask permission to transfer some of your records. If you anticipate this you may save time be securing a copy of previous records or having them mailed to my office. This requires written permission from you and may take a couple of weeks, so plan ahead.

CANCELLING If you are unable to keep your appointment or are going to be late, please call my office as soon as possible. This courtesy allows me to be of service to other patients. A charge will be made for repeated broken appointments.

EMERGENCY CARE If you need urgent care after hours, call my office telephone number and my exchange will locate me. If I am not available, I will always have available a colleague in whom I have full confidence. In a true emergency, it is best to go to the emergency room at Childrens' Hospital, where the physician on duty will begin treatment and call me or my available substitute.

TELEPHONE CALLS Feel free to call the office if you have questions regarding your condition, medication, treatment, or test results. My nurse can often answer questions and arrange prescription refills. She may wish to consult me before answering your question, or may feel I should talk to you. When it is necessary to speak to

me personally, I will return your call as soon as conditions permit. There is no charge for telephone consultations.

FEES Charges for my personal services are determined by the time required and vary with the complexity of the problem. My fees are competitive with other area internists. Please do not hesitate to ask to see my fee schedule nor to discuss my fees if you have any questions.

BILLING We do not like to send bills, and the costs of paperwork and postage affect my fees. I encourage and request payment for routine services at the time of your office visit, and accept cash or check. If the complexity of the visit requires higher fees and you cannot pay at the time of your visit, billing arrangements can be made.

INSURANCE We will provide you with special forms at the end of your visit which will enable you to complete your own insurance form and will give you a record for income tax purposes. The receptionist can help you in whatever way necessary to complete your insurance. We look to the patient for payment of the bill. Your insurance company will reimburse you directly for any payments made to this office, and will pay more promptly to the patient than to the doctor. This helps reduce office costs and results in more time for patient care and saving to you. If you have Medi-Cal, we assume responsibility for collecting fees. Difficulty involved in producing duplicate copies of these forms is such that a fee must be charged for such copies.

LABORATORY—X-RAY We do a limited amount of tests in the office. The majority of tests are done either at a private laboratory or at one of the nearby hospitals. We will instruct you when and where to go for these tests. The laboratory or hospital will bill you directly for these services. ENCLOSE THEIR BILLS WITH MY BILL WHEN FILING FOR INSURANCE REIMBURSEMENT.

CONFIDENTIALITY Your medical records are strictly private. No information will be given to your employer, friends, relatives or other physicians without your permission. The only exception to this is when required by law, as in industrial cases, assults, etc.

DOCTOR—PATIENT RELATIONS Relations between patients, doctors, and office personnel are best when based on mutual understanding and respect. I make a special effort to explain everything to you. If ever you have questions, or if something is not clear, do not hesitate to ask. If you have any suggestions or complaints regarding my services, fees, or personnel, please tell me so that I may better serve you.

Please, no smoking or eating in the waiting area.

number to make his own appointment. Since referring physicians are a valuable source of patients for a practice, every effort must be made to accommodate the patient as soon as possible.

Disruption of the Scheduling System

A schedule can be disrupted for a variety of reasons and you must be prepared to adapt to unplanned events. The common causes of scheduling disruptions are the following:

- Patient failure to keep appointments;
- Patient cancellations;
- Delayed arrival of the physician; or
- Physician absence because of emergency.

Each disruption requires different handling, but they have one thing in common: the disruption should be kept to a minimum, and the patient's needs and comfort should be foremost in your mind.

Patient failure to keep appointments

Handling technique.   Occasionally patients will fail to keep an appointment without notifying the office. As noted in the description of the appointment book, this patient action is termed *no show*. Anyone can inadvertently miss an appointment. If you contact the patient or the patient calls the office you should be courteous and understanding and schedule another appointment. If the situation occurs repeatedly you will have to explain diplomatically the problems that result. It may be effective to explain that when you do not know that the reserved time will be free, you cannot offer the time to another patient. When repeated failure to keep appointments interferes with proper care of a patient, the physician may choose to dismiss him. The legality of this situation is discussed in Chapter 5, and the technique is discussed in Chapter 11.

Recording.   It is vital that any failure to keep an appointment without notification be recorded in the appointment book as previously discussed. It should also be recorded in the patient's chart. Each document verifies the other.

Patient cancellations

Rescheduling.   When a patient cancels an appointment you should attempt to reschedule it during the same telephone call. This will allow you to maintain continuity of care for the patient and to maintain your scheduling system. Rescheduling at the time of the cancellation gives you immediate access to the time required and the reason for the appointment. This will reduce the time spent on the call.

Notations.   Cancelled appointments should be noted in the appointment book and the patient's chart along with the date of the rescheduled appointment. These notations help you in documenting a patient's cooperation or lack of cooperation in participating in his own care.

Use of time.   If the appointment is cancelled enough time in advance, the appointment time can be offered to another patient. If it is a late cancellation the time may serve as a buffer against unplanned-for patients or used to accomplish other duties.

Delayed arrival of the physician

Reasons and staff notification.   Physicians can be delayed in arriving at the office for a variety of reasons related to their work. An operation may begin and end late because of scheduling difficulty at the hospital, the physician may remain with an emergency patient until an ambulance arrives, or a medical society meeting may run overtime. These delays are understandable and relatively infrequent. The important issue is that the physician notify the office staff of the delay as soon as it is evident and estimate the time of arrival so that the staff can make adjustments. You may have to remind the physician occasionally of the importance of staff notification.

Notifying patients.   Given a valid reason for the delay, patients usually respond with understanding, especially if it is not a common occurrence. They realize that the situation was beyond your control.

You will need first to explain the situation to the patients who have already arrived in the office. Some medical assistants find this an uncomfortable duty. Remember that patients respond well to a frank explanation; it is highly preferable to sitting in the reception room guessing at the cause of the delay. Your next step is to attempt to reach patients by telephone in the order that they are scheduled to arrive at the office. Patients in transit to the office will have to receive an explanation of the situation when they arrive. The remaining patients can be notified at home or work before leaving for the appointment. Each patient should be offered the options of waiting for the physician to arrive or rescheduling an appointment on another day. Because of your experience, you will be able to help the patient decide. If an operation is delayed once it may happen again, and the doctor waiting for an ambulance at a patient's home may have to accompany the patient to the hospital. A medical society meeting will end relatively quickly, because each physician has an office to attend. In any case, patients should be aware that the remainder of the day is likely to run behind schedule.

Physician called away from office

It is possible for physicians to be called out of the office after office hours have begun. This might be for a medical emergency or perhaps to deliver a baby. Whatever the reason, it will disrupt the office schedule. The same procedure is followed in this situation as when the physician is delayed in arriving at the office.

REFERRAL APPOINTMENTS

Your responsibilities will include assisting patients who are referred from your office to another office or agency for consultation, diagnostic studies, or hospitalization. Patients feel protected in their own physician's care and will feel somewhat insecure when referral is necessary. They will ask questions such as "What is the other doctor like?" "Will the procedure hurt?" and "Will the treatment work?" You should be able to reassure patients requiring referral as well as assist with the arrangements.

You must be careful, however, that your reassurance is based on accurate information. When patients ask what the other physician is like, they are asking for a comparison with their primary physician. You should be discreet and nonjudgmental and focus on the patient's benefit. You might say, "Dr. Smith is less talkative than Dr. Adams but just as conscientious." If you know a procedure is painful say, "Yes, there is some discomfort involved, but the procedure is important and the staff will help you stay as comfortable as possible." Patients will appreciate your honesty, and it builds their trust in you. You must be extremely careful with questions about the outcome of treatment. Patients with questions seeking a promise of cure should be redirected to the physician. You might respond with a question such as, "Did Doctor Adams talk with you about the treatment? If you still have questions the doctor will be glad to speak to you again before you leave." Each type of referral involves certain scheduling responsibilities and options.

Physician Consultation Scheduling Options
Patient schedules appointment

Patients who wish to schedule their own appointment with the consultant should be given, in writing, the name, address, and telephone number of the consulting physician. A preprinted patient re-

ferral slip can be given to the patient with this information and other data the consultant might want (Figure 9.7). If known, you can also give the name of the administrative assistant in the consultant's office. The patient will feel that the transition is more personal. You might also place a brief call to the consultant's office so that the patient's call will be expected.

Assistant schedules appointment

If you make the appointment for the patient you may be able to expedite the process and reduce the patient's stress. The medical assistant in the consultant's office might be persuaded to supply an earlier appointment when speaking to another medical assistant rather than the patient. Showing preference to a medical assistant over a patient is not appropriate behavior, but it can exist. Rather than reacting negatively, remember that the patient's well-being is the important issue. You should develop and maintain rapport with other office personnel, because it will be to a patient's benefit. Once the appointment is scheduled you can note the information on a patient referral slip (Figure 9.7).

Physician schedules appointment

There will be occasions in which it is urgent that the patient be seen by the consultant as soon as possible, perhaps even the same day. If the medical assistant is unsuccessful in obtaining an appointment, another approach may be necessary. This option involves the referring physician speaking directly with the consulting physician, and it should be reserved for special situations. This approach is usually very effective in acquiring the necessary patient services.

Diagnostic Studies (Outpatient)
Appointment scheduling

Diagnostic studies are frequently scheduled for patients at other offices or agencies. You will usually be responsible for scheduling these studies because of the medical terminology that is often involved.

Scheduling information

When calling an office to schedule a diagnostic study you should first identify yourself and the physician's office you represent and state the name of the study you want to schedule. The diagnostic office assistant may need to retrieve a special appointment schedule. Next you will need to supply certain information that you have gathered before

Figure 9.7
Consultation referral
slip.
Courtesy Histacount Corp,
Melville, NY.

Date_____

To: Dr._____

_____

This will introduce my patient,

_____

For:

☐ Diagnosis   ☐ Treatment

☐ Case history has been forwarded to you under
separate cover.

Remarks:

_____

_____

_____

_____

Dr._____

FORM No. 120   **DCM** *HISTACOUNT CORPORATION* MELVILLE, NEW YORK 11746

placing the call, including the following information about the patient:

- Name;
- Age or date of birth;
- Insurance carrier; and
- Suspected diagnosis or reason for study.

The patient will need a referral slip. You may keep blank slips on hand (Figure 9.8), or diagnostic offices may provide you with preprinted forms with their name, address, and telephone number. You fill in the date and time of the appointment and the study to be performed.

Patient instructions

Many diagnostic studies require preparation of the patient in advance of the examination. This might be a special diet, fasting, or preparation with medication. Most diagnostic offices will provide you with preprinted forms that you can give to and review with the patient. If the diagnostic office is in your building or nearby, the patient can be di-

rected to stop at the office for instructions and, if needed, preparatory substances. The latter option will save you time and provide the opportunity for the patient to meet the diagnostic office assistant.

Hospitalization
Elective and emergency admissions

Elective hospitalization refers to an admission process that is preplanned and may be necessary for certain diagnostic studies, treatment, or surgery. An emergency admission is based on the criteria discussed in scheduling emergency office appointments. Either you or the physician will schedule an emergency admission. If the patient is first examined in the office you will generally make the hospital arrangements. As in any scheduling situation, certain information must be available before the call is placed, and you must be prepared to supply information to the patient.

Figure 9.8
Diagnostic referral slip.
Courtesy Histacount Corp, Melville, NY.

```
┌──────────────────────────────────────────────────┐
│                                                    │
│  LABORATORY REQUEST      DATE_____           │
│                                                    │
│  TO_____           │
│                                                    │
│  _____           │
│                                                    │
│  RE:_____           │
│           PLEASE DO THE FOLLOWING TESTS            │
│                                                    │
│  ☐ R.B.C. & HGB._____            │
│  ☐ W.B.C. & DIFF._____            │
│  ☐ SED. RATE_____             │
│  ☐ RH FACTOR & BLOOD TYPE_____            │
│  ☐ BLOOD SUGAR_____             │
│  ☐ N.P.N._____            │
│  ☐ URINE ANALYSIS_____             │
│  ☐ PREGNANCY_____             │
│  ☐ B.M.R._____            │
│  ☐ E.K.G._____           │
│  ☐ FECES FOR_____            │
│  ☐ C.S.F. FOR_____            │
│  ☐ CULTURE OF_____             │
│  ☐ OTHER_____             │
│  _____          │
│  _____          │
│                                                    │
│              DR._____           │
│                                                    │
│  FORM NO. 113    HISTACOUNT CORPORATION, MELVILLE, L.I., N.Y. 11746 │
└──────────────────────────────────────────────────┘
```

Information needed by admissions office

The admissions office personnel will often be your first contact with the hospital. The information needed to schedule a hospital admission usually includes the following:

- Admitting physician's name and the names of any other physicians involved in the patient's care;
- Patient's name and date of birth;
- Admitting diagnosis;
- Patient's social security number;
- Patient's insurance carrier;
- Insurance ID number;
- Room preference, such as private, semiprivate, smoking, nonsmoking;
- Prior admissions and date of last admission;
- Possible prior authorization requirement; and
- Insurance carriers telephone number.

The patient's medical record should provide you with all of the necessary information.

Surgical cases

When a patient is being admitted for elective surgical treatment you will need to contact the operating room secretary first. You cannot determine the date of admission before you know the date that the surgery can be scheduled. In some instances, the patient can be admitted to the hospital the morning of the surgery; in other cases the patient is admitted the day before surgery. The operating room secretary will need to have the following information:

- Surgeon's name;
- Procedure planned;
- Time the procedure is expected to take;
- Anesthesia requested;

Figure 9.9
Hospital admission request.
Courtesy Histacount Corp, Melville, NY.

ALVIN MYLES JONES, M. D.
965 WALT WHITMAN ROAD
MELVILLE, N. Y. 11749
——
HAMILTON 1-1200

HOSPITAL ADMISSION REQUEST   DATE_____

TO_____

REQUEST THAT_____AGE_____SEX_____

ADDRESS_____

BE ADMITTED ON_____•_____TO ☐ PRIVATE ☐ SEMI-PRIVATE ☐ WARD
                  DATE   HOUR

PREFERRED LOCATION_____FOR APPROXIMATELY_____DAYS

DIAGNOSIS_____

CONTEMPLATED TREATMENT ☐ MEDICAL   ☐ SURGICAL   ☐ CARDIAC

☐ SPECIAL NURSES CONTEMPLATED_____ ☐ NOT CONTEMPLATED ☐ WILL ADVISE
                          NUMBER

IMMEDIATE ORDERS_____

_____ SIGNED_____

- Name of assistant surgeon for major cases; and
- Patient's name, age, and sex.

Once the surgery is scheduled you may call the admissions office. If it is an emergency situation the patient is admitted first, and the operation is scheduled as soon as possible. Operating rooms are prepared to handle emergency cases 24 hours a day.

Instructions to patients

Patients to be admitted to the hospital are naturally anxious and will need your help during the process. Your calm and organized manner will reassure the patient. First you will provide the patient with written or preprinted referral slips (Figure 9.9), which should include the following information about the hospital:

- Name;
- Address;
- Telephone number; and
- Check-in time.

Patients will also ask you questions regarding various hospital policies. It will be helpful if you familiarize yourself with some basic information about the hospitals frequently used in your practice. You can anticipate inquiries about billing, insurance deductibles, prepayments needed for the uninsured, and visiting hours.

Patients may need to be advised about what they should bring with them to the hospital. Few items are actually needed. These include robe, slippers, personal hygiene items, and some diversional materials (books, writing materials). If the patient is scheduled for surgery you should be prepared to tell them that prior to admission, certain routine procedures will be performed, including the following:

- Chest x-ray examination;
- Laboratory tests;
- Electrocardiogram;
- Visit from the anesthesiologist; and
- Special skin preparations.

If the patient knows that these procedures are routine, anxiety can be greatly reduced.

In all referral procedures the importance of

communication cannot be overly stressed. Taking time to explain an activity to patients will make them more comfortable and make the process smoother for everyone.

VISITORS OTHER THAN PATIENTS

From time to time you can expect visitors other than patients to arrive at the office requesting to see the physician. Predetermined office policy will dictate the manner in which each visitor will be handled. Protocol for certain types of visitors follows.

Physicians

When another physician arrives at the office, the caller should be announced and escorted immediately to the physician's private office. If the physician is in an examining room with a patient, the caller should be seated in the private office and the physician in the treatment room notified of the guest's arrival. The physician will either leave the treatment room to speak with the visitor or tell you how soon he or she can see the visitor. You can then tell the visitor the waiting period.

Pharmaceutical Representatives

Representatives from pharmaceutical companies are frequent visitors to medical offices and agencies. Many will simply drop in and some will call in advance to see what the best time to see the physician would be. Physicians usually have an established policy about seeing pharmaceutical representatives. Some *never* see them; if this is the case you must politely inform the representatives of the policy. Physicians who see pharmaceutical representatives usually prefer to limit the visit to a brief call, perhaps 5 minutes. You will be responsible for setting the visit limits. The representatives are aware of this and will respond to your cue. You need

only say, "The doctor can see you for a very few minutes." Since the "reps" want to be able to call again, they will respect the limits.

Sales Representatives

Sales representatives will call and can be seen by the person responsible for routine purchases. Major purchases are usually decided by the physician, but the representative is usually greeted by the medical assistant who will gather the basic information to pass on to the physician. Details of purchasing will be discussed in Chapter 11. Your responsibility at this point is to know that the representative must be screened by you before approaching the physician.

Family Members and Friends

Although physicians often discourage the habit of family or friends dropping into their office it occurs occasionally. When it does the person should be greeted politely and the physician notified. If the physician's office is available the caller may be seated there to wait for the physician.

Former Patients

It is a source of pleasure to a physician when a former patient drops in to say hello and share some news. The visitor is usually very aware of the physician's schedule and does not wish to interrupt. This patient-caller should be asked to wait in the reception area while you check to see if the physician is available. If at all possible, the physician will usually try to see the caller. If it is impossible to interrupt the physician or if the physician is away from the office, the caller will understand. You should tell the caller that you will make certain the physician knows of the visit, and you should offer to take a message.

Conclusion

The medical assistant is the pivotal person in developing and maintaining a time management system. This administrative system involves planning for expected and unexpected events and, most impor-

tantly, tactfully dealing with many people in the office and in outside facilities. Managing scheduling systems is a challenging and rewarding experience.

Review Questions

1. At the most, how long should a patient have to wait in the reception area before seeing the physician? What are your responsibilities to the waiting patient?
2. What should time management accomplish?
3. What callers can you expect to a medical office, and how should they be handled?
4. What role does the medical assistant play in a caller's first impression of a medical office? What are the medical assistant's responsibilities in creating a good first impression?
5. Describe an ideal reception area.
6. Evaluate the four types of appointment systems and their relationship to time management.
7. Describe the basic equipment for an appointment system and for scheduling referral appointments for patients needing consultation with another physician, diagnostic studies, or hospitalization.
8. Describe the methods of handling visitors other than patients to the medical office, including other physicians, pharmaceutical representatives, sales representatives, family or friends, and former patients.

Chapter 10

Records Management

- Purpose of a records management system
- Contents of a medical record
- Filing equipment and supplies
- Filing systems

- Filing procedures
- Record deletions and corrections
- Record protection
- Retention of medical records
- Informal record systems

Objectives

On completion of Chapter 10 the medical assistant student should be able to:

1 Define the terms listed in the vocabulary.

2 Define and state the purpose of a medical records management system.

3 List the subjective and objective patient data contained in a medical record.

4 Describe the four organizational divisions of a medical record.

5 List and describe the equipment and supplies necessary to a filing system.

6 Define the four types of filing systems.

7 State and describe the five steps of the filing procedure.

8 Describe the process of making deletions from a medical record; state the reasons for and technique of making corrections in a medical record.

9 Describe the techniques for protecting medical records.

10 Discuss opinions on the retention of medical records.

11 Describe the assistant's responsibility for the informal record systems, including master calendars, tickler files, correspondence, financial records, and physician's personal records.

Vocabulary

chronological Arranged in the order of time.

confidential Information to which a person may be privy and cannot be shared without the express authorization of the person to which it pertains.

cumulative Growing in number by repeated additions.

derogatory Tending to discredit or belittle.

diplomatic Skillful in the conduct of affairs.

retention The act of keeping in one's power or possession.

scrutiny Close inspection or examination.

subpoena A written order commanding a person to appear in court.

Receiving, processing, and gathering papers in an orderly manner for storage are necessary functions in every business. Records management is the development and maintenance of a systematic method of fulfilling these functions. The management of medical records is a responsibility that should be orderly and systematic. The main purpose of keeping accurate and complete medical records is to assist in giving the best possible care and treatment to the patient. Therefore attention to the details of records management requires the special attention of the medical assistant.

PURPOSE OF A RECORDS MANAGEMENT SYSTEM
Provision of Optimum Care
Single location of data

One factor in providing the best possible medical care is having all of the information regarding a patient in one place. That place is the patient's individual medical chart. Every patient's chart is ideally stored in a single location, the filing cabinet or record-storage area. If patient information is systematically stored in a known, single location, it will be readily available to the physician and personnel when it is needed.

Continuum of information

The medical record provides the medical staff with a chronological history of a patient's care, illnesses, injuries, responses to treatment, and general condition at all stages throughout the relationship with the physician. Patients frequently forget various events and responses to particular medications, and the physician cannot possibly remember the details of care given to each individual because of the numbers of patients that he or she cares for over the course of a career. The well-maintained record provides a detailed and logical sequence of events to the benefit of both the patient and the physician.

Provides data from various sources

The office medical record is developed around the observations and notations of the physician based on conversations with and examinations of the patients. In addition, the record serves as a storage unit for information from a variety of sources. The outside sources of medical information include reports from laboratory and diagnostic facilities of examinations requested by the physician, detailed information gathered if the patient is hospitalized, consultations requested of other physicians, and records of other health care providers who have treated the patient. This cumulative information assists the current physician in the continuing care of the patient.

Rapid Information Retrieval

Proper development, maintenance, and storage of patients' medical records allows for rapid retrieval of information. There are many instances when the speed at which patient data can be located and transmitted will affect a positive outcome for a patient in need. Consider the situation of a child brought to an emergency room after ingesting a parent's prescription medication. The parent, concerned about getting care for the child, leaves for the emergency room without the medication bottle and cannot remember the name of the drug. When your office is contacted, the speed with which you can provide the information could be vital to the survival of the child.

Legal Protection
Protection of the patient

Confidentiality. The proper maintenance and storage of patients' medical records will provide for the confidentiality of the information contained in them. You should think of the record as the person, and the same privacy you would provide for the patient should be provided for the record. This will create an atmosphere in which the patient can feel confident in being totally frank with the physician.

Protecting patients' identities. The protection of your patients and their records should always be your first thought when *any* inquiries are made about them. Some requests will be perfectly innocent and should be handled diplomatically. For example, one patient may notice another person leaving the doctor's office and inquire, "Was that Sam Johnson? I haven't seen him in years. Do you have his number? I'd really like to call him." Since you may not confirm the patient's name or release the telephone number, you might reply, "I am sorry Mr. Simpson, I cannot give out anyone's phone number, just as I would not give out yours to anyone without your permission." With this type of statement, you have not confirmed or denied the departing patient's identity and have subtly educated the patient on confidentiality.

When a subpoena for a medical record is delivered in person, the server must present it to the medical assistant along with a check to cover the cost of processing the chart. If it turns out that the person is not a present or former patient, the check is retained and the subpoena is returned after the assistant signs a form stating that no records are available. In an effort to cut costs, some subpoena firms call an office in advance to inquire if records are available. This is a method of determining if an individual is under the physician's care. If you respond that you have a record for that patient, you

Figure 10.1
Records release form.
Courtesy Colwell Systems, Inc, Champaign, Ill.

RECORDS RELEASE

Date_____

To _____

_____

I hereby authorize you to release to

_____

_____

any information including the diagnosis and records of any treatment or examination rendered

to me during the period from_____to_____

_____
SIGNATURE

_____
WITNESS

NO. 3341 COLWELL CO CHAMPAIGN. ILL

---

are breaching confidentiality. The appropriate response would be, "If you will forward the subpoena, I can check our files."

Release of records. The release of patients' records was discussed in Chapter 5, including the few instances in which certain information can be provided without the patient's consent. In all instances for which consent is required, the patient's permission should be obtained in writing. Most offices keep a supply of preprinted forms with blanks for the appropriate information (Figure 10.1).

Protection of the physician

Documentation of care provided. The patient's medical records provide the primary documentation of the evaluation, examination, treatments, and conclusions determined by the physician. Entries in medical records should be written clearly and legibly. Physicians cannot be expected to remember previous impressions or treatments prescribed and must depend on the accuracy of the record. Should a legal issue be raised regarding the care or condition of a patient, the medical record is usually the first source of information evaluated.

Permanent protection. A medical record is a lasting proof of care and is credible regardless of the time elapsed since an entry was made. Since a lawsuit may be filed years after an event, the record is considered more reliable than the physician's memory. For the record to provide protection, it must be carefully prepared and maintained.

Legal Considerations
Entries

Unalterable. The entries in a medical record are unalterable. In other words, notes written in a patient's medical record cannot be changed or removed. Should an error be recognized, a specific technique should be used to correct. If records are handwritten, all notations should be made in a neat and legible manner. This technique will be discussed later in this chapter.

Authorized personnel. Because of the importance of the medical record, office policy should be established indicating which personnel are authorized to make entries in a patient's record. As a professional medical assistant you will undoubtedly be responsible for medical records, including entry making. You must always keep in mind the importance of the medical record for patient care and for legal purposes.

Entries to be avoided

A thoughtless comment in a patient's chart could give the impression that the physician is uninterested in the care or prejudiced in his or her opinion of the patient. This impression can influence the credibility of the physician and the quality of care provided. Humorous or sarcastic remarks should never be written in a patient's record. Physicians and assistants should also take care not to attempt to describe another physician's findings or treatments. Information provided by the patient can be enclosed in quotation marks to indicate the source. If more information is required, the patient can sign a records release so that the other physician's records can be acquired.

Statistical Information

Physicians may wish to gather and evaluate data on the effectiveness of a treatment plan or follow the course of several patients with the same diagnosis. Medical records can provide this information, which can be abstracted and maintained in a separate file. The increasing use of computers to store records and abstract data is a great help with statistical information. You should remember, however, that this information, whether abstracted by you or a computer, is still confidential and must be protected.

CONTENTS OF A MEDICAL RECORD
Patient Data
Demographic data

The first step in developing the patient's record is to gather demographic data from the patient on his first visit to the office. This information will be used initially to introduce the patient to the physician and subsequently to contact the patient if necessary, to establish the accounting records, and to assist with insurance billing. The information most often requested includes the following:
- Full name;
- Date of birth;
- Sex (name may not be indicative);
- Complete home address;
- Home telephone number (or number where messages can be left);
- Marital status;
- If married, spouse's name or next of kin;

- Occupation, employer and work address and telephone number;
- If married, spouse's work information;
- Insurance carrier and identification numbers;
- Insurance carriers address;
- Referral source;
- Social Security number;
- Driver's license number; and
- Name of reference who does not live with you to contact in emergency.

Changes in social attitudes regarding independent identity may cause a married patient to decline to provide information about a spouse. This wish must be respected, but you could explain that the information is for notification purposes, particularly in the event of an emergency, and not an assumption of dependence. Some patients may refuse to give their Social Security number or driver's license number. This too must be respected, since it will be difficult to explain that the information is requested for purposes of tracing the patient in the event an account is not paid.

Methods of patient registration. The demographic information may be obtained by two methods: (1) a patient-completed form or (2) an oral interview.

A patient-completed registration form may be one of your own design or may be selected from those offered by office-supply companies (Figure 10.2). The form, on a hard writing surface such as a clipboard, is handed along with a pen or pencil to the patient on his arrival in the office. The patient is asked to complete the form and return it to the receptionist. The form may be put into the record as written, or the information may be typed onto a patient-history form.

Gathering demographic information by interview is a more personal technique, but you must be careful to provide privacy during the interview. The data may be handwritten and subsequently transcribed onto the history sheet or typed as the information is acquired.

Each method has advantages and disadvantages, which are noted in Table 10.1.

Personal and medical history. The personal history, including social habits and family history, and medical history are necessary to prepare a foundation for the physical examination and subsequent treatment. Historical information can also be gathered by patient-completed forms or by interview. Details of the information gathered and the forms used are discussed in Chapter 18.

Reason for visit. The patient may have given the reason for the visit at the time the appointment was made but is usually asked again at the begin-

Figure 10.2
Patient registration form.
Courtesy Histacount Corp,
Melville, NY.

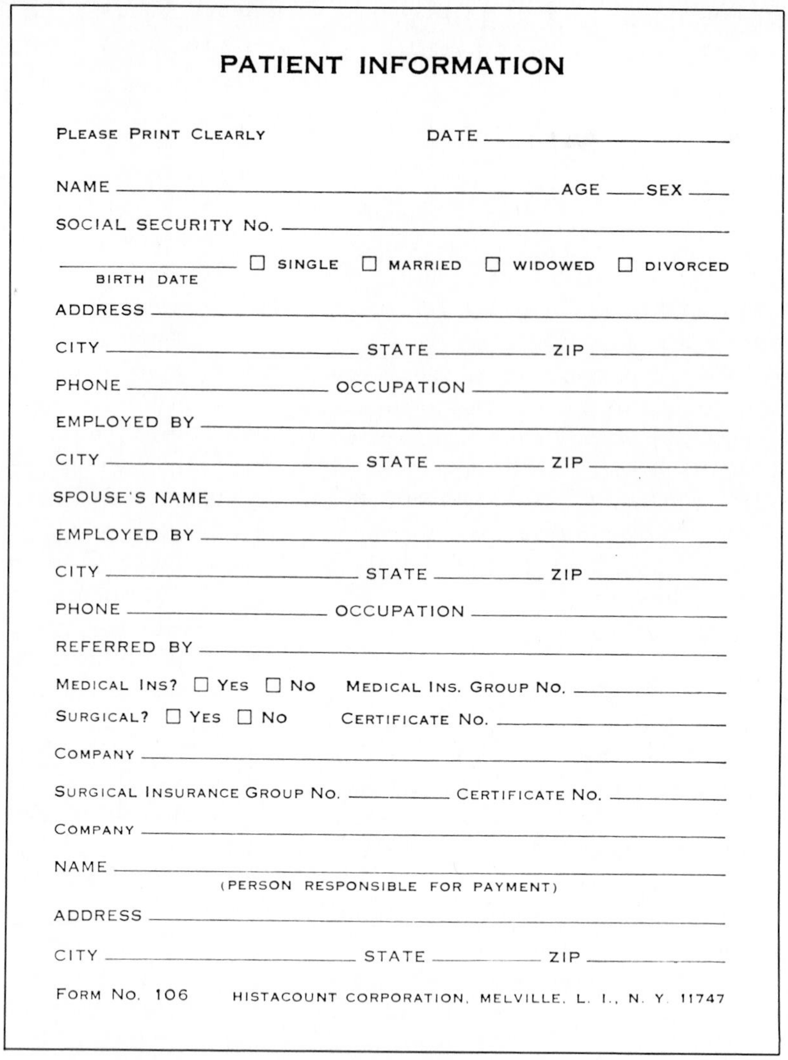

PATIENT INFORMATION

PLEASE PRINT CLEARLY　　　　　　DATE _____

NAME _____AGE ____ SEX ____

SOCIAL SECURITY No. _____

_____ ☐ SINGLE ☐ MARRIED ☐ WIDOWED ☐ DIVORCED
BIRTH DATE

ADDRESS _____

CITY _____ STATE _____ ZIP _____

PHONE _____ OCCUPATION _____

EMPLOYED BY _____

CITY _____ STATE _____ ZIP _____

SPOUSE'S NAME _____

EMPLOYED BY _____

CITY _____ STATE _____ ZIP _____

PHONE _____ OCCUPATION _____

REFERRED BY _____

MEDICAL INS? ☐ YES ☐ No　MEDICAL INS. GROUP No. _____

SURGICAL? ☐ YES ☐ No　CERTIFICATE No. _____

COMPANY _____

SURGICAL INSURANCE GROUP No. _____ CERTIFICATE No. _____

COMPANY _____

NAME _____
(PERSON RESPONSIBLE FOR PAYMENT)

ADDRESS _____

CITY _____ STATE _____ ZIP _____

FORM No. 106　　HISTACOUNT CORPORATION, MELVILLE, L. I., N. Y. 11747

Table 10.1
Advantages and disadvantages of patient registration method

	Advantages	Disadvantages
Patient-completed forms	Saves employee time	Patient's handwriting may be illegible
	Patient may be more relaxed	Patient may not understand questions
		Impersonal
Oral interview	Provides time to establish rapport with the patient	Requires employee time
	Assures that all questions are answered completely	May increase patient nervousness
	Information typed onto permanent record ensures clarity	

ning of the visit. This information is recorded in the patient's own words (see Chapter 18).

Objective data

The objective entries in a medical record are based on observations made during the course of examining the patient and through reviews, diagnostic studies, and subsequent care. Objective findings and conclusions include the following:

- Physical measurements;
- Physical examination findings;
- Diagnostic study reports;
- Diagnosis and prognosis;
- Treatment plan; and
- Outcome of treatment.

All of the items listed are developed during the course of evaluation and treatment visits. Each subject is discussed in Chapters 17 and 18.

Organization of the Medical Record

Each office will develop a procedure for the organization of a medical record that suits the needs of personnel working with the record and the personal preference of the physician. Many prefer to divide the chart into subsections, with each subsection maintained in chronological order and secured with a paper clip. Staples should be avoided because of the damage they cause to individual sheets when they are removed or replaced to add new sheets.

Physician's notes

The physician's notes begin with the information history and initial evaluation. Subsequent visits are noted on sheets titled *Progress notes*. The date is stamped on the notes to indicate the date of each visit. Some physicians prefer that progress notes, the first section encountered when the chart cover is opened, be maintained in reverse chronological order, with the sheet describing the most recent visit on top and the oldest entry on the bottom. This avoids having to turn multiple sheets to locate the space to begin notations for the present visit.

Diagnostic and hospital records

The next section in the medical record contains diagnostic studies. This section is frequently referred to by the physician for monitoring the patient's condition or progress and in discussions with patients regarding their care. Diagnostic reports are usually stored in chronological order with the most recently dated report at the back of the section.

Some of the subsections preferred are as follows:

- Progress notes;
- Consultations;
- Laboratory;
- X-ray;
- Operative reports;
- Correspondence; and
- Prescriptions or medications.

Correspondence

The correspondence section contains letters and narrative reports from physicians or facilities that have provided care for the patient in the past. Correspondence from the patient can also be included in this section. Patients often send the physician cards from vacation spots or announcements of special events in their lives. Retaining these items in the record will serve as a reminder for the physician to mention the greeting or event on the patient's next visit.

Insurance forms

The fourth section of the patient's record contains copies of insurance forms prepared by the administrative assistant. It is particularly important to retain copies of Medicare and Medicaid forms, which might be subject to inspection and are necessary for documentation of services. Some offices store insurance forms in separate chronological files, but this can be time consuming. If you need to compare the record with the form, you will have to retrieve information from two sources.

FILING EQUIPMENT AND SUPPLIES
Storage Cabinets

Medical records may be stored in a variety of cabinets designed to protect the record while allowing easy access and retrieval. Filing cabinets are available in pull-out drawer–style, shelf-style, and open filing–style systems.

Shelf-type cabinets have either stationary or pull-out shelves. When purchasing a pull-out drawer cabinet or shelf cabinet, you must be sure that it has full suspension, which is a built-in mechanism that allows you to slide out only one drawer or shelf at a time. This is a safety factor that prevents the cabinet from tipping forward. Figure 9.2 shows a stationary shelf-type file. Open files are simple frames with dividers that hold files without any means of closure (Figure 10.3).

Drawer- and shelf-type filing cabinets have the advantage of being tightly closed, which provides

Figure 10.3
Open filing cabinet.

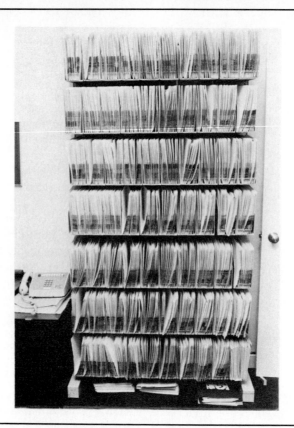

dust-free and fireproof storage. Cabinet locks, which are optional, provide maximum security for records.

Guides
Dividers

Dividers are available to assist you with rapid location and retrieval of records. They are available for alphabetical, numerical, geographical, and subject filing systems. Dividers allow you to subdivide major headings into segments of your choice.

OUTguides

An office with several employees and physicians may find that time is lost each day attempting to locate charts that are being used in various areas within the office. Although the practice should be discouraged, it is also possible that a physician may take a chart out of the office to dictate a report or compare it with hospital records. OUTguides are firm paper inserts in the shape of a chart cover or an actual folder that is left in place of a record removed from the files. The OUTguide has prelined spaces to note the file name, date removed, by whom, and to what location. The chart

is then easily located, saving the staff time and frustration.

Folders

Folders, or chart covers, are manila forms designed to store and protect the forms and documents of an individual's medical record. Each record is stored in a separate folder.

Folders are available in two basic styles: top-tab, used most conveniently in drawer-type filing cabinets, and side-tab, for the shelf-type cabinet. Either style folder is available with color-coded tabs (Figure 10.4). Color coding is discussed under alphabetical filing systems later in this chapter.

Labels
Cabinet

The doors of drawer and shelf-type filing cabinets have small frames for cards that identify the contents. The card may be labeled with the first and last names, numbers, or letters of the folders in the drawer.

Figure 10.4
Tab folders, color coded.

Folders

A label must be affixed to the tab of each file folder for the purpose of identification and easy retrieval. Chart labels are available pregummed on rolls or on sheets. The name should be accurately typed on both sides of the label, last name first, before it is affixed to the tab.

FILING SYSTEMS
Alphabetical

The alphabetical filing system is the easiest and most commonly used system for organizing patients' records. Labeled folders are arranged in the same sequence as the letters of the alphabet. The filing cabinet is divided to accommodate each letter, and the divider guides also supply subdivisions for letters that typically include more charts than others. For example, you will notice that many charts appear in the section *A*. Divider guides may be positioned for both the first and second letter of the last name at various intervals, for example, *A*, *Ad*, *Al*, and *Ap*. Other letters such as *I*, *O*, and *Z* usually do not hold many charts and are therefore not subdivided.

Using the alphabetical system of filing will be the easiest in a medical practice, since it is the most common and for many the easiest method to learn. The one drawback to this system is encountered by rapidly growing practices, in which charts are added to each section, and the space provided for each alphabetical section has to be expanded periodically. This usually involves shifting all of the charts in the system to redistribute the space.

Color coding

Color coding is the technique of using predetermined colors to assist in the rapid location of files and the avoidance of misfiling records. The selected colors may be incorporated into the folder tabs or, for economical reasons, may be added by attaching labels edged in various colors to the tabs. The greatest advantage of color coding is the assistance it provides in locating a chart that has been misfiled.

To initiate a color-coding system you first select the colors to be used and then determine the letters of the alphabet that will be represented by the various colors. Your color code is then applied using the *second* letter of the last name of each patient, because if the first letter were used you would have large sections of the cabinet displaying the same color. By using the second letter you reduce the *number* of charts displaying each color in each section, and all the colors are repeated in each alphabetical segment (Figure 10.4).

Your color code reference card may read as follows.

If the *second* letter of the last name is:	The folder or label color is:	As in:
A, B, C, D	BLUE	KANE OBEN ECKHART IDOR
E, F, G, H	RED	BENSON UFUS AGERMAN CHAN
I, J, K, L, M	GREEN	HINES BJORN AKERMAN CLAYBORN EMERSON
N, O, P, Q	YELLOW	INORSON BORDEN EPSON AQUINAS
R, S, T, U, V, W, X, Y, Z	PURPLE	BRAVERMAN ESTERLY OTTER PULVER AVER EWELL OXLEY AYERS IZUNO

You can see that if you missed *Inorson* as *Imorson*, the chart with the yellow tab for the *N* would stand out next to the green tabs, which represent *M*.

Color coding can also be used to indicate type of insurance, the patient's primary physician in a multiple-physician practice, or patients with certain diagnoses under study. The primary alphabetical color system remains unchanged, but the additional identification may be added with removable clip-tabs or small strips of colored tape. Your instructor will be able to demonstrate the technique for you.

Numerical

In numerical filing, materials are primarily categorized by number and secondarily by an alphabeti-

cal cross-reference. Each new patient is assigned a number in sequence. A cross-reference is established after the number has been assigned. Either an index card or ledger card is arranged alphabetically and followed by the previously assigned numerical code. Office computers can also store and arrange this information for you. The advantages of the numerical system are its capacity for expansion without rearrangement of the cabinets as in alphabetical filing and clear identification of individuals with similar or identical names. You will usually encounter this system in hospitals, large clinics, or group-practice situations.

Geographical

Filing according to the patient's place of residence is a technique reserved for major clinics or medical centers and must be cross-referenced by an alphabetical system. This system may be used in facilities wishing to gather statistical data or trying to locate a disease process within a geographical area. It is, in fact, a method more commonly used in business than medicine. Although you will rarely encounter this system, you should know that it exists.

Subject

Subject filing may be used for patient records as a cross-index if the physician is interested in gathering statistics on various disease processes. You will use subject filing in the business aspect of the practice for keeping information and correspondence in appropriate categories. Folders are prepared and labeled to store information on subjects such as equipment maintenance contracts, office policies, office procedures, workmen's compensation injury reports, and so forth. These folders may be kept in a file drawer in the administrative assistant's desk for easy access.

FILING PROCEDURES

Every item arriving in the office that pertains to a patient or to business must eventually be processed for filing. It is in your best interest to approach this task in an orderly and systematic manner to limit the time involved and to assure the accurate disposition of the material.

A filing system usually includes the following steps:

- Examination;
- Indexing;
- Coding;
- Sorting; and
- Storing.

These steps should be carefully developed and then be outlined in the office procedure manual.

Examination
Filing indicator

When an item arrives at your desk for filing, you must first check for a predetermined indicator that it has been reviewed by the physician. This is particularly important for diagnostic reports and consultations that will require patient follow-up. The indicator to file is often the physician's initials in an agreed-upon location, such as the upper right-hand corner of the document.

You will also be reviewing business correspondence for filing. This may be initialed with instructions to follow before the document is stored, such as "check the cost of maintenance contract last year." You will then check for the information requested, attach it to the correspondence, and return the document to the physician. You will eventually receive it back with further instructions.

Condition of an item

Any item ready for filing should be checked for unnecessary clips, staples, or tears in the document. Before processing, the clips and staples should be removed and the tears mended with tape to prevent further damage to the document.

Indexing

Indexing is a method of determining the destination of each document to be filed. Diagnostic studies usually arrive with the patient's name near the top of the record. Other correspondence may have an *RE:* line that will tell you the person or subject, but some may have information buried in the body of the document.

Coding

After determining the name or subject of a document, it must be highlighted in some manner. This activity is called coding. You could write the indexing factor in the upper right-hand corner of the page or circle or underline it where it appears in the document. Whatever method you choose you must use it consistently, since others responsible for sorting and storing the documents will depend on the code for guidance.

Sorting

The fourth step in a filing procedure is sorting, a method of subdividing the documents. Since most filing is associated with patient's records, which are typically filed alphabetically, the alphabetical method will be discussed here.

Major headings

The documents to be filed each day are first sorted by the first letter of the last name. This provides you with a crude series of major subheadings. If you have a large, private work area on which the documents can be placed in separate stacks alphabetically, you can accomplish your sorting in this manner. If space is limited, you may use a sorting aid. Commercial desk sorters are instruments that have a series of sturdy dividers attached at one end and that are open at the other end to allow you to insert your documents. The dividers are staggered, so that when the instrument is flat on the desk each tab with the individual letter of the alphabet is visible. The effect is similar to the one you would see if you horizontally spread a deck of cards so that the number or letter would be visible along one edge of each card. Each divider is deep enough to hold many standard-size sheets of paper without obstructing the sorting tabs.

Once you have completed sorting by major headings, all items in each letter of the alphabet must be indexed.

Alphabetical indexing

The final step of sorting, alphabetical indexing, is a method of organizing documents in the order in which the folders are placed in the filing cabinet. Standard indexing rules like the ones developed and maintained by the American Records Management Association are used in most businesses, including medical practices.

Rules of indexing.   Indexing is based on dividing a name into units. Units are numbered beginning with 1. Three units are usually sufficient for the average medical practice. The rules are collectively summarized in Table 10.2. A more detailed description is presented here.

1. Persons' names are indexed with the last name as Unit 1, the given (first) name as Unit 2, and the middle name or initial as Unit 3. For example, John C. Jones is indexed as:

Unit 1	Unit 2	Unit 3
Jones	John	C.

2. Once in units, the names are read from left to right, compared, and then placed in alphabetical order with the first letter that is different becoming the next order for filing. Thus Jones, Jane A. will be filed before Jones, John C., because the *a* in *Jane*

Table 10.2
Summary of indexing rules

Rule on	Name	Unit 1	Unit 2	Unit 3
Proper names	John C. Jones	Jones	John	C.
Proper names given in:				
Initials in place of a given name	J. Jones	Jones	J.	
Initial as first name with middle name provided	J. Charles Jones	Jones	J.	Charles
Hyphenated names	Sylvia Clayton-Moore	Claytonmoore	Sylvia	
Apostrophes	Morton's Pharmacy	Mortons	Pharmacy	
Prefixes	Claude de Mason	Demason	Claude	
	Elizabeth D. Mac Adams	Macadams	Elizabeth	D.
Abbreviations	Mary St. John	Saint	John	Mary
	Wm. C. Cosgrove	Cosgrove	William	C.
Titles	Dr. Mary A. Smith	Smith	Mary	A. (Dr.)
Seniority	Henry R. Adams, Jr.	Adams	Henry	R. (Jr.)
Married women using husband's name	Mrs. John C. Smith (Helen J.)	Smith	Helen	J.
Government offices	Federal Justice Department	United	States	Justice
Banks	First Interstate of Tulsa	Tulsa	First Interstate	Oklahoma

is the first letter that is different alphabetically before the *o* in *John*.

3. Initials used in place of a first name are considered a unit and placed before a spelled-out name. Thus Jones, J., or Jones, J. Charles is placed before Jones, John C.

4. Any hyphenated name is considered a single unit; the hyphen is disregarded. Thus Clayton-Moore, Sylvia, is indexed as:

Unit 1	Unit 2
Claytonmoore	Sylvia

5. Apostrophes are disregarded in indexing. Thus Morton's Pharmacy is read as *Mortons Pharmacy*.

6. Names with prefixes are filed as one unit, ignoring the space between the prefix and the name. Thus Claude de Mason is read and indexed as:

Unit 1	Unit 2
Demason	Claude

7. Abbreviated portions of names are read and indexed as if written in full. Thus Mary St. John is indexed as:

Unit 1	Unit 2	Unit 3
Saint	John	Mary

and Wm. C. Cosgrove is indexed as:

Unit 1	Unit 2	Unit 3
Cosgrove	William	C.

8. The prefixes Mac and Mc may be filed in one of two ways: (a) You may use individual dividers to indicate a separate section for all *Mc's* and another for all *Mac's*. These would become a subsystem within the files where the name following the prefix becomes the first indexing unit. Following the *Mac* divider, the names MacDonald, MacAndrew, MacHenry in proper order would be indexed as:

Unit 1	Unit 2	Unit 3
Adams	Elizabeth	D.
Donald	Joseph	
Henry	Sharon	L.

Mc would be the next divider and include names organized in the same way as those under *Mac*. The dividers will then resume the normal alphabetical order. (b) You may disregard the prefix and treat it the same as indicated in Rule 5. Thus MacDonald, MacHenry, and MacAdams would be read, indexed, and filed thus:

Unit 1	Unit 2	Unit 3
MacAdams	Elizabeth	D.
MacDonald	Joseph	
MacHenry	Sharon	L.

9. Titles and seniority indicators either preceding or following a name should be disregarded. These are noted on the record only so that you can address the person properly. Thus Dr. Mary A. Smith and Henry R. Adams, Jr. are indexed as:

Unit 1	Unit 2	Unit 3
Smith	Mary	A. (Dr.)
Adams	Henry	R. (Jr.)

10. Married women who have adopted their husband's surname are indexed using the woman's given name. Thus, for example, put the file under Mrs. Helen J. Smith, not Mrs. John C. Smith (Helen J.).

11. Government offices are indexed by level of government. This is first stated by nationality, then department, bureau, and division, which will require additional units. This knowledge is used more often in locating information in a telephone directory. Thus Federal Justice Department, Bureau of Narcotics and Dangerous Drugs is indexed as:

Unit 1	Unit 2	Unit 3	Unit 4
United	States	Justice	Narcotics

12. Banks are indexed by city, bank name, and state. Thus First Interstate of Tulsa is indexed as:

Unit 1	Unit 2	Unit 3
Tulsa	First Interstate	Oklahoma

13. Persons' surnames that can be mistaken for given names should be cross-indexed by placing an OUTguide or blank folder in the incorrect site. For example, John R. James should be properly indexed thus:

Unit 1	Unit 2	Unit 3
James	John	R.

The mistaken site marker for this patient should read:

Unit 1	Unit 2	Unit 3	
John	James	R.	SEE
James	John	R.	

Storing

The final step in the filing procedure is the storing of the documents. Your responsibility is to see that the items are placed in the proper folder, the proper section within the folder, and in proper chronological order within the section. You must also see that the folder is replaced in the proper position in the filing cabinet.

RECORDS DELETIONS AND CORRECTIONS
Deletions

Deletions are sometimes made in medical records in an effort to keep the file as concise and orderly as possible and to reduce the overall storage space required for medical records. Who determines what can be deleted is a very serious statement that should be declared in the office policy manual.

Only the physician should decide what specific material may be deleted from an office medical record. Medical assistants should never take it on themselves to make such a decision, even if an exact duplicate of a report is already in the record. The physician should always be consulted in cases of items that are not discussed in the policy manual.

It is recommended by most medical associations that information regarding documents removed from patient charts either be microfilmed or retained in a permanent storage area.

Delegated staff actions

Once a decision has been made on what material may be deleted, the physician may designate certain staff members to complete the procedure. This will usually be the administrative assistant. Should the physician decide to complete the task personally, the assistant should not take it negatively. Most physicians are rightfully very cautious with records because of their legal importance and because the physician is ultimately responsible for the contents and condition of the record.

Typical material deleted

The material that may be safely deleted from the medical record includes the following:

- Duplicates of diagnostic studies;
- Normal hospital studies over 3 years old; the hospital will have the originals if needed; retain any abnormal reports; and
- Insurance forms over 3 years old.

Individual progress notes or pages of notes should never be deleted from a medical record. Entry errors may be corrected as described later in this chapter.

Protecting confidentiality

Extreme care must be taken to make sure that material discarded from the patient's chart is disposed of properly. No one should be able to discern the patient's name or connect the name with a report when it is discarded. The best method is to completely destroy the document by burning or shredding. The other option is to tear the document carefully into very small pieces.

Corrections
Reasons for corrections

Occasionally it is necessary to make a correction in the progress notes of a patient's record. This occurs when incorrect data is recorded in the patient's record or an entry is made in the wrong chart. Incorrect data might be discovered while, for example, recording a patient's weight as 103 pounds and noting that it was recorded as 156 pounds on a previous visit. One of the notations must be incorrect. The fact should be rechecked and the entry corrected. Data can be recorded in the wrong chart if, for example, you have several charts in your hands at one time and inadvertently make an entry intended for the chart of one patient in the progress notes of another. Again, a correction is in order.

Correction technique

Any information noted in the chart, whether factual or not, becomes part of the permanent record. You must *never* attempt to obliterate a chart entry. If an error in charting is discovered you should do the following:
1. Strike a single line through the error.
2. Date and initial the strikeout.
3. If the problem is incorrect data, enter the correct information directly below the strikeout. Date and initial the entry.
4. If the entry is made in the wrong chart, follow Step 1 and note "Recorded in chart by error. Information transferred to chart of John C. Adams."
5. Date and sign the strikeout and explanation.

Step four is vital for legal purposes, because it can be verified. It is not considered a breach of confidentiality.

RECORDS PROTECTION
Records Temporarily Out of File Cabinet

The common reasons for taking a record out of the filing cabinet and the methods of monitoring its whereabouts using OUTguides were discussed earlier. However, you must protect and pay particular attention to medical records that are out of the office because they were subpoenaed. Most subpoenas require that the original document be submitted. If you *must* send a record out, be certain to photocopy at least the doctor's progress notes, since they can never be replaced.

Most subpoena services are prepared to microfilm a record in your medical office, although they may not volunteer the option. You should ask if it is possible, particularly for a sizeable record. You then avoid the possibility of losing the record in the mail and the additional cost of photocopying.

Keep a list of charts that must be sent out, the date they are sent, and to whom they are sent. If they have not been returned in 10 days, contact the subpoena service and ask them to locate the record and notify you of when it will be returned.

After Office Hours

At the end of each day all possible records should be returned to the filing cabinet for security purposes. As you leave the office, the cabinets should be closed and, if possible, locked. This will prevent scrutiny by maintenance-service personnel and will preserve them in case of fire.

Transfer of Files
Active to inactive status

Each office will establish a policy on when a record should be considered inactive and transferred to storage. In most situations this will depend on the following:
- Age of the chart (time since last visit);
- Type of practice; and
- Space available in the "active" filing cabinets.

Many offices find that 2 years since the last visit is an appropriate span for considering a record for storage. The other two elements are strictly individual.

Protection of transferred files

When a chart is transferred to inactive status, it may be stored on the premises or at some other location. In either case a list of inactive charts should be retained in the office to avoid unnecessary searching. A small file box containing 3 × 5 cards may be the most efficient technique of noting inactive charts, because the cards can be easily alphabetized when new names are added. Using OUTguides for this purpose would defeat the objective of saving space in the filing cabinet.

RETENTION OF MEDICAL RECORDS
Period of Retention
Options

There are ongoing debates about the amount of time records should be retained after certain events. These events include the following:

- Treatment of a minor;
- Closure of a case;
- Death of a patient;
- Retirement of the physician; and
- Death of the physician.

Opinions will vary from one state to another and by whether the opinions are those of an attorney, a medical association, or a management consultant.

When care involves a minor, the record should always be kept at least until the child becomes an adult and thereafter until local statute of limitations runs out.

Closure of a case, as in a specialist's care, may warrant destroying a chart after a given period of time. Most agree that the chart should be retained for at least 10 years.

After the uncomplicated death of a patient, some suggest that the chart be retained through the statute of limitations and then destroyed.

In the event of a physician's retirement, the charts of deceased patients may be destroyed after a selected period of time following the death. Following appropriate notification, as discussed in Chapter 5, the records of living patients may be transferred to the physician continuing the practice or to a physician of the patient's choice on receipt of a written authorization.

On the death of a physician, the patient's records are put under the care of a custodian of records, often the physician's spouse or a former employee who is willing to perform the duties involved. The disposition of the record is similar to the method that follows a physician's retirement.

General advice

Because of the increasing frequency of professional liability suits and the variations in statutes, many authorities are beginning to agree that the only safe option on record retention is retaining them forever. In other words, medical records should never be destroyed. If the physician retires or dies, the requested records should be forwarded and the others retained by the physician or his or her heir.

Storage Sites

Inactive records may be stored in specifically designed file storage boxes in a storage area on the office premises, with a professional storage company, or on microfilm. On the premises is the ideal option for an ongoing practice, because inactive records may be needed from time to time. Professional storage facilities are appropriate if the physician has retired or died, but this option causes re-

trieval problems for an active practice. Microfilm is an ideal option from the perspective of saving space, but it is relatively expensive.

INFORMAL RECORD SYSTEMS
Master Calendars

Medical assistants usually develop informal record systems to help them efficiently accomplish their varied responsibilities.

A master calendar, usually one that displays a month at a glance, allows you to list well in advance items and events that recur annually on the same date every month. You may then preplan the time necessary to deal with the events and assist the physician with notification of upcoming financial needs. The categories and the items included in master calendars are presented in Table 10.3 without further explanation, since the details are discussed in the various chapters of Part Two of this book. This list is offered now to alert you to the items and to demonstrate the integration of various duties.

Tickler Files

The common term for a file system designed to remind you of patients or events that require follow-up is a *tickler file*. The tickler file may take various forms, but it is always based on chronological order.

The most commonly used tickler file is maintained in a small file box containing 3×5 cards and dividers for each month of the year (Figure 10.5). At the beginning of each month, the cards in that section are pulled out, and the necessary action is taken. Each card will contain a separate activity or patient's name and the reason the card is in the file. Most often the cards are used to recall patients for routine examinations, such as physical examinations or annual Pap smears. You can notify the patient by telephone or mail. Once the appointment is made, the card may be inserted behind the divider for the same month the next year.

Some medical assistants prefer to use a desk calendar (Figure 10.6) as a tickler file. This can work very well if you are able to accomplish all the items noted on a given day. If not, you must take time to rewrite them on a subsequent day.

Medical Correspondence not Related to Patients

Every office receives a certain amount of correspondence that is medical in nature but unrelated

Figure 10.5
Tickler file.
Courtesy Colwell Systems, Inc,
Champaign, Ill.

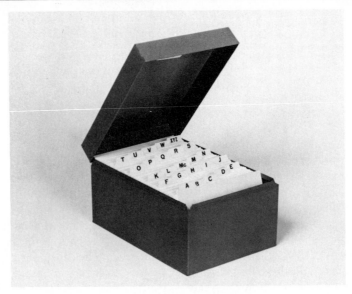

Table 10.3
Common items on a master calendar

Insurance premiums due	Routine payments	Renewal dates	Tax dates	Meetings	Holidays
Property	Salaries	Medical licenses	Federal tax deposits	Annual conventions	Traditional holidays
Life	Rent				
Health	Janitorial services	Narcotics licenses	State and federal quarterly taxes	Committees	Religious holidays
Professional liability	Leased equipment	Association membership	Annual state and federal tax filing (April 15)		Legal holidays
Disability	Laundry service Medical-surgical supplies	Subscriptions			

to individual patients. This correspondence can be stored by subject in separate folders for ready access. Materials that you will receive could be classified under the following headings:

- Professional associations;
- Physician's personal file (correspondence with friends and colleagues);
- General medical information such as Food and Drug Administration bulletins, drug company bulletins, and communicable disease statistics; and

- Business correspondence.

Correspondence regarding the business operations of the office also need to be retained in subject folders for future reference. These files might have the following titles:

- Rental agreements;
- Leased equipment;
- Maintenance contracts; and
- Bills to be paid.

Figure 10.6
Desk calendar.
Courtesy Colwell Systems, Inc,
Champaign, Ill.

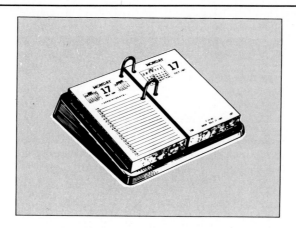

Financial Records

The permanent financial records must be stored in a secure and safe location, preferably a fireproof cabinet. These records include the following:

- Checks;
- Bank statements;
- Accounting ledgers;
- Bank deposit receipts; and
- Patient account records.

If these items have been used during the course of the day, they should be returned to their storage site before the office is closed.

Physician's Personal Records

Monitoring the physician's personal records is generally not your responsibility, but you may be asked to maintain a master list of the storage location of certain items such as the following:

- Wills;
- Property deeds;
- Insurance policies; and
- Contracts.

Most commonly these are stored in bank safety-deposit boxes.

Conclusion

The importance of a systematic approach to records management cannot be overly stressed. Records provide documentation for all medical care provided and for all business transactions.

Your role is fundamental to the development and maintenance of an effective and efficient records management system.

Review Questions

1. State the five major purposes for an organized records management system.
2. What options do you have in registering a new patient in your office? What information do you collect?
3. How would you organize the physician's notes in the medical record? How would you organize the diagnostic and hospital reports, correspondence, and insurance forms?
4. Develop a filing system based on the equip-

ment, possible systems, and procedures described in this chapter.
5. Who can decide what material to delete from a record? What material can usually be deleted?
6. What actions would you take to protect medical records temporarily out of the filing cabinet, after office hours, and when transferring files to inactive status?
7. How long should a medical record be retained? How can it be stored?

8. List some of the items you might include on a master calendar regarding insurance premiums, routine payments, renewal dates, tax dates, and meetings.
9. What is a tickler file? How does it work?

10. What techniques are used to store medical correspondence not related to patients, business correspondence, and financial records?

SUGGESTED READINGS

American Medical Association: Medicolegal forms with legal analyses, Chicago, 1981, The Association.

Campbell, C: Medical record management, ed 7, Berweyn, IL, 1981, American Medical Records Association

Johnson MM, and Kallaus NF: Records management, ed 2, Cincinnati, 1974, South-Western Publishing Co.

Chapter 11

Written Communication

- Importance of written communication
- Outgoing communication
- Incoming communication

Objectives

On completion of Chapter 11 the medical assistant student should be able to:

1 Define the terms listed in the vocabulary.

2 Discuss the importance of written communication.

3 List and describe the equipment necessary to produce outgoing written communications.

4 Discuss the four basic communication skills.

5 List and describe the three acceptable styles for letters and the 12 possible parts of a letter.

6 Describe the types of correspondence generated by the administrative medical assistant and the four basic steps followed in preparing the correspondence.

7 List the five Postal Service suggestions for preparing envelopes and describe the folds used for three different envelopes.

8 Contrast the four classes of mail.

9 Describe the five special services provided by the Postal Service.

10 Discuss the methods of handling five problems encountered with outgoing mail.

11 Discuss the four elements that should be included in office policy regarding incoming mail.

12 Describe the types of incoming mail, the proper sequence for stacking items, and the equipment needed to accomplish the task.

13 Discuss the medical assistant's role in annotating or responding to correspondence.

14 Describe the method of handling incoming mail when the physician is absent from the office.

Vocabulary

affidavit A written statement signed, as under oath, to affirm the truth of a document.

affix To attach.

annotate To reduce a written communication to a limited explanatory statement.

bond paper A superior quality paper with a firm surface used for correspondence.

confidential Private or secret.

consultation report The decision and plan determined necessary for the care of an individual.

correspondence An exchange of letters as a means of communication.

narrative An account of an observation or event in writing.

organizational title The official position of an individual within the structure of a business or company.

proofread To review a written work for errors.

stationery The paper and envelopes required for writing.

transcription The act or process of converting notes or dictation to a complete, typed form.

Written communication is the unspoken exchange of ideas between individuals who in many instances have never met one another. The manner in which communication to and from a medical practice is handled will affect the efficiency of the office.

IMPORTANCE OF WRITTEN COMMUNICATION
Method of Conducting Business

Written communication is the most common method of conducting business. There are plans to eliminate the need for traditionally written and transmitted communication in the not too-distant future. Information will be instantly transferred from one computer terminal to another, and if a record is needed, the computer will prepare a copy of the message. But for now, letters must still be dictated, transcribed onto stationery, and mailed to the person with whom you wish to communicate.

Provides a Permanent Record

Written communication provides a permanent record to document opinions or business transactions. Some communications will be stored in the patient's record to assist with his care; others will be put in business files. Should a question arise over an issue, a written document can settle the dispute. Communication pertinent to an office and copies of all communications from an office should be retained for future reference.

Outgoing correspondence

Any communication from an office produces an impression of you and your employer based on the quality of the letter. Individuals who have never met you will be forming opinions about you from your letter. It is very important that correspondence from your office be accurate and clearly stated to avoid misunderstandings and a possible negative effect on the office.

Incoming correspondence

Correspondence that arrives at your office must be handled in a timely fashion, that is, as soon as possible. Most incoming items require some action or response. You will be responsible for evaluating and processing the communications with particular attention to those that regard patients.

OUTGOING COMMUNICATIONS
Types

The most common communications that are sent out from a medical office are the following:
- Consultation reports;
- Narrative reports to insurance companies or social service agencies; and
- Business (nonmedical) letters.

The first two categories represent the bulk of the correspondence and relate to patient evaluations and care. The third category relates to services and purchases required to maintain the facility.

Equipment

Certain basic equipment is necessary to generate effective correspondence and process it for mailing. The production equipment includes the following:
- A typewriter or word processor;
- Dictation equipment;
- Correcting fluid or paper; and
- Dictionaries (standard and medical).

Processing equipment includes the following:
- A postage scale; and
- A postage meter or stamps.

For efficiency, all equipment should be located close to the administrative medical assistant's desk.

Word processors or typewriters

A word processor is a specialized computer that handles a variety of typing and editing functions. There are two basic sets of equipment that can be purchased or leased to provide word processing services for an office. One set includes an electronic typewriter and a television-type screen. The typewriter provides the keyboard to enter information onto a computer disk for storage and onto the screen for you to proofread before printing the permanent copy. Once the material is ready to your satisfaction, the typewriter becomes the printer. This set of equipment has the advantage of allowing you to use the typewriter independently or in conjunction with the computer processor. The other equipment set option includes a small keyboard that is similar to a typewriter keyboard, a viewing screen, and a printer. This set functions the same as the other one except that the typewriter cannot be used independently.

Word processors are increasing in popularity, particularly in offices that generate a large amount of correspondence and reports. Since many reports are redundant, with only minor wording changes, a word processor can significantly reduce the amount of typing that is required. The basic letter or report can be stored on tape cassettes or disks and displayed on the screen as needed. The variable information can be inserted before printing. After printing, the variable information can be removed so that the basic format is ready for the next use.

Other advantageous features of word processors include the following:
- Personalization of multiple letters;
- Rapid drafting or revision of lengthy documents;
- Adding, deleting, or moving words, phrases, sentences, or paragraphs without retyping the entire page or document;
- Automatic realignment of margins; and
- Automatic alignment of figures, tables, or graphs for statistical reports.

Word processing equipment can be purchased or leased for use in the office or facility. Should the employer not wish to acquire the equipment, there are word processing services available, some limited to medical services. These services often return the finished report within 24 hours and guarantee complete confidentiality. Since you may be involved with word processors, either through direct use or through a service, it is in your best interests to familiarize yourself with their potential functions and operations. You can anticipate increasing use of word processors as technology advances and prices are reduced.

Otherwise, the typewriter is the basic writing equipment to use in preparing correspondence. Your typewriter should be kept in good condition. Many offices keep a service maintenance contract that covers their typewriters to keep them in the best working order. Typewriters are available with pica (large) or elite (small) type. Many newer typewriters are single-element machines, which means they print using a movable ball rather than individual characters. This element eliminates the need for a movable carriage, allowing the typewriter to rest

in a more compact space. Elements are also available with a dual-pitch option, which allows the change from pica to elite type at will.

Some typewriters have regular keyboards and utilize the white correcting sheets. Others have a self-correcting key utilizing a lift-off tape; still others will incorporate a new feature called word spell, which allows for the verification of correct spelling. Many typewriters now incorporate a limited amount of memory for letters or reports that are frequently produced with minor changes.

Dictation equipment

Few physicians prefer to have assistants with shorthand skills these days. The vast majority prefer electronic dictating equipment. There is a large variety of equipment available. Many physicians use the smaller hand-held recorders that are voice activated and utilize microcassettes. This allows the physician to carry the microrecorder with them, using it as they see patients and visit hospitals, to dictate notes as they travel to and from facilities.

Correcting fluid or paper

If you do not have a self-correcting typewriter, you will need correcting fluid or paper to correct occasional typing errors.

Dictionaries

A standard dictionary and a medical dictionary should be readily available to check the spelling of words of which you are uncertain or to check whether you are using a word in the correct context. The new word spell computer-like dictionaries are available for checking the spelling of words, some of which carry from 60,000 to 500,000 words.

Postage scale

The amount of postage affixed to outgoing mail is based on the weight of each item. To be certain of the weight and avoid mail returns for additional postage, use a postage scale which are available at any business stationery store.

Postage

Offices with a high volume of mail often prefer the convenience of a postage meter. You can arrange to lease a postage machine and meter from several firms that can install the equipment and instruct you in its use. The serial number of the meter is registered with the post office.

When the meter is taken to the post office, a prepaid, set amount of postage is keyed into the meter by a postal employee, and a tamperproof seal is attached. You then set the meter for the desired postage and simply insert the envelope, or you may insert postage tape if the item to be sent is bulky. The display window that indicates the postage available will be reduced each time the meter is used. When the postage is depleted you must return the meter to the post office to be replenished, or you may now send a check for postage and within a day or two call a special number with your postage code. You will then receive a special code to key into the postage meter. This will then reset the meter to include the new postage amount. This avoids numerous trips to the Postmaster. Or, for the cost of postage plus a service fee, a postal representative will service the equipment at your office.

Some offices prefer to avoid the meter-leasing fee by periodically purchasing stamps. If you do not have a high volume of mail, this method may work well. Postage stamps may be purchased at the post office or by mail for a minimal service charge.

Letter service

The Postmaster and other larger mailing firms now offer either overnight delivery or twenty-four-hour delivery service. This service can be extremely useful and valuable when mail must reach its destination very quickly. Each of these services has a specially made envelope and mailing label to quickly identify this mail.

Stationery
Quality

The stationery selected for formal correspondence should be of high quality so that it will make a good impression. The quality of paper is determined by grades or by the weight of the paper. The materials used in making paper, wood pulp or cotton fiber, also affect its appearance. Business stationery is usually within the 16- to 24-pound weight range and contains at least 25% cotton fiber.

Size

Most offices purchase stationery in two sizes. The standard size letterhead ($8\frac{1}{2} \times 11$ inches) is considered the basic stationery for business letters and formal reports, with envelopes matching in size, weight, and fiber content. Brief, informal letters are usually sent on $7\frac{1}{4} \times 10\frac{1}{2}$ inch letterhead called *monarch* or *executive size* stationery, also with ap-

propriate-sized envelopes. The informal stationery should match the standard size in weight and fiber.

Embossed vs. engraved letterhead

The stationery letterhead can be applied in two ways. Engraving impresses each letter and number into the stationery—if you pass your fingertips over the engraved letterhead, it will feel flat. Embossing raises the letters and numbers above the surface—an embossed letterhead will feel "bumpy" to the touch. Embossing is considered the more elegant letterhead and is more expensive.

Second sheets and copies

Lengthy correspondence that requires a second page is continued on a plain sheet that matches the letterhead in quality. A copy of each letter is retained in the office, and additional copies are sometimes required for other persons interested or involved in the subject of the correspondence. "Copy sheets" are also available; they are much lighter in weight than the originals, and one margin is marked vertically in red letters with the word *copy*. The use of copy sheets has been greatly reduced in favor of the use of photocopy equipment.

Communication Skills
Spelling

Correct spelling is vital to the impression transmitted by written communication. If you know you have difficulty with spelling or are occasionally in doubt about a word, use the appropriate dictionary. Extreme care should be taken to spell all names correctly. The addressee's title and address should be verified if you are in doubt.

Punctuation

Standard methods of punctuation should be used throughout all correspondence. If the salutation of the letter is formal, stating the addressee's title or courtesy title (Mr. or Ms.) and last name only, it is followed by a colon. If the salutation is informal, using the addressee's first name, it is followed with a comma.

Transcription

Skill in transcription is developed primarily through practice and concentration. The quality of transcription may be influenced by the quality of dictation, but experience usually compensates for halting dictation.

Editing and proofreading

On especially important communication or communication that is still in the developmental stages, you may want to make a rough draft first. This draft is typed on utility-quality paper. Form is ignored, and the draft is double-spaced throughout to allow room for comments or changes. Comments and changes at this stage are referred to as *editing*. Once the draft is acceptable, the material can be prepared in final form.

Letter Styles
Physician's preference

The choice of which style to use in office correspondence is usually based on the physician's preference. If the physician does not show a preference, you may choose the style best suited to the practice and most convenient for the volume of correspondence.

Acceptable styles

Blocked.   In the blocked letter style, the dateline, subject line, complimentary close, and typed signature begin at the center point of the page. All other parts of the letter begin at the left-hand margin. For an example of this style, see Figure 11.1.

Semi-blocked.   The semi-blocked style is basically the same as the blocked style with the exception that the beginning line of each paragraph in body of the letter is indented five spaces. For an example of this style, see Figure 11.2.

Full blocked.   In the full blocked style all lines or all parts of the letter begin at the left-hand margin. For an example of this style, see Figure 11.3.

Parts of a Letter
Letterhead

The embossed or engraved letterhead is normally centered near the upper edge of the page and usually includes the physician's or agency's name and address and often the telephone number and practice specialty.

Dateline

The dateline indicates the date that the correspondence was transcribed and is placed two line spaces below the letterhead. The month should be spelled out in full, not abbreviated, followed by the day, a comma, and the year in four digits. The international order of writing the dateline, day first, then the month, and finally the year, is not considered appropriate.

Inside address

The inside address contains three and possibly more lines, all of which are flush with the left margin. It is placed a minimum of four single-line spaces below the dateline; more space is appropriate if needed to center the letter attractively. The inside address includes the following, listed in the order in which they should appear:

- Addressee's name;
- Organizational title, if appropriate;
- Company name, if appropriate;
- Street address or post office box number; and
- City, state, and zip code.

The addressee's name is preceded by a courtesy title such as *Ms., Mr., Dr.,* or *Prof.* If the addressee is a physician the courtesy title is omitted, and the initials *M.D.* follow the name.

Subject line

Placed two line spaces below the inside address, the subject line is usually centered regardless of the letter style used. This line is intended to alert the reader to the reason for the letter; centering it commands attention. The subject, frequently a patient, is preceded by *Re:* which means *regarding*. The subject line may be underlined for further emphasis.

Salutation

The salutation is a greeting to the addressee. It is placed two lines below the inside address or the subject line, whichever is lower. The greeting may be formal or informal. Each begins with the word *Dear,* followed either formally by a courtesy title and the addressee's last name or informally by the addressee's first name. If a physician is greeted formally, the courtesy title is not abbreviated *(Dr.)* but spelled out *(Doctor)*. Occasionally your employer will strike out a formally typed salutation to a colleague and write in the addressee's first name. This is a recognized technique of "personalizing" the correspondence.

Body of the letter

The body of the letter is begun two lines below the salutation, according to the style you have chosen:

Second-page heading

If a second page is necessary to complete a communication, it should have a heading for identification in case it is separated from the first page. The heading should include the addressee's name, the date, the page number, and the subject if it was

Figure 11.1
Example of blocked letter style.

RICHARD C. OSWALD, M.D.

2385 Bayor Road
Brookline, MA 02146

May 10, 1984

Robert C. Parsons, M.D.
Women's Clinic
240 Woodside Road
Boston, MA 02134

Re: Mary O'Malley

Dear Doctor Parsons:

I saw our mutual patient, Mary O'Malley, in my office today for a follow-up examination. As you are aware, she has been taking Dyazide, one tablet daily.

On physical examination: Weight 106 pounds. Blood pressure supine 120/80 in the right arm, pulse 86; standing 108/72 in the right arm, pulse 90. Lungs were clear to auscultation and percussion. Carotids were normal. There was no jugular venous distention present. Peripheral pulses were full, equal, and symmetric. Extremities revealed no edema, cyanosis, or clubbing.

An electrocardiogram, a copy of which is enclosed, was within normal limits.

I will be seeing Ms. O'Malley again in 3 months. If you have questions, please call me.

Sincerely,

Richard C. Oswald, M.D.

RCO:ep

Enclosure

used on page one. The heading for page two of a letter might read as follows:

Robert C. Parsons, M.D.   May 10, 1989
Re: Mary O'Malley   Page Two

Complimentary close

The complimentary close is the method of ending a communication, and the closure selected should be in keeping with the tone of the salutation. A for-mal letter should be closed *Very truly yours* and an informal one *Sincerely, Warm regards,* or *Best wishes.* The closure is placed two lines below the last line of the body of the letter, in the position appropriate to the style.

Typed signature

The typed signature is placed four lines below and flush with the complimentary close.

Figure 11.2
Example of semi-blocked style.

RICHARD C. OSWALD, M.D.

2385 Bayor Road
Brookline, MA 02146

May 10, 1984

Robert C. Parsons, M.D.
Women's Clinic
240 Woodside Road
Boston, MA 02134

Dear Doctor Parsons:

Mary O'Malley

   I saw our mutual patient, Mary O'Malley, in my office today for a follow-up examination. As you are aware, she has been taking Dyazide, one tablet daily.

   On physical examination: Weight 106 pounds. Blood pressure supine 120/80 in the right arm, pulse 86; standing 108/72 in the right arm, pulse 90. Lungs were clear to auscultation and percussion. Carotids were normal. There was no jugular venous distention present. Peripheral pulses were full, equal, and symmetric. Extremities revealed no edema, cyanosis, or clubbing.

   An electrocardiogram, a copy of which is enclosed, was within normal limits.

   I will be seeing Ms. O'Malley again in 3 months. If you have questions, please call me.

Sincerely,

Richard C. Oswald, M.D.

RCO:ep

Enclosure

Reference initials

The reference initials are placed two lines below the typed signature. The physician's initials are capitalized, and the transcriber's are in lower case. The initials are separated by a diagonal slash or a colon.

Enclosure or carbon copy notation

If the letter is accompanied by additional materials you will indicate this by stating *enclosure:* two lines below the reference initials. If others are to receive a copy of the letter, the initials *cc:* are noted two lines below the reference initials or the enclosure line, whichever is last. The notation *cc:* is followed by the name or names of those receiving a copy. If multiple copies are sent, the names are listed one below the other in alphabetical order or order of rank.

Signature of the sender

The physician will sign the letter after reviewing it for content and accuracy. If for some reason the physician is not available to sign the communication but instructs the transcriber to send it on com-

Figure 11.3
Example of full blocked style.

RICHARD C. OSWALD, M.D.
2385 Bayor Road
Brookline, MA 02146

May 10, 1984

Robert C. Parsons, M.D.
Women's Clinic
240 Woodside Road
Boston, MA 02134

Re: Mary O'Malley

Dear Doctor Parsons:

I saw our mutual patient, Mary O'Malley, in my office today for a follow-up examination. As you are aware, she has been taking Dyazide, one tablet daily.

On physical examination: Weight 106 pounds. Blood pressure supine 120/80 in the right arm, pulse 86; standing 108/72 in the right arm, pulse 90. Lungs were clear to auscultation and percussion. Carotids were normal. There was no jugular venous distention present. Peripheral pulses were full, equal, and symmetric. Extremities revealed no edema, cyanosis, or clubbing.

An electrocardiogram, a copy of which is enclosed, was within normal limits.

I will be seeing Ms. O'Malley again in 3 months. If you have questions, please call me.

Sincerely,

Richard C. Oswald, M.D.

RCO:ep

Enclosure

pletion, the transcriber can sign the physician's name, and follow it with a slash and the transcriber's initials. The transcriber may also insert a line two spaces below the typed signature stating, *dictated but not read,* which relieves the physician of complete responsibility for communication errors.

Correspondence Generated by Administrative Medical Assistant

Much outgoing office communication is the responsibility of the medical assistant. The skill and timeliness with which this communication is handled will reflect on the assistant and ultimately on the physician. Each letter that leaves a medical office reveals subtle information about the intelligence, ability, and efficiency of the writer.

Some of the medical assistant's correspondence responsibilities might include the following:
- Responses to patient inquiries on administrative procedures;
- Exchanges with suppliers and business associates;
- Account collections; and
- Exchanges with insurance companies.

Because of the importance of written communication, planning should be an integral part of each letter.

Preparing a Letter

Preparing a letter or any communication involves the following four basic steps:
- Organizing the information;
- Drafting a reply;
- Editing the rough draft; and
- Preparing the final draft.

It is a natural inclination to attempt to save time by bypassing some of these steps, but doing so rarely saves time and often results in lost time. The most important step is organizing the information. Note the word is *organize,* not *gather;* the information to be used in correspondence must be set down in a logical manner that can be easily followed by the reader.

Having the necessary information in the proper order will allow the other steps to be accomplished easily. You will note the similarity to the steps used by the physician when developing an important communication. A rough draft allows you to see your statements more clearly. Always review your own work critically, as if you were the recipient rather than the writer.

Preparing the Envelope

The proper preparation of the envelope is important for the correspondence to reach the addressee quickly. A business envelope is prepared with the sender's name and address printed in the upper left-hand corner. The addressee's name, company name, street address or post office box number, and city, state, and zip code should be typed on the face of the envelope.

Special notations

Special notations, such as *Attention: Ms. Adams* or *Personal,* should be placed in the lower left-hand corner on the face of the envelope.

In an effort to speed mail processing with the use of automated envelope readers, the Postal Service offers some suggestions for preparing the envelope. A sample of these guidelines follows:
1. When using the No. 10 envelope (business-letter size), you should begin typing the address 12 lines from the top and four inches from the left edge of the envelope. On smaller, standard-size envelopes (No. 6¾) begin the address down 12 lines from the top and 2½ inches from the left edge.
2. Use capital letters throughout the address.
3. Eliminate all punctuation.
4. Identify the state according to the standard two-letter state code (see Appendix D).
5. The last line of the address must contain the city, state, and zip code in 22 total spaces, including blanks between words. Since the state abbreviation, the zip code, and the spaces between the city and state and the state and zip code total 9 digit-spaces, the letters of the city must not exceed 13 digits. Approved abbreviations have been developed for cities with lengthy names.

The Postal Service expects to introduce their system in 1984. To reduce confusion, the *National Zip Code Directory* includes sections on abbreviation and instructions for mailing. When the automated system is introduced, instructions can be expected via direct mail to each business customer.

Folding Letters
Tri-fold for no. 10 envelope

Letters on standard business-size (8½ × 11) stationery are folded in thirds beginning at the bottom. The top is then folded down from the top. When completed, there will be three sections or two creases. The crease made by folding the top down is the edge to insert into a No. 10 envelope.

Tri-fold for no. 6¾ envelope

Letters or forms on standard-size sheets that must be inserted into No. 6¾ envelopes are folded in three motions that will produce the creases. The lower edge of the paper is lifted up and toward the top until the edges and corners match. The crease you make will produce a sheet folded in half. Next lift the right-hand edge and fold one third of the way across the page. Then lift the left-hand edge and fold over the previous one-third segment. The last crease made is the first inserted into the envelope.

Folding for window envelopes

The fold required for envelopes with windows is a tri-fold that resembles pleating. It is used for most statements that you receive in the mail. The first fold is made by lifting the bottom edge and creasing at one third of the length of the sheet. The correspondence is then placed face down and the free edge is lifted up and back so that the inside address is facing you. The sheet is then placed in the envelope with the inside address facing the window. Before sealing the envelope turn it over and be sure the entire name and address are visible through the window.

Affixing Appropriate Postage

Determine the weight of the item to be mailed with the aid of a postage scale. For first-class mail the first ounce is one fee, and each subsequent ounce is several cents less. Do not incorrectly calculate the total postage by multiplying the total ounces by the cost of the first ounce. Determine the total weight in ounces, subtract 1 ounce, and multiply by the fee for subsequent ounces. Add this amount to the fee for the first ounce to determine the total postage due. Affix the postage by meter or in stamps to the upper right-hand corner on the face of the envelope.

Classes of Mail
First class

First class mail includes rapidly processed correspondence such as handwritten or typed letters, postal cards, postcards, and business mail.

Second class

Newspapers and periodicals (magazines, journals) are mailed at second-class (reduced) rates under a special permit issued to publishers of printed materials that come out at least four times a year. The public can mail single copies of books or other printed materials at second-class rates if the item weighs less than 16 ounces. Items over this weight are mailed at fourth-class rates.

Third class

Third-class mail consists of unsealed or marked and sealed matter that weighs less than 16 ounces. This category includes circulars, booklets, catalogs, and so forth. Third-class mail is commonly called advertising mail.

Parcel post

Fourth-class mail is commonly referred to as parcel post and consists of all mailable matter that weighs 16 ounces or more and is not considered first-class or second-class mail. The upper limits of parcel post are 70 pounds or a total of 100 inches in combined length and circumference. Fourth-class mail must be packed and wrapped carefully because of the rough handling it receives.

Remember any package must be sealed with regular or reinforced packing tape approved by the postal service. Packages sealed with twine, string, masking tape, or cellophane tape will be rejected.

If in doubt about the proper class or most efficient way to send an item, call the local postal service information number. A postal employee will assist you.

Special Services
Certified mail

For a fee in addition to the regular postage, certified mail provides a record of delivery that is retained at the addressee's post office for 2 years. A return receipt, signed by the addressee or addressee's agent, can be acquired and returned to the sender to verify that the item was received. Another fee is charged for this service.

Registered mail

First class and priority mail may be registered if the contents are valuable. The value of the item is declared by the sender. The fee for this service is based on the declared value of the item, and the sender is given a receipt that must be retained until the item is received by the addressee. A return receipt may also be included with this service for an additional fee. If registered mail is lost or damaged in transit, the Postal Service will pay the declared value up to $10,000 if the item is not also insured by another source. If commercial insurance is carried on the item, the Postal Service can pay up to $2,000 in a coordinated effort with the insurance company to pay for the total value of the item.

Insured mail

Third-class and fourth-class mail may be insured against loss and damage up to $400. The insurance fee is based on the stated value of the item.

Express mail

Express mail is a fast intercity delivery system geared to the special needs of business and industry for fast, reliable transfer of time-sensitive documents and products. Overnight delivery is guaranteed, with 95% reliability.

The following are the five service options for express mail:

- Door to door—item is picked up at sender's office and delivered to addressee's office;
- Door to destination airport—item is picked up at sender's office and delivered to airport in addressee's city, where it is picked up;
- Sender's airport to addressee—item is taken by sender to nearest airport for direct dispatch to addressee;
- Airport to airport—item is dispatched to and retrieved from respective airports; and
- Regular express mail service—mail taken to designated postal facilities by 5:00 PM may be picked up at addressee's designated postal facility at 10:00 AM or delivered to addressee's office by 3:00 PM the next day.

Mailgrams

Mailgrams are a special service offered jointly by the Postal Service and Western Union. Messages charged by 100-word units may be dictated by telephone to Western Union, which transmits them to the destination city for next-day delivery by the Postal Service.

Special Problems
Change of address

If the office or agency site is to be changed, the Postal Service should be notified at least one month in advance. This will assure that mail is forwarded without delay. If the office moves to another city, you must sign a form accepting responsibility for the cost of forwarding all mail other than first-class items.

If you wish to locate an addressee who has moved without notifying the office, you should note *address correction requested* on the envelope. If the post office can forward the mail, the new address is noted on a card and returned to the sender with postage due for the service. This is money well spent if you are attempting to collect a large outstanding account.

Nonstandard mail

Extra postage will be required for items deemed nonstandard in size by the Postal Service. Since the criteria for determining nonstandard size involve minute and confusing measurements, many manufacturers of odd-sized envelopes place a notice in the spot where postage is to be placed stating *extra*

postage required. The fee schedule can be obtained from the Postal Service.

Tracing lost mail

If you believe that a piece of first-class, registered, certified, or insured mail is lost, you should notify the post office and complete the required forms. When reporting the loss you should bring along any receipts associated with the item.

Recalling mail

If you wish to intercept a mailed item before it is delivered to the addressee, you may make a written request, accompanied by an identically addressed envelope, to the local post office. If the letter is already in transit, the postmaster will attempt to intercept the item at the destination post office. Any expenses incurred, such as for long-distance telephone calls or telegrams, are the sender's responsibility.

Nonmail items dropped into mailbox

Should you inadvertently drop a nonmail item into a mailbox and you wish to retrieve it because of its value, a special procedure is required. Notify the Postal Service immediately, using the emergency number if after business hours. The Postal Service will take the location of the mailbox, your name, and the type of item lost. A "special pickup" will then be ordered. The person handling your call will advise you to wait at the mailbox and give you the approximate waiting time. When the driver arrives, the entire contents of the box will be collected, and the driver will advise you where you will be able to retrieve the item. Do not ask the driver for it; it is temporarily the property of the Postal Service.

Be prepared to provide a detailed description of the item and to sign affidavits before recovering the item.

INCOMING COMMUNICATIONS
Office Policy

Each medical office establishes a policy regarding the processing of incoming mail. This should include a statement about who is to process the mail, what may or may not be opened, how the mail is routed within the office, and where prepared mail is to be left for the physician.

Usually the administrative medical assistant will be responsible for processing all incoming correspondence. In the event that he or she is away from the office, a predetermined alternate employee will fulfill the responsibility. The alternate employee should be trained and prepared before he or she is needed.

Opening the mail

Office policy should be established regarding what mail can and cannot be opened and examined by the medical assistant. Usually items marked *Personal* or *Confidential* are left sealed and opened only by the addressee. The physician may also indicate specific items, such as bank statements or attorney correspondence, that are to remain sealed.

Routing incoming mail

Routing mail means separating it by addressee. Once this is accomplished, the items are either placed in a predetermined spot for pickup or delivered to the appropriate person. The larger the office or agency, the more formal the routing system will be.

Physician's mail

Each physician will have a preference about where the mail should be placed until it can be reviewed. The primary consideration is privacy, and the mail, opened or closed, should be placed out of the line of vision of callers to the office. Most physicians will want the mail placed on their desk.

Sorting Mail
Types of incoming mail

Mail is usually sorted and stacked according to class, with first-class mail on top. Following this technique, you or the physician will encounter the most important items first. If the mail has been properly sorted and stacked, the items you can expect to see, from top to bottom, will be as follows:
- Special delivery items or Mailgrams;
- Business correspondence;
- Payments from patients;
- Medical reports;
- Personal mail;
- Periodicals or newspapers;
- Pharmaceutical literature or samples; and
- Advertisements.

Equipment for Handling Mail

The equipment you will need to process incoming mail includes a letter opener, paper clips, a date stamp, and a stapler.

The letter opener should be firm, narrow, and sharp enough to slide under the sealing flap of an envelope and separate it without leaving ragged edges. Paper clips should be clean and without rough edges, since they are used to group pieces of correspondence that arrive in the same envelope. You will want to avoid soiling or tearing the paper.

Some offices use a date stamp to indicate on an item the date and time that it arrived in the office. This will assist you in evaluating the efficiency of the methods you use in responding to items that require an answer.

A stapler will be needed for securing small items enclosed in a letter or similar items that will be stored together, such as a series of laboratory reports made on the same day.

Processing Mail
Opening mail

The process of opening mail will be completed more efficiently if there is adequate working space and the necessary equipment is close at hand.

Presort the mail into separate stacks of mail you may not open, first-class mail, and so forth. All envelopes to be opened can then be placed facedown with the seals pointing the same direction so that each piece is in a ready position for insertion of the letter opener. After each item has been opened, it can be placed face up for the next step in the process. Mail for other employees can be set aside in the envelope for routing. Next, each item of correspondence for the physician or you is systematically removed from the envelope, and if the sender's address is not on the correspondence it is clipped to the envelope. Each letter is reviewed for needed action and to be sure that indicated enclosures are included. Missing enclosures should be noted on the correspondence, and the sender should be notified. Each item is then stamped with the date, if this is the office policy, and routed.

Annotation

Some physicians prefer that the medical assistant thoroughly review each piece of correspondence, highlighting the key points by underlining them in a highly visible color or briefly summarizing them in the margin. This process is called annotation, and it saves the physician a great deal of time. If the correspondence relates to a patient or previous communication, the necessary documents should be retrieved and attached to the current letter.

Responding to inquiries

As you gain experience with correspondence, you may be delegated the responsibility of responding to some inquiries without the physician's direction. This too will save time for the physician, and accepting the responsibility will enhance your value to the health care team.

Mail processed by the medical assistant

Beginning early in your career, you will be expected to handle certain items and inquiries that arrive in the mail. These responsibilities will include handling insurance forms and inquiries, payments from patients, pharmaceutical samples, and supply ordering. The details of handling these items are discussed in the various appropriate chapters.

When Physician is Away

When the physician is away from the office for meetings or vacations, you will need to adjust your technique of handling the mail. First, you will need to know precisely where the physician is and how to get in touch with him or her. Second, each piece of mail must be evaluated for the urgency of a requested response. The physician will need to be contacted regarding correspondence that cannot await his or her return.

Items that can await the physician's return but require an interim response will be handled by you. If the mail includes a notification of a meeting that will take place before the physician's return, you should notify the organization or meeting chairman to obtain an excused absence. Requests for reports, conferences, or records may be deferred, but the requester should be notified that the physician is away and will fulfill the request on his or her return. All mail needing the physician's attention should be stored in a safe and private location until it can be reviewed.

Conclusion

Developing skill in handling the various aspects of written communication will help you as an individual and project a positive image of you and your employer to patients and business contacts. Written communication requires constant attention, because it provides permanent documentation of events and transactions on details that you could not possibly remember. Constant monitoring of the system will assure its efficiency and effectiveness.

Review Questions

1. Why is written communication so important to a business?
2. What equipment is needed to prepare correspondence and process it for mailing? What is the purpose of each piece of equipment?
3. What skills will help you in preparing correspondence?
4. Prepare a letter in full-blocked style and label the 12 parts of the letter.
5. What steps will you take when preparing correspondence?
6. How will you determine which class of mail is correct for an item you are preparing to send?
7. What special services does the Postal Service provide?
8. Name and describe four problems you might encounter with outgoing mail.
9. Develop an office policy for handling incoming mail.
10. List in order the sequence in which you would stack incoming mail, beginning at the top of the stack.
11. How will you process the mail when the physician-employer is away from the office on vacation?

SUGGESTED READING

Strunk W Jr and White EB: The elements of style, ed 3, New York, 1979, Macmillan Publishing Co, Inc.

Chapter 12

Billing Systems

- Accounts receivable
- Data necessary for effective billing
- Billing services
- Billing considerations
- Credit and collection policies
- Collection system
- Special collection problems

On completion of Chapter 12 the medical assistant student should be able to:

1 Define the terms listed in the vocabulary.

2 Describe the importance of accounts receivable and the medical assistant's responsibilities to the office and patients with regard to the billing system.

3 List the basic information needed from the patient and the information provided by the office to form the foundation of an effective billing system.

4 List and describe the three basic in-office methods and the two methods from outside the office of providing bills to patients.

5 Compare the three options for computerized services.

6 Discuss the special considerations necessary for preparing a patient's statement, selecting a billing cycle, billing minors, or billing third-party payers.

7 Describe the reasons for establishing a credit and collection policy, the methods of informing patients of the policies, and the medical assistant's role in effective collection of accounts.

8 Discuss the three major components of an account collection system and the elements of each.

9 State the five special collection problems and the methods of managing each situation.

Vocabulary

accounts receivable A figure that represents the total dollars due to the physician who has provided services or goods.

asset Anything of value that belongs to a person or business and can be evaluated in dollar amounts.

computer memory bank The section of a computer that accepts the information you enter (type) into it and stores the data until you need it.

credit An extension of time allowed a customer or client to pay after a service has been provided.

data An organized collection of facts that can be analyzed and used to produce reports or documents.

debtor A person who owes money to an individual or a business.

emissary A person who acts as the representative or agent for another individual, particularly when diplomacy is needed.

intermediary Situated or coming between; acting as a harmonizing agent.

third party Someone other than the provider or the recipient of a service.

Patient billing systems provide the foundation for all financial functions and indeed for the survival of a medical practice. Payment for medical services is the source of income for the physician and, ultimately, for you.

ACCOUNTS RECEIVABLE

Accounts receivable is the term used to indicate in a dollar amount the medical services provided that still need to be paid for by patients. The figure that represents accounts receivable is the *total* amount due from all patients combined. The efficiency of the office billing system is often decided by the amount of the accounts receivable record.

Medical Assistant Responsibilities
To office

The primary responsibilities of the medical assistant in relation to the billing system are to maintain accurate billing procedures and to collect outstanding accounts receivable. The ability of the health care team to continue to provide medical services depends on the income generated by those services. The process is a complete cycle that must be monitored constantly for potential breaks.

To patients

The medical assistant primarily responsible for billing has the responsibility of educating the patient. This often involves explaining specific items noted on individual statements, since patients may be confused by the terminology or concerned about the fee. The educational process should actually begin before medical services are provided, at which time the medical assistant can explain to each new patient the office policy on fee establishment, account collection, and credit. Specific techniques of patient education will be discussed later in the chapter.

DATA NECESSARY FOR EFFECTIVE BILLING

To establish a billing system you will need two specific blocks of information. One of these is provided by the patient, and one is generated by the physician and the medical assistant.

Patient Information

Gathering information from the patient is the first step in establishing an account and integrating the patient into the billing system. This information includes:
- Patient's name, spelled correctly;
- Name of the person responsible for paying if other than the patient;
- Complete billing address (home);
- Complete medical insurance information; and
- Data for collection purposes.

The first four items are self-explanatory. The fifth, collection data, involves information that might be helpful in evaluating the patient's ability to pay or in locating a patient "lost to the practice," that is, difficult to trace. Collection data include employment status, name and location of employer, and unique identifying numbers such as Social Security or driver's license numbers. The method of obtaining all billing information was discussed in Chapter 10 (Figure 12.1).

Office-Generated Information

Once an account is established and medical services are begun, the remaining data needed to produce a bill will be generated by the physician and introduced into the billing system by the medical assistant. This information, known as transaction data, includes the following:
- The date of the visit or procedure;
- The five-digit insurance billing code that identifies each specific medical service;
- The fee for the service; and
- The diagnosis, stated and possibly in code.

Without both kinds of information—that provided by the patient and that generated by the provider—a statement of services cannot be sent.

BILLING SERVICES
In-office Billing Procedures
Typed statements

In the past, statements for medical care services were individually typed by the medical assistant each month. The process was extremely time consuming and eliminated the possibility for the medical assistant to assume more challenging responsibilities. This system is all but outmoded today ex-

Figure 12.1
Patient registration form.
Courtesy De A Eggers and Associates, San Rafael, Calif.

PATIENT REGISTRATION FORM

DATE

PATIENT ACCOUNT NUMBER

☐ **NEW**   ☐ **CHANGE**

PLEASE TYPE OR PRINT CLEARLY — (DR. CODE – R.D. CODE – CARRIER CODE FOR OFFICE USE ONLY)

PATIENT INFORMATION

PATIENT'S NAME - LAST, FIRST, MIDDLE INITIAL	DATE OF BIRTH	SEX	SOCIAL SECURITY #
	Mo Day Yr	☐Male ☐Female	

ADDRESS — STREET, APT. NO.	DOCTOR CODE	REFERRING DOCTOR	R D CODE
	EMPLOYER		

CITY	STATE	ZIP	TELEPHONE — HOME	TELEPHONE — OTHER

RESPONSIBLE PARTY FOR BILLING

NAME - LAST, FIRST, MIDDLE INITIAL	☐SAME AS ABOVE	PATIENT RELATIONSHIP TO RESPONSIBLE PARTY ☐SELF ☐SPOUSE ☐CHILD ☐OTHER

ADDRESS - STREET, APT. NO.	CITY	STATE	ZIP
	TELEPHONE - HOME	TELEPHONE - OTHER	

INSURANCE

PRIMARY INSURANCE CARRIER NAME, TELEPHONE	CARRIER CODE	POLICY/ID#	GROUP#

INSUREDS NAME - LAST, FIRST, MIDDLE INITIAL	☐SAME AS ABOVE	EMPLOYER	EMPLOYER PLAN COVERAGE ☐YES ☐NO

ADDRESS - STREET, APT. NO.	PATIENT RELATIONSHIP TO INSURED ☐SELF ☐SPOUSE ☐CHILD ☐OTHER
	TELEPHONE - HOME	IF CHAMPUS ☐ACTIVE ☐RETIRED ☐DECEASED

CITY	STATE	ZIP	SOCIAL SECURITY #	BRANCH OF SERVICE:

SECONDARY INSURANCE CARRIER NAME, TELEPHONE	CARRIER CODE	POLICY/ID#	GROUP#

INSUREDS NAME - LAST, FIRST, MIDDLE INITIAL	☐SAME AS ABOVE	EMPLOYER	EMPLOYER PLAN COVERAGE ☐YES ☐NO

ADDRESS - STREET, APT. NO.	PATIENT RELATIONSHIP TO INSURED ☐SELF ☐SPOUSE ☐CHILD ☐OTHER
	TELEPHONE - HOME	IF CHAMPUS ☐ACTIVE ☐RETIRED ☐DECEASED

CITY	STATE	ZIP	SOCIAL SECURITY #	BRANCH OF SERVICE:

Please remember that insurance is considered a method of reimbursing the patient for fees paid to the doctor and is not a substitute for payment. Some companies pay fixed allowances for certain procedures, and others pay a percentage of the charge. It is your responsibility to pay any deductible amount, co-insurance, or any other balance not paid for by your insurance.

IN ORDER TO CONTROL YOUR COST OF BILLINGS, WE REQUEST THAT OUR CHARGES FOR OFFICE VISITS BE PAID AT THE CONCLUSION OF EACH VISIT.

If this account is assigned to an attorney for collection and/or suit, the prevailing party shall be entitled to reasonable attorney's fees and costs of collection.

To the extent necessary to determine liability for payment and to obtain reimbursement, I authorize disclosure of portions of the patient's record.

I hereby assign all medical and/or surgical benefits, to include major medical benefits to which I am entitled including MediCare, private insurance, and other health plans to:

This assignment will remain in effect until revoked by me in writing. A photocopy of this assignment is to be considered as valid as an original. I understand that I am financially responsible for all charges whether or not paid by said insurance. I hereby authorize said assignee to release all information necessary to secure the payment.

SIGNED _____ DATE _____

cept in practices that involve a limited number of patients. Practices of this type either do not require much income or charge a substantial fee for each service.

Another consideration in the use of this billing system is the changes that have occurred in the education of the professional medical assistant. Today's medical assistants are prepared to assume a wide variety of duties, and their time and talents would be wasted on this type of billing system.

Ledger cards

Ledger cards are forms printed on firm paper that are designed to record the financial activity of an individual patient. The card provides spaces for the patient's name and address and then a series of columns in which to .record the date and type of transaction and the current balance due. Transactions may be typed or handwritten onto the ledger card as they occur so that the balance in the last column is always current.

Ledger cards used alone are processed monthly by the medical assistant, who must photocopy each ledger card with a balance, fold the copies, insert them along with a return envelope into a window envelope, affix the postage, and mail them. It is possible to lease equipment that will fold, stuff, seal, and apply postage automatically, but it is relatively expensive. It might be wiser to apply the money to a billing service that will also assist you with cumulative accounting information and status reports to help monitor the efficiency of the billing system. Discussion of these systems follows.

Pegboard systems

Pegboard systems are unique in that they allow you to retain control of your billing system within the office while adding insurance and accounting features. Because it can perform several functions at once, the pegboard is also referred to as the Write-It-Once system.

The term *pegboard* is derived from the appearance of the equipment used to hold the various forms. The board is made of lightweight metal and is appropriately sized for the average desk. The pegs extend down the left-hand edge to hold the corresponding perforations on the accounting sheets.

Pegboard systems are still very popular in medical offices because they eliminate the need to write the same information several times to achieve the results the pegboard gets with one writing.

The cost to establish a pegboard system can vary from approximately $200 to $750, depending on the features you select and the printing fees.

The basic system shown in Figure 12.2 includes the following:
- Patient charge slip and receipt;
- Ledger cards;
- Journal page; and
- Folding pegboard.

You may choose to include a feature commonly called the *superbill* (Figure 12.3). This multicopy slip is a patient charge slip, a receipt, and a form that the patient can use to bill his own insurance carrier. You may select from standard superbills or design one to meet your needs. The initial imprinting adds to the cost of establishing the system and is proportional to the superbill design.

You can see the advantageous role the superbill can play in saving you the time that would be spent billing patients' insurance carriers. The overall cost of the system can be quickly recovered in time that might otherwise have been spent collecting past-due accounts.

Alternative Billing Services
Microfilm billing

Microfilm billing is a service that may be used in conjunction with ledger card- or pegboard-type systems. A representative of a microfilm company comes to your office at least once a month and uses a portable microfilm camera to photograph each of your ledger cards that has an active balance. The filming process generally takes no more than 20 minutes. The film is then forwarded to the company plant for processing.

Once the film is developed, statements are printed, stuffed along with return envelopes, and mailed directly to the patients. If requested, collection or recall messages may also be included.

Microfilming allows the personal aspect of maintaining ledger cards while eliminating the chore of processing them. An added benefit is the protection of your accounts receivable records, because a microfilm copy of your ledger cards is retained at the company. Should anything happen to your account cards the company can supply you with the information to reconstruct them.

Computerized services

As a practice grows, caring for greater numbers of patients or perhaps adding more physicians to the group, the billing system will need to be updated. Manual systems, such as typed statements or ledger cards, may be too time consuming to be profitable. Computer systems or services are becoming recognized as an efficient alternative. There are four basic computerized billing services that readily

Figure 12.2
Pegboard display.
Courtesy Colwell Systems, Inc, Champaign, Ill.

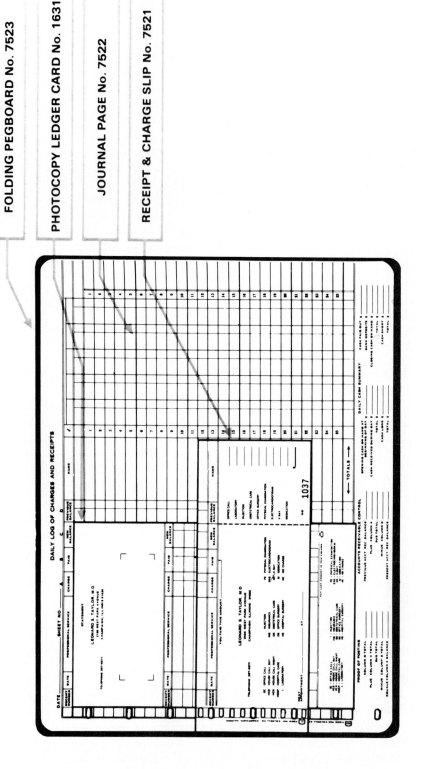

FOLDING PEGBOARD No. 7523

PHOTOCOPY LEDGER CARD No. 1631

JOURNAL PAGE No. 7522

RECEIPT & CHARGE SLIP No. 7521

pegboard saves space on desk.
(Folding board only 8¾" x 11")

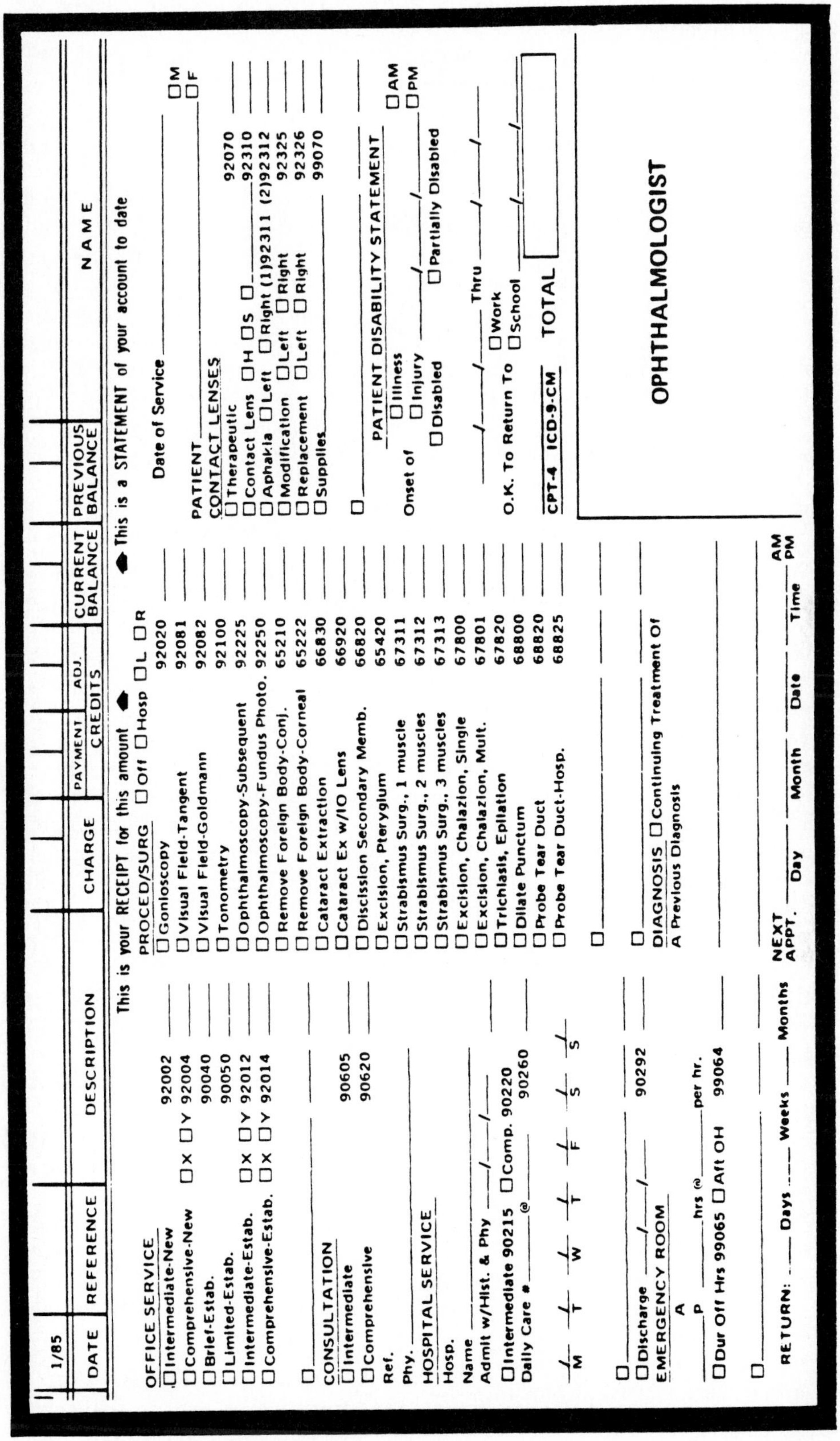

Figure 12.3
Superbill.

DATE	REFERENCE	DESCRIPTION	CHARGE	PAYMENT	ADJ. CREDITS	CURRENT BALANCE	PREVIOUS BALANCE	NAME

1/85

This is your RECEIPT for this amount ◆ □ Off □ Hosp □ L □ R

◆ This is a STATEMENT of your account to date

PROCED/SURG

□ Gonioscopy	92020
□ Visual Field-Tangent	92081
□ Visual Field-Goldmann	92082
□ Tonometry	92100
□ Ophthalmoscopy-Subsequent	92225
□ Ophthalmoscopy-Fundus Photo.	92250
□ Remove Foreign Body-Conj.	65210
□ Remove Foreign Body-Corneal	65222
□ Cataract Extraction	66830
□ Cataract Ex w/IO Lens	66920
□ Discission Secondary Memb.	66820
□ Excision, Pterygium	65420
□ Strabismus Surg., 1 muscle	67311
□ Strabismus Surg., 2 muscles	67312
□ Strabismus Surg., 3 muscles	67313
□ Excision, Chalazion, Single	67800
□ Excision, Chalazion, Mult.	67801
□ Trichiasis, Epilation	67820
□ Dilate Punctum	68800
□ Probe Tear Duct	68820
□ Probe Tear Duct-Hosp.	68825

OFFICE SERVICE

□ Intermediate-New	92002
□ Comprehensive-New □ X □ Y	92004
□ Brief-Estab.	90040
□ Limited-Estab.	90050
□ Intermediate-Estab. □ X □ Y	92012
□ Comprehensive-Estab. □ X □ Y	92014

CONSULTATION

□ Intermediate	90605
□ Comprehensive	90620

Ref.
Phy.

HOSPITAL SERVICE

Hosp.
Name
Admit w/Hist. & Phy
□ Intermediate 90215 □ Comp. 90220
Daily Care # @ 90260

M T W T F S S

□ Discharge 90292
EMERGENCY ROOM
A
P hrs @ per hr.
□ Dur Off Hrs 99065 □ Aft OH 99064

RETURN: ___ Days ___ Weeks ___ Months

Date of Service _____

□ M
□ F

PATIENT _____

CONTACT LENSES

□ Therapeutic		92070
□ Contact Lens □ H □ S □		92310
□ Aphakia □ Left □ Right (1)	92311	(2)92312
□ Modification □ Left □ Right		92325
□ Replacement □ Left □ Right		92326
□ Supplies		99070

□ _____

PATIENT DISABILITY STATEMENT

Onset of □ Illness □ AM
□ Injury □ PM
□ Disabled □ Partially Disabled

_____ / _____ Thru / _____

O.K. To Return To □ Work
□ School

CPT-4 ICD-9-CM **TOTAL** [   ]

OPHTHALMOLOGIST

DIAGNOSIS □ Continuing Treatment Of A Previous Diagnosis

□ _____

NEXT APPT. ___ Day ___ Month ___ Date ___ Time ___ AM PM adapt to a medical practice: (1) batch systems, (2) full-service systems, (3) on-line systems, and (4) in-house mini or microprocessors. When a practice uses a computer system, each patient is usually assigned an account number. This number then becomes another element in the transaction data and must be used to process any transaction for that patient.

Batch systems. The "batch" method of computerized billing involves compiling all new patient information, each day's transactions (that is, charges, payments, plus adjustments, and minus adjustments). The "batch" may be made up of one copy from the superbill or charge slip of each patient seen during the day. These will be clipped together with an adding machine tape for all of the charges for the day. An additional group of forms will be used to record all of the payments and adjustments for the day. Again, these should be clipped together with an adding machine tape totalling all payments and adjustments. When the "batch" arrives at the computer billing company, a data entry operator will enter the data into the physician-client data bank.

Full-service system. The full-service system of computerized billing involves the same data collection compilation as the batch. Usually with this type of service the service bureau will process all charges, payments, or adjustments and will produce all statements, insurance forms, reports, and recall notices. The practice will be provided with the reports as agreed upon with the physician-client. The service bureau will proceed to monitor all patient accounts with the patient and/or third-party payer. With this type of system the service bureau follows the account through collection. Usually the payments will be received and recorded by the physician's office, with the service bureau receiving a percentage of the collected income for this service. A variation of this might be that the service bureau charges the physician-client by the number of transactions recorded per month.

On-line systems (in-house terminal with direct transmission). On-line computer systems do not eliminate the need for writing out the transaction data. There must always be a source document, that is, a charge slip or payment record. The office is equipped with a computer terminal. A cathode ray tube (CRT) screen usually rests above the terminal; this may be one or two pieces. Together they look like a typewriter with a small television screen. This is linked to a computer that may be in a building many miles away from your office. There are two methods of connecting the CRT with the computer. One method may be to dial a specific number at the computer center. You will wait to hear a high-pitched tone. You will then place the receiver into what is called a "modem." This modem then links the CRT with the computer. The other method is called "hard wire," which means that the CRT and the computer are directly connected and may be used as needed. No matter which method is utilized, you will need a "password" to communicate with the computer processing unit. Each physician-client will be provided with a password or series of passwords. After typing the password, you will be allowed to communicate with the computer. Anything keyed (typed) into the computer usually appears on the screen within a few seconds. This is how each patient transaction is recorded. You may also request to see data previously stored in the computer, and it will appear on the screen (Figure 12.4).

Mini-microprocessor. The basic equipment of mini-microprocessors includes the CRT, terminal, computer, memory bank, and a printer. The printer allows the office to print on paper the data input into the computer. This is considered an in-house system and does not require that there be outside connection by telephone.

BILLING CONSIDERATIONS

Regardless of the type of billing service used, there will be many considerations that must apply. If you work as the practice receptionist, you will often be responsible for obtaining all information needed to complete accurate billing.

Statement Preparation

It is important to the office records and particularly to the patient that the data on the statement be completely accurate. Any error in the information will be upsetting to the patient and will require corrective measures for the office records. Accuracy must be assured for all elements of transaction data but particularly for the procedure code and the fee.

It is also important that the itemization of the services provided be precise and easily understood. If the statement is clear, it will minimize the number of telephone calls to the office requesting explanations.

Billing Cycle
Planning and preparation

Generally, the term *billing cycle* refers to the time lapse you select to occur between statements. To

Figure 12.4
Computerized billing equipment.
Courtesy Pacific Medical Center,
San Francisco, Calif.

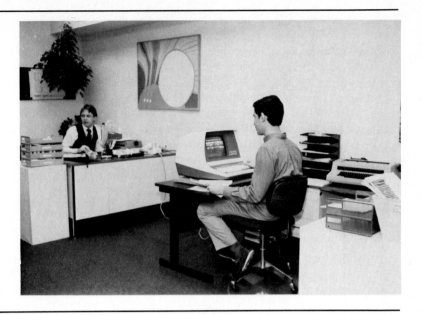

initiate the cycle you should select the date on which you want the statement to arrive at the patient's home. Financial consultants frequently suggest that statements arrive 3 to 5 days before the end of the month to take advantage of first-of-the-month paydays. Next, determine the cut-off date. The cut-off date represents the last day of patient transactions that will appear on the statement. Each billing system requires a different number of days to prepare the statements for mailing. If you will be typing 25 statements, a 1-day task, your cut-off date will be the day before the statement should arrive. Microfilm and batch computer services usually require 5 days, therefore the cut-off date will be 5 working days before the delivery date. Depending on the cycle you have chosen, and the demands of your billing service, you can plan the advance time needed to prepare or submit the data needed for statements.

Cycles based on practice needs

The once-a-month billing cycle is the most common in medical practices. Physicians and medical assistants find this system the least disruptive and the most amenable to advance planning.

Intermittent-cycle billing refers to the technique of billing predetermined segments of the accounts receivable at various times throughout the month. This system is usually used by companies with credit-card customers because of the extremely large volume of statements they handle. The account segments are usually decided alphabetically. An office might decide on four monthly billings, so that cycle 1 statements would be sent to patients whose names begin with the letters *A* through *F*, cycle 2 statements to those whose names begin with *G* through *L*, and so forth.

The major advantage to intermittent-cycle billing is that the income payments occur relatively evenly throughout the month. Once-a-month cycles tend to generate the greatest amount of income during the first week after statements are received, and income dwindles down to nothing the week before statements are to be sent. The disadvantage to intermittent-cycle billing is that the medical assistant responsible for the billing system feels constant pressure about meeting deadlines and handling patient financial issues.

Billing Minors or Third-party Payers
Minors

Billing for services provided to minors requires special attention to certain legal details. You will be expected to make determinations on financial responsibility and appropriate preparation of statements.

Determination of responsible party. Since a minor cannot legally be held responsible for any financial statement, you must determine at the time of the *first* visit the person legally responsible for the child. You must remember that this is not always the child's parents; even children with living parents can be in the legal guardianship of another person. You might pay particular attention to the child who is brought in for care by someone other than a parent. If you are billing an insurance company for the minor, please note that many states have implemented the coordination of benefits "birthday rule." Except for cases of dependent children of divorced or separated parents, the rule stipulates that the health plan of the person whose birthday falls earlier in the year (month/day/not year) will pay first and the plan of the other person covering the dependent will be the second payer.

If the persons with the two plans covering the same dependent have the same birthday, the plan of the person who has had the coverage longer is the primary payer.

If either of the two plans has not adopted the "birthday rule" (that is, if one of the plans is in another state), the rules of the plan without the "birthday rule" will determine which plan is primary and which is secondary.

Address statement to responsible party. The account and the statement should not be addressed to the minor, even with a *c/o—in care of* notation naming the responsible party. The appropriate method is to fully address the statement to the responsible party with an *Re:* notation naming the minor.

Separated or divorced parents. A legal determination of custody and legal responsibility will have been made in the case of a child of divorced or legally separated parents. The parent with legal custody is responsible for the child's debts. In the event of joint custody, the parents are jointly responsible.

Emancipated minors. Individuals who are 16 years of age or older but not yet 18 who live outside of their parents' residence, and who are independent financially are legally responsible for the debts they incur.

Third-party payers

In some instances an individual or organization will request that a patient be given a special examination or evaluation. The one who requests the service accepts financial responsibility and is termed the *payer*. Since the payer is not the patient or the physician, he is considered a third party in the arrangement, thus the term *third-party payer*. Some of the organizations or individuals in this classification are discussed in the sections that follow.

Examinations requested by insurance companies. Insurance companies frequently request the services of an independent physician, one unknown to the patient, for an objective evaluation of his health status or a determination of the degree of disability.

Worker's Compensation cases involve individu-als who are injured or acquire an illness in the course of their job. Financial settlements are often determined on the basis of the opinion of the physician. Some physicians even limit their practices to Workmen's Compensation cases, and their fees are paid by the Workmen's Compensation insurance company.

Individuals who apply for life insurance or who are to be insured as a benefit of their jobs are often given physical examinations that are paid for by the insurance company.

Examinations requested by social services. Some claims for federal disability benefits are made by individuals with complex problems. In an effort to determine the degree of disability, social services agencies may pay a physician for an independent evaluation. This is particularly likely to occur if the claimant disagrees with a previous determination by the agency.

Examinations requested by attorneys. Physicians may examine a client or claimant at the request of either the plaintiff or the defense attorney. In criminal cases, the request may come from the prosecutor. The fee is paid by the attorney who requests the examination.

Examinations ordered by the court. Numerous cases have occurred, particularly in custody battles, where one parent is trying to prove that placing the child with the other parent is detrimental to the child's welfare. Thus a judge may order either a physical or psychological evaluation of the child and/or the parents. Usually the judge will stipulate who is responsible for payment of the evaluation. You will then coordinate billing with the attorney or attorneys for the designated responsible party.

CREDIT AND COLLECTION POLICIES
Reasons for a Policy

The subject of credit, the accumulation of debt, and the collection of accounts is a delicate situation that must be handled tactfully and legally by the medical assistant. An established policy will guide the medical assistant in this important function.

The most important reasons for a policy are that it does the following:

- Establishes guidelines for informing patients of payment procedures;
- Standardizes the information given by all employees to all patients; and
- Reduces the overall costs to all patients by avoiding the expense of repeated billing and possibly collection agency fees.

Methods of Informing Patients
Patient information pamphlet

Some physicians choose to convey their policy to patients in writing by providing them with an informative pamphlet. Other physicians may be timid about discussing financial issues in the pamphlet. They should be reminded of the importance of finances to the office, and the subject should be discussed frankly. Since the pamphlet will discuss a number of policies, a discussion of finances will not look out of place.

Personal discussion

The other method of introducing the patient to office credit policies is to discuss policies privately with the patient at the time of the first visit. It is interesting to note that the medical assistant, rather than the physician, is often viewed as the financial manager. This perception can be used to the benefit of the office, since the patient perceives the discussion as taking place with a person of authority.

Discussion reinforcement. It may be effective to reinforce the office policy by giving the patient a copy of the policy pamphlet after the discussion. The patient can read it at his leisure and keep it for future reference. The pamphlet also eliminates a patient claim of lack of knowledge of the policy.

Medical Assistant's Influence on Collections

Management of the billing system includes the collection of unpaid and overdue accounts. The medical assistant's effectiveness in account collection depends on his or her attitude when explaining the office policy on accounts with overdue balances. It is important that the conversation be conducted diplomatically and in a routine, matter-of-fact manner. You should convey a positive and nonthreatening attitude based on the assumption that all fees will be paid and that your reason for the discussion is merely to describe the office policy on billing and credit.

COLLECTION SYSTEM
Current Accounts Receivable

The most effective techniques in managing accounts that represent money owed to the office are to give close attention to each account as each fee is entered and also to make the patient aware of it.

Charge slips or superbills

Using a charge slip or a superbill is one method of making patients immediately aware of the fees incurred during a visit. The slip is given to patients by the administrative assistant at the end of each visit to hold as a receipt or to submit to their insurance company for reimbursement. Since the slip includes the charges of the day and any outstanding amounts due, patients are reminded of the total amount due to the office. Personally receiving the slip from the medical assistant subtly reminds patients that the staff is equally aware of the balance due.

Payment at time of visit

Many offices or agencies request payment at the time services are rendered. This is possible in some types of practices, such as internal medicine, pediatrics, or family practice, in which the fee is predictable. It may not be possible when major fees for services are involved, such as in surgery or orthopedics, and the patient usually cannot be expected to be financially prepared.

If office policy directs you to collect at the time of service, you will need to be diplomatic but direct with the patient. Since the policy will have been described to the patient in an information pamphlet or discussed in advance of the first visit it will not be a surprise, but it may need reinforcing. It is particularly important if the patient is to be seen only once or is an out-of-town visitor. Some offices post a sign, clearly visible to waiting patients, that states "Payment is expected at the time service is rendered." Another technique is to remind the patient of the fee when he stops at your desk with the superbill that the physician has signed after checking off the appropriate services. After you have calculated the fee from a prepared list corresponding to the service codes you may return the slip to the patient and simply state, for example, "The charge for today, Ms. Smith, is $20.00." The message is clear yet professional.

Charge cards

Credit cards have become a common method of acquiring and paying for goods and services. Some cards, such as Visa and Mastercard, are known as bank cards and can be used for many things. Responding to patient requests and the wish to improve collections, some physicians accept bank cards as a method of payment for services. When the charge slip is sent to the card company, the physician is paid the amount due minus a fee (1% to 3% of the total due) for the card company's services. The card company must then collect the amount due from the person who charged the ser-

Figure 12.5
Federal Truth in Lending
Statement.
Courtesy Colwell Systems, Inc,
Champaign, Ill.

LEONARD S. TAYLOR, M.D.
2100 WEST·PARK AVENUE
CHAMPAIGN, ILLINOIS 61820

TELEPHONE 352-7658

FEDERAL TRUTH IN LENDING STATEMENT
For professional services rendered

Patient _____

Address _____

_____

Parent _____

1. Cash Price (fee for service) $ _____

2. Cash Down Payment $ _____

3. Unpaid Balance of Cash Price $ _____

4. Amount Financed $ _____

5. FINANCE CHARGE $ _____

6. Finance Charge Expressed As
   Annual Percentage Rate   _____

7. Total of Payments (4 plus 5) $ _____

8. Deferred Payment Price (1 plus 5) $ _____

"Total payment due" (7 above) is payable to _____
at above office address in _____ monthly installments of $ _____
The first installment is payable on _____ 19 ____ , and
each subsequent payment is due on the same day of each consecutive month
until paid in full.

_____   _____
    Date   Signature of Patient; Parent if Patient is a Minor

FORM 9402 COLWELL SYSTEMS, INC. CHAMPAIGN, ILLINOIS

vices. All credit card companies charge the patient interest or finance charges on the amount due.

Billing patients for services

In practices in which patients are allowed to accumulate the charges for services and are billed at the end of the cycle, you will need to inform them of the policy associated with this method. Patients must understand that this is an added service and that the account should be paid in full each month.

While physicians are always willing to recognize special situations and accept partial payments each month until the account is paid off, usually without a finance charge, the practice should not be encouraged. If a finance charge is to be added to the unpaid balance the patient must be notified in advance, in writing, based on the "Truth In Lending" laws (Figure 12.5).

Some patients will feel that it is acceptable to wait for payment from insurance companies and expect you to keep track of their claims. You must explain that help with filing patients' insurance claims is an added service, and that you cannot act as an intermediary between patients and their insurance companies. Doing so could become very time consuming, and some insurance companies feel that your inquiry is a breach of client confidentiality. You may print a simple statement explaining this on the back of the patient's receipt or superbill.

Aging Accounts Receivable
Definition of aging

Aging is a term applied to the technique of classifying each account with a balance due by the length of time the amount has been owed to the office. Since statements are usually sent once a

Billing Systems *Chapter 12*

month, the aging segments are stated in terms of 30, 60, 90, and over 90 days, averaging all months out to 30 days each.

The amount on a patient's statement that represents new services provided during the present month are classified as current or "this-month" charges. The day statements are sent to patients for current charges is day one or the day aging begins. If the charges have not been paid by the time the next statement is sent, the account is considered 30 days old because the patient has had 30 days in which to pay the fees. Each time statements are sent and the fees have not been paid the amount ages 30 more days. You might think of it as you do your birthday; you become age one by starting to count from the day you were born. A financial account reaches a new category by counting from the day the statement was first sent.

Reasons for aging accounts

Evaluating system. Separating accounts into aging categories allows you to see at a glance the effectiveness of your collection system. Once each account has been classified and the appropriate dollar amount of each account has been entered in the correct category, you will be able to calculate the total amount due in each aging bracket. You may also determine the percentage each age category represents.

Statistics, in the form of dollar totals and percentages, help you and the physician decide if your collection techniques are working. The largest percentages should be in the current month's charges, next largest in the 30-day category, and so forth; the smallest percentage should be in the "over 90 days" group. Collection experts agree that you can consider a problem to exist if 10% or more of the accounts receivable are 90 days or older. The office accountant can help you and the physician determine appropriate percentages for each category and make changes in the collection system to improve the situation.

Alerting personnel. Aging techniques will alert you to the specific accounts that require your attention. Using a form such as the one shown in Figure 12.6 is one method you can use to make this determination easily and to note the specific action taken to collect the account. Collection techniques will be discussed later in this chapter.

Methods of aging

Aging by hand. If you use an in-office billing system, such as typed statements or ledger cards, you will need to age the accounts by hand. This can be accomplished by using a sheet such as the one shown in Figure 12.6.

As you can see, it is possible for one account to have amounts due in several age categories if charges for services provided in various months remain unpaid. Figure 12.7 demonstrates how the dollar amounts shown in Figure 12.6 were determined. Any partial payment made is subtracted from the *oldest* portion of the account. When the $20 was paid on 11-15-84, it was applied toward the $70 debt incurred on 9-12-84, only partially reducing the oldest segment of the account.

To complete the process you will need to determine the total dollars represented in each column and calculate the percentages they represent. The dollar totals are acquired by simply adding together each amount in each column. The percentages are determined by separately dividing the total of each column by the accounts receivable total. The formula is as follows:

$$\frac{\text{Age category total}}{\text{All accounts receivable total}} = \text{Category percentage}$$

Example:

$$\frac{\$500}{\$5,000} = 10\%$$

In other words, if your accounts receivable total is $5,000 and your 90-day-old accounts total is $500, 10% of the total accounts receivable has been overdue from patients for 90 days.

Computer systems. If you use a computer-assisted billing service, the computer will produce an aging report for you upon your "demand" or request. This report is separate from the report of all accounts and may list only those accounts with balances 30 days old or older. If an account has only current amounts due, it will usually be listed as a current account. There are many variations as to the configuration of this report by the computer systems.

Account age and collectibility

Experience has shown that the longer an account exists without any payment being made on it, the less likely it is that the account will ever be collected. Some experts feel that if an account reaches 90 days without any payment there is only a 50% chance that any of the money will *ever* be collected. This will vary depending on the general state of the economy and sometimes the location of the practice. For example, in a town that depends on one industry, a plant strike that suddenly puts everyone out of work will influence the payment of

Figure 12.6
Accounts receivable age analysis.
Courtesy Colwell Systems, Inc, Champaign, Ill.

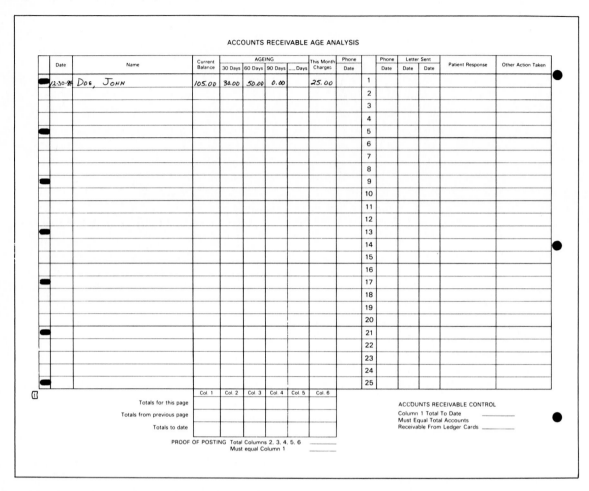

bills. If the decision is between rent and food or the physician's bill, the latter will be ignored. A practice in this environment may want to set a stricter policy on cash at the time of service to prepare for such potential problems. Although such an event represents the extreme, it serves as a reminder of the need for constant attention to the accounts receivable situation.

In addition, everyone is aware that each day a dollar is worth less than it was the day before. Therefore each day that elapses until a bill is paid means that, in the end, less than the amount charged will actually be collected.

In general, accounts should be considered for beginning collection attention at approximately 45 days of aging—prior to the third statement.

Collection Techniques
Legal considerations

When you are attempting to collect overdue accounts there are certain legal limitations on your collection methods that you must observe. These limitations exist to protect the patient. If you must contact debtors at their place of employment because their mail is being returned or their telephone has been changed without a forwarding number, you must observe extreme caution. If the debtor's calls are screened you must not reveal to anyone other than the debtor the reason for the call. Merely state your name and ask for the person you need to speak with.

If you contact debtors at work you must respect the fact that they may not have adequate privacy

Figure 12.7
Patient account
card.
Courtesy Histacount Corp,
Melville, NY.

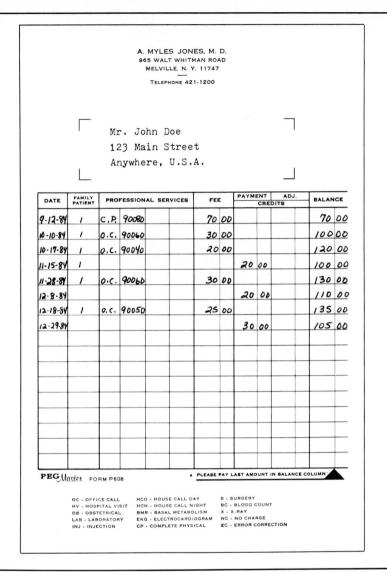

to speak with you. When this is obvious to you because of the answers they give or you detect an effort to conceal the conversation, such as whisper-
ing, you should retreat, telling the patient you understand but must discuss the problem. Leave your
name and telephone number and firmly but politely state that it is important the call be returned.
Persisting in the call when it may jeopardize the
patient's privacy or job can result in legal action
against the caller for harassment.

   If you must contact the reference sources of patients to locate them, the same considerations apply. Revealing to the reference the reason for calling is also considered a breach of confidentiality.

Collection goal

The primary goal of account collection policies is
to keep the percentage of accounts receivable 60
days and older as low as possible. It is also important to develop collection procedures that will meet
this goal in the most tactful and discreet manner
and with as little staff time as is possible to perform the task efficiently. Each office uses different
specific techniques. You will need to experiment to
determine which techniques will work best in your
situation. Sometimes a combination of techniques
is necessary. It may be impossible for the patient to
pay in full, in which case you must be flexible and
willing to arrange a payment schedule. Collecting

an account in a series of payments is preferable to not collecting it at all. Any collection contact and subsequent information or arrangements should be noted in writing, and the patient should be made aware of the notation. This reinforces your seriousness in following through.

Personal interview

You may choose to speak to the patient in person as a first attempt to collect an account. This may be possible on a follow-up visit to the office. As always, the discussion should be tactful and diplomatic but factual. You must be certain to conduct the interview in absolute privacy and allow the patient the opportunity to explain any extenuating circumstances. Mutually acceptable payment schedules should be noted in the accounting record and the patient should be aware of the notation.

The personal interview is time consuming if you have many accounts to deal with. It is dependent on the patient's arrival in the office and contingent on the opportunity of private time with the patient when it is convenient for you. It will also necessitate a reminder note placed on the chart so that the opportunity is not forgotten and inadvertently missed.

Telephone

Most collection specialists believe the use of the telephone is the most effective technique in managing the collections system. Because you can approach most patients as you encounter them on your list of telephone calls to make, you remove the element of chance while retaining the advantage of personal contact. Patients often respond more quickly to personal contact than to written notices. The legal considerations of telephone contact have previously been discussed and must be observed.

Written notices

Personal notes. Sending a special note to each patient with a delinquent account is costly, particularly in terms of employee time. However, handwritten notes on the statements have proven to be very effective. If an individual letter is written it should be tactful and direct, requesting that the amount due be paid or the patient contact the office to make arrangements. You will be signing the letter, noting "Administrative assistant to Dr. Jones" or your appropriate title below your typed signature. The wording of personal collection letters should be checked with the physician, since ultimately the letters represent him or her.

Preprinted form letters. Most medical office suppliers can provide you with a five-part series of collection notices that increase in forcefulness of message (Figure 12.8). The most gentle is used for the first attempt to collect; the last is used when all attempts have been exhausted and the account is about to be referred to professional bill collectors. The appropriate notice is sent with the statement from the office or separately, 10 days after the statement, as a reminder.

Messages on statements. Microfilm and computer billing services can print collection messages directly on the monthly statements. The possible messages are similar to but briefer than the preprinted cards. The intensity of the message is chosen by a predetermined code that advises the service of the message you want.

Collection agencies

When to use collection agencies. When all in-office collection techniques fail, a decision must be made whether to refer the account to a collection agency. If a patient indicates a willingness to pay but was a temporary hardship, the physician commonly holds the account pending payment. However, if the debtor has not made *any* attempt to contact the office and explain the situation or work out a payment plan, the account may be turned over to a collection agency.

Responsibility for agency actions. Physicians usually want to be involved in the decision of which accounts are turned over for collection and which collection agency will be used, because they can be held legally responsible for the techniques used by the agency. Collection agencies or bureaus must observe the same legal restrictions discussed earlier. Therefore it is vital that physicians choose a conscientious and reputable collection agency. Some local medical societies develop their own collection bureaus to assist physicians, because this gives them greater control over collection techniques. Other medical societies will evaluate the local collection bureaus and recommend or endorse one that is determined to be appropriate for handling the particularly delicate accounts associated with medical practices.

Fees associated with agencies. All collection agencies charge a fee for collecting delinquent accounts. Until recently it was not uncommon for an agency to retain 50% of the amount collected as its fee. However, agencies found that their high fees prevented many physicians from turning over accounts or caused them to wait until it was too late to collect anything. To encourage account referrals

Figure 12.8
Preprinted collection notices.
Courtesy Colwell Systems Inc, Champaign, Ill.

M_____19____

_____

Did you forget that check you were going to mail us last month? Please consider this a gentle reminder of your obligation to this office in the amount of $_____, due since _____.

Your prompt remittance will be appreciated.

3621

M_____19____

_____

Our office records show that you received $_____ worth of professional services and that this sum has been due us since _____. If there are considerations we should know about, please telephone or stop in the office. Problems can always be worked out when good faith exists. Get in touch with us at once—*or better yet, send your check in full.*

3622

M_____19____

_____

Please let us hear from you about the $_____ for which we have sent you monthly reminders since last _____. If you cannot make full payment, a check on account will protect your credit rating. We want to be understanding, *but need your cooperation—now.*

3623

M_____19____

_____

We've been as lenient as we can about that delinquent account of yours but have had no response from you. You will please send full payment at once, or arrange for *definite settlement—* before _____. Otherwise we will have no choice but to turn this matter over to an outsider for collection as provided by law.

Balance due $_____

3624

FINAL NOTICE

M_____19____

_____

Your account has been allowed to run much longer than normal credit practices permit. If this were the usual commercial account, legal action would already have begun.

You will consider this your final notice. Unless you can make full payment, or arrangements for payment, within the next _____ days, your account will be turned over to an outside agency.

The amount due us is $_____.

3625

within a reasonable period of time, collection agencies have developed various sliding scales or flat rates. A sliding scale means that the larger the dollar value of the account, the lower the percentage retained by the agency. Flat rates are based on the number of accounts referred rather than the dollar amount collected.

Patient care after collection action

An office policy must be established on the future association between patients and physicians after serious collection problems. Most physicians choose between two options: (1) terminating the physician-patient relationship or (2) requiring cash payment at the time services are rendered.

SPECIAL COLLECTION PROBLEMS
Disputed Charges
Medical assistant responsibility

A disputed charge can exist when the patient does not agree with the amount billed or is billed for services not rendered. The latter may occur when you inadvertently post a visit for one patient to the account of another patient. The patient being charged will usually call the error to your attention. You must verify the error and post the visit to the proper account. Regardless of the billing service you use, you should immediately type and send a statement to the patient who should have received the bill. Otherwise an additional 30 days will elapse before the correct patient is billed.

Seeking the physician-manager's advice

When the disputed charge relates to the amount billed for a service that was performed, the patient usually feels that the fee is too high. You may attempt to discuss it with the patient and explain that the fee is usual for the area and approximately the amount charged by similar physicians. If you feel that the patient is still uncertain, you can offer to discuss it with the physician for the patient or suggest that the patient speak directly with the physician. It is usually better if you act as the patient's emissary with the physician. Physicians often feel uncomfortable discussing fees and will offer to lower a charge rather than discuss it. If you can privately discuss the issue with the physician you can evaluate it objectively and without pressure. Each case must be examined separately, and if the patient's request is valid or brought on by in-

ability to pay you may determine an appropriate adjustment.

Medical society intervention

If a serious dispute exists, patients or physicians may request an objective determination from the local medical society. Most medical societies have a professional relations committee that will examine all of the pertinent facts, including the physician's records, and make a decision about the charges. The physician must abide if the decision is to reduce the charge.

Claims Against Estates

If a patient's account has an outstanding balance at the time of the patient's death, you must file a claim against the estate to be paid. The form to be filed is called a creditor's claim and is merely an itemization of the charges, the total amount due, and the physician's signature. The physician's signature must be notarized, witnessed, and verified by a notary public before the claim is submitted for payment.

Filing a creditor's claim

Once a creditor's claim has been completed in triplicate, all the copies must be submitted for payment. A photocopy should be retained in your files. If you know the deceased patient's attorney or estate executor the claim may be submitted to him. Otherwise, the claim should be filed with probate clerk of the county in which the patient lived. This should be done within the time specified by the county.

You will suspend your regular billing of the patient's account but must monitor the amount due from the estate. The executor or county clerk will notify you if funds are available to pay all or part of the claim. If you have not been notified within 60 days, you should inquire and follow up on the claim.

Bankruptcy

Bankruptcy is filed under federal laws when a business or individual has debts that exceed assets. The local division of the federal court will notify you in a legal document when a patient files bankruptcy under either Chapter 11 or Chapter 13 of the bankruptcy laws. Both attempt to reorganize and settle the filer's debts, but Chapter 13 protects a wage earner by preventing claimants from putting a lien on the wages. Putting a lien on the wages would defeat the purpose of reorganization, which is to evaluate all of the debtor's assets and if possible prepare a schedule to pay off the existing debts. Wages are considered part of the assets.

When you are notified of bankruptcy proceedings you are advised of the amount the debtor claims to owe the physician. If you agree with the amount you simply await the court's decision. If not, you must appear at the hearing or submit a notarized document itemizing the charges and balance due. In either case, you must immediately suspend direct billing of the patient and await the court decision. A physician's bill represents an unsecured debt, one not backed by a specific asset, and it is often dismissed. If it is paid, payments may be at a nominal monthly rate, and it may take years to settle the account. Since you must accept the court's decision, you cannot collect by any other means, and you do not have to bear the cost of billing services, you should view these payments as better than the alternative.

Options to Sue
Small claims court

If all billing and collections methods have been conducted properly, the patient exhibits no intention to pay the debt, and you cannot determine any extenuating circumstances for nonpayment, the physician may consider filing a suit in small claims court to recover the money. Small claims courts are for claims of a limited amount, presently under $1,000. The limit changes periodically to remain in proportion to the cost of living. It is usually sufficient to cover a physician's claim.

The advantage of a small claims suit is the elimination of legal fees. The physician and the debtor state their own cases to a judge, who makes a decision and notifies each party of the binding court order within a short period of time. The physician often wins these suits.

Attorney-directed suit

Physicians rarely resort to a civil lawsuit handled by an attorney to collect an outstanding debt. This type of suit is very costly, often costing more than the debt that is owed, and not worth the time necessary to complete the process. On occasion physicians will have their attorneys write a letter to try to collect a debt. This may be effective, since it implies that further legal action is possible, and a letter will definitely cost less than a lawsuit. In every case, however, the physician must consider the value of the amount to be collected in relation to the cost of collecting it. If there is little to gain the account might best be written off the accounts receivable records as a bad debt, that is, uncollectible.

Loss of Accounts Receivable Records

The details of accounts receivable are vital to the financial survival of a medical office or agency. If you utilize microfilm, an outside computer billing service, or an in-house computer system that has back-up tapes kept off premises or out of the office, and the records are lost, you can reconstruct the accounts, aging, and total due. If other billing methods are used and no copies of the records exist outside of the office, the loss of the accounts receivable data could be devastating. Since loss by fire or flood is possible, if unlikely, insurance is available against these events for a nominal fee. The insurance company will base the insurance premium on the average accounts receivable. You will need to report the accounts receivable amount monthly during the first year of the policy so that the company can determine an appropriate premium rate.

The insurance carrier may require the logical precaution of storage in a closed, insulated metal cabinet and proof that security was observed if a claim is made. You will need to develop the habit of always returning the records to the storage area each evening before closing the office.

Conclusion

Every aspect of billing and collection, from acquiring the data necessary to produce a bill through explaining policy, charges, and managing special problems, requires your attention, tact, and understanding of available services. Special attention should be paid to the everchanging laws that are designed to protect the rights of consumers and providers of services.

Review Questions

1. What are accounts receivable? What must you do to manage these accounts?
2. List and describe the minimum information necessary to establish a patient's account; list the information you or the physician must supply.
3. What billing services can you use in your office to produce bills to patients? How does each one work?
4. What should you keep in mind when preparing statements and when selecting a billing cycle?
5. What is different about billing minors and third-party payers? Where should the bills be sent for each?
6. How does a credit and collection policy help you in your work? How can you inform patients of these policies?
7. List and describe the four methods of collecting current accounts receivable. What could you say to encourage a patient to pay at the time of the visit?
8. What is accounts receivable aging and how is it done by hand? Determine the age of the account entries as of 10-15-89 if the following visits were posted: 7-12-89, $40; 7-18-89, $25; 8-22-89, $25; 9-8-89, $20; and 10-12-89, $25; and payments were $40 on 8-15-89 and $20 on 9-8-89.
9. When should you become concerned with the age of an account?
10. What legal considerations should you keep in mind when attempting to collect an overdue account? State and describe the five methods you can use when collecting overdue accounts.
11. What are your responsibilities when a charge is disputed, when the debtor dies, and when the debtor files bankruptcy?

SUGGESTED READINGS

Doyle JJ and Dennis RL: The complete handbook for medical secretaries and assistants, ed 2, Boston, 1978, Little, Brown & Co.

The American Medical Association: The Business Side of Medical Practice, Chicago, 1979, The Association.

MediCare Explained, Chicago, 1986, Commerce Clearing House.

Chapter 13

Insurance

- Insurance defined
- Medical practices and insurance
- Patient health insurance
- Types of health insurance plans
- Methods of payment
- Sources of insurance
- Controlling utilization

- Filing insurance claims
- Methods of monitoring claims to be processed
- Processing claim forms
- Helping patients with insurance
- Insurance protection for the medical practice

Objectives

On completion of Chapter 13 the medical assistant student should be able to:

1   Define at least the terms listed in the vocabulary.

2   Discuss the purpose of health insurance and the patient's responsibility when using the coverage for health care services.

3   List the five methods of access to health insurance and the six types of health plans available.

4   List and describe the three components of a physician's profile.

5   Compare and contrast assignment of benefits by the patient to the physician and acceptance of assignment by the physician.

6   List and describe the three government-mandated sources of insurance and the four sources of private plans.

7   Discuss utilization review and the role of the medical assistant in the process.

8   List the equipment needed to file insurance claims.

9   List and discuss the three methods of monitoring claims to be filed.

10   List the four major reasons for the return of insurance claims for reprocessing.

11   Describe techniques for helping patients file their own insurance claims.

12   List and describe the four general classifications of insurance needed to protect the medical practice.

Vocabulary

assignment of benefits The transfer of one's right to collect an amount payable under an insurance contract.

benefit The amount payable by the carrier toward the cost of various covered medical or dental services.

broker (insurance) An individual licensed by the state to sell insurance who represents multiple insurance companies rather than a single firm.

capitation rate A fee determined by a prepaid health plan applied to each person insured and expected to cover the expenses of providing necessary health care for one year.

carrier A term applied to companies that provide insurance to protect individuals from financial loss.

claim A demand presented to an insurance company to pay for services provided for an insured.

clause An element of a contract that states a single feature or restriction of the document.

copayment The portion of a service fee that the insured must pay.

deductible An amount the insured person must pay before policy benefits begin.

experience rate The number of claims submitted for payment of services compared to the total number of individuals covered by an insurance policy.

fee for service The method of billing by a physician in private practice, whereby the doctor charges for each professional service performed.

fiscal year A 12-month period that begins on the same predetermined date each year and is selected for financial purposes.

indigent A person unable to secure the financial means to meet his basic needs.

insured A person protected against financial loss by an insurance policy.

intermediary An insurance company or organization capable of processing claims for another payer.

mandate A law or order from a legislative government body.

Medicaid A health insurance program sponsored by both the federal and state governments. The program is state specific with general federal guidelines to be followed. Medicaid is an assistance program and is available in all states in various forms.

peer An individual or group that is similar to another individual or group; professionally, an individual with the same educational preparation and credentials as another.

policy A document or contract that describes the insurance coverage for an individual or a property.

private sector The business and industry owned and operated by private citizens.

provider Supplier, physician, or the one providing services to the insured (patient).

public sector The area of operations that is controlled by a government agency and funded by public money.

reimbursement Payment to an individual for expenses previously paid.

subscriber Individual named as the primary person covered by an insurance policy.

variance Deviation from the expected.

Insurance is an integral part of everyone's life, so you can definitely expect to encounter various types of insurance in the course of your professional responsibilities. It will help you organize your work if you understand the purpose, potential, and methods of processing transactions covered by insurance policies.

INSURANCE DEFINED

Insurance is protection against financial loss caused by possible but unplanned events that can affect an individual or business. Depending on the protection you want or anticipate needing, insurance can be acquired from two sources: private companies or, in special situations, government agencies.

Premiums are the fees you must pay to be protected by an insurance policy. Premiums are determined after consideration of several factors by the insurance company. These include the likelihood that the insured will need financial reimbursement, the likelihood that an event will occur, and the company's past experience with claims. Premiums are determined for a fixed period of time, usually one year in advance, and may be paid all at once or divided into partial payments to be made throughout the coverage period. The policy is evaluated at the end of the period to determine if the premium should be adjusted. Excessive claims against an insurance policy may result in an increase in an individual premium. If the insured is part of a group, that is, several people who need the same type insurance, the cost of protection can be shared, since members of the group will make varying demands on the policy.

MEDICAL PRACTICES AND INSURANCE

It is rare that a patient seeking care in your medical office or agency will not have some form of health care coverage. Patients may be part of a group plan where they work, may be protected at work by another policy in case they are injured or become ill because of their job, may have a personal health insurance policy, or may be protected by a government program.

You will also encounter various insurance policies that are acquired to protect the office or agency against financial loss. It is important for you to understand the types of insurance policies your office purchases so that you will know to which company to submit a claim in the event of a loss. The possible insurance policies protecting a business are classified as property insurance, legal liability insurance, criminal loss insurance, and package policies. Insurance for the business will be discussed later in the chapter.

PATIENT HEALTH INSURANCE
Purpose

The purpose of patient health insurance is to defray or reduce the amount of personal money that an individual must pay for health care services. Health insurance is a relatively new form of protection that is becoming increasingly necessary because of the constant rise in the cost of health care. Health insurance has evolved to keep pace with the increasing cost of complex health services and the personnel who provide them.

Some people will require extensive health care services while others will need few or none. Since it is impossible to predict future needs, health insurance is purchased in the event that services are necessary. The insurance carrier estimates the total claims that will be made during the period covered by an insurance policy, and the cost is then shared, in the form of a premium, by *all* the people insured by the company.

Patient's Responsibility
Knowing coverage

Each individual or group insurance policy is unique. A policy may be written to cover only some services or a broad range of possible health needs. Ideally patients will have read their insurance plan literature and understand which services are covered by the insurance company. Unfortunately, this is not always the case. Because each plan is different, you must avoid making statements such as, "I'm sure your insurance will pay for this," when you cannot be sure it will. You must also avoid the time-consuming task of reviewing a patient's insurance literature to determine the coverage. You might misinterpret it and assure a patient that a service is covered when it is not. Patients will undoubtedly feel differently toward you when they discover that they must pay for services they thought the insurance company would cover. Instead, you should tell patients that since each contract is different it would be better if

they called their insurance carrier to find out what will be covered.

Insurance information card. Patients with health insurance coverage are issued identification cards, which usually state the following:
- The name of the carrier;
- The patient's name;
- The patient's group and personal subscriber identification number;
- Where to submit claims;
- A brief description of covered services; and
- Telephone number for prior authorization.

Unfortunately, it is rare that subscribers or patients will truly understand their insurance coverage.

Patients who have an independent plan rather than one through a group of their choice are still assigned a number. This number indicates to the carrier that they are an independent subscriber.

You should request to see the identification card of all insured patients at the time of the first visit and make a photocopy of the card for your records. The photocopy will provide verification in case a number is transposed on the record or an insurance claim form. The patient's insurance should be verified periodically, especially when you recheck the patient's address, telephone number, and employment information. If the patient's place of employment changes you can expect the insurance coverage to change, and the patient may not remember to show you the new card.

Insurance verification. If you are working in a practice that provides services that frequently come under the major medical portion of the policy (that is, hospital services, surgery, obstetrics, psychiatry, and so on) it is important that the insurance be verified. Identify yourself and the physician, indicate the patient's name, subscriber name, and all identifying numbers (Figure 13.1).

Understanding payment methods

Do not assume that patients will understand the details of working with insurance companies and their payment methods. In fact, most patients are intimidated by insurance companies' methods. Your office policy and procedure manuals will assist you in working with patients on insurance matters.

Patient responsibility for bills. Except for the situations discussed in Chapter 12 in which a third party pays 100% of the cost of care, patients must understand that they are ultimately responsible for all charges. This means that you will need to explain to patients carefully, personally, through an

Figure 13.1
Questions to ask when verifying a patient's insurance.
Courtesy De A. Eggers & Associates, San Rafael, Calif.

When verifying a patient's insurance, ask the following questions:
- Name of person with whom you are speaking, first name and last name.
- Is there a deductible?
- How much?
- Has it been met?   Yes   No
- Are all the services we are providing covered under major medical?
- Are services covered under basic benefits?
- What are the benefits for inpatient services:
- What are the benefits for outpatient services?
- At what percentage do you reimburse?
- Is that of fee or UCR?
- If UCR, can you give me an idea on what the patient can expect to be reimbursed on our charge of ?
- Is there a yearly maximum for this type of service?
- If so, has any been used? How much?
- Is there a lifetime maximum?
- If so, has any been used?   How much?
- Insurance company name:

- Address for mailing insurance claim:

- Telephone number
- Name of person who verified the coverage.
- Date of coverage verification.   By whom:

information folder, or through a combination approach, that the contract for care is between the physician and the patient. Therefore the agreement to pay for services is between the physician and the patient, not between the physician and the insurance company. A separate relationship exists between the patient and the insurance company. Patients are responsible for all charges, whether they are reimbursed by the insurance company or not.

Role of office personnel.   The role you will play in helping patients recover their money from insurance companies was discussed in Chapter 12 but bears repeating. You should not attempt to act as an intermediary between patients and their insurance carriers. Doing so is time consuming and does not allow patients the opportunity to learn from the experience. You might keep the claims inquiry numbers of the major local insurance carriers on file to give to patients; this will indicate to them

that you are not uninterested in their needs.

Assisting with billing insurance.   Most office medical assistants will assist patients with billing their insurance carriers by automatically providing the data necessary to file a claim, either in the monthly statement or on a superbill given at each visit. Many offices also complete the appropriate insurance forms for patients. This is an extra service provided for patients, not an automatic right of the patient. Some patients have several insurance policies and rely on the medical assistant to file a variety of forms for them. This can become a problem, particularly if the forms are brought or sent in at different times. If this is done, the chart or financial records must be retrieved several times for one patient.

To discourage this practice, offices can provide several copies of the superbill at one time, and each can be sent to a different company. Another alternative is to charge for completing insurance forms.

Figure 13.2
Example of letter indicating routine waiver of deductible and co-insurance
amounts.
Courtesy De A. Eggers & Associates, San Rafael, Calif.

PROGRAM MEMORANDUM

Reprinted HCFA - BO A/B   Health Care Financing
Transmittal No. A-85-4   Administration
            B-85-3

                                                    Date: MARCH 1985

SUBJECT: Routine Waiver of Deductible and Coinsurance Amounts

It has been recently brought to our attention that the volume and seriousness of the cases involving the routine waiver of deductibles and coinsurance by certain physicians and suppliers has grown dramatically. As a result, we believe there is a need at this time for carriers to aggressively seek out instances of routine waiver and to make specific reductions in charge screens for these providers.

As you know, current program instructions (section 5220 of the MediCare Carriers Manual) indicate that a billed amount that is not reasonably related to an expectation of payment should not be considered as the "actual charge" for processing a current claim or determining customary charge screens. Carriers have been expected to thoroughly review all situations that come to their attention when a physician or supplier routinely and consistently waives the collection of deductibles and coinsurance to determine whether their actual and customary charges should be reduced.

It appears, however, that carriers have not actively sought out specific instances of routine waiver, and that specific reductions in actual and customary charges once a routine waiver has been discovered have not been made on a consistent basis.

While we are developing a stronger range of sanctions against those who routinely waive deductible and coinsurance amounts, we believe carriers currently need to aggressively seek out instances of routine waiver and diligently enforce existing sanctions. Among other actions, carriers should review any advertising by suppliers designed to waive MediCare deductibles and coinsurance and alert such providers that they are in potential violation of the law, at risk of having their customary charges reduced and an overpayment assessed, and subject to criminal prosecution by the Department of Justice.

The American Medical Association states that charging for completing insurance forms is not unethical. It suggests, however, that if you wish to charge it is in the best interest of public relations that the first form be completed at no charge and that a nominal fee be charged for subsequent forms billing for the same procedures.

Responsibility for unpaid portion. Most insurance policies are written based on an 80/20 ratio. This means that the insurance company will pay 80% of the allowable charges and that the patient can expect to be responsible for 20% of the total charges. In reality this is not always the end result, and you will need to explain why to the patient. The word *allowable* is the key to understanding the situation.

Most often the physician's fee and the fee allowed by the insurance company for an individual procedure are not equal; the allowed fee will usually be less. The dollar and percentage differences caused by this situation mean that the patient will be paying more than expected. You may need to use an example to explain the situation. Whatever method you use will need to convey to patients that they are responsible for the total amount billed, not the amount allowed by the insurance company. The one exception to this rule will be discussed under Medicare payment options.

Health Care Financing Administration (HCFA). Memorandum No. 85 (Figure 13.2) requires that the physician supplier make a reasonable attempt (three billings) to collect the difference (from the subscriber) between what was paid by the insurance carrier and the original bill. HCFA mandates that if a physician or a supplier consistently writes off the difference between the paid amount and the billed amount, then the carrier, private or public, should reduce that provider's profile to the accepted payment amount. For example, if the physician's fee for a particular service is always $1,000, the carrier allows $800 and pays $640. If the physician accepts the fee of $640 as payment in full and the carrier finds out, then the physician's fee for that service with that carrier now has become $640, since the physician accepted that fee as payment in full.

TYPES OF HEALTH INSURANCE PLANS
Access to Health Insurance
As an individual

Anyone with the money to pay the insurance premium can contract with a carrier for any insurance plan available. Premiums for individual plans generally cost more than other policies but allow each individual to select the plan he wants.

As part of a group

Patients can gain access to group insurance plans in a variety of ways. The most common group is formed by people who work together or belong to the same labor union. Other group plans are available through education or social organizations formed to meet a common goal.

Worker's Compensation

Worker's Compensation is statutory insurance, that is, required by law. Each state directs that every employer with a certain number of employees (the minimum varies from state to state) must provide an insurance policy that will pay for all medical care needed to treat injuries or illnesses that are the result of the job. The employer pays the insurance premium.

Special automobile insurance

Many automobile insurance policies include a clause to cover injuries incurred as a result of an automobile accident. This clause is usually referred to as bodily injury coverage. People may pay for this type of insurance to provide coverage for the passengers in their car, regardless of who causes the accident, or for the occupants of any other vehicles if the insured is responsible for the accident.

Government plans

Medical care coverage is available to certain segments of the population through government-sponsored plans. Medicare is a federal plan that provides for the care of people age 65 or older and for people of any age who are permanently disabled. Medicaid is federally mandated but administered by each state. It provides for the care of the indigent in need of medical care. Finally, the Civilian

Health and Medical Program of the Uniformed Services (CHAMPUS) and the Civilian Health and Medical Program of the Veteran's Admistration (CHAMPVA) provide health care coverage for active-duty military personnel and their dependents in some circumstances and also for retired military personnel. The eligibility for and processing of the various types of health insurance will be discussed later in this chapter.

Available Health Plans

There are many possible components of a health insurance policy, and the insurance subscriber may select one or more of these components when developing a health coverage policy. Each component will be briefly described in the section that follows.

Basic benefits

A basic health plan will provide varying coverage for patients using the nonsurgical services of a physician for office, hospital, home, and emergency room visits. Also a basic plan usually covers diagnostic studies (laboratory and radiological). Most basic plans do not cover routine physical examinations, eye examinations, family planning services, or medically necessary equipment such as artificial limbs. They may have a maximum annual benefit allowed stated in dollar amounts, such as "X-ray examinations covered to a maximum benefit of $400 annually." Plans that state maximum benefits allowed regardless of possible complications are referred to as indemnity plans.

Major medical

Major medical plans are often acquired to supplement basic benefits or are offered as a combined plan and provide coverage to a much higher dollar amount. This type of plan is occasionally still referred to as *catastrophic* insurance, although you should avoid the phrase because of its very negative implications. Major medical coverage begins where a basic plan leaves off, paying for expenses incurred because of a very serious or prolonged illness. These plans frequently cover many of the items disallowed by the basic coverage.

Hospitalization

A health plan that provides for inpatient services in an acute-care facility is often termed a *hospitalization policy*. This plan will pay for the basic hospital services of bed, board, and staff nursing care at a predetermined rate, usually for a two-bed room. If patients want a private room, they must personally pay the rate difference between a two-bed (semiprivate) room and the private accommodations. If the private room is medically necessary, for example, to prevent the spread of infection, the insurance company will pay the difference. In addition, the plan pays for all services necessary to diagnose or treat an illness or injury including medications, x-ray examinations, laboratory studies, operating room, and rehabilitation therapy.

Surgical

Surgical coverage provides for the services of a surgeon and, for major operations, an assistant surgeon. Surgeons may bill for surgery provided in their offices, for outpatient hospital surgery, and for surgery requiring hospitalization of the patient. The most noticeable gap between billed and allowed fees occurs in surgical cases, and you should be able to discuss this with patients.

Income protection

Some companies offer a policy that will provide patients with a steady income for a specified period of time in the event that they must be hospitalized. The plans vary but usually pay even if the patients are receiving sick pay from work and include the period of time in the hospital and the at-home recovery time designated by the physician. These policies will help with living expenses and may also help fill the gap between billed and allowed fees.

Companion plans

Many insurance companies offer plans designed to pick up the payment of the 20% not paid by conventional insurance plans. These companion plans are available to the patient or subscriber as a supplement to Medicare. However, many of these plans incorporate exclusions or limitations that are not usually apparent to the patient or subscriber. Thus the subscriber must be very cautious to check out all of the exclusions on their plan. Frequently the patient will expect you to know and understand the exclusions or limitations of their plan.

Special risk insurance

Insurance policies are available that will pay patients a fixed amount each week when hospitalized or temporarily incapacitated by a specific disease. The diseases covered are usually cancer or heart attack.

Insurance experts believe that special risk insurances are rarely worth the premiums paid over a long period of time. The emotional response to certain diseases, however, will entice people to acquire special insurance. Although you should not advise patients on the type of coverage they should purchase, you may suggest that they check with an insurance agent or broker about the long-term benefits of various plans.

METHODS OF PAYMENT
Physician Fee Profile

You will often hear physicians refer to their *profile* when discussing patient-care insurance payments. A profile is a numerical image of physicians' patterns of charging for various services as monitored by insurance companies that are billed for reimbursement. The individual profiles physicians refer to represent usual fees. Comparative profiles are developed from all fees submitted by any physician in the geographical area for each service code. These profiles set the standards for customary and reasonable (UCR) standards and determine the maximum charges an insurance carrier will allow.

Usual fees

Usual fees for each physician are calculated by computer and represent the fees routinely charged by a physician for each service. The profile is calculated by a computer for a specific period of time, usually one year. This becomes the base year that determines the fees paid. Physicians may feel that the system is unfair to claimants, because the base year may be several years earlier than the one in which the services are billed.

Fees may change over time because the costs of maintaining an office will increase, requiring more income. If you wanted to determine a physician's usual fee you would select a specific period of time, at least one year, and check the fees for a specific procedure at the various times throughout the year. The fee that occurs most often is the usual fee. For example, if your survey reveals charges for a specific procedure to include $10, $12, $12, $14, and $16 the usual fee would be $12.

Customary fees

Fees are considered customary if they fall within the upper and lower profile limits for physicians of the same specialty or practice type who practice within a geographic area determined by the insurance company. If the upper limit profile is $18 for a specific service code and the lower limit is $14, the physician who submits a bill for $16 will have the fee recognized as customary.

Reasonable fees

Fees are commonly declared reasonable if they meet the criteria for usual and customary fees. In some cases, there can be multiple problems that make the services more complex and warrant a higher fee. Physicians submitting a higher-than-average fee should attach a statement and documents to support the extra fee. The claim will be reviewed by a panel of the physician's peers, and the appropriate fee will be determined.

Resource based relative value study (RBRVS). In 1988 Congress allotted some $2.5 million to Harvard to establish a relative value for each procedure performed. This is very similar to the Relative Value Study that was established several years ago by the CMA and the FMA. At one time the FTC (Federal Trade Commission) considered the RVS as price fixing and ruled it illegal. However, the Medicaid programs continue to reimburse under a unit value because the states are exempt from FTC rulings. If the RBRVS is adopted, it is expected that reimbursement to physicians and suppliers of medical services will be more equitable nationwide.

Assignment of Benefits

When there is an option, an assignment of benefits is an instruction to the insurance carrier about where to send the insurance payment.

Assignment by patient to physician

Method of assignment. Most individual and group insurance plans will automatically reimburse the patient if they do not receive specific instructions to do otherwise. To speed the reimbursement process and protect income by having the carrier pay the physician directly, many offices and agencies have patients assign the benefits to the provider. This may be accomplished by having patients sign an assignment of benefits form, the assignment section of an insurance form, or a superbill designed with an assignment section. To incorporate all areas of the policy, the assignment should stipulate to include major medical (Figure 13.3). In many states this ensures that both the basic policy benefits and the major medical benefits will be paid to the physician.

Patient instructions. The assignment of benefits by the patient to the physician does *not* absolve the patient of future financial responsibility. You will need to explain to patients that they will be billed and considered responsible for the difference between the amount charged by the physician and the amount paid by the insurance company.

Physician accepts assignment

Physician's choice. In some instances, physicians may choose to accept assignment. This indicates that the physician will expect all payments from all carriers, other than those programs where the physician is an enrolled (or contract) provider, to be paid directly to the physician. The physician, in this instance, is required to make a reasonable attempt to collect the balance of the amount originally billed from the subscriber or responsible party. In box 13 of the standard claim form, the insurance biller should either have the subscriber sign or indicate "Signature on File." There is an area on each insurance form near the place where the physician signs the document which states "Accepts assignment" followed by boxes to check yes or no. With Medicare claims it is mandatory that one of the boxes be marked.

When the physician accepts assignment, the insurance company determines the allowed fee and pays the physician the percentage the carrier stipulates based on the insured's policy benefits. The physician is then expected to bill the patient the amount not paid by the carrier. Only in the State of Massachusetts is the physician expected to accept the insurance carrier's part as payment in full when the physician accepts assignment. The physician may accept the insurance carrier's payment as payment in full if it is evident that the patient is living on a fixed income or is experiencing a period of financial hardship. If this is the case, the physician's office is required to have a "Waiver Due to Economic Hardship" signed. This may also occur if the patient is another physician or a member of his or her family. In this instance the balance is adjusted due to "Prior Agreement."

No-option situations. There are certain instances in which physicians do not have a choice on assignment; by accepting the patient they agree to the fee paid by the insurance company or intermediary as payment in full. This occurs with Worker's Compensation cases, Medicaid or Medicare-Medicaid patients, and certain Blue Shield plans if the physician is a participating provider.

SOURCES OF INSURANCE
Government-Mandated Plans
Medicare

Medicare was established in 1966 through an amendment to the Social Security Act. It is available for the aged or disabled and is designed to assist patients with a major portion of their medical bills.

Figure 13.3
Assignment of benefits and what it means.
Courtesy De A. Eggers & Associates, San Rafael, Calif.

When you accept the assignment of benefits from either MediCare or CHAMPUS, the check will come to you and you are agreeing that you will accept as total payment what the government recognizes or allows. Example: Charge is $100.00, MediCare or CHAMPUS recognizes $80.00 and pays you $64.00. You may bill the patient the difference between $64.00 and the $80.00, but you must write off the difference between the $80.00 and $100.00.

When you do not accept the assignment of benefits, then the check goes to the patient and you may collect the full $100.00.

With other insurance companies, when you accept the assignment, it only means that the check comes to you. You still have the right to collect the full amount of the charges.

SAMPLE:

ASSIGNMENT OF BENEFITS:

I hereby assign all medical and/or surgical benefits, to include major medical benefits to which I am entitled, including Medicare, private insurance, and any other health plans to:

This assignment will remain in effect until revoked by me in writing. A photocopy of this assignment is to be considered as valid as an original. I understand that I am financially responsible for all charges whether or not paid by said insurance. I hereby authorize said assignee to release all information necessary to secure the payment.

SIGNED:_____DATE:_____

ASSIGNMENT OF BENEFITS: I hereby assign all medical and/or surgical benefits, to include major medical benefits to which I am entitled, including MediCare, private insurance and any other health plans to:

This assignment will remain in effect until revoked by me in writing. A photocopy of this assignment is to be considered as valid as an original. I understand that I am financially responsible for all charges whether or not paid by said insurance. I hereby authorize said assignee to release all information necessary to secure the payment.

SIGNED: DATE:

Eligibility. Citizens become eligible for Medicare benefits beginning with their sixty-fifth birthday and should register with a local Social Security office at least three months before that date. Medicare is also available to individuals of any age who have been declared permanently disabled and have been receiving financial disability assistance for two years. Determination of eligibility is ultimately made by program evaluators.

Benefits. *Hospital services* are provided under Part A of the Medicare program and are paid from a fund contributed to by the self-employed or by working individuals and their employers. These contributions are in the form of a tax levied under the Federal Insurance Contributions Act (FICA). Anyone eligible for Medicare may receive Part A benefits. Railroad employees and some federal-government employees are not part of the Social Security system and receive their old-age hospital benefits from other sources. Railroad retirement funds administer their Medicare separately from Social Security Medicare; federal employees have an independent benefits program.

Physician medical services are provided under Part B of Medicare, a voluntary program that requires the payment of a monthly premium. The monthly premium is nominal when compared to other insurance and is usually withheld from monthly Social Security checks.

For people who are still employed past the age of 65 and whose employer has more than 20 employees, the employer must provide an employee with the same insurance coverage as provided to other employees. This then makes that insurance carrier the primary coverage and Medicare the secondary coverage. If the primary carrier pays more for the service than Medicare would allow in the first place, then there will be no further payment from Medicare. Should the patient retire or terminate employment, the process reverses and Medicare again becomes the primary carrier. It is best to request that the patient provide the physician's office a letter stating the date of retirement or the date termination will be effective.

SSI (Social Security Income) patients qualify for Medicare benefits even though they are not over age 65. In such cases it has been determined through physician documentation that the patient has suffered two or more years from either a physical or mental illness. In many instances patients will not have worked enough to have contributed sufficient funds into the Medicare program to qualify for benefits. Such patients will be qualified to utilize benefits through their parents.

Immigrants/aliens may also qualify for Medicare benefits if they are over age 65 and have resided in the United States for more than 5 years. If the patient has not resided in the United States for five years, request that the patient secure a form from the Social Security Office stipulating the date the patient will be eligible for Medicare benefits.

Physician options and responsibilities. Physicians have the option of participating in the Medicare program. If the physician chooses to participate, then the physician's office must file all claims to Medicare and must accept assignment of benefits for all claims. If the physician chooses not to participate, then he or she has the option of accepting assignment on some claims but not on others. If a physician chooses not to participate and provides elective surgical services that are over $500, the physicians's office must apprise the pa-

tient of the fee for the surgery, the amount Medicare is expected to pay, and what the expected amount due from the patient will be. This must be in writing and acknowledged with the patient's signature. Medicare may request proof of such acknowledgement (Figure 13.4).

Whether or not the physician chooses to participate, there may be some services that are either not a benefit of the Medicare program or may not be considered "medically necessary" by Medicare. In either case the physician's office is required to so notify the patient that Medicare may consider the service not a benefit of the program or not medically necessary; see attached example of form that must be signed (Figure 13.5). Should the physician's office not apprise the patient of this information, the Medicare program may consider the lack of such notification to the patient to be an attempt to defraud the government.

Other situations considered by Medicare to be fraud are:
- False representation with intent to gain;
- Billing for services not rendered;
- Duplicate billing;
- Upgrading/using procedure codes higher than services actually rendered; and
- Receiving "kickbacks" from labs or imaging facilities.

The Medicare program has various methods for compiling the above data:
- Computer comparison of billings for that practice;
- Beneficiary complaints;
- Physician employee complaints; and
- Anonymous phone calls.

Any of the above may result in the following for the physician:
1. Sanctions:
   - One year to lifetime from the Medicare or Medicaid program;
   - Notice published in local newspapers for 3 weeks after sanction; and
   - Notice published in the national bulletins.
2. Civil monetary penalty law:
   - Assessment of up to twice the amount of the fraudulent portion of the claim.
3. Civil suit.
4. Criminal suit (imprisonment).

Medicaid

Indigent aid. Medicaid is available to assist persons who qualify to acquire necessary medical care. It is available to eligible persons who have no access to care or to those who have Medicare but

Figure 13.4
How to calculate the Medicare estimated payment for elective surgery and the
Medicare beneficiary obligation.
Courtesy De A. Eggers & Associates, San Rafael, Calif.

How to Calculate the Medicare Estimated Payment For Elective Surgery and the Medicare Beneficiary Obligation

1. Your actual charge for the service.   _ _ _ _ _
   (If less than $500 no notification to the patient is necessary.)

2. The Medicare approved charge.   _ _ _ _ _
   This is the lowest of your actual charge, your customary charge, or the area
   prevailing charge. (If you have accepted assignment on a claim for the
   same service, the Medicare approved charge was provided to you. If you
   do not know this information, contact your carrier.)

3. Enter the difference between your charge and the Medicare approved
   amount (line 1 minus line 2).   _ _ _ _ _

4. Enter the 20% coinsurance on the Medicare allowable charge.   _ _ _ _ _

5. The beneficiary's out-of-pocket expense.   _ _ _ _ _

You must provide the beneficiary the information on lines 1, 2 and 5. (Assume that the $75
deductible has been met.)

Draft Notice to the Patient

Date:

Because I do not plan to accept assignment for your case, federal law requires me to provide
you information on the amount that I intend to charge you for your surgery, the amount that
Medicare will pay you, and the amount (including the Medicare required coinsurance) that
you will be responsible for. (You may have other insurance that will cover all or part of this
difference.)

Type of Surgery: _____
Estimate of my Fee: _____   (from line 1)
What Medicare should pay: _____   (from line 2)
The Out-of-Pocket costs for which
    you will be responsible: _____   (from line 5)
(Including Medicare required coinsurance)

You should obtain your patient's signature on this form and retain it in your records.

---

are unable to pay the difference between allowed Medicare fees and the total cost of coverage.

Combined effort.   Medicaid is a cooperative arrangement between each state and the federal government that was initiated by the Social Security amendments of 1966 and receives its authority from Title XIX of Public Law 89-97. The federal government provides a major portion of the funds for the program, with the remainder of the funds provided by each state. In addition, each state accepts the responsibility for administering the program.

State responsibilities.   Each state makes independent determinations on details of the Medicaid program regarding an applicant's eligibility, services available through the program, and maximum payments that will be made to providers for services rendered. Each state issues to eligible pa-

Figure 13.5
Statement of denial of Medicare services.
Courtesy De A. Eggers & Associates, San Rafael, Calif.

Medicare will only pay for services that it determines to be "reasonable and necessary" under section 1862 (a) (1) of the Medicare law. If Medicare determines that a particular service, although it would otherwise be covered, is "not reasonable or necessary" under the Medicare program standards, Medicare will deny payment for that service. I believe that, in your case, Medicare is likely to deny payment for:

Date: Reason: Service: Fee: Signature:

_____ _____ _____ _____ _____

I have been notified by my supplier that he or she believes that in my case Medicare is likely to deny payment for the items or services identified above, for the reason # stated. If Medicare denies payment I agree to be personally and fully responsible for payment.

_____
Patient Signature

1. Medicare does not usually pay for this many visits or treatments.
2. Medicare usually does not pay for this service.
3. Medicare usually pays for only one nursing home visit per month.
4. Medicare usually does not pay for this injection.
5. Medicare usually does not pay for this many injections.
6. Medicare does not pay for this because it is a treatment that has yet to be proved effective.
7. Medicare does not pay for this office visit unless it was needed because of an emergency.
8. Medicare usually does not pay for services by more than one physician during the same period.
9. Medicare does not pay for this many services within this period of time.
10. Medicare usually does not pay for more than one visit per day.
11. Medicare usually does not pay for such extensive procedures.
12. Medicare usually does not pay for like services by more than one physician of the same specialty.
13. Medicare usually does not pay for this equipment.
14. Medicare usually does not pay for this lab test.

tients an official identification card, some with a series of removable labels, each month that they remain eligible. Although each state administers a Medicaid program, the state may use different terminology for the name of the program, thus leading to confusion by the medical assistant when out-of-state patients refer to Medicaid programs in their states by different names. Medicaid may be referred to as Medical Assistance, Public Assistance, DPW, Welfare, Medicaid, Title XIX, Medi-Cal (California), SAMI (Nevada), and ACCESS (Arizona).

Physician options and responsibilities. Physicians have an option as to whether they choose to accept Medicaid patients. An office policy should be established and the guidelines for accepting Medicaid patients made known to all employees. Physicians may accept patients with the Medicare/Medicaid combination, they may choose to accept

Medicaid patients only on referral from another provider, only from the hospital Emergency Department when they are on rotation, or only for consultation.

Many times the physician will have to restrict the percentage of Medicaid patients in the practice, since patients with Medicaid frequently require a much greater level of service and the low reimbursement for services can be almost prohibitive (as low as 30% of the physician's usual fee). Physicians must then write off the unpaid portion. In other words, physicians who accept Medicaid patients must accept the state's schedule as payment in full and may not bill the patient for the remaining unpaid portion. Many states have imposed stringent guidelines on the actual billing requirements, prior authorization requirements, and/or time-frames for claims submission. Consequently, the additional paper work and staff time required makes the reimbursement amount virtually negligible.

If it is office policy not to accept Medicaid patients, you will be responsible for screening new patients and informing them of office policy. You may be able to suggest physicians who accept Medicaid or refer individuals needing care to the county medical society, where a list of physicians who accept Medicaid is kept.

If Medicaid patients are accepted, you will need to check identification cards before the first visit each month. At this time you should photocopy the card for your records. You will also need to keep abreast of program changes and covered services, which are usually communicated in printed bulletins mailed periodically to all providers. Also be careful to bill according to the very specific program rules unique to each state.

CHAMPUS

CHAMPUS is the abbreviation for Civilian Health and Medical Program of the Uniformed Services. This is a congressionally funded, comprehensive health benefit program designed to provide families of uniformed services personnel and service retirees a supplement to medical care in military and public health service facilities. Beneficiaries may receive a fairly wide range of civilian health care services, with a significant share of the cost or amount paid for by the federal government. Usually these patients seek care from military medical facilities near their homes. However, there are times when they can seek care through a private physician's office or hospital. When beneficiaries live within a 40-mile radius of a military facility where they could receive the same level of service or the same service, they must provide the physician's office with a Form DD1251, "Non-availability Statement," from either the commanding officer of the military facility or the CHAMPUS advisers.

CHAMPUS eligibility. Public Law 569, passed in 1956 and subsequently expanded in 1966 by the Military Medical Benefits Amendment Act, allows treatment in nonmilitary facilities for select individuals. CHAMPUS benefits are available for the following:
- Dependents of military personnel;
- Military retirees;
- Dependents of military retirees; and
- Dependents of deceased military personnel or deceased retirees.

Benefits. CHAMPUS allows eligible beneficiaries to receive many types of inpatient and outpatient services through private-sector providers.

These services are paid for in part by the federal government. The payment schedules are similar to those of private insurance in that they have a deductible and copayments that are the patient's responsibility. After the deductible is paid, which is currently $50 per patient with a combined total per family of $100, dependents of military personnel are responsible for a copayment of 20%; all others eligible for benefits pay a 25% copayment.

CHAMPVA

CHAMPVA was established in 1973 for the spouses and dependents of individuals permanently disabled or dead as a result of service-related duties. Once eligibility is established and cards are issued, potential patients may seek care from private-sector providers.

Claims for CHAMPUS and CHAMPVA services must be filed either on the CHAMPUS 500 Form (section 13.9) or on the HCFA 1500 Standard Claim Form (Figure 13.8). The top half, items 1 through 18, is to be completed and signed by the patient or his legal guardian; the bottom half, items 19 through 32, is to be completed by the medical assistant; and item 33 is to be signed only by the physician. A signature stamp or the medical assistant's signature as the physician's representative may not be substituted for the personal signature of the physician.

The benefits and payment schedules for CHAMPVA patients are the same as for CHAMPUS patients. As with other government programs, the rules are relatively rigid and may change periodically. The official manual on eligibility, services, and billing is available through your regional CHAMPUS office or by writing to O'CHAMPUS Fitzsimmons Army Base, Aurora, CO.

Worker's Compensation

Availability. Every state possesses its own individual Worker's Compensation law, and the basic purposes of each law are the same: that employees who are injured or become ill as a result of their employment will have adequate means of support if they are unable to work and that they will be free from the cost of any medical services.

Employers must provide for these benefits and usually do so through a Worker's Compensation policy paid for solely by them. Since the guidelines in each state vary, be aware of those unique to your area. For example, some states do not require that employers have coverage if they employ fewer than 10 persons.

Administered by state. The laws of each state indicate who is eligible for Worker's Compensation benefits but usually leave the determination to the physician treating the patient. If an employer, insurance company, or the state is in doubt about a patient's claim, they may request a determination from the Worker's Compensation Board or Industrial Relations Board.

The Worker's Compensation Board also establishes a fee schedule that sets the maximum amount payable for each health care service. The maximum amount allowed is usually less than the physician's standard fees. However, physicians who accept a Worker's Compensation case, sometimes referred to as an "industrial" case, agree to accept the predetermined fees. In essence, they are accepting assignment.

Insurance coverage. Some employers who have a relatively low risk of an employee suffering an injury or illness prefer to pay necessary expenses directly in the event that they occur. These employers are referred to as self-insured. In this situation the bills for services are sent directly to the employer. Most often, however, the employer acquires a specific insurance policy to cover such events. The annual premium is relatively low and calculated according to the combined salaries of covered employees and the previous experience rate.

Claims made. It is important to remember that claims may be made for any illness or injury that is the result of a job or the work environment, regardless of cause and including employee carelessness. Before Worker's Compensation laws were passed in the 1930s, the attitude prevailed that employees should protect themselves. However, the laws presume employer responsibility and guide employers in educating and providing a safe environment for employees.

Benefits to patients. Patients with work-related injuries or illnesses have a right to expect payment of all necessary medical services including hospitalization, rehabilitation, and occupational therapy. Patients will also receive their routine salary during the period that they are unable to work. In cases of permanent disability, a hearing is held and a settlement determined. This settlement represents the total compensation for the illness or injury. In the event of a work-related death, the Worker's Compensation Board will determine the total benefits to be paid to the survivors.

Filing claims. There are two types of forms that are necessary to file Worker's Compensation claims. The first time a physician sees a patient in a Worker's Compensation case, the physician must complete a Doctor's First Report (Figure 13.6).

You will probably be responsible for acquiring the information for items 1 through 11 on this form. The information may be typed or written in by hand.

Be as precise as possible when acquiring this information. The employee may be uncertain of the Worker's Compensation insurance carrier or confuse it with his private health insurance carrier. If there is any doubt, call the employer's personnel department. Also pay particular attention to item 11, the patient's statement of the cause of the injury or illness. It should be written in the first person in the patient's own words, and in quotes for the greatest validity.

For example, the entry might read: "I was entering the cafeteria when I slipped on a wet spot. I twisted my left ankle outwardly before I fell to the ground."

The entry should *not* read: Twisted left ankle laterally after contact with wet spot on cafeteria floor.

The form should then be clipped or stapled to the front cover of the chart to alert the physician of the need to complete the form. The physician's notes for items 12 through 20 are usually handwritten.

Each state establishes the time limits within which Worker's Compensation cases must be reported. Employers must notify the insurance company, often within 48 hours, on a special form that details the circumstances and conditions at the time the claim originated. Physicians must also file timely reports, usually withn five days of the patient's first visit.

After the physician completes the initial report, type an original and four copies of the claim. These will be distributed as follows:

- The original and one copy to the insurance carrier;
- One copy to the employer;
- One copy to the state compensation board; and
- One copy retained for the physician's files.

If only one visit is required, prepare a statement immediately and submit it with the Doctor's First Report. If several visits are involved, which will be indicated on your initial report, send your routine office statement for subsequent visits. If the visits are beyond the original estimate or complications develop, submit a Doctor's Monthly (or Final) Report and a bill. In any case *all* bills must be sent directly to the employers, if self-insured, or to the insurance carrier directly. Patients must never be billed for any services for care in a work-related case.

Figure 13.6
Doctor's First Report form for Worker's Compensation cases.

**DOCTOR'S FIRST REPORT
OF
OCCUPATIONAL INJURY
OR ILLNESS**
STATE OF CALIFORNIA

Immediately after first examination, mail original to insurer or self-insured employer. Failure to file a doctor's report is a misdemeanor (Labor Code 6413.5). In addition, in the case of diagnosed or suspected pesticide poisoning, you are required to: Send one copy of this report directly to the Division of Labor Statistics and Research, P.O. Box 603, San Francisco, CA 94101; send one copy to your local health officer; notify your local health officer by telephone within 24 hours.

A. INSURER

		DO NOT WRITE IN THIS SPACE
1. **EMPLOYER NAME**		
2. Address: No. and Street City Zip		
3. Nature of business (e.g., food manufacturer, building construction, retailer of women's clothes)		

4. **PATIENT NAME** (First name, middle initial, last name)	5. Sex ☐ Male ☐ Female	6. Date of birth	
7. Address: No. and Street City Zip	8. Telephone number ( )		
9. Occupation (Specific Job Title)	10. Social Security Number		
11. Injured at: No. and Street City	County		
12. Date and hour of injury or onset of illness	13. Date and hour of first examination or treatment	14. Date last worked	15. Have you (or your office) previously treated patient? ☐ Yes ☐ No

16. **HISTORY** (History of injury or onset of illness. If occupational illness, specify exposures, chemicals and/or compounds.)

17. **MEDICAL FINDINGS** (Use reverse side if more space is required and for remarks, if any.)
A. Subjective complaints

B. Objective findings

X-ray and laboratory findings (State if none.)

C. Diagnosis (If occupational illness, identify etiologic agent.)

18. Are your findings and diagnosis consistent with history of injury or onset of illness?   ☐ Yes   ☐ No
If "No", please explain.

19. Is there any other current condition that will impede or delay patient's recovery?   ☐ Yes   ☐ No
If "Yes", please explain.

20. **TREATMENT**	Treatment Rendered	Further treatment required? ☐ Yes ☐ No
☐ Office ☐ Hospital out-patient ☐ Hospital in-patient		Physical therapy? ☐ Yes ☐ No
If in-patient, Give Hospital Name and Location	Date admitted	Estimated stay

21. **WORK STATUS**

Is patient able to perform usual work? ☐ Yes   ☐ No

If no, give date when you estimate patient will be able to return to:
Usual work: Modified work:

DOCTOR (name and degree) (Type or print)   No. and Street   City   Zip

Doctor's Signature   IRS Number   Telephone number ( )   Report Date

FORM 5021 (Rev. 2)
(May 1980)

**PLEASE SUBMIT YOUR REPORT WITHIN FIVE DAYS OF YOUR EXAMINATION
DELAY IN SUBMITTING THIS REPORT MAY CAUSE A DELAY IN BENEFITS TO YOUR PATIENT**

CAM Ⓤ D OSP

Private Plans
Blue Cross

History. The original concept of Blue Cross was the result of the economic distress of the nation's hospitals when the Great Depression of the 1930s left them with empty beds and unpaid bills. The American Hospital Association has played a major role in the development of Blue Cross, and today there are over 200 nonprofit Blue Cross plans throughout the United States that provide financial assistance for a variety of health care services.

Possible plans. Depending on the area of the country, Blue Cross plans may be available for coverage of hospital, medical, or surgical services or for any combination of the three. In addition, Blue Cross has developed a "Companion Care" plan that provides supplementary benefits to patients who have Medicare. Several companion options are available, including those that pay for Medicare deductibles and the 20% for hospitalization not paid by Medicare.

Eligibility. It is possible to acquire Blue Cross insurance as an individual or as part of a group. Individual plans cover one person and, if appropriate, his family. Group plans are available through employers or associations for employees or members and their families. The primary insured person is the subscriber, and eligible family members are dependents. If the insurance is an employment benefit, the employer may pay all or a major part of the subscriber's premium; if dependents are covered, the employee pays the additional coverage, often through payroll deductions.

Benefit payments. When a physician's services are billed to Blue Cross and the patient signs the authorization, payment of the carrier's portion will be sent directly to the physician. The patient is responsible for the remainder of the fee. If the patient assignment is not signed, the benefits check will be sent to the patient, often with both the patient and physician listed as payee. Theoretically this check would require both signatures to be cashed, but if this is not enforced, the physician may have difficulty recovering the payment.

Blue Shield

History. Like Blue Cross, the first Blue Shield organizations were born of the Depression and the need of physicians to protect their incomes. Blue Shield plans are also nonprofit and are local or statewide corporations. There are approximately 100 Blue Shield plans covering over 40% of the U.S. population. Because the original intent was to pay for physicians' services, Blue Shield plans were known as physicians' service organizations. Blue Shield has since diversified, like Blue Cross, and dropped the word *physician* from its title. Blue Shield is no longer considered physician sponsored.

Possible plans. Blue Shield offers the same options available through Blue Cross including a Medicare companion plan to supplement both Parts A and B of the Medicare program

Eligibility. Blue Shield is also available under individual and group contracts that are paid for in the same manner as Blue Cross. As is usually the case, a group plan premium is less costly for the subscriber.

Payment. Blue Shield develops fee profiles on physicians just as other insurance companies do. These profiles influence the determination of UCR fees.

Physicians may elect to be members of the local Blue Shield organization. As members they agree to accept the UCR fee as payment in full for services on some specific plans; other plans may allow the physician to bill the patient up to the shown allowed amount on the Explanation of Benefits (EOB). Patients of Blue Shield physician-members are responsible, however, for the annual deductible and for services that are not covered. Nonmembers' services will also be covered, but the patient can be billed for the difference between the UCR payment and the physician's actual fees in addition to the deductible and services that are not covered. Payment is automatically sent to physician-members and is sent to nonmembers if the patient signs the assignment. Otherwise the payment is sent to the patient.

Independent insurance carriers

Development. Currently there are approximately 1,000 private insurance companies that provide a variety of health policies. After World War II independent insurance carriers entered the health care field because of public need and the improvement of the insurance industry. The rapid advances in medical technology and the accompanying sharp escalation of medical care costs motivated the public to find a way to protect itself against the expenses. The relative prosperity of the economy at the same time allowed the insurance industry to introduce broad forms of insurance coverage, including major medical, that were previously unavailable.

Commercial companies may offer service plans, which pay on the UCR schedule, or indemnity plans, which pay a fixed amount for various injuries or treatments. The greater the amount of the indemnity or benefits, the higher the premium.

Plans available. An individual health insurance plan is purchased directly by the individual receiving the benefits. The policy is issued to the individual and/or eligible dependents. The individual health policy may also be obtained by an individual by converting from a group plan when the individual has terminated with the employer who contracted for group health coverage (as determined under COBRA legislation passed in 1987). Usually an individual plan will have higher premiums with fewer benefits, as compared with the same group plan.

Group health plans. A group health plan is a plan purchased for individuals by an employer or administrator of an association. This plan is written for any group of participants and their eligible dependents under a single policy issued to the employer or group. Individual certificates of membership in the group plan are issued to the individuals and dependents with equal coverage to each person in the plan.

Commercial health insurance carriers. Commercial health insurance carriers are for-profit companies that provide group and/or individual plans. These plans are paid for in the form of premiums. Coverage and benefits of an insurance plan underwritten by a commercial carrier will vary widely from plan to plan and carrier to carrier. The type and amount of payment will also vary greatly. The plans are governed by the state insurance commissioner since they include both life insurance and medical insurance.

Eligibility. Carriers have many methods and guidelines to determine eligibility; each contract or policy may have different requirements.

Reimbursement. Payment of benefits through policies held with independent carriers is generally made directly to the insured and not to the provider of care unless the patient authorizes an assignment. The patient is responsible for the physician's entire bill regardless of what the insurance policy pays.

Prepaid health plans

Development. By the early 1970s the federal government recognized the dramatic increases in health care costs and the public pressure to do something about them. In addition, while health insurance programs generally paid for services required for illness or injury, few would cover preventive services. In evaluating possible solutions, the government identified prepaid group practice

as one mechanism that had a proven record in controlling costs. Doctor Paul Ellwood, a presidential advisor, coined the phrase *health maintenance organization* (HMO), and federal support was proposed to create a national network of HMOs.

In 1973 the federal HMO Act (Public Law 93-222) was signed into law. It authorized federal funds for five years to establish and develop new HMOs. According to this law, an HMO provides or arranges for a comprehensive range of inpatient and outpatient health care services based on a fixed, prepaid fee. If the HMO is administered properly and its services provided appropriately, the plan will function within the budget. If not monitored properly the plan will go over budget and have to provide care throughout the premium period without reimbursement, since the reimbursement rate was calculated in advance. This puts the emphasis on keeping patients well and treating them early, hopefully preventing the need for major medical care.

Methods. By 1978 the HMO laws had been amended twice to promote the survival of the concept. Further grants were made available to qualifying groups wishing to continue or develop efficient HMOs. Under this concept, physician services may be delivered through three possible modes, which are described here.

Staff model. Physicians involved in the staff model type of HMO work in a group-practice clinic that is owned by the HMO and that employs its own physicians on a salaried basis.

Group model. Physicians who work in a group practice clinic enter into an agreement to provide services to the HMO subscribers. Based on a medical service agreement, the physicians' group accepts as fee for service a predetermined capitation rate. This means that each month the group receives a flat fee for each subscriber to the HMO. Some members will not see the physicians at any time during the month while others will require many services. If the capitation rate has been calculated properly and the physicians carefully select the methods of care, the physicians should be able to provide all needed services and still earn an income. Involved physicians may continue to treat nonmembers of the HMO on the usual fee-for-service basis.

Individual practice association (IPA). The IPA model is a legal entity that is organized and operated by physicians to promote the preservation of the private-practice concept. Through this mechanism, physicians join together to enter into contractual arrangements with other parties, such as

Figure 13.7
Criteria for evaluation
of modified HMOs,
PPOs, and/or IPAs.
Courtesy De A. Eggers &
Associates, San Rafael, Calif.

Criteria for Evaluation of Modified HMOs, PPOs, and/or IPAs

1. If you sign up, how long is the period you are committed to before you can change your mind?
   A. Six months
   B. One year
   C. Longer
2. Do you pay a fee to joint?
   A. If there a one-time fee?
   B. Is it a fee to be paid annually?
   C. If a group practice, is every member of the practice required to joint?
   D. Must each physician pay for a fee or is there a flat fee for the whole group?
3. How much paperwork is required for the office staff?
4. Must all patients have second opinions for surgery? For psychiatric care?
5. Can the physician refer outside the panel of providers or contracting hospital if deemed necessary?
6. What are the utilization review guidelines?
7. What are the reimbursement rates for fees?
   A. By unit?
   B. By RVS?
   C. Which year of RVS?
8. Which coding system do they use, CPT, HCPCS, DSM III?
9. What recourse is available for slow reimbursement by each of the entities?
10. Is an appeals process utilized if you do not like the way the claim is processed?
11. Does the provider of service have a say so or is there an open vote required for any major moves by the board of directors?

HMOs and other prepaid health plans, to provide medical services from private offices and in hospitals to a specific population of subscribers. Membership in an IPA does not limit a physician's practice to the treatment of patients covered under an IPA or HMO contract. As the individual IPA physicians provide services to the HMO subscribers, they submit their claims to the IPA for reimbursement on a predetermined fee-for-service basis. The fund available to pay for care is also based on a capitation rate. If care has been provided prudently, the funds will be adequate to pay all claims submitted throughout the prepaid time period; if not, physicians must continue to provide care without reimbursement. This is termed an *at-risk* form of insurance, because the *physician* is at risk of not being paid; the patient is not at risk, because care must be provided without prejudice.

Preferred provider organization (PPO). The PPO concept is a legal entity that has been organized by a variety of promoters (hospitals, physicians, insur-

ance carriers, and other groups). Through this mechanism, physicians and hospitals join together to enter into contractual arrangements with other parties, such as employers, unions, and associations, to provide medical services in private offices and in hospitals to that specific population of enrollees or subscribers. Membership in a PPO does not limit a physician's practice to the treatment of patients covered under the PPO contract. As the PPO physicians and hospitals provide services to the PPO subscribers, they submit their claims to the specific entity for reimbursement on a predetermined fee-for-service basis. The funds available to pay for care are also based on a predetermined rate. If care has been provided prudently, the funds will be adequate to pay for all claims submitted throughout the paid time period. If not, the physicians and hospitals must continue to provide care without reimbursement. This is another type of at-risk form of medical coverage, since the physician and hospital are at risk of not being paid.

The physician should evaluate each contract (be it a modified HMO, IPA, or PPO) very carefully before agreeing to participate (Figure 13.7). The assistant must be aware that with many of these contracts there is a greater burden of paperwork placed on the insurance assistant and many variations of requirements for second opinions, prior authorizations, and predeterminations prior to treatment.

Medical assistants and HMOs. As a professional medical assistant you may choose to work in an HMO. If you work in a group or IPA type practice, you will use both fee-for-service and HMO billing techniques. Each HMO functions according to a unique set of rules as long as it meets the federal criteria as an organization. If you are working in a practice associated with an HMO, familiarize yourself with the details of billing for services. Some group and IPA models require that a small deductible, $1 to $3, be paid by the patient for each visit.

CONTROLLING UTILIZATION
Reasons for Controls
Monitoring quality of care

The rapidly growing variety of available health care services and the number of providers has caused many groups to be concerned with the quality of health care being given. These groups include patient advocates, providers (peers), and the federal government. They are seeking methods of monitoring the care patients receive and the need for ancillary services based on the premise that each individual has the right to the best care possible.

Cost containment

Hand in hand with the need for quality control is the growing concern over the costs of medical care. The availability of insurance and facilities has sometimes resulted in the overuse or improper use of health care services.

In 1972 the federal government took the initiative in attempting to control the costs of medical care, since a large portion of those costs was paid for by government programs. The Social Security Act was amended to allow the formation of professional standards review organizations (PSROs) to monitor both the quality and cost of health care services provided with government funds. Other payers have since become equally interested in controlling the cost of health care.

Involvement in Utilization Review
Government insurance programs

Through the PSROs the government has established certain mechanisms to control costs under the common term *utilization review* (UR). The purpose is assurance and documentation that care is necessary and is provided at the appropriate level. The UR activities with which you will come into contact involve prior authorization for elective hospitalization and concurrent review during hospitalization.

Prior authorization. When a patient is to be admitted to a hospital for elective (nonemergency) medical or surgical care, permission must be obtained in advance of the admission. A review coordinator or physician associated with the PSRO will, based on the information provided, make a determination on the necessity of hospitalization. If the services can be safely provided in an outpatient setting, the request for hospitalization will be denied. Outpatient services cost much less than inpatient care and therefore are encouraged.

Concurrent review. Briefly, concurrent review is a method of monitoring patients who have been admitted to the hospital for care. Their charts are reviewed on admission and every few days thereafter to determine if they need to stay in an acute-care hospital or if their care can be continued at a nursing facility or at home.

HMOs

Primary care. Utilization review is built into the HMO concept from the perspective of centralized control. Many HMOs conduct patient care through a concentration on primary care. Each patient selects or is assigned a primary care physician who manages the patient's needs and refers patients to specialists or for hospitalization as needed. This helps monitor activity and, since other services may not be paid without primary physician referral, avoids unnecessary services or self-referral by patient to specialists.

Emphasis of care. Care through HMOs stresses health maintenance and preventive care. It is based on the principle that patients should seek care before problems begin or before they require major care. Through early intervention care can be provided at a reduced cost and on an outpatient basis rather than at costly, inpatient hospital rates.

Other insurance companies

Employer's request. Since employers pay a majority of the health insurance premiums for their employees, they are now requesting stricter guidelines by the carriers. Insurance premiums are steadily rising due to increased utilization of services. In other words, patients request and use more sophisticated services than may be considered necessary for appropriate, effective care. In an effort to curb health care costs, employers are encouraging insurance carriers to assist in the containment of health care costs. Many times this results in carriers requesting that certain types of services be reviewed by a utilization review organization prior to authorization being given to proceed with the planned treatment. Some insurance carriers are attempting to educate patients regarding proper utilization: putting an emphasis on primary care physicians to direct patient care, including all referrals to specialists, and monitoring hospitalization to minimize the length of stay.

Second opinion for elective surgery. Some insurance companies are requiring a second opinion when elective surgery is recommended. When surgery is recommended the patient must be seen by another surgeon, who is selected by the insurance company. If the second surgeon concurs with the original recommendation the surgery may be performed by the original surgeon. If there is disagreement between the surgeons, the insurance company may chose not to pay for the procedure or may request a third opinion. The insurance company will pay the entire fee for the second opinion. The second-opinion physician is strictly an independent consultant and may not accept the patient for treatment, even if the patient prefers him or her.

Medical Assistant's Role in Utilization Review
Knowing restrictions

The government and private insurance restrictions for cost containment will vary from one area to another. Learn the rules and regulations that apply in your area and be alert to the changes that take place. Government agencies and insurance companies will usually mail announcements to each physician's office regarding any program changes. Have a system arranged with your employer to assure that these announcements are shared with all employees.

Necessary permissions

If advance permission is needed for certain referrals or hospitalizations, you will be responsible for filing the proper forms and notifying the appropriate agencies or facilities. Being aware of the necessary advance steps and following established procedure will make the process simple and reduce the stress on you and on patients. These rules need not interfere with other responsibilities if you have planned an efficient procedure.

Hospital reviewers

On occasion you may receive a telephone call from the hospital utilization review coordinator. He or she will need to speak with the physician for information regarding a hospitalized patient. The coordinator works with the physician to see that the patient does not stay in the hospital any longer than is medically necessary. If the patient needs convalescent care, the hospital discharge planner will locate an appropriate facility and notify the physician of the planned transfer. These services provided by hospital personnel relieve you of duties that in the part were often performed by medical assistants working with family members.

FILING INSURANCE CLAIMS
Claim Form
Government and Blue Cross and Blue Shield

In some instances claim forms for Medicaid may be supplied by the intermediary. However, for Medicare, Blue Cross, Blue Shield, CHAMPUS, and CHAMPVA the provider of service is expected to utilize the HCFA 1984 version of the uniform claim form (Figure 13.8). The Medicare intermediary usually assigns each physician a provider number; Medicaid, Blue Cross, Blue Shield, and sometimes (depending on the geographic location) CHAMPUS (Figure 13.9) will utilize the same provider number. When a claim is filed the intermediaries use this number to enter data into their computers.

Intermediaries are making an effort to standardize the various claim forms. This will help when filing claims for patients, because each data section will be in the same location on each form regardless of the intermediary.

Worker's Compensation

Doctor's First Report and Monthly Statement forms for Worker's Compensation claims may be obtained from the local Department of Industrial Relations or from the individual insurance company that will be paying for the case. The forms supplied by the insurance company may be preprinted with the company name and address; those supplied by the Department of Industrial Relations provide space for you to insert the insurance company information. While the latter requires one more step, it may be the most convenient, because

Figure 13.8
Medicare form (HCFA-1500). **A**, Front.

Figure 13.8, cont'd
Medicare form, (HCFA-1500). **B.** Back.

HEALTH INSURANCE CLAIM FORM

REFERS TO GOVERNMENT PROGRAMS ONLY

MEDICARE AND CHAMPUS PAYMENTS: A patient's signature requests that payment be made and authorizes release of medical information necessary to pay the claim. If item 9 is completed, the patient's signature authorizes releasing of the information to the insurer or agency shown. In Medicare assigned or CHAMPUS participation cases, the physician agrees to accept the charge determination of the Medicare carrier or CHAMPUS fiscal intermediary as the full charge, and the patient is responsible only for the deductible, coinsurance, and noncovered services. Coinsurance and the deductible are based upon the charge determination of the Medicare carrier or CHAMPUS fiscal intermediary if this is less than the charge submitted. CHAMPUS is not a health insurance program and renders payment for health benefits provided through membership and affiliation with the Uniformed Services. Information on the patient's sponsor should be provided in those items captioned "Insured"; i.e., items 3, 6, 7, 8, 9 and 11.

SIGNATURE OF PHYSICIAN OR SUPPLIER (MEDICARE AND CHAMPUS)

I certify that the services shown on this form were medically indicated and necessary for the health of the patient and were personally rendered by me or were rendered incident to my professional service by my employee under immediate personal supervision, except as otherwise expressly permitted by Medicare or CHAMPUS regulations.

For services to be considered as 'incident' to a physician's professional service, 1) they must be rendered under the physician's immediate personal supervision by his/her employee, 2) they must be an integral, although incidental part of a covered physician's service, 3) they must be of kinds commonly furnished in physician's offices, and 4) the services of nonphysicians must be included on the physician's bills.

For CHAMPUS claims, I further certify that neither I nor any employee who rendered the services are employees or members of the Uniformed Services (refer to 5 USC 5536).

No Part B Medicare benefits may be paid unless this form is received as required by existing law and regulations (20 CFR 422 510).

NOTICE: Any one who misrepresents or falsifies essential information to receive payment from Federal funds requested by this form may upon conviction be subject to fine and imprisonment under applicable Federal laws.

NOTICE TO PATIENT ABOUT THE COLLECTION AND USE OF MEDICARE AND CHAMPUS INFORMATION

We are authorized by HCFA and CHAMPUS to ask you for information needed in the administration of the Medicare and CHAMPUS programs. Authority to collect information is in section 205(a), 1872 and 1875 of the Social Security Act as amended and 44 USC 3101, 41 CFR 101 et seq and 10 USC 1079 and 1086.

B

The information we obtain to complete Medicare and CHAMPUS claims is used to identify you and to determine your eligibility. It is also used to decide if the services and supplies you received are covered by Medicare or CHAMPUS and to insure that proper payment is made.

The information may also be given to other providers of services, carriers, intermediaries, medical review boards and other organizations or Federal agencies as necessary to administer the Medicare and CHAMPUS programs. For example, it may be necessary to disclose information about the benefits you have used to a hospital or doctor.

With the one exception discussed below, there are no penalties under Social Security or CHAMPUS law for refusing to supply information. However, failure to furnish information regarding the medical service rendered or the amount charged would prevent payment of Medicare or CHAMPUS claims. Failure to furnish any other information, such as name or claim number, would delay payment of the claim.

It is mandatory that you tell us if you are being treated for a work related injury so we can determine whether worker's compensation will pay for treatment. Section 1877(a) (3) of the Social Security Act provides criminal penalties for withholding this information.

MEDICAID PAYMENTS (PROVIDER CERTIFICATION)

I hereby agree to keep such records as are necessary to disclose fully the extent of services provided to individuals under the State's Title XIX plan and to furnish information regarding any payments claimed for providing such services as the State Agency, or Dept. of Health and Human Services may request. I further agree to accept, as payment in full, the amount paid by the Medicaid program for those claims submitted for payment under that program, with the exception of authorized deductibles and coinsurance.

SIGNATURE OF PHYSICIAN (OR SUPPLIER): I certify that the services listed above were medically indicated and necessary to the health of this patient and were personally rendered by me or under my personal direction.

NOTICE: This is to cerfity that the foregoing information is true, accurate, and complete.

I understand that payment and satisfaction of this claim will be from Federal and State funds, and that any false claims, statements, or documents, or concealment of a material fact, may be prosecuted under applicable Federal or State laws.

PLACE OF SERVICE CODES:

1 – (IH)	–	Inpatient Hospital
2 – (OH)	–	Outpatient Hospital
3 – (O)	–	Doctor's Office
4 – (H)	–	Patient's Home
5 –	–	Day Care Facility (PSY)
6 –	–	Night Care Facility (PSY)
7 – (NH)	–	Nursing Home
8 – (SNF)	–	Skilled Nursing Facility
9 –	–	Ambulance
0 – (OL)	–	Other Locations
A – (IL)	–	Independent Laboratory
B –	–	Other Medical/surgical Facility
C – (RTC)	–	Residential Treatment Center
D – (STF)	–	Specialized Treatment Facility

TYPE OF SERVICE CODES:

1	– Medical Care
2	– Surgery
3	– Consultation
4	– Diagnostic X-Ray
5	– Diagnostic Laboratory
6	– Radiation Therapy
7	– Anesthesia
8	– Assistance at Surgery
9	– Other Medical Service
0	– Blood or Packed Red Cells
A	– Used DME
M	– Alternate Payment for Maintenance Dialysis
Y	– Second Opinion on Elective Surgery
Z	– Third Opinion on Elective Surgery

Figure 13.9
CHAMPUS/CHAMPVA form.

CHAMPUS/CHAMPVA CLAIM FORM
For services or supplies provided by civilian sources except Institutions
Read cover instructions and the back of this form before completing and signing!

Form Approved
OMB No.
022-RO382

Patient/Sponsor Information (Items 1 through 18 to be completed by the beneficiary/patient or sponsor)

1. PATIENT'S NAME (Last name, First name, Middle initial)

2. PATIENT'S DATE OF BIRTH
MONTH   DAY   YEAR

7. SPONSOR'S NAME (Last name, First name, Middle initial)

3. PATIENT'S ADDRESS (Street, city, state, ZIP code)

4. PATIENT'S SEX
☐ MALE   ☐ FEMALE

8. SPONSOR'S SOCIAL SECURITY NO. OR VA FILE NO.   9. VA STATION NO.

PHONE NO. (Include area code)

6. PATIENT'S RELATIONSHIP TO SPONSOR
☐ SELF   ☐ SPOUSE
☐ NATURAL or   ☐ STEPCHILD
   ADOPTED CHILD
OTHER (Specify):

10. SPONSOR'S DUTY STATION OR ADDRESS FOR RETIREES

5. MILITARY/VA IDENTIFICATION CARD
CARD NO.

ISSUE DATE   EFFECTIVE DATE   EXPIRATION DATE
MONTH DAY YEAR   MONTH DAY YEAR   MONTH DAY YEAR

15. IS CONDITION WORK RELATED?
☐ YES ☐ NO
MILITARY SERVICE RELATED?
☐ YES ☐ NO
AUTOMOBILE ACCIDENT RELATED?
☐ YES ☐ NO

PHONE NO. (Include area code)

11. SPONSOR'S BRANCH OF SERVICE
☐ USA ☐ USAF ☐ USMC ☐ USN
☐ USCG ☐ USPHS ☐ NOAA ☐ VA

12. SPONSOR'S GRADE/RANK

14. DO YOU HAVE OTHER HEALTH INSURANCE? ☐ YES ☐ NO
IF YES, ENTER NAME OF OTHER PLAN OR PROGRAM:

13. SPONSOR'S STATUS
☐ ACTIVE DUTY   ☐ RETIRED   ☐ DECEASED

ADDRESS

CITY   STATE   ZIP

16. INPATIENT/OUTPATIENT CARE
☐ OUTPATIENT ☐ INPATIENT-EMERGENCY ☐ INPATIENT HOSPITAL-OUTSIDE 40 MILE RADIUS
☐ INPATIENT-SKILLED NURSING FACILITY ☐ INPATIENT-OTHER
☐ INPATIENT HOSPITAL-WITHIN 40 MILE RADIUS (ATTACH DD FORM 1251)

14a. TYPE OF COVERAGE:
☐ EMPLOYMENT (GROUP)   ☐ MEDICAID   ☐ STUDENT PLAN
☐ PRIVATE (NON-GROUP) ☐ MEDICARE   ☐ OTHER:

17. DESCRIBE CONDITION FOR WHICH YOU RECEIVED TREATMENT. IF AN INJURY, NOTE HOW IT HAPPENED.

14b. OTHER IDENTIFICATION NUMBER   14c. EFFECTIVE DATE
MONTH DAY YEAR

14d. OTHER PROGRAM THROUGH EMPLOYMENT?
EMPLOYER NAME:

18. SIGNATURE OF PATIENT OR AUTHORIZED PERSON, CERTIFIES CLAIM INFORMATION AND AUTHORIZES RELEASE OF MEDICAL OR OTHER INSURANCE INFORMATION. READ INSTRUCTIONS AND BACK OF THIS FORM BEFORE SIGNING.
SIGNED: DATE: RELATIONSHIP TO PATIENT:

Physician/Other Provider (Items 19 through 33 are to be completed by the physician or other provider.)

19. NAME, ADDRESS & PHONE NO. OF REFERRING PHYSICIAN

20. NAME & ADDRESS OF FACILITY WHERE SERVICES RENDERED (other than home or office)

☐ PRIVATE PRACTICE or ☐ UNIFORMED SERVICES

21. PROVIDER OF SERVICES
☐ ATTENDING PHYSICIAN
☐ OTHER

22. HOSPITALIZATION INFORMATION
MO DAY YEAR   MO DAY YEAR
ADMITTED   DISCHARGED

23. LAB WORK OUTSIDE YOUR OFFICE?
☐ YES ☐ NO CHARGES:

24. DIAGNOSIS, SYMPTOM OR NATURE OF ILLNESS OR INJURY, RELATE DIAGNOSIS TO PROCEDURE IN COLUMN "D" BY REFERENCE TO NUMBERS 1, 2, 3, or DX CODE
1.
2.
3.

25. A. DATES OF SERVICE MO/DAY/YEAR	B. PLACE OF SERVICE	C. PROCEDURE CODE IDENTIFY:	D. DESCRIBE PROCEDURES/SUPPLIES FOR EACH DATE. SUBMIT REPORT EXPLAINING UNUSUAL SERVICES OR CIRCUMSTANCES	E. DIAGNOSIS CODE	F. CHARGES	LEAVE BLANK

26. PATIENT'S ACCOUNT NO.

29. PHYSICIAN'S OR OTHER PROVIDER'S NAME ADDRESS, ZIP CODE & PHONE NO (INCLUDING AREA CODE)

G. TOTAL CHARGES
$

30. AMOUNT PAID BY BENEFICIARY
$

31. AMOUNT PAID BY OTHER INSURANCE
$

27. PROVIDER'S SOCIAL SECURITY NO.

32. AGREEMENT TO PARTICIPATE (READ BACK OF THIS FORM)
☐ YES   ☐ NO

28. PROVIDER'S EMPLOYER I.D. NO.

33. SIGNATURE OF PHYSICIAN OR OTHER PROVIDER (READ BACK OF THIS FORM BEFORE SIGNING)
SIGNED: DATE:

*PLACE OF SERVICE CODES
1 — (IH) — INPATIENT HOSPITAL
2 — (OH) — OUTPATIENT HOSPITAL
3 — (O) — DOCTOR'S OFFICE

4 — (H) — PATIENT'S HOME
5 — (DCF) — DAY CARE FACILITY (PSY)
6 — (NCF) — NIGHT CARE FACILITY (PSY)

7 — (NH) — NURSING HOME
8 — (SNF) — SKILLED NURSING FACILITY
9 — (AMB) — AMBULANCE
0 — (OL) — OTHER LOCATIONS

A — (IL) — INDEPENDENT LABORATORY
B — (OF) — OTHER MEDICAL/SURGICAL FACILITY
C — (RTC) — RESIDENTIAL TREATMENT CENTER
D — (STF) — SPECIALIZED TREATMENT FACILITY

CHAMPUS FORM 500 JUNE 1978

you will have to keep only one set of each form rather than sets of forms for each insurance company that refers patients for care.

Independent insurance companies

Each insurance company has a claim form of its own design, although each company requires the same basic information. Patients insured by independent companies will bring or send in the forms supplied for them.

When asked to file claims to independent insurance companies, you will find that the variations in the forms will require more of your time. The time spent on independent claims can be reduced by using a universal claim form (Figure 13.6) or a superbill. Using this method the patient or insured will fill out the patient information portion of the independent claim form. You will prepare the provider portion of a universal claim or a superbill and give it to the patient. The patient attaches the provider information to the independent insurance company's form and submits the claims for processing. This method will save you time to devote to other duties and will reinforce patients' responsibilities for the financial aspects of their care.

Other Equipment
Writing instruments

When filling out claims or reports to submit to insurance intermediaries, the typewriter is the preferred instrument. It provides clear, unmistakable characters that can be easily read. If forms or superbills are prepared by hand, use a pen that will imprint the information clearly through all copies. It is important that you print rather than use cursive handwriting, because printing reduces the possibility of misreading.

Adding machine or calculator

Except in situations in which your statements and forms are prepared by computers, confirm the totals of fees submitted on each claim form. The amount totals should be checked twice to be certain that they are correct, if using a calculator that does not produce a printed record on tape of the figures that were entered. If a tape is produced, enter the data once and compare the entries on the tape, item-by-item, with the entries on the form.

Code books

To standardize billing and simplify data on insurance forms the Health Care Financing Administration (HCFA) now authorizes the use of the HCFA Universal Claim Form 1500. HCFA also deter-

mines the codes for procedures and diagnoses that are required for medical claims processing. Effective January 1988, HCFA required that on all government claims that procedures would not only require a narrative, but also require the use of the CPT-4 procedure coding. CPT stands for Current Procedural Terminology, which is a descriptive listing of terms identifying codes for reporting medical services and procedures performed by a physician. The purpose of the terminology is to provide a uniform language that will accurately designate medical, surgical, and diagnostic services and will thereby provide an effective means for reliable, national communication among physicians, patients, and third-party payers.

CPT was initially developed by the American Medical Association (AMA) in 1966 through the Committee on Insurance and Prepayment Plans (CIPP). It began as a four-digit system of standard terms, provisional eponyms, and descriptors.

Since the first edition, CPT has been expanded to five-digit codes with a series of two-digit modifiers. CPT is currently in its fourth edition and is published and updated annually.

Coding system

All health insurance programs utilize some form of a coding system. It is envisioned that at some point in the future all health insurance claims processing will utilize the same national coding system. The use of a national procedure coding system would not only improve administrative and operational function by providing the common language but would facilitate important national/regional data collection.

In an effort to formulate this uniform coding system, the federal government, through activities of the HCFA, in cooperation with the AMA and the Insurance Association of America, formulated the Health Care Financing Administration Common Procedural Coding System (HCPCS).

HCPCS follows the AMA CPT-4 architecture in that it employs a five-digit code and a series of two-digit modifiers. But, unlike CPT-4, HCPCS also contains an additional series of five-character codes (an alpha followed by four numericals). HCPCS is comprised of the following three distinct levels of procedure codes plus the series of modifiers:

Level 1. The current procedural terminology, fourth edition (CPT-4), a listing of descriptive terms and identifying codes for reporting medical services and procedures, is the basis for reporting most medical/surgical services performed by physicians. The CPT-4 was devised and is maintained by the AMA.

Level 2. The Health Care Financing Administration developed additional alpha-numeric codes (A0000-V5999) to identify nonphysician (supplier) as well as additional physician services and procedures not found in the CPT-4.

Level 3. Where there is no appropriate national code assignment (level 2 or 2 codes) for a given service or procedure, the Medicare carrier has the option of assigning an alpha-numeric code within the range (W1000-Y9999). These codes allow the carrier the flexibility to code a particular service/item that may be unique to that service area or only seen in that local level at this time. HCFA evaluates level 3 codes from all carriers periodically to determine if a national code should be assigned. It is therefore possible that services and procedures in the local code category will be moved to the national category and assigned a different number.

Relative value studies (RVS)

Relative value studies, such as the California Relative Value Study (CRVS), are designed to describe medical/surgical services specifically for reimbursement purposes. The CRVS was first developed by the California Medical Association in 1956 to identify services rendered by physicians and to assign unit values to indicate the relativity within each individual section of the services described.

The CRVS was updated periodically to maintain its suitability for continued use in a changing scientific environment and economy. In the mid-1970s the Federal Trade Commission ruled that the use of the relative values were in violation of price fixing regulations and are therefore no longer to be promulgated. The procedure description feature of the CRVS, however, has survived and was updated as recently as 1985. It is now known as the California Standard Nomenclature. The Florida Medical Association, however, has continued to publish the FRVS, the most current edition being the 1986 FRVS. It is available to all states through the Florida Medical Association.

Diagnostic coding

International Classifications of Diseases (ICD). The International Classification of Diseases, ninth revision, Clinical Modification (ICD9-CM), is based on the official version of the World Health Organization's ninth revision, International Classification of Diseases. This modification replaces the eighth revision of the International Classification of Diseases, adapted for use in the United States (ICDA-8) and the hospital adaptation of the ICDA (H-ICDA).

ICD9-CM is used to serve as a classification of morbidity data for indexing of medical records, medical care review, and ambulatory and other medical care programs as well as basic health statistics.

The ICD9-CM is published in three volumes. Volume 1 provides a tabular listing of diagnoses, symptomatology, and health-related conditions. Volume 2 is an alphabetical index of diseases. Volume 3 is both a tabular and alphabetical index of diagnoses or diseases.

Diagnostic and Statistical Manual, Third Edition (DSM-III). The *Diagnostic and Statistical Manual* is a diagnosis coding system utilized primarily by psychologists and by psychiatrists. DSM-III was developed by the American Psychiatric Association's Task Force on Nomenclature and Statistics.

The codes in DSM-III are compatible with the ICD9-CM; however, additional diagnostic information is included, which is specific to the psychiatric specialty and is also used for data collection purposes.

Modifiers. The use of modifiers permits a provider to indicate the circumstances under which a procedure as performed differs from the description by the use of a five-digit code.

There are five reasons to use modifiers: (1) they eliminate the need for a lengthy report; (2) they give a more accurate description of services; (3) they may increase or decrease the fee; (4) they may indicate a component of service or adjunctive service; and (5) the physician's fee profile will not be affected as a result of fees being reduced in certain cases.

Use modifiers when (1) the service or procedure being rendered has both a professional and a technical component or either one; (2) the service or procedure is performed by more than one physician and/or in more than one location; (3) the service or procedure has been increased/reduced; (4) the service or procedure was repeated; (5) part of the service was performed in conjuction with another service; or (6) unusual events occurred.

Modifiers are added as suffixes to the procedure code where it is required to give additional information regarding the circumstances, setting, patient condition, and so on. As with procedural coding, national and local modifiers are utilized.

In addition to the two-digit modifiers identified in the CPT-4, further two-digit alpha-numeric and two-digit alpha modifiers are assigned nationally.

These national modifiers are in ranges A1-V9, and AAVZ. Where there is no appropriate CPT-4 national modifier, carriers will assign a two-digit alpha-numeric or alpha modifier to identify certain billings. Local modifiers are in ranges W1-Z9 and WA-ZZ.

Medical records

The medical record of each patient for whom a claim is filed will be needed. The record should give easy access to all the necessary personal and medical data, including current insurance information.

Accounting information

To complete a claim form, the accounting information from the patient's ledger card or from computer billing printouts will be needed. This information includes the date services were provided, the procedure code, and the charges for the service.

Medicaid proof

For patients using Medicaid, a copy of each month's card should be retained with the record copy of the claim form in case verification of the Medicaid number is required by the intermediary. Only in the state of California does one have to affix a copy of a Proof of Eligibility (POE) to the claim form. For California an original MEDI label must be affixed to the claim for the following services—psychology, optometric, audiology, podiatry, chiropractic, sterilization procedures, cosmetic procedures, physical therapy, occupational therapy, or speech therapy. It is to the medical assistant's advantage to always photocopy the Medicaid form with the appropriate form attached. Also tape the label on the form with nonglare tape (Figure 13.10).

METHODS OF MONITORING CLAIMS TO BE PROCESSED
Forms to be Filed

To avoid overlooking or losing claim forms that must be processed, set up separate file folders for each type of insurance you handle. The method you choose will depend on the volume of forms you process. Doctor's First Reports for Worker's Compensation should always be kept with the patient's record and be processed immediately after the first visit because of the legal requirements.

For all other claims, select the appropriate form as the patient arrives for a visit or when you are notified that the physician has seen a patient at an-

other facility. Office patients should sign the authorization to release information and authorization to pay at the time of the visit. The form should then be dated and placed in the folder(s) in chronological order. Then process the forms, in the order in which they were initiated, at preplanned times during each filing period.

Insurance Log

You may develop a log for insurance forms to be processed. It can consist of a single sheet in a spiral notebook with separate columns for the patient's name, type of insurance, date entered in log, and date completed. An alternative way to develop a log is to maintain separate sheets in a ring binder with one sheet set aside for each type of insurance. Each sheet can be divided into columns for the patient's name, date entered, and date the form is completed and sent. If an insurance log is used, you may choose one of these methods or design a log that fits the needs of your office or agency.

Claims Processed Daily

Superbills allow claims to be completed on a daily basis, because the form is given to the patient at the time of each visit and the patient becomes responsible for submitting the claim. If you process claim forms for patients and have a limited patient volume or adequate numbers of personnel, you may be able to process the forms on a daily basis. The appropriate form may be attached to each patient's chart as it is prepared for the visit. The physician may sign the form and insert the diagnosis after seeing the patient and completing the progress notes. When the chart is returned to the assistant, the remaining necessary information can be entered on the form and the form sent to the proper insurance intermediary. If other visits are scheduled for the same illness or injury, place the partially completed form in the record and retain it until the series of visits is completed.

PROCESSING CLAIM FORMS
Forms Completed by Office Staff
Necessary equipment

If some or all of the insurance forms are completed by the administrative office personnel, there is a minimum amount of equipment needed to complete the job. Supplies of forms from companies with which you communicate regularly should be kept on hand. Since universal claim forms can be

Figure 13.10
Professional supplier claim form used in California.

FASTEN HERE

DO NOT STAPLE IN BAR AREA

PROVIDER NAME AND ADDRESS

ROBERT K CEMORE MD
490 POST STREET #234
SAN FRANCISCO CA

1. CLAIM CONTROL NUMBER   F.I. USE ONLY
2. MEDI-CAL PROV. NO.   CHECK
00A1344320   5
3. MEDICARE PROV. NO.   DIGIT
6. ZIP CODE
94120

PROFESSIONAL/SUPPLIER CLAIM FORM

4. ☐ MEDI-CAL
5. ☐ MEDICARE

AFFIX LABEL HERE   AFFIX LABEL HERE

Elite Pica 7 (415) 567 2276 ◄ PROVIDER PHONE NO.   PLEASE TYPE ALL REQUIRED INFORMATION   Elite Pica
Typewriter Alignment

PATIENT'S COMPLETE NAME, AND ADDRESS
8 THOMAS J TAYLOR
1146 46TH AVENUE
SAN FRANCISCO CA 94122

9 MEDICARE NUMBER   10 SEX M/F M   11 WAS CONDITION RELATED TO EMPLOYMENT N   12 DATE OF ONSET   13 TAR CONTROL NUMBER
14 MEDI-CAL I.D. NUMBER 38609457355511   15 CODE   16 DATE OF BIRTH 122324   PATIENT ACCOUNT NUMBER TAYLOR
17 SERVICES RELATED TO HOSPITALIZATION FROM 06019- 18 THRU 06089- 19 EMER. CERT. 20 OTHER COV. 21 BILLING LIMIT 1 22 ATTACH-MENTS 23 D.M.E. CODE 24 MEDICARE STATUS 0

28 OTHER HEALTH INS. COV.-ENTER NAME OF POLICY HOLDER, PLAN NAME, ADDRESS AND POLICY NO. 25 PATIENT'S PHONE NUMBER (AREA)
NAME & ADDRESS OF FACILITY WHERE SERVICES WERE RENDERED (IF OTHER THAN HOME OR OFFICE) 27 FACILITY PROVIDER NO.
MARIN GENERAL HOSPITAL GREENBRAE   HSC90016F

29 OUTSIDE LAB   30 LABORATORY NAME AND ADDRESS

31 NAME OF REFERRING PROVIDER   32 REFERRING PROVIDER NUMBER

PRIMARY DIAGNOSIS DESCRIPTION
33   34 PRIMARY ICD-9-CM 930 8   35 SECONDARY DIAGNOSIS DESCRIPTION   36 SECONDARY ICD-9-CM

DESCRIPTION	BILLING PROVIDER CHARGE FOR OUTSIDE LAB SERVICES		DELETE	DATE OF SERVICE	PLACE OF SERVICE	FP/ CHDP	RENDERING PROV. NO. IF OTHER THAN BILLING PROV.	PROCEDURE CODE MOD	QUANTITY	SERVICE CHARGES
37	38		39 ☐1	40 06029-	41 3	42	43	44 65222	45 1	46 875 00
47	48		49 ☐2	50 MM DD YY	51	52	53	54	55	56
57	58		59 ☐3	60 MM DD YY	61	62	63	64	65	66
67	68		69 ☐4	70 MM DD YY	71	72	73	74	75	76
77	78		79 ☐5	80 MM DD YY	81	82	83	84	85	86
87	88		89 ☐6	90 MM DD YY	91	92	93	94	95	96
97	98		99 ☐7	100 MM DD YY	101	102	103	104	105	106
107	108		109 ☐8	110 MM DD YY	111	112	113	114	115	116

REMARKS/EMERGENCY CERTIFICATION STATEMENT:

117 BLOOD PINTS   BLOOD DEDUCT 118   119 TOTAL CHARGES 875 00
120 MEDICARE DEDUCTIBLE   121 MEDICARE CO-INSURANCE   122 MEDICARE PAID
123 MEDICARE DISALLOWED   124 PATIENT'S SHARE OF COST   125 OTHER COVERAGE   126 DEDUCTIONS
127 DATE OF EOMB   128 DATE BILLED   129 NET AMOUNT BILLED 875 00
130   131   132   133   134   135 TOTAL CHARGES
136 AMOUNT PAID
137 ANY UNPAID BALANCE DUE

SIGNATURE REQUIRED FOR EMERGENCY CERTIFICATION   / / DATE

PATIENTS OR AUTHORIZED PERSON'S SIGNATURE (READ BACK BEFORE SIGNING). I authorize the release of any Medical Information necessary to process this claim and request payments of Medicare Benefits either to myself or to the party who accepts assignment.
138   SIGNED   DATE

This is to certify that the information contained above is true, accurate, and complete and that the provider has read, understands, and agrees to be bound by and comply with the statements and conditions contained on the back of this form.
139 SIGNED   06129-
Signature of provider or person authorized by provider to bind provider by above signature to statements and conditions contained on this form.

140 ☐ I DO ACCEPT ASSIGNMENT
141 ☐ I DO NOT ACCEPT ASSIGNMENT

40-1C 12/87

SEE YOUR PROVIDER MANUAL FOR ASSISTANCE REGARDING THE COMPLETION OF THIS FORM.

FORWARD TO APPROPRIATE F.I.

substituted for most insurance carriers' forms, you may wish to use this option. The universal form reduces the amount of searching you must do to locate the various spaces in which information is to be entered. You will also need the patient's account information, the patient's medical record, a calculator or adding machine, and pens.

Medical assistant's responsibilities

You will be expected to complete as much of the claim form as possible from the medical record and patient account information. These are the components of filling out the HCFA 1500 Universal Claim Form (Figure 13.8).

1. Check the available program box at the top of the form. If more than one insurance program is involved (for example, Medicare and Medicaid), check more than one block.

Patient and insured subscriber information

Block 1–Patient's name. Copy the spelling of the patient's name exactly as it appears on the subscriber's insurance identification card. For Medicare beneficiaries, request the red, white, and blue Medicare card. For Medicaid information, enter the last name first, then the first name followed by the middle initial in Block 1.

Block 2—Patient's date of birth. Indicate month, day, and year, if available.

Block 3—Insured's name. If the patient is covered by employment-related health insurance, show the full name of the employed person. This name should also appear in Block 9.

Block 4—Patient's address. Give the patient's current mailing address (include apartment number and zip code). Please furnish patient's telephone number if available. If the patient resides in a convalescent facility or nursing home, indicate the name of the facility in addition to the address.

Block 5—Patient's sex. Check the appropriate box.

Block 6—Insured's Medicare number. Copy the health insurance claim number exactly as it appears on the Medicare card. Include *all* letters. Do not enter a Medicaid number here; see Block 9. When Medicare is secondary, identify the patient by name and health insurance claim number in Block 9.

Block 7—Patient's relationship to insured. If the patient has health insurance based on his/her own or spouse's current employment, check the appropriate box.

Block 8—Insured's group number. If the patient has employment-related health insurance, show group number or name.

Block 9—Other health insurance coverage. Indicate patient's Medicaid identification number for crossover claims or policy number for other coverage if Medicare is primary.

If Medicare is secondary payer because of employment-related insurance, show the patient's name and health insurance claim number. If this insurance is based on spouse's employment, also show his/her name and health insurance claim numbers.

If Medicare is a secondary payer because of employment-related insurance (ESRD or working aged), enter the name and health insurance claim number of the policy holder and the name and address of the employer plan.

If Medicare is the secondary payer because of automobile no-fault liability insurance, show the name and address of the automobile no-fault liability insurer.

Block 10—Was the condition related to. Check the appropriate box or boxes.

Block 11—Insured's address. If the name in Block 3 is different from the name in Block 1, show the complete mailing address of the insured. For crossover claims, affix stickers, if appropriate, in this block.

Block 12—Patient's or authorized signature. Obtain the signature of the beneficiary or an authorized representative. If a lifetime signature has been obtained (Figure 13.3), indicate patient's payment authorization on file.

Physician or supplier information

Block 14—Date of accident. If charges were incurred because of an automobile accident, enter the date the accident occurred.

Block 15—Date patient first consulted you for this condition. Indicate the date the patient first consulted you for the condition for which services are now being billed.

Block 19—Name of referring physician or other source. The name and complete address of the referring physician is required by Medicare for consultation; independent laboratory charges submitted without a diagnosis; independent radiology billing submitted without a diagnosis; billings by physicians administering antigens supplied by another source; podiatric routine foot care; physical therapy by a therapist in an independent practice; prosthetics/orthotics; eye appliances; psychological testing; ambulance; desirable medical equipment (DME); nonphysician ECG/chest x-ray; outpatient speech pathology; occupational therapy; audiology testing; and portable x-ray.

Block 20—For services related to hospitalization, give hospitalization dates. This item should be completed when medical services are rendered as a result of or subsequent to related hospitalization.

Block 21—Name and address of facility where services are rendered. The facility name and city must be listed if the services were performed in a place other than an office or home. Facilities included are independent lab; ASC; HAASC; dialysis centers; CORF; SNF; NH; and hospitals.

Block 22—Was laboratory work performed outside your office. If laboratory work is being charged on this bill, this item must be completed. If work was performed outside of the physician's office, the "Yes" box should be checked and the amount charged for the service entered. If more than one laboratory service was performed outside the physician's office, show the dollar amount charged the physician by the laboratory for each individual test on the right of column 24D. If the physician's charge is the same as the amount charged by the laboratory (this is mandatory for Medicare), the charges should be shown in 24E with a statement, "Actual charge made by laboratory to physician for the test."

Blocks 21 and 22 must be completed for all laboratory work performed outside the physician's office. If no work is performed outside the physician's office, you must stamp on the claim "No purchased diagnostic test."

Block 23A—Diagnosis or nature of illness or injury. Describe the nature of the illness or injury treated. ICD-9-CM diagnosis coding is required in most states for relating this information; however, a narrative should be utilized. Also use this block to identify Medicare as a secondary payer, ESRD beneficiary, working age, or accident. For ESRD patients, indicate if the patient is in training for self-dialysis.

Block 24A—Date of service. Enter the month, day, and year for each procedure. If "from" and "to" dates are shown for a number of identical services, the number of days or units for these services should be entered in column F. Use a separate line for each month. Do not include two months together on the same form particularly during the months of December of one year and January of the next year.

Block 24B—Place of service. Use one of the following place of service codes listed on the reverse side of the claim form.

POS code	Place of service
IH	Inpatient hospitalization (acute)
OH	Outpatient hospital (includes ambulatory surgical centers [ASC]; hospital-affiliated clinics and dialysis centers, emergency services, CORFs)
IKC	Independent kidney center
O	Office (includes free-standing physician-directed clinics)
H	Home (includes rest homes and residential care facilities or nonnursing facilities)
IL	Independent laboratory
SNF	Skilled nursing facility
NH	Nursing home
OL	Other location

When billing for laboratory services, the following guidelines will apply:

Circumstances	POS Code
Lab service performed at physician's office	O
Lab service purchased from another physician who maintains a lab in his/her office	OL
Lab service purchased from an independent lab	IL
Lab service performed by independent lab, sample taken from a hospital inpatient	IH

Block 24C—Fully describe procedures, medical services or supplies furnished for each date given.

A. Identify the appropriate procedure code and modifier (S) for each service.

B. Include a narrative description along with the appropriate procedure code and modifier.

C. Do not use, if at all possible, alone without coding. It is preferred to use an unlisted procedure code. Include operative report, discharge summary, consultation report, or other pertinent documentation.

D. Operative report should always be included when the surgical procedure or procedures is unusual or complex; when there is no corresponding procedure code or modifier and is described as a by-report or unlisted procedure; and when surgeries involved co-surgeons and/or team surgery.

E. For anesthesia services, indicate the time in hours and minutes. Include applicable modifiers.

F. When billing for monthly capitation payments, indicate MCP in this block. Also use this block to identify "temporary patient" when renal-related services are furnished to ESRD patients dialyzing away from the usual setting.

Block 24D—Diagnosis code. ICD-9-CM codes are to be used in this field and may be entered to relate the date of service and procedures performed in the appropriate diagnosis when there is more than one diagnosis shown.

Block 24E—Charges. The charge for each listed service must be entered. If laboratory services were performed outside the physician's office, each lab service must be listed with the laboratory's charge and the physician's charge.

Block 24F—Days or units. Indicate the number of services, the number of days of services, or the number of units involved.

Block 24G—TOS (Type of service). Leave this field blank. Disregard type of service code listing on the reverse side of the claim form. It is not required at this point.

Block 25—Signature of physician or supplier. Signature of the provider/authorized representative. Note: Include date.

Block 26—Assignment. Check "yes" or "no" box to indicate assignment choice. Providers who have signed the participation agreement with the Medicare program will have all claims processed as assigned. If neither box was checked on the straight Medicare claim and the biller is not participating, the claim will be processed as assigned. Note: On Medicare/Medicaid cross-over claims the provider must accept assignment to receive residual payments.

Block 27—Total charge. Indicate the total charges for all services billed on the claim.

Block 28—Amount paid. Indicate any amount paid by the patient; if none, enter 0. This block must be completed on a Medicare assigned claim. If billing Medicare as a secondary payer, the amount paid by the primary insurer must be entered there.

Block 29—Balance due. Provide any unpaid balance due. This must be completed on a Medicare assigned claim.

Block 31—Physician's or supplier's name, etc.. Give the full name, address, and telephone number of the physician or supplier. Include provider number.

Block 32—Your patient's account number. Optional.

Block 33—Your employer ID number. SSA number or employee number.

If there are items that do not apply to the particular case being reported you may leave them blank. It is not necessary to indicate N/A (not applicable). If there are some questions you cannot answer from the resources available, put a check with red ink next to the item as a quick locater when you review the forms with the physician.

Once you have completed as much of each form as possible, clip the forms to the appropriate patient's chart and present them to the physician for review and signature. When the physician is finished with them, the forms can be separated from the chart and the copies placed in the appropriate section of the patient's medical record. The originals are then prepared for submission to the insurance carrier. Some services require supporting documents such as operative, pathology, or narrative reports. Once each form is ready, it should be mailed to the appropriate insurance intermediary.

Avoiding Returned Claims
Advantages

If claims are improperly processed, insurance companies will return them for resubmission. It is to the advantage of your office to avoid this step if possible. Claims that can be processed on receipt by the carrier will improve the accounts receivable figures in the office, because they will be paid faster. This is particularly true of major fees for complicated diagnostic and treatment services. Avoiding returned claims also reduces the work load of the administrative personnel. If a claim is returned, you will have to determine the reason for the return, retrieve the appropriate records, and resubmit the corrected form to the insurance company.

Common reasons for returned claims

There are four common reasons that forms are returned from the insurance carrier to the physician's office. They are the following:

- Erroneous or missing data;
- Missing attachments;
- Incorrect carrier; and/or
- Illegibiligy.

Erroneous or missing data. Before you submit insurance forms to the insurance carrier for processing, spend an extra moment to double-check that all data are present and correct. The trouble spots often involve the following:

- Missing or incorrect insurance identification numbers;
- Incomplete or missing diagnosis;
- Missing physician's signature;
- Missing or incorrectly multiplied fees for services; and/or
- Dates of treatment that do not correspond with support documents.

The limited time you spend confirming these items

will save time in the end by avoiding returned claims.

Missing attachments. Claims for certain services require the submission of documents to support or decribe the claims made by physicians. Although insurance carriers may not include a statement of this requirement with the claim forms, you should assume that the documents are necessary. Always submit support documents necessary to support unusual services or By Report (BR) procedures; these may include unusually complex consultations, treadmill reports, extensive operative reports, and pathology reports for cases involving malignancies, since the fees will be much higher than in cases of benign pathology.

Incorrect carrier. Claims submitted to the incorrect insurance carrier will delay payments because of the time spent trying to determine the patient's eligibility before the claim is returned. Most errors of this type can be avoided by frequently checking with patients about the status of their insurance coverage. Most insured individuals have their policies reviewed and updated once a year through their employment, and the employer may even change insurance companies at a review. However, since patients may not remember to tell you of any changes, you must take the responsibility of checking.

Illegibility. Insurance forms and superbills that are handwritten require special attention to legibility. If completing these forms by hand you should print, using a pen that will imprint through all copies. If the physician writes in the diagnosis and there is any doubt that it can be clearly understood, you may reprint it, enclosed in parentheses and immediately following the physician's notation.

Remaining Current on Claims Processing

The methods used to process insurance claims are changing rapidly because of the use of computers, and the information required on claims will also change as cost-containment mechanisms are introduced. You will need to keep abreast of these changes, and several resources are available to help in this endeavor. There are four commonly available resources, and there are others that you will become aware of in your area. The four common sources of information are as follows:

- Bulletins from insurance carriers. Some major carriers, especially Blue Cross, Blue Shield, and Medicare-Medicaid intermediaries, send routine updates on claims processing. These

updates should be read on arrival and retained for future reference.
- Articles in *The Professional Medical Assistant,* the official journal of the American Association of Medical Assistants.
- Professional relations representatives from Medicare and Medicaid.
- Courses that provide updated information.
- Local medical societies offer useful information in their organization magazines and may hold periodic "brown-bag" lunches to inform office personnel of recent administrative changes, including insurance billing.

You will want to take advantage of all available resources to keep current on the methods necessary to have claims processed in the least possible time.

HELPING PATIENTS WITH INSURANCE
Filing Their Own Claims

When possible it is to your advantage to encourage patients to file their own insurance claims. Since patients may not submit claims in a timely manner, you will need to instruct them that they must pay at the time of service or on receipt of their statement rather than waiting until the insurance company pays. You will also need to spend some extra time educating patients in the process, but doing so will save time in the future.

The most appropriate claims that can be filed by patients involve simple services, such as office or hospital visits for medical care. Claims that require supporting documents should be filed by office personnel, because it is inappropriate to give patients copies of operative reports, pathology reports, and so on.

Superbills, discussed in Chapter 12, are the simplest method of providing patients with the information they need to file claims. You may have the filing instructions printed on the back of the form to reinforce the verbal instructions given to patients. An alternative is to produce a statement with all the necessary information, including diagnosis. This can be accomplished with handwritten or computer statements.

Answering Patients' Questions

Patients may ask questions regarding their current health insurance or insurance they are considering. This is time consuming and beyond the scope of your responsibility, but be prepared to offer patients the courtesy of suggesting information resources to them.

The most frequent inquiries will involve whether or not the patient's insurance will cover a service or procedure and how much of the cost the insurance company will pay. Since insurance cards contain minimal information, you should not attempt to make any statement about the coverage. Instead, suggest that patients contact their insurance company or their employment personnel office, where there is usually an employee involved with health benefits.

Another common question about health insurance involves insurance options. The patient may ask either "What is the best insurance I can get?" or "I have been offered two plans at work—which one would be better for me to take?" It is not appropriate for you to attempt to answer these questions, but you can suggest that patients need to acquire the insurance that will best meet their personal needs. You might suggest that they contact an insurance broker who can compare policies for them and help them assess the various options.

The final common question patients ask involves what they should look for in insurance coverage. You can suggest that they contact the major reputable insurance companies, where representatives should be willing to answer questions and supply literature. Contacting an insurance broker, who will have access to information about policies from many companies, is an alternative to contacting insurance carriers independently. You can suggest that patients read a policy carefully, check the policy limits, and ask their agent questions before purchasing insurance.

INSURANCE PROTECTION FOR THE MEDICAL PRACTICE
Reasons for Insurance

Physician-employers will need to obtain insurance coverage for various aspects of the medical practice. The basic reason for insurance in a medical practice is the same as the reason for insurance in any situation: to protect against personal financial loss. Your responsibilities for the various insurances required will probably be limited to storing and retrieving policies and reminding the physician when the premium is due.

Policies should be stored in a safe, fireproof environment. The most common location is in a safety deposit box in a local bank. If policies are kept on the office premises they should be kept in a fireproof cabinet, preferably locked for additional security. To make policy retrieval easy, you should keep a master list of all office insurance policies in an accessible place in your work area. The list should include the following information:

- Type of policy;
- Insurance company;
- Policy number; and
- Annual renewal date.

Since policies are only in effect if insurance premiums are paid, you will need to establish a means of assuring that payment dates are not missed. The easiest method is to use a master calendar or tickler file. Insurance companies typically send renewal notices in advance of the due date but if the notice should be lost, either before or after reaching your office, you should have a back-up reminder system. The date noted in the reminder file should be two to four weeks before the renewal date. If you have not received a renewal notice by two weeks before the renewal date, contact the insurance company or the office insurance broker.

Classification of Insurance

Although you will not be responsible for the investigation or acquisition of insurance policies for the office, it is to your professional and personal advantage to understand the basics of protective insurance. Insurance policies are classified as follows:

- Property insurance;
- Criminal loss insurance;
- Legal liability insurance; and
- Package policies.

Medical offices usually have one or more of these policies to protect the physician from financial loss.

Property insurance

There are many possible policies that can be purchased to protect against property loss; only the more common will be described here.

Damage to owned building and contents provides basic coverage for loss from fire and may be extended to include loss from vandalism or malicious mischief. The latter is often necessary, since medical offices are common targets for burglars in search of cash and drugs.

Consequential loss coverage can be very important to a medical practice, since the loss of property or contents may result in loss of the ability to conduct business during the course of rebuilding property or replacing furnishings or equipment.

Broad-form coverages may be a method of attempting to cover a practice for all of the items just discussed and all other potential risks, but you should be aware that most policies still include some exclusions such as floods, earthquakes, and tornadoes. Careful reading of insurance policies is always wise but is particularly important with this type of coverage.

Special area needs will depend on the area in which the practice is located. Insurance may be obtained for specific possible needs, such as protection against loss to hurricane, earthquake, or flood. In areas where there is a high risk of these events, the insurance premium can be expected to be particularly high.

One thing to keep in mind when acquiring property insurance is that the policy can be written at actual cash value or for replacement value. Replacement value is more appropriate, because inflation will make the cost of replacing any item higher than it was at the time of purchase.

Criminal loss insurance

Criminal loss in a medical practice usually relates to the loss of funds or property from theft by employees. Protection against this type of loss is classified as fidelity bonds, which can be purchased in three forms. Individual fidelity bonds protect the employer against losses from any dishonest act by an employee. An application for this type of bond must be completed by each employee. The employees will then be named individually with the insurance bonding company. Scheduled fidelity bonds may be purchased to cover individual employees or specific positions for a stated dollar amount. A blanket fidelity bond covers all employees automatically, regardless of position, for a dollar limit established by the employer. The blanket bond has the additional advantage of payment for the loss even if the responsible employee cannot be identified.

Legal liability

Comprehensive general liability. Comprehensive general liability is a broad form of coverage designed to protect the policy holder from financial losses to injury caused by a condition or defect on the premises or by operational hazards. It also provides protection for building owners against claims as a result of conditions created by renters. This is a policy similar to the public liability commonly held by homeowners and renters, except that the dollar amounts for a business are generally higher because of the number of people who visit the office.

Professional liability. Professional liability was discussed at length in Chapter 5 under medicolegal considerations. The professional liability insurance carried by physicians to cover their acts and omissions and those of their employees is basically related to claims for bodily injury and issues related to patient care.

Worker's Compensation. States have mandated that insurance coverage be provided for employees in the event that they are injured or become ill in the course of their work. In many states the physician-employer can also be covered under the same policy as the employees, since the physician is subject to the same exposure. Although some states do not require coverage from employers with fewer than 10 employees, most medical practices carry Worker's Compensation regardless of the number of employees because of the possible exposures in a medical environment.

Excess liability and umbrella policies. Excess liability and umbrella forms of legal liability coverage are available to provide coverage for unexpected claims or events. Excess liability extends the dollar coverage provided by basic liability policies to assist with exceptionally large claims. An umbrella policy may be purchased to serve as "catch-all" coverage to protect the policyholder against all of the possible hazards not covered by or excluded from basic liability policies.

Conclusion

The subject of insurance is extensive and evolutionary. Types of insurance coverage and the addition to policies of cost-containment requirements will influence the methods you use to remain knowledgeable about the subject so that effective and efficient insurance processing procedures can be maintained. Continued monitoring of office policy and procedures will assure the least disruption of reimbursement for services and the efficient control of policies required to protect the medical practice.

Review Questions

1. Describe in your own words how you would explain to patients their responsibilities regarding their health insurance.
2. Explain three of the several types of coverage available.
3. How would you explain to a patient the difference between assignment of benefits by the patient and acceptance of assignment by the physician?
4. What is the difference between Medicare and Medicaid? What is the difference between CHAMPUS and CHAMPVA?
5. Who is eligible for Worker's Compensation?
6. Describe Medicare's role as a secondary payer.
7. Describe how the need for adequate documentation affects utilization review.
8. Describe in logical sequence an efficient method of processing insurance claims for patients.
9. What will patients need to file their own insurance claims?
10. What types of insurance policies are needed to protect the medical practice? What are your responsibilities with regard to office policies?

SUGGESTED READINGS

American Medical Association: Current Procedural Terminology, ed 4, Chicago, 1989, The Association.

International Classification of Diseases, Ninth Revision, Clinical Modification (ICD9-CM), Pittsburgh, 1988.

Source Book of Health Insurance Data, 1982-83, Update 1984, Washington DC, 1984, Health Insurance Association of America.

Chapter 14

Computers in the Health Environment

- Understanding computer language
- How computers function
- Needs assessment
- Hardware/software

Objectives

On completion of Chapter 14 the medical assistant should be able to:

1 State five ways in which a medical office can utilize a computer system.

2 Explain reasons why a physician might use a computer system.

3 Define computer terminology and abbreviations.

4 Recognize which reports are the most valuable to the practice.

5 Review the cross-check computerized insurance claim forms.

Vocabulary

acct type Account type.

adj Adjustment.

alpha order In alphabetical order.

appt Appointment.

backup A duplicte file to protect information.

basic A programming language.

batch processing When data is handled by an outside source and later returned to the client.

baud The speed of the communication between devices, usually the CRT and the CPU.

boot starting up the computer.

byte Usually 6 or 8 bits, it is the unit of symbolic transfer; each character, number, or letter is one byte.

cartridge disk A disk in a convenient cartridge form.

chip An integrated circuit.

cobol A business-oriented computer language.

continuous form Forms or paper that are pin-fed.

CPU Central processing unit; the heart of the computer.

crash When the system becomes inoperative.

CRT Cathode ray tube.

cursor A lighted mark that indicates your place on the CRT.

data entry Input of information.

database Accumulation of files in the CPU.

debug Eliminates problems.

default Values supplied by the system when none are entered.

directory Table of contents of a file system.

disk A flat plate or cartridge used as a memory device.

disk drive Operates the disk.

diskette A storage medium similar to a disk but in soft form, may be called a floppy disk.

dot matrix The use of dots to form letters and numbers.

download Sending of information from one system to another.

dun A message placed on delinquent billing statements.

field A part of the record used for specific information (name - - - - - - - - -).

file Collection of records of the same type and format.

format Arrangement of data or records in a file.

hardcopy Printed copy on paper (for example, an insurance form).

hard disk Memory storage unit in rigid form.

hardware The equipment

headcrash Hardware failure that damages the disk.

index A fast means of locating specific data.

input Data to be entered.

key To enter data on a keyboard.

line printer A device that prints in lines instead of individual characters.

line surge A severe increase in voltage that can cause damage to the computer.

load Transfer data or a program to execute data.

login To use your identification password.

mainframe Large central computer.

megabyte One million bytes.

memory Data in computer.

menu A listing of function or programs.

microcomputer Small compact computer.

minicomputer A medium-powered computer.

modem A communication device that allows the computer to use telephone lines to access other devices.

network A system of interrelated computers.

on-line Using CRTs with direct link to a computer off-site.

operating system An internal software language to control the hardware.

output Data or information delivered by the system after processing.

password User identification to allow access to the system.

powerdown The sequence of steps to shut down a computer.

powerup The sequence of steps used to start a computer.

printer Device that produces hardcopy.

program A sequence of instructions for the computer.

purge To eliminate data.

screen What is visible on the CRT.

scrolling Moving data up or down on the CRT.

sector One area on a disk.

sort To sequence data according to specified instructions.

source code Original program code that is translated to an object code for computer use.

system A package of instructions designed to complete specified tasks.

timeshare Multiple users on the same system.

transaction An action between the data entry operator and the computer.

word processing A system for writing, editing, and storing information (letters, reports, etc.).

SOFTWARE APPLICATIONS

Computer systems have many applications in the medical office. The most prevalant is the medical billing system for producing statements, insurance forms, a compilation of accounts receivable, and collection of the accounts. The computer system may also be used to record the accounts payable, produce checks to pay invoices, and maintain a general ledger for the practice. Many systems will also incorporate payroll, production of payroll checks, and the information required for government reporting. Also available with many systems is the appointment system. This system allows the practice to maintain appointment scheduling within the system instead of keeping an appointment book. This is extremely helpful when there are more than two physicians in a practice.

Medical Billing Systems

Of the many computer systems available to the medical practice, there are three principal types: in-house, batch, and on-line.

In-house system

The office or in-house computer is equipment that can be purchased or leased. The system is usually utilized by a single physician or by a group practice.

Batch system

The "batch" method of computerized billing involves compiling all new patient information and each day's transactions (that is, charges, payments, plus adjustments and minus adjustments). The "batch" may be made up of one copy from the superbill, charge slip, or document for each patient seen during the day. These will be clipped together with an adding machine tape for all of the charges for the day. An additional group of forms will be utilized to record all of the payments and adjustments for the day. Again, these should be clipped together with an adding machine tape totaling all payments and adjustments.

When the "batch" arrives at the computer billing company, a data entry operator will enter the data into the physician-client's data bank. Normally the data will be picked up on a weekly basis by a messenger and delivered to the processing center. The processing center then feeds the information into the computer system. These types of processing units can usually accommodate a large number of offices with greater flexibility, as it normally has a larger computer, more memory, and more extensive programming available. The user may pay the computer firm a monthly fee for each active account and may also pay a basic charge for the processing of the forms, statements, reports, and recall notices. There are also firms available in certain areas that will not only process all information, but will also pursue each patient account through payment from the insurance carrier or patient. These firms are normally paid a percentage of the dollars collected.

On-line system

This system is an in-house terminal with direct transmission. On-line computer systems do not eliminate the need for writing out the transaction data. There must always be a source document, that is, a charge slip or payment record. The office is equipped with a computer terminal. A cathode ray tube (CRT) screen, consisting of one or two pieces, usually rests above the terminal. Together they look like a typewriter with a small television screen. There is a link with a computer that may be in a building many miles from your office. There are two methods of connecting or linking the CRT terminal with the off-site computer. One method may be to dial a specific number at the computer center and waiting to hear a high-pitched tone. At the sound of the tone, place the receiver into what is called a modem. This modem links the CRT terminal with the computer. The other method is what is called "hardwire," which means that the CRT terminal and the computer are directly wired and may be used as needed. No matter which method is utilized a "password" is needed for you to communicate with the computer processing unit. Each physician-client will be provided with a password or a series of passwords. After typing your password, you will be allowed to communicate with the computer. Anything keyed (typed) into the computer usually appears on the screen within a few seconds. This is how each patient transaction is recorded. You may also request to see data that has been previously stored in the computer and it will appear on the screen.

EVALUATION OF THE PRACTICE NEEDS
Converting to Computer

The decision to convert from a manual system to a computer is usually made by the physician. However, physicians have become aware that they must enlist the aid of computer-literate personnel in the practice or an outside consultant in determining the true needs of the practice. Most advisers on the subject will still recommend that the physician allow the office staff to give their opinions and suggestions. There are usually numerous reasons why a physician will elect to go into a computerized billing system. Some are:
- Office efficiency may be increased;
- The overall cost is lower than manual processing of information;
- Better management control and more current information will be available;
- The physician may expand the practice more conveniently;
- Collections may be improved; and
- Records are more secure.

Before a computer system is implemented, the physician's office will need to review and evaluate all business aspects of the practice.

Once a particular computer system and set of applications is acquired, it can be difficult to make changes. The physician will frequently request the assistant's suggestions to determine applications the practice should implement. The assistant should be aware that many times the purchase of a system can be disastrous if certain criteria are not considered.

Criteria
Consider current environment

List the positive and negative points of the practice's current system. A list of efforts needed to coordinate the office's current system should also be developed.

The assistant will need to help the physician determine applications necessary for the practice, that is, billing/accounts receivable, appointment scheduling, payroll, general ledger, accounts payable, word processing (for medical records, or research), and patient reporting systems.

A major consideration for any practice should be about the location of the CPU within the facility as well as how many CRTs will be needed.

The medical assistant and the physician will need to request information regarding hardware, system software, growth capabilities, maintenance, training, installation, costs, security, and a myriad of other details. It is to the advantage of the assistant and physician to request an evaluation of needs by an outside consulting firm that does not have a business connection with the vendor who is attempting to sell the system to the physician. The medical assistant can assist the physician by requesting to see the system in operation in three other locations and speak with the medical assistants in those practices.

Data entry

Each computer system has its own method of data entry codes whether by letters or numbers. However, some of the codes required for a medical billing system are fairly standard. For diagnosis, the current coding required is the ICD9-CM (International Classification of Diseases, ninth revision—Clinical Modification). (The ICD9-CM is published by ICD9-CM, Box 360121, Pittsburgh, PA 15250-6121.) For procedure codes or the description of services rendered, the Current Procedural Terminology (CPT-4) five-digit code system is used. For Medicare claims there is also the Health Care Procedural Coding System (HCPCS) as developed by the Health Care Financing Administration. Some states also utilize the relative value study (RVS), which is a method of five-digit procedure codes with unit values. Each medical practice must be aware of the capability of using these codes in the system chosen.

When a physician secures a computer system, the computer replaces the manual or pegboard bookkeeping system. To illustrate the input and output from a computer system, samples will be shown throughout this chapter. Output is shown as daily, weekly, and monthly. Various reports utilized are described in detail in the following section.

Forms

Forms used for a computerized billing system normally are connected together in what is called pinfeed. While the medical assistant should be familiar with all of the following forms, not all offices will use every form since the data overlaps.

Patient information sheet (see Figure 12.1)

The patient information sheet establishes all insurance and billing information for the patient.

Charge slip (Figure 14.1)

The charge slip or fee ticket is usually personalized to the practice. It is basically the key to any successful billing system and triggers everything automatically, including the third-party insurance form.

The assistant fills in the patient's name, date of service, patient's account number, and any change of insurance information. The assistant then places the charge slip on the front of each patient's medical chart before his/her visit. The physician simply checks or circles the indicated services and diagnosis, writes in the fee, and hands the charge slip to the patient. The patient then arranges payment at the front desk or payment desk. The assistant keys the data into the computer with pre-set codes and the computer does the rest; that is, the computer generates a statement and/or a completed insurance form(s) and incorporates the data into daily, weekly, and month-end financial analysis of the practice.

Because the charge slip is customized to fit the particular practice, usually just circling the procedure codes is required for most patients. However, the physician can write in a new diagnosis in the open area of the charge slip. The assistant then completes this by filling in the correct diagnosis codes from the ICD9-CM. The practice can revise the charge slip whenever office requirements change. Charge slips are often used with the pegboard bookkeeping system.

Other information

Most computer companies have a variety of forms to handle the input of additional information obtained after the patient information sheet has already been submitted; such data may include the following:

- Information changes, used when there is a change in the patient's address, insurance coverage, or employment status;
- Hospital charges, used when the physician makes hospital rounds (Figure 14.2);
- Payment/adjustment form, used to show what monies have been received from patients and/or insurance carriers, and adjustments for portions not paid or allowed by Medicare or Medicaid (Figure 14.3); and
- Recall notice, a notice to remind a patient that it is time to return to the practice for a recheck (Figure 14.4).

Reports
Transaction list

The transaction list is a daily control report that defines each day's charges, payments, and adjustments. It is used for balancing each day's transactions. Usually the system must balance with the day's input prior to generating this report.

Figure 14.1
Charge slip form.
Courtesy De A. Eggers
& Associates, San
Rafael, Calif.

ACCOUNT NO.	DR. NO.	PATIENT ACCOUNT #	MEDI-CAL STICKER	DATE
130,				

PATIENT NAME			MEDICARE/SOCIAL SECURITY NO.	CONDITION	SEX	BIRTH DATE
LAST	FIRST			Injury 1 ☐ Injury 2 ☐ Pregnancy 3 ☐	M ☐ F ☐	

PATIENT ADDRESS			TELEPHONE	
STREET	CITY AND STATE	ZIP CODE	AREA	NUMBER

GUARANTOR OR SUBSCRIBER		POLICY NO.	GROUP NO.	COVG. CODE	RELATION
LAST	FIRST				Self 1 ☐ Spouse 2 ☐ Child 3 ☐

INSURANCE CO. NAME	INSURANCE CO. ADDRESS

From Empl.	New Illness	New Ill. Date	INJURY	INJ. DATE	HOW INJURED	PREG. DATE
Yes ☐ No ☐	Yes ☐ No ☐		Auto 1 ☐ Other Home 2 ☐ 3 ☐			

HOSP.	Admit Date	Disch. Date	OUTSIDE LABORATORY WORK			PATIENT REFERRED	
			AMOUNT	NAME	LOCATION	DOCTOR	CITY
			Yes ☐				

DIAGNOSIS

		M.D. Assessment	CONT. CASE
4140 Coronary Artery Dis.	428 Cardiac Failure		Yes ☐ No ☐
401 Hypertension	434 Cerebral Vascular		Type of Service
395 Aortic Valve Dis.	425 Cardiomyopathy		Surg. ☐
394 Mitral Valve Dis.	7469 Congenital Heart		Asst. Surg. ☐
396 Mitral/Aortic Valve	427 Cardia Arrhythmia		Anesth. ☐
416 Pulmonary Heart Dis.			RECALL DATE
426 Cardiac Conduction	4292 Cardiovascular Specf. DX		

PLACE OF TREATMENT: 1- I.P. Hosp.   2- O.P. Hosp.   3- Office   4- Home   6- Laboratory   7- ECF   8- Nursing Home

DESCRIPTION	Code		Unit Mod	AMOUNT	PT	DESCRIPTION	Code	Unit Mod	AMOUNT	PT
Comprehensive New Exam	01	90020			3					
Brief Exam	03	90040			3					
Limited Exam	04	90050			3					
Intermediate Exam	05	90060			3					
Extended Exam	06	90070			3					
Comp Yearly Re-exam	07	90080			3					
Comprehensive Re-exam	08	90085			3					
Comprehensive Consult	09	90620								
Unusual Consult	10	90630								
Hospital										
Hospital Admit	11	90220			1					
Hospital Admit Limited	12	90215			1					
Brief Hospital Exam	13	90240			1					
Limited Hospital Exam	14	90250			1					
Intermed Hosp Exam	15	90260			1					
Extended Hosp Exam	16	90270			1					
Electrocardiogram	17	93000			3					
Rhythm Strip	18	93040			3					
Blood Pressure	19	90040	24		3					
Combined rt and lt Cath	20	93526			1					
Combined rt Cath	21	93527								
Combined lt ht Cath	22	93547								
Combined rt and lt	23	93549								

PAYMENT: ☐ CASH   ☐ M/C   ☐ VISA

ASSIGNMENT OF BENEFITS: I hereby assign all medical and/or surgical benefits, to include major medical benefits to which I am entitled, including Medicare, private insurance and any other health plans to:

This assignment will remain in effect until revoked by me in writing. A photocopy of this assignment is to be considered as valid as an original. I understand that I am financially responsible for all charges whether or not paid by said insurance. I hereby authorize said assignee to release all information necessary to secure the payment.

SIGNED: _____   DATE: _____

Figure 14.2
Hospital charges form.
Courtesy De A. Eggers & Associates, San Rafael, Calif.

AS   JK   KC   WTA   RC   BB   GG   EK

HOSPITAL PATIENTS WEEKDAYS: ROOM # _____

PT. NAME _____

INSURANCE(S) _____

REFERRING M.D. _____

ADDRESS & TEL. _____

_____

ADMIT DATE:_____ DIS. DATE: _____

DIAGNOSIS _____

PT. NAME _____   ROOM NO._____

SURGERY:	43.32 MVR	45.91 Aort. aneur. rep.
	43.33 TVR	45.92 Cong. heart dis.
45.81 ACB	43.34 Double valve	45.99 Other surgery:
43.31 AVR	45.00 Pacemaker	Specify:

DATE	FOLLOW UP		ADMISSIONS		CONSULTATIONS	
M	H: 1 2 3 4 5 6	7 8 9		C: 1 2 3 4 5	NC
	H: 1 2 3 4 5 6	7 8 9		C: 1 2 3 4 5	NC
T	H: 1 2 3 4 5 6	7 8 9		C: 1 2 3 4 5	NC
	H: 1 2 3 4 5 6	7 8 9		C: 1 2 3 4 5	NC
W	H: 1 2 3 4 5 6	7 8 9		C: 1 2 3 4 5	NC
	H: 1 2 3 4 5 6	7 8 9		C: 1 2 3 4 5	NC
T	H: 1 2 3 4 5 6	7 8 9		C: 1 2 3 4 5	NC
	H: 1 2 3 4 5 6	7 8 9		C: 1 2 3 4 5	NC
F	H: 1 2 3 4 5 6	7 8 9		C: 1 2 3 4 5	NC
	H: 1 2 3 4 5 6	7 8 9		C: 1 2 3 4 5	NC
	H: 1 2 3 4 5 6	7 8 9		C: 1 2 3 4 5	NC
	H: 1 2 3 4 5 6	7 8 9		C: 1 2 3 4 5	NC

SCHEDULE RETURN VISIT _____

TYPE OF BILLING: (circle one)

   A. Standard
   B. Accept MediCare (full)
   C. Accept assignment & patient 20%
   D. Discount (specify %)_____
   E. Special instructions_____

M.D. Assessment: (circle one)

   1. High 2. Medium 3. Low 4. Unknown

RC 12/8

FOLLOW UP CHARGES

H1 90240   F/u Brief   (**-10)
H2 90250   F/u Limited (11-15)
*H3 90260 F/u Intermed.(16-27)
H4 90270   F/u Extended (28-30)
H5 99150   Detention   (30 +)
      (report needed)
H6 90292   Final Day

ADMISSIONS

H7 90200   Limited
H8 90215   Intermediate
*H9 90220 Regular

Procedures & Dates:

CONSULTATIONS

C1 90600   Brief
C2 90605   Limited
C3 90610   Intermed.
*C4 90620 Regular
C5 90630   Complex
NC *****   No Charge

Weekly transaction list (Figure 14.5)

Some computer systems have audits to help discover an error such as posting to a wrong account. The weekly listing provides information on all patients who received services that week, a compilation of all charges, payments, and adjustments.

Month-end report (Figure 14.6)

The month-end report is issued at the end of each month to bring all active accounts up-to-date. It lists all medical and financial transactions within the month, notes each patient's current balance, notes the date the last statement was sent to the patient, and notes the date on which the last insurance form was produced. It also summarizes charges, payments, and adjustments for the month.

Cumulative report

The cumulative report can provide the same information in alphabetical sequence monthly, biyearly, yearly, or longer. This report can provide the practice with total in-office account control

Figure 14.3
Payment/adjustment form (see p. 217).

PROVIDER NAME: _____

DATE: _____

ACCT#	PATIENT NAME	CODE	DESCRIPTION	Adjust Patients Balance		CASH	BANK#	AMOUNT
				(−)	(+)			
1								
2								
3								
4								
5.								
6.								
7								
8.								
9								
10								
11.								
12								
13								
14.								
15.								
16								
17.								
18								
COLUMN TOTALS						A		B

TOTAL DEPOSIT $ _____
(A + B)

PAYMENTS
01 Rec'd On Account
02 Blue Cross Payment
03 Blue Shield Payment
04 Medicare Payment
05 Medi-Cal Payment
06 Insurance Payment

ADJUSTMENTS
07 Medicare Write-Off
08 Medi-Cal Write-Off
09 Industrial Write-Off
10 Accept Ins Assignment
11 Sent to Collections
12 Courtesy Discount
13 Refund
14 Posting Error (+)
15 Posting Error (−)
16 Adjustment (−)

Figure 14.4
Recall notice form.

```
FROM   Sam B. Good, M.D.
       1234 Anywhere Street
       San Francisco, CA 94102




          Mr. Goodnight:

          Please call the office for an appointment to check your
          Hypertension.  The office number for Consulting Cardiology
          Associates is 415-234-9000.  We look forward to hearing
          from you.

                                    Sincerely,
                                    Sam B. Good, M.D.


               TO    Charles Z. Goodnight
                     4445 Bush Street, #405
                     San Francisco, CA 94118
```

and yields an invaluable, day-by-day record of the accounts receivable.

Aged listing (Figure 14.7)

The aged listing report provides the practice a listing of all outstanding patient accounts by classification (private insurance, Worker's Compensation, Medicare, Medicaid, etc.) It will provide a listing of patient name, responsible party, telephone number, date of last payment, and amount outstanding for 30, 60, or 90 days. This report is extremely beneficial in providing data necessary to allow for collection follow-up.

Provider production report (Figure 14.8)

The provider production report provides in-depth information regarding total charges, payments, and adjustments by the physician. It is particularly useful in practices where there are several physicians. This report allows physicians to track by month the amount of revenue generated by each physician.

Procedure report (Figure 14.9)

The procedure report can usually be generated weekly, monthly, or by any given time frame. It de-

tails which procedure codes are being most frequently used by the practice during a given period of time.

Report generator

Most comprehensive computerized billing systems are capable of generating specialized reports for the needs of a particular practice; that is, the obstetrician-gynecologist who wants a monthly report listing all pregnant patients as well as their due dates.

Patient statement (Figure 14.10)

Most computerized billing systems produce an itemized billing statement each month. Normally a monthly statement is produced for each member of the family, showing charges, payments, and the balance due. A computerized statement usually shows a breakdown of the amounts due, which are delinquent, and number of days delinquent. This information is always important from the standpoint of collecting the accounts. Some computer billing systems will produce statements by family. Normally the computer company provides the paper product to produce the statements.

Figure 14.5
Weekly transaction list.

WEEKLY TRANSACTION LISTING   GROUP 225

Date 06/01/89

Acct#	Patient	Date	Procedure	Description	ICD9	Amount	Payment
10025	Alvarez	05/01/89	90350	Limited Visit (SNF)	250.0	60.00	
10003	Boudreaus	05/01/89	90060	Intermediate Exam	414.0	50.00	
10005	Bowen	05/02/89	90060	Intermediate Exam	465.9	50.00	
10006	Cabalquint	05/02/89	90060	Intermediate Exam	466.0	50.00	
10009	Callie	05/02/89	90050	Limited Exam	560.0	43.00	
		05/02/89	36415	Veni-Puncture	560.0	12.00	
10089	Dunlap	05/03/89	90020	Comprehensive NP	414.0	128.00	
		05/03/89	93000-YB	EKG	414.0	52.00	
		05/03/89	89205	Occult Blood	414.0	10.00	
		05/03/89	36415	Veni-Puncture	414.0	12.00	
10123	Hazel	05/03/89	90060	Intermediate Exam	250.0	50.00	
10114	Hudson	05/03/89	90060	Intermediate Exam	465.9	50.00	
10023	Kassel	05/03/89	90060	Intermediate Exam	560.0	50.00	
		05/03/89		Payment received			
		05/03/89		Travelers Pmt 4/8/89			50.00-
10021	Ridell	05/03/89		MCare 4/25/89			26.40-
10022	Ruther	05/03/89		Prud. Pmt 4/5/89			15.60-
							225.00-

05/28/89 Accounts Receivable   16,895.77

                Charges   617.00
                (+) Adjustments   0.00
                Payments   317.00
                (-) Adjustments   0.00

06/01/89 Accounts Receivable   17,195.77

Figure 14.6
The month-end report.

```
MONTH END REPORT                          GROUP 225              Page 15
06/01/89

Acct#   Patient        Balance/Aging Mess.   Date      Procedure   Description        ICD9    Amount

10025   Alverez        Bal    121.00  A E    05/01/89  90350       Limited Visit SNF  250.0   60.00
        Emmanuel       Type Pri Pay     *
        2141 Alemany   Prv.    61.00
        SF, CA         Smt 05/01/89
        922-9505       Ins 05/01/89 #1N/CI

10003   Boudreaus      Bal     50.00  M C     05/01/89  90060       Intermediate Exam  414.0   50.00
        Andrea         Typ M/Caid
        24 Buss St     Prv.       0
        SF, CA         Smt
        445-2345       Ins 05/05/89 #1

10089   Dunlap         Bal    202.00  T R     05/03/89  90020       Comprehensive NP   414.0  128.00
        Dizzy          Typ Ind                05/03/89  93000-YB    EKG                414.0   52.00
        16 Smith       Prv.       0           05/03/89  89205       Occult Blood       414.0   10.00
        SF,CA          Smt                    05/03/89  36415       Veni-Puncture      414.0   12.00
        567-9083       Ins 05/03/89


Previous Accounts Receivable:         139,234.78
        Charges                                    25,908.00
        (+) Adjustments                                22.50
        Payments                                   13,223.50
        (-) Adjustments                             1,040.00

06/01/89 Accounts Receivable:         150,901.78


* (30),  ** (60),  *** (90) All or part of balance is past due
```

Figure 14.7
The aged listing report.

```
AGED ACCOUNTS RECEIVABLE                              GROUP 225

06/01/89

Acct#    Patient                 0-30     31-60     61-90      Total      Telephone

10025    Alverez, Emmanuel      60.00     61.00               121.00     922-9505
10003    Boudreaus, Andrea      50.00                          50.00     445-2345
10005    Bowen, Hoss            50.00               75.00      125.00     443-1254
10006    Cabalquint, Maria      50.00     50.00              100.00      123-4321
10009    Callie, Slim           55.00     55.00               55.00      322-2134
10089    Dunlap, James         202.00                         202.00     567-9083
10230    Hazel, Hazel           50.00               27.00      77.00     456-7898
10114    Kassel,Bob                                335.00     335.00     456-9090
10023    Lemming, Rebecca                        1,000.00   1,000.00     456-8970
10021    Ridell, James                            80.00      80.00      657-6890
10022    Ruther, Dana                             25.00      25.00      567-9876


GRAND TOTAL                    517.00    166.00  1,569.00   2,242.00
```

Patient ledgers

Some computer companies provide, as an optional feature, a ledger for each patient account if requested by the physician. Usually this is unnecessary, however, as the reports provide all information required for each account.

Recall notice

Most computer billing companies provide a recall notice that can be generated as needed to remind patients that they are due for an appointment. These notices can be sent out by the computer company or by the assistant.

The medical assistant's role

With nearly all medical office computer systems, the medical assistant will be the principal operator. Normally the equipment is located near the "front desk," where much of the patient communication is ongoing either by telephone or by patients coming into the office. Terminals and printers should be located to protect the confidentiality of what they display. Food, drinks, cigarette smoke, ashes, and dust should be kept at a minimum around the computer components.

The primary function of the medical assistant is to key all new data into the computer, to retrieve information on the screen or printer in answer to patient or physician questions, and to initiate and handle the periodic printouts, such as statements, insurance forms, and daily records.

Flow of Information

The flow of information to the medical assistant for entry into the computer is much the same as for a manual system. A new patient is registered by keying the same type of information into the system that is normally typed on a ledger card. A patient account number is assigned by the assistant and/or the computer. This number is used to identify the patient in the computer. Charge slips are the source of what happens during an office visit, the procedure(s) performed, and charges for the visit. Payments from the patients are the source of information for receipts.

Data entry by the assistant

Data entry is accomplished by keying the data as it is received. Most computer systems make this easy by prompting with helpful messages that tell the operator what to do next at each step.

First, a "main menu" of the major functions of the system is displayed on the screen and the operator simply selects the desired function by entering the code number as shown on the screen (Figure 14.11). Once into the function, the screen indicates the required information for the selection. The operator normally has an opportunity to check all transactions before completing the entry. Incorrect data is easily corrected by different methods; however, all systems allow for error correction. Once the operator completes all data entry, he/she balances all charges, payments, and adjustments to

Figure 14.8
The provider production report.

PROVIDER PRODUCTION REPORT   GROUP 225

Date: 01/01/89

Provider		Total	%	Private Pay	%	Industrial	%	Medicaid	%	Miscellaneous	%
01	Chg	3,464.00	100	2,658.00	76.7			806.00	23.3		
	+Adj	210.00	100	210.00	100.0						
	-Adj	94.20	100					94.20	100.0		
	NET	3,579.80		2,868.00	80.1			711.80	19.9		
	Pmt	574.05	100.0	388.00	67.6			186.05	32.4		

**********PRODUCTION TOTALS AND SUMMARY**********

Calculated Using 56 Transactions

	Chg	3,464.00		2,658.00	76.7			806.00	23.3		
	+Adj	210.00		210.00	100.0						
	-Adj	94.20						94.20	100.0		
	NET	3,579.80		2,868.00	80.1			711.80	19.9		
	Pmt	574.05		388.00	67.6			186.05	32.4		

Figure 14.9
The procedure report.

```
PROCEDURE REPORT                          GROUP 225

    06/01/89                              Times    Total Amount

    90000    Brief New Patient Exams        12       3,245.00
    90010    Limited New Patient             3         535.00
    90020    Comprehensive New Patient      23       6,789.00
    90040    Brief Office Exam              85       5,656.00
    90050    Limited Office Exam            27       1,234.00
    90060    Intermediate Office Exam       88       5,909.00
    90070    Extended Office Exam            2         200.00
    90220    Comp. Hospital Admit           10       2,220.00
    90250    Limited Hospital Exam          13       1,155.00
    90260    Intermediate Hosp Exam          7         700.00
    93000    EKG                            14         752.00

    89205    Occult Blood                    7          70.00

    36415    Veni-puncture                  10         100.00

    TOTAL SERVICES                         301      28,565.00
```

Figure 14.10
Patient
statement.

```
0233 10683                STATEMENT       Tax ID:94-24444444
Robert B. Clean, M.D., Inc.               License: 00G12380
2333 Clay Street, #999                    Pulmonary
San Francisco, CA 94120

Business  Office (415)457-1668
```

ACCOUNT NUMBER	PREVIOUS BALANCE	PRESENT BALANCE
10683 ***	25.00	267.75
USE THE ENCLOSED ENVELOPE. AND MAKE PAYMENT TO	DATE	06/01/89

```
Robert B. Clean, M.D., Inc.          Re: Sammy H. Class
2333 Clay Street, #999               Sammy H. Class
San Francisco, CA 94120              2345 Bay Street
                                     San Francisco, CA 94133
```

ACCOUNT NUMBER	PREVIOUS BALANCE	PRESENT BALANCE	30 DAYS PAST DUE	60 DAYS PAST DUE	OVER 90 DAYS PAST DUE
10683 ***	25.00	267.75			267.75

DATE OF SERVICE	CPT-4	DESCRIPTION	ICD9-CM	AMOUNT
11/16/88	90020	Comprehensive New Pt	491.0	175.00
11/23/88	90060	Intermediate Office Exam	491.0	60.00
12/28/88	90060	Intermediate Office Exam	491.0	60.00
12/28/88	94001	Spirometry	491.0	45.00
01/04/89	90050	Limited Office Exam	491.0	45.00
01/04/89	90730	Flu Vac	491.0	15.00
12/04/88		Ins. Pd. 11/16/88		157.25-

```
            Patient: Sammy H. Class
```

DATE	06/01/89	YOUR PRESENT ACCOUNT BALANCE IS	267.75

```
Robert B. Clean, M.D., Inc.          Keep for tax records
1333 Clay Street, #999
San Francisco, CA 94120
```

Figure 14.11
The main menu can be set up to access various billing functions.

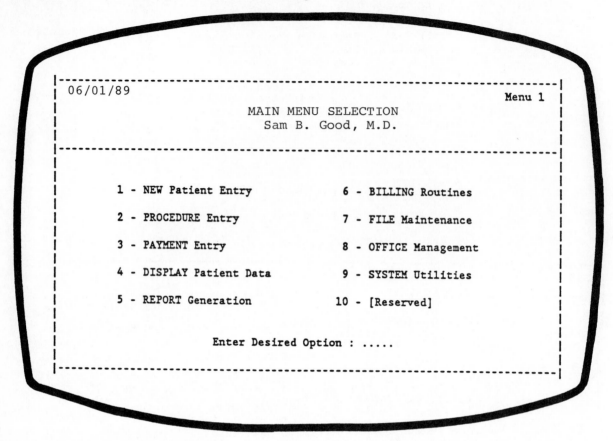

```
| 06/01/89                                               Menu 1 |
|                     MAIN MENU SELECTION                       |
|                      Sam B. Good, M.D.                        |
|                                                               |
|                                                               |
|         1 - NEW Patient Entry        6 - BILLING Routines     |
|                                                               |
|         2 - PROCEDURE Entry          7 - FILE Maintenance     |
|                                                               |
|         3 - PAYMENT Entry            8 - OFFICE Management     |
|                                                               |
|         4 - DISPLAY Patient Data     9 - SYSTEM Utilities      |
|                                                               |
|         5 - REPORT Generation       10 - [Reserved]           |
|                                                               |
|                                                               |
|                 Enter Desired Option : .....                  |
|                                                               |
```

the system before asking the system to perform an audit of the accounts. Once the system has audited the accounts, the operator should not be able to change information regarding charges, payments, or adjustments without explaining the reason for the adjustment. This creates what is known as an audit trail, which provides justification for every write-off and/or adjustment of an account balance.

System operation

Most major operations of a computer system are fairly simple. However, it is not as easy to replace a computer operator as it is a typist. Therefore it is wise within any practice for more than one person to learn how to operate the equipment so that all the speed and convenience of the system is still available during periods of vacations and illness. If

there is only one medical assistant in the office, the physician or the physician's spouse should at least have some familiarity with the system.

It is also important to have prompt and competent repair service. If the equipment fails, it usually means the suspension of many business functions and doing without stored information until the repairs are completed. This can be absolutely critical in the medical office.

The most reasonable solution is to accept the "maintenance contract" most computer companies provide at the time of purchase for both hardware and software. This not only protects the buyer against sizeable repair expenses, but also allows for an organized system for supplying experienced labor and parts for repair. You might remind the physician to insist upon some assurance of either "same" or "next day" service.

Conclusion

Individuals choosing a career in medical assisting will find themselves in a challenging profession that provides many, oportunities to demonstrate acquired skills. Almost every aspect of business is confronted within the medical office. No other profession provides such a diverse and varied background. Should the medical assistant choose to work in another environment, all skills would be an asset to the individual.

Review Questions

1. Describe the most common application of software for the medical office.
2. Describe an in-house system.
3. Describe a batch system.
4. Describe an on-line system.
5. Should office personnel have any input regarding the type of computer system needed for the office?
6. Name three reasons a physician may consider changing to a type of computer system.
7. List the types of software applications.
8. What should a vendor propose regarding growth capabilities?
9. What should the physician's office expect regarding maintenance service?
10. Should the physician request training of staff?
11. What should the physician indicate on the "charge slip"?
12. Describe the most commonly available reports for a physician's practice.
13. Describe the use of a recall notice.
14. Describe the administrative medical assistant's primary function with the computer.
15. Describe the information displayed on a "Main Menu."

SUGGESTED READINGS

American Medical Association: The business side of medical practice, Chicago, 1979, The Association.

Code it right, Salt Lake City, 1988, Med-Index.

Covel, AG: So you're going to buy an office computer, Prof Med Assist, March/April 1982, pp 16-17.

Sellars, D: Computerizing your medical office: agenda for you and your staff, Oradell, NJ, 1983, Medical Economics.

Should you computerize, TEC Helix, 1984.

Chapter 15

Fundamentals of Banking and Bookkeeping

- Banking systems
- Bookkeeping

Objectives

On completion of Chapter 15 the medical assistant student should be able to:

1 Define the terms listed in the vocabulary.

2 Discuss the basic functions of banking and the medical assistant's responsibility for interaction with the bank.

3 Describe the uses and parts of a check.

4 List and describe the seven types of checks.

5 Describe efficient policies for accepting checks, including types and uses of endorsements, and policies for accepting cash payments.

6 Discuss techniques of preparing bank deposits accurately and depositing funds in the bank.

7 Discuss the three major reasons that checks are returned from a bank and the procedures for processing returned checks.

8 Describe the techniques for preparing checks for accounts payable and storing the supporting documents.

9 Develop an effective and efficient policy for systematic bill paying.

10 State the reason for reconciling a bank statement and an efficient related policy.

11 Reconcile a bank statement.

Vocabulary

ABA number The number printed in the upper-right corner of a check to identify the location of the bank at which the check is to be redeemed.

accounts payable A record of the outstanding debts that are to be paid, usually by a specific date.

accounts receivable A record of the dollar value of services provided for which payment is expected.

check A written order to a bank to pay the bearer or presenter with the amount stated.

credit An accounting entry that reduces the amount due on an account; acknowledgment of a payment of a debt.

debit An accounting entry that increases the amount due on an account.

magnetic ink character recognition A series of numbers and characters printed in unalterable ink at the bottom of a check, including the checking account number of the payer and the amount of the check;

these numbers are subsequently "read" by a machine for speedy processing.

payee The person named as the individual to whom the stated amount of a check is payable.

payer The person who signs the check to release the funds to the payee.

reconcile To make consistent or compatible; in banking, to make the necessary adjustments on a bank statement or check register to make the figures consistent.

The independent subjects of banking and book-keeping are presented together to reinforce the fact that the two are interrelated. Each area involves accounts receivable and accounts payable, and the status of accounts receivable affects the ability to respond to the needs expressed in accounts payable. While the responsibility for the banking and bookkeeping functions may be assigned to different employees, teamwork and an understanding of both are required for efficiency.

BANKING SYSTEMS
Basic Elements
Functions of banking

The basic banking functions that you will encounter involve the following activities:

- Depositing funds;
- Withdrawing funds;
- Reconciling statements; and
- Using auxiliary services.

The funds deposited to checking and savings accounts are principally generated from the collection of accounts receivable. Funds are withdrawn by check or transferred from savings to checking for distribution and are used to pay business-related accounts payable. The distribution of funds must be conducted in a systematic manner, because the records are needed by the practice accountant and are subject to examination by government tax agencies. Statements of the checking account are sent from the bank every month and must be reconciled immediately to verify the funds available to the practice. In addition to the basic services, banks offer other services such as safe deposit boxes, loans, and retirement plans that may be needed by a medical practice.

Employee Responsibility

Your role in maintaining control of bank functions cannot be overemphasized. Attention to the smallest details will simplify all subsequent functions of reconciliation of funds and eventually the bookkeeping activities. The status of the banking and bookkeeping has an impact on all of the basic functions needed to provide patient care. The availability of personnel, facilities, and equipment is dependent on financial security.

Checks

Checks have become the foundation for most banking services and virtually all business transactions. A check is a written order for the transfer of money (Figure 15.1). Checks are provided for a charge by the bank where funds are held in a checking account. Regardless of the bank, all checks include certain basic components, some preprinted with information that will not change.

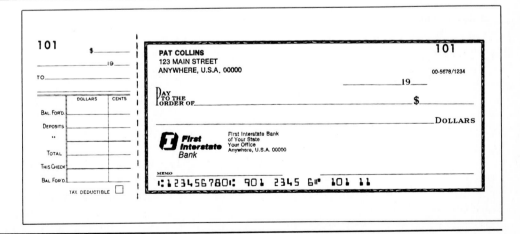

Figure 15.1
Standard check with stub.
Courtesy First Interstate Bank, Los Angeles, Calif.

Checks include the following information or space to enter information:

- Preprinted name and address of payer;
- Preprinted sequential number of check;
- American Bankers Association (ABA) number;
- Space to enter date check is written;
- *Pay to the order of* line and space to enter name of payee;
- Space to enter amount of check in number form;
- Space to enter amount of check in writing;
- Space for authorized signature of payer;
- Preprinted name and address of bank; and
- Magnetic ink character recognition (MICR) figures for bank processing of check.

All of the blank spaces must be filled in before a bank will process a check for payment.

Types of checks

You are most familiar with the standard form of bank check, which is supplied in pads and used by the public in completing daily transactions. Checks can be provided in other forms, however, and you should be familiar with them.

Cashier's checks are written by a bank on a bank form that represents guaranteed payment. The funds for payment of the check are debited from the payer's account at the time the check is written. A service charge is usually added.

Certified checks are similar to cashier's checks in that the funds are guaranteed, but certified checks are written on the payer's own check form and verified by the bank with an official stamp. The stamp indicates that the bank certifies the availability of the funds.

Limited checks are written on forms that are preprinted with a figure representing a maximum dollar amount for which the check can be written or a time limit during which the check is valid. This type of check is often used for payrolls or insurance payments.

Money orders represent guaranteed payment, because they are purchased for the cash value of the order plus a service charge. Domestic money orders can be purchased from post offices, banks, and authorized agents in retail stores. International money orders can be acquired in U.S. dollars to be cashed in foreign countries.

Traveler's checks are preprinted with stated dollar amounts and represent assurance of payment to the payee, since they are prepaid. They provide space for the signature of the payer to appear twice on the face of the check. One space on each check is signed at the time of purchase in the presence of the seller; the other space is signed at the time the

check is cashed. This precaution is to protect the payer in the event that the checks are stolen, because the payee can easily compare the signatures.

Voucher checks (Figure 15.2) provide three separate sections for complete information about the details of the transaction represented in the check. The upper portion of the face of the check is the standard form, and the lower portion of the face provides room for details of the transaction, such as payroll deductions, reason for the check, or the bookkeeping account to which the check is to be credited. Once the check is completed, the face portion is detached and forwarded to the appropriate payee, the carbon is discarded, and a second sheet remains with the payee as a duplicate copy of the transaction. Supporting documents, such as receipts or invoices, can be attached to the copy for a complete, permanent record.

Accepting checks for accounts receivable

An office policy should be established to guide you with decisions about accepting checks for payment of accounts receivable. You will find that the majority of outstanding bills are paid by personal checks to be drawn on the bank accounts of patients. This is common and acceptable business practice.

There are other checks that you may wish to avoid, because the payer is unknown to you. These are known as *third-party* checks, because the payee is the third person in the process. A third-party check is one that is written by an unknown party to the payee, in this case your patient, who wishes to release the check to you for payment of an outstanding balance. Since you do not have contact or experience with the payer, you increase the risk that funds are not available to pay the face value of the check.

Government or payroll checks are another form of third-party check. You may be inclined to accept these checks, because the payer appears reliable. You will find, however, that the amount of the check is frequently larger than the amount owed. This will require you to either refund the overpayment in cash or issue an office check for the difference, requiring additional work for you and increasing the risk of financial loss.

Occasionally, patients will send checks for payment that result in an overpayment on an account. This may occur if the check was written for the incorrect amount or an insurance carrier made a payment since the patient's statement was sent. You can handle this situation by either returning the incorrect check to the patient and requesting that a new check be written for the correct amount

Figure 15.2
Voucher check.
Courtesy First Interstate Bank, Los Angeles, Calif.

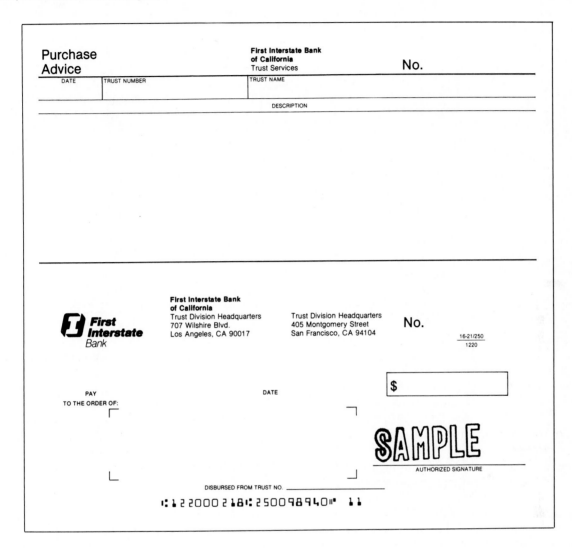

or depositing the check in the office account and writing a refund check to the patient for the amount of the overpayment. The second option is considered the soundest business practice, since it assures payment of the account.

Finally, checks with the notation *in full* or *paid in full* written on the face indicate that patients understand that their account will have zero balance once the check is recorded. You will need to be certain that this is correct before depositing the check. By depositing a check with this notation, you are acknowledging that it is correct; if it is not correct you may have difficulty collecting the balance due.

Endorsement of checks

A check must be endorsed to transfer the access to funds from one person to another. This is accomplished by signing or rubber-stamping the back of the check in ink, at the left end, and perpendicular to the bottom of the check. Endorsements are regulated in all states by the Uniform Negotiable Instrument Act. Checks may be transferred to several individuals, as noted in the discussion of third-party checks. If a check is made payable to the physician but there is an error in the spelling of the name, have the physician sign his or her name as written on the face of the check, followed by the endorsement stamp.

Figure 15.3
Receipt book.

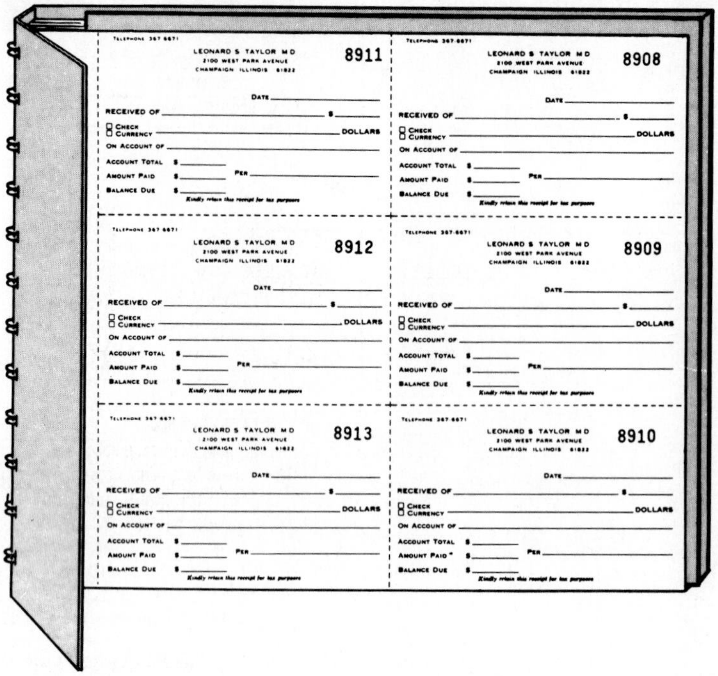

Accepting Cash Payments

Patients will occasionally pay cash for services. When accepting cash, you need to be very careful that both you and the patient agree on the amount involved in the transaction. You should always count the payment in the presence of the payer. The ascending total amount should be spoken aloud as each bill is counted, and the total amount restated to the patient for acknowledgment. You should then write a receipt for the patient, preferably using a receipt book that produces a copy that can be retained by the office as a permanent record (Figure 15.3). The original of the receipt is given to the patient.

Deposits to Checking Accounts
General policies

Policies and procedures will vary from office to office, but there are some considerations that need to be incorporated into the routines in any business. When working with incoming funds, you should do the following:

- Keep daily receipts (cash and checks) in a single, safe location;
- Prepare and make deposits daily;
- Compare deposit slip total with day sheet;
- Keep duplicates of deposit slips in office;
- Keep bank receipts of deposits; and

- Record deposit total in checkbook or master calendar.

While cash and checks are in the office, they should be stored in a location that is not accessible to anyone other than employees. For additional security the deposits should be made daily, especially if cash is involved. Most branch banks have locations that are convenient enough to include this activity in the daily routine. To assure accuracy, you should compare the daily credits to accounts receivable with the total on the deposit slip. If they do not match, you will need to retrace the individual items to determine if they match. Discrepancies often occur because of transposed numbers or an item omitted from one of the records. Duplicate deposit slips are automatically produced if the pegboard system is used. If you use the deposit slips provided by the bank, you may photocopy the slip before submitting it to the bank and retain the copies in chronological order. An alternative is to keep a stenographer's notebook and use carbon paper to imprint a copy of the deposit slip as you complete it onto consecutive pages of the book. After the deposit has been made, you can attach the bank deposit receipt to the corresponding page in the notebook to be retained as proof to check against deposits recorded on the monthly statement. And finally, you must know the balance in the account on a daily basis. This can be accomplished by add-

Figure 15.4

Checking account deposit slip.
Courtesy First Interstate Bank, Los Angeles, Calif.

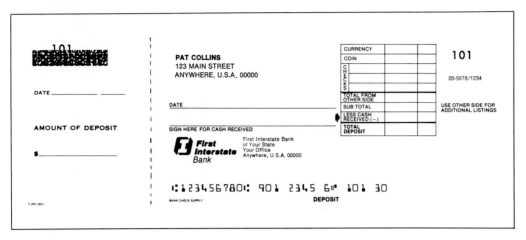

ing each deposit to the current balance on the check stubs or, if you use voucher checks, by keeping a master calendar on which you enter all deposits and checks written daily (Figure 15.4).

Completing the deposit slip

The deposit slip is the method of indicating to the bank the total dollar value in cash and checks to be credited to the depositor's account (Figure 15.4). All entries on the deposit slip must be clearly printed in ink to assure that they can be recorded correctly at the bank. The top section of the slip is devoted to the cash portion of the deposit. The total amount in currency (bills) is entered separately from the total amount in coins. The next section is for checks. Each check is recorded separately on numbered lines. The left-hand section of the check section provides space to record the ABA number of each check. If room is available, you may wish to note the last name of the payer above the ABA number to assist with locating errors. Directly opposite the ABA number is a section to enter the amount of the check in dollars and cents. Space is provided at the bottom of the slip for the total amount of the deposit. Double-check the total on an adding machine or calculator; the amount should equal the total receipts from your day sheet.

If the totals of the deposit slip and day sheet do not agree, search for the error that can occur in either document. First, recheck your addition. If the totals remain the same, check each item on the deposit slip to be sure you did not transpose any numbers. Next, subtract the lesser number from the greater to determine the amount of the error and search for the missing item in that amount. The error can be one of omission, when an item is not recorded on the day sheet or the deposit slip, or one of commission when an entry is recorded twice.

Methods of deposit

Deposits can be accomplished in three ways: in person, by mail, or in commercial night depositories. Automatic teller machines are not adaptable to business practices because they can only deal in cash; businesses must transact all business by check to have a permanent record. Making deposits in person is the most direct method, and the teller immediately provides a receipt to verify the transaction. If you deposit by mail, cash payments cannot be included because of the risk of loss or theft. Mail deposits also delay credit to the account for at least 24 hours while the item is in transit. Some prefer this method, however, because it can be completed at the end of the business day and include all transactions. An alternative to mailing that fulfills this objective is the use of the night depository. Bank clients with business (commercial) accounts can obtain a key to the night depository and a set of bags with security locks. Deposits can be prepared at the end of the day and brought to the bank after hours. Bags dropped in the night depository rest in a locked safe until bank employees retrieve them the next day. Your deposit is recorded and a receipt placed in the bag, which you may claim during bank business hours.

Figure 15.5
Returned item notices. **A,** Checking. **B,** Savings.
Courtesy First Interstate Bank, Los Angeles, Calif.

A

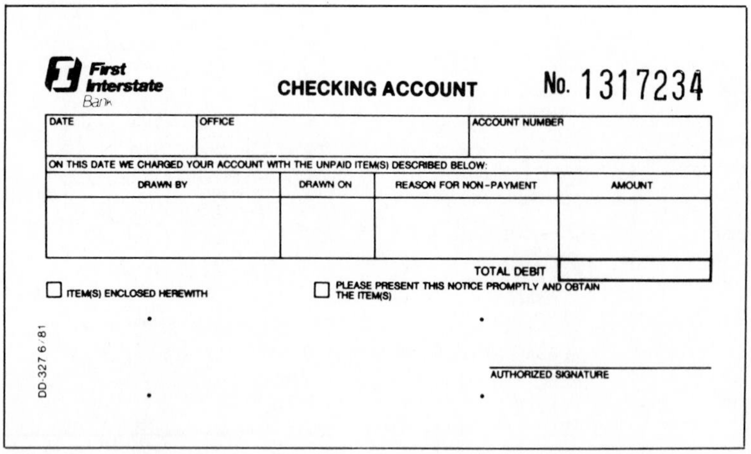

First Interstate Bank CHECKING ACCOUNT No. 1317234

DATE	OFFICE	ACCOUNT NUMBER

ON THIS DATE WE CHARGED YOUR ACCOUNT WITH THE UNPAID ITEM(S) DESCRIBED BELOW:

DRAWN BY	DRAWN ON	REASON FOR NON-PAYMENT	AMOUNT
		TOTAL DEBIT	

☐ ITEM(S) ENCLOSED HEREWITH ☐ PLEASE PRESENT THIS NOTICE PROMPTLY AND OBTAIN THE ITEM(S)

AUTHORIZED SIGNATURE

DD-327 6/81

B

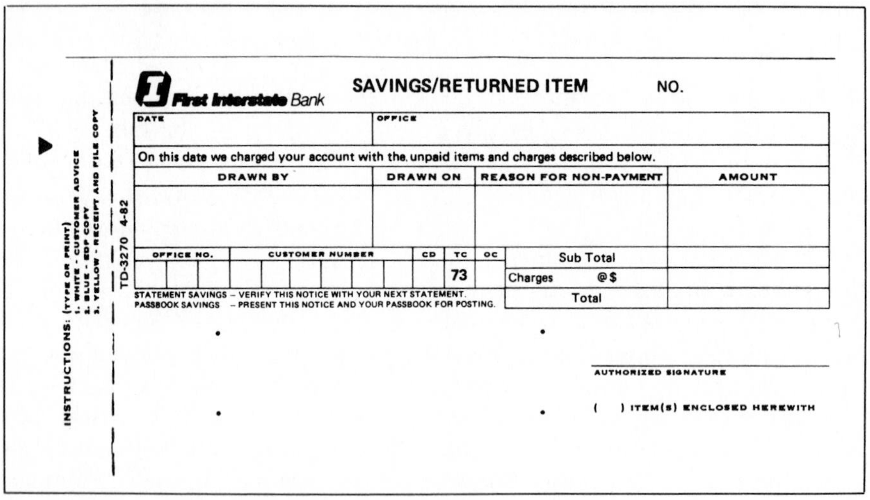

INSTRUCTIONS: (TYPE OR PRINT)
1. WHITE - CUSTOMER ADVICE
2. BLUE - EDP COPY
3. YELLOW - RECEIPT AND FILE COPY

TD-3270 4-82

First Interstate Bank SAVINGS/RETURNED ITEM NO.

DATE	OFFICE

On this date we charged your account with the unpaid items and charges described below.

DRAWN BY	DRAWN ON	REASON FOR NON-PAYMENT	AMOUNT

OFFICE NO.	CUSTOMER NUMBER	CD	TC	OC		
					Sub Total	
			73		Charges @$	
					Total	

STATEMENT SAVINGS – VERIFY THIS NOTICE WITH YOUR NEXT STATEMENT.
PASSBOOK SAVINGS – PRESENT THIS NOTICE AND YOUR PASSBOOK FOR POSTING.

AUTHORIZED SIGNATURE

( ) ITEM(S) ENCLOSED HEREWITH

Returned Checks

Occasionally, checks deposited for processing will be returned to the depositor by the bank. When a check is returned by the bank to the depositor it will be accompanied by a returned item notice (Figure 15.5). This may occur for a variety of reasons, many of which you can identify before depositing and thereby avoid the extra bookkeeping required when an item is rejected.

Before submitting a check to the bank, you should examine all entries on the face for completeness and accuracy. The common errors are as follows:

- Date missing;
- Payee's name missing;
- Signature missing; and
- Disagreement of amount in numerals and amount written out.

If the date or payee's name is missing, you may fill them in; if the signature is missing or there is disagreement of amounts, the check must be returned to the payer. The bank will also reject a check that is not endorsed. Double-check the back of each check to be certain that the item has been stamped or signed.

The final reason for the bank to return a check is difficulty with the payer. This is something you cannot predict or prevent. Returned checks in this group will be stamped with an explanation, usually one of the following:

- Refer to maker;
- Not sufficient funds (NSF); and
- Other.

Refer to maker indicates that you should contact the payer for an explanation. This notation may be because of a stop-payment order or a problem with

Figure 15.6
Savings account deposit slip.
Courtesy First Interstate Bank, Los Angeles, Calif.

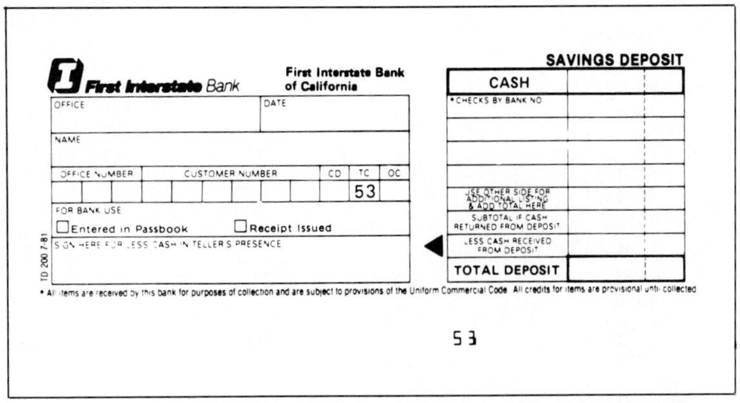

the transfer of funds. *NSF* indicates that the payer's account does not contain sufficient funds to pay the amount stated on the check. *Other* is rarely noted, but when it is there may be problems such as illegibility or a signature that does not match the one on file with the bank.

Action on returned checks

Checks that are incomplete or include errors can be handled in several ways. You can return the check to the payer with an explanation and request a new check, advise the payer that you will hold the incorrect check until a replacement arrives, or advise the patient to bring a correct check on the next visit if it is within the next few days.

When a check is returned with a *Refer to maker* or *NSF* notation, telephone the payer immediately. The payer may explain that an error was made and request that the check be resubmitted for payment. To accompish this, cross out the notification stamp, write the word *resubmit* on the face and back of the check, and prepare a new deposit slip. You might want to call the payer's bank to verify that the funds are available before resubmitting the check.

If you have any doubts about the credibility of the check or if the patient is relatively new to the practice and you do not have a credit history, you may wish to pursue more aggressive collection measures. You may request that the patient send payment in the form of a cashier's check or money order or make payment by cash in person. In any case, hold the returned check until you receive the alternate payment. If payment is not received after attempts to work directly with the patient, notify the patient that you will transfer the account to a collection agency and do so.

Deposits to Savings

Funds not needed for current accounts payable should be transferred to savings, because the funds in savings will earn interest. It is also a sound business practice to retain sufficient funds to maintain a practice for at least two months, in the event that income ceases for any reason.

Transfer of funds from a commercial checking account to a commercial savings account should be done by check. It assures the safety of the funds and provides a record of the transaction to be posted in the ledger accounts. The savings account deposit slip (Figure 15.6) is completed in the same manner as a checking account deposit slip. The check ABA number is entered in the right-hand column and the check amount in the space provided. You may wish to maintain a copy of the deposit slip for office records in the same manner as you do the checking account deposit slips.

The permanent record for a savings account is a passbook. You will take this book with you to the bank when conducting a transfer involving a savings account, and the bank teller will make a notation of the transaction. The passbook provides an up-to-date statement of deposits, interest earned, withdrawals, and account balance.

Cash Disbursement

Cash disbursement is a common bookkeeping term for the distribution of funds to creditors. The use of the word *cash* can be confusing, because if it is taken literally, you would infer that cash is used to pay outstanding bills. In a business, you should consider the term *cash* to be synonymous with *check*. Only checks should be used for the disbursement of funds, because they provide proof of

Figure 15.7
Write-It-Once check
writing system.
Courtesy Histacount Corp,
Melville, NY.

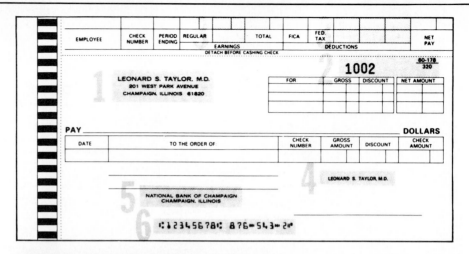

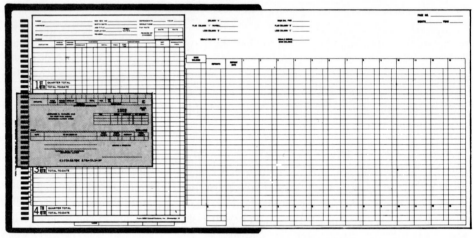

payment, produce a permanent record for documentation for tax purposes, and reduce the likelihood of embezzlement.

Check writing techniques

Although the basic components of checks are the same, the technique you use in preparing checks for signature will vary slightly with the type of check used. Your office may use a write-it-once system, prenumbered checks with the stubs, or prenumbered voucher checks that produce a carbon copy.

Write-it-once system. Check writing systems have been developed that produce a check and a disbursement register through a carbon strip on the back of the check. This produces a record of the payee, date, check number, and net amount of the check (Figure 15.7). The remaining columns of the register are used to charge the expense to the appropriate account. Each check register contains space to record 25 checks.

Checks with stubs. When using checks with stubs, fill out the stub portion first. This portion includes the following:
- Date check is written;
- Payee's name;
- Beginning account balance;
- Amount of check; and
- New balance (previous balance minus amount of current check).

Completing the stub first ensures that the information available is an accurate reflection of the balance of funds in the bank account. You should double-check the mathematical results for accuracy and write the new balance in the appropriate spot on the next stub in preparation for the subsequent check.

Voucher checks without stubs. Although voucher checks produce a carbon copy for a permanent record, you will need to develop a method of monitoring the daily bank balance. On a calendar with a 1- or 2-inch box for each date, enter the beginning balance each day, add the total of the daily deposit, subtract the total of all checks written each day, and arrive at the daily ending balance.

Method of completing checks. Checks must be written with materials that cannot be altered. They should be handwritten in ink or typewritten. Another option is to write out all information except the net amount of the check, which may be imprinted by a machine that perforates the paper. Any of these methods is acceptable. Write-it-once systems require the check to be handwritten. Checks with stubs may be typewritten if the check is detached from the stub, but you must be careful to complete the stub information. Voucher checks may be handwritten, using a pen that will imprint the copy, or typewritten for assured legibility.

In most cases, the checks will be prepared by you and presented to the physician-employer for signature. Complete the date, payee's name, check amount in numerals and handwriting, and memoranda portion with invoice numbers, if applicable. Any supporting documents and the envelope in which the check will be mailed should be attached before presenting the check for signature. The signee should verify the amount of the check with the document, usually an invoice or statement.

Errors on checks. There will be occasions when an error is made in the preparation of a check. If the error is major, such as writing the name of the payee on the line provided for the handwritten dollar amount, the check becomes invalid. You will need to strike a line across the entire face of the check and write the word *VOID* in large letters on the face in ink. The check is retained as proof of its invalid status. If the error is minor, such as writing the number *74* when you intended *84,* you may change the *7* to *8;* the authorized signee must initial the change.

Support documents. Support documents are important to provide proof of payments made on valid business expenses and are subject to auditing by the federal Internal Revenue Service. These documents include invoices, statements for supplies and services, and vouchers for salaries and expenses. You will need to develop a method of retaining the supporting documents indefinitely and in an orderly manner. For stub or write-it-once systems, you can note the check number and date paid on each document and store the documents for each month in an envelope or manila file. The file can be stored with the corresponding monthly statement that will arrive from the bank. Supporting documents can be attached directly to the corresponding copy of voucher-type checks. The checks can then be arranged in batches by month and stored with the appropriate bank statement.

Account holds

On rare occasions you will be notified by the bank that a hold has been placed on the checking account. This usually relates to a deposited item for which the bank needs assurance of redeemability. The check may be for an unusually large amount or from a bank in another geographical location. Hold means that the bank will not credit your office's account until the check has been processed and paid by the payer's bank. Your office's bank will indicate the specific period of time that the hold will be in effect, and until that time has elapsed you must treat that dollar amount as unavailable funds. You may not write checks that would involve those funds until the hold has been lifted.

Systematized bill paying

Policy. A policy should be established to assure that accounts payable are administered in an orderly and timely manner. The timetable established will depend on the size and needs of the practice. Checks can be written weekly, biweekly, semimonthly, or monthly. The schedule choosen should be followed consistently; it will allow for budgeting the funds necessary to meet the schedule. The policy should also indicate the person responsible for preparing the checks and maintaining the documents and who is authorized to sign checks. In some practices only one signature is necessary to legally transfer funds; in others two signatures are required for all checks or for those over a predetermined dollar amount.

Policy exceptions. You will encounter situations that require deviation from the schedule established for accounts payable or offers that make it advantageous to make an exception. Some suppliers offer a discount on their statement if the bill is paid within a certain number of days from the date of the statement, usually 10 days. Others may offer a discount if payment is included when the order is placed or may require that payment be made in advance. Take advantage of the discounts offered even if it means preparing a check on a nonscheduled day. Payments required with orders may also necessitate deviation from the schedule if the order cannot be delayed.

Master calendar. A master calendar of recurring debts will be helpful in preparing a check-writing schedule and planning a budget for the practice. There are certain items that are predictable on a monthly or periodic basis. These include the following:

- Rent or mortgage payments;
- Janitorial services;
- Telephone charges and related services;
- Laundry;
- Medical-surgical supplies;
- Office supplies;
- Automobile payments;
- Insurance policy premiums; and
- Taxes.

By maintaining a master calendar or reminder system you will be able to plan for the needed funds and make transfers from savings to checking if necessary.

Invoices and statements. You will also need to develop a system of storing and checking invoices and statements that are held until the scheduled payment dates. Maintaining a set of manila folders will assure that these items are not lost or overlooked. One folder can be labeled *Invoices* and used for storing the slips that arrive with supplies delivered or are left by individuals providing services for the office. Other folders can be labeled *Statements* or labeled with specific dates if bills are to be paid on a schedule, such as the fifteenth and thirtieth of each month. When a statement arrives, the appropriate invoices are retrieved and compared. The invoice numbers and the dollar amount should correspond with those listed on the statement. If there is any discrepancy, the biller should be contacted. The statement can then be stored in the appropriate statement folder until payments are made. Invoices should be retained even after payments are made, because they provide details of individual pricing, which do not appear on statements and can be used for future comparison.

Bank Statements
Purpose

Banks provide monthly statements of checking accounts that are used to determine if any errors have been made in office or bank accounting notations and to confirm the financial status of the account. The statement includes the debits and credits noted by the bank and is accompanied by checks that have been processed and paid to creditors by the bank. The returned checks allow you to ascertain checks that have not been paid and may not have reached their intended destination.

Policy

Statements usually arrive on or about the same date each month. Office policy should include the directive that bank statements should be reconciled as soon as possible after arrival and may indicate a specific date by which this should be accomplished. It should also be office policy that the statement be reconciled by a person other than the one who makes deposits or prepares the checks for signature. This is a standard business practice designed to prevent embezzlement.

Parts of a statement

Bank statements may vary in appearance, but they all contain certain basic information (Figure 15.8, *A*). The face of a statement includes the following information:

- Closing date;
- Caption;
- List of checks processed; and
- List of deposits.

The caption is a synopsis of the activity that has taken place during the month up to the closing date and includes the beginning balance, total value of checks processed, total amount of deposits made, service charges, and ending balance of the account. The checks processed by the bank may be listed by check number, by the date they were paid, or by both, but the listing always includes the dollar value of the check. Finally, deposits are noted by the date the bank recorded the deposit and the dollar amount credited.

The back of bank statements is printed with the regulations governing the responsibilities of both parties, the instructions for reconciling the statement, and a worksheet for accomplishing the reconciliation.

Reconciling the statement

The task of reconciling a bank statement can be relatively simple if it is approached in an orderly manner. Working with the face of the statement, first compare the beginning balance of the current statement with the ending balance of the previous statement. They should always agree. Next, compare the deposits noted by the bank with your records or receipts, placing a check mark next to each correctly recorded deposit. Deposits submitted toward the end of the month may not be posted by the closing date of the statement. The deposits not credited but recorded in your office records for the calendar month involved should be noted in the appropriate space on the back of the statement.

Next, compare the face value of the checks enclosed with the corresponding value of the checks noted on the statement, again placing a check mark next to the correctly listed ones. The returned checks should then be put in numerical order. You will be able to determine which checks are outstanding by the numbers missing from the sequence. Each outstanding check is listed by number on the back of the statement (Figure 15.8, *B*), the dollar value of each is traced through the check stubs or copies, and the amount is entered on the worksheet. Separately add and total the deposits not credited and the outstanding checks.

The final steps in reconciling the statement are according to a standard procedure which is as follows:

1. Note the ending statement balance.
2. Add the total deposits not credited.
3. Determine the subtotal of step 1 plus step 2.
4. Subtract the total checks outstanding.
5. Note the final total.

Next, identify the balance in the checkbook or on the master calendar for the last date of the month to be reconciled, subtract any service charges imposed by the bank, and adjust for any debit or credit entries made during the month. The total ar-

Figure 15.8
Bank statement. **A**, Front.

A

```
The Complete Statement®
DIRECT INQUIRIES TO                    (790) ACCT NO.                    ——        15
                                            (PER)                                   X

                                      First
                                      Interstate
                                      Bank

                                                                    ——  ——
                                                                              31
                                                                             1 1
                                                                  PAGE      1
                                      THIS STATEMENT DATE    AUGUST 31, 1982
                                      NEXT STATEMENT DATE SEPTEMBER 30, 1982

CHECKING ACCOUNT
                                      SUMMARY
        BEGINNING BALANCE. . . . . . . . . . . . . . . . . . .        721.35
            TOTAL DEPOSITS/CREDITS. . . . . . . . . . . . . . .      2,250.00
            TOTAL CHECKS/DEBITS . . . . . . . . . . . . . . . .        921.11
            SERVICE CHARGES . . . . . . . . . . . . . . . . . .          5.75
        ENDING BALANCE . . . . . . . . . . . . . . . . . . . .      2,044.49

        MINIMUM BALANCE ON 08-27 . . . . . . . . . . . . . . .        109.74
        AVERAGE BALANCE. . . . . . . . . . . . . . . . . . . .        485.00

                        CHECKING ACCOUNT TRANSACTIONS

    CHECKS

    CHECK NO  DATE PAID        AMOUNT      CHECK NO  DATE PAID        AMOUNT

        2401    08-13           80.00        2423    08-09           33.47
        2415*   08-03           38.31        2424    08-13           16.81
        2417*   08-02           35.57        2426*   08-25           40.00
        2418    08-13           25.00        2427    08-23           20.89
        2419    08-10           29.20        2429*   08-27           29.24
        2420    08-11          325.00        2430    08-27           30.00
        2421    08-10           10.00        2431    08-31           19.50
        2422    08-09           28.12

    DEPOSITS

    DATE        AMOUNT        DATE        AMOUNT        DATE        AMOUNT

    08-12       250.00        08-30     2,000.00

    ELECTRONIC FUNDS TRANSFERS AND DESCRIPTIVE TRANSACTIONS

    DATE      TYPE OF TRANSACTION                      WITHDRAWALS      DEPOSITS

    08-04  CASH WITHDRAWAL    FI CARD   ATM NO 0688        20.00
    08-16  CASH WITHDRAWAL    FI CARD   ATM NO 0688        40.00
    08-17  CASH WITHDRAWAL    FI CARD   ATM NO 0688        20.00
    08-23  CASH WITHDRAWAL    FI CARD   ATM NO 0688        40.00
    08-30  CASH WITHDRAWAL    FI CARD   ATM NO 0642        40.00

                    Notice: Please see reverse side and any accompanying statement(s) for important
                    information Examine this statement carefully and report any irregularities promptly
```

Continued.

Figure 15.8, cont'd
Bank statement. **B,** Back.

B

How to use
The Complete Statement

How to balance your checkbook:

1. Subtract the monthly service charge and any other charges not previously deducted from your checkbook balance.
2. Add to your checkbook balance each Balance Plus Deposit Order and Automatic Deposit.
3. Add Interest Paid, if you have a Checkbook Interest Account.
4. List and total the amount of all deposits entered in your checkbook that are not shown on the statement in the space provided for "Deposits Not Credited."
5. Compare and check off each paid check against your checkbook record. List and total all checks you have not checked off in the space provided for "Checks Outstanding." Note: An asterisk (*) next to any check listed on the reverse means there has been a break in the numerical sequence of your checks.
6. Perform the indicated steps in the "Statement Reconciliation" section.

If your checkbook and bank statement do not balance:

- Review last month's reconcilement to make sure any differences were corrected.
- Check additions and subtractions in your checkbook.
- Compare the amount of each check and deposit with the amount recorded in your checkbook and on this statement.
- Make sure all outstanding checks have been recorded under "Checks Outstanding."
- Make sure that each paid check you received with your statement has been recorded in your checkbook.
- Make sure that Day & Night Teller® and Day & Night Telephone Banking transactions (if any) are listed.

Deposits Not Credited		Checks Outstanding			
Date	Amount	Date	Amount	Date	Amount
Total $		Total $		Total $	

Statement Reconciliation

Statement Ending Balance	$
Add: Deposits Not Credited	+ $
Subtotal	$
Subtract: Checks Outstanding	– $
Total Should Agree With Your Checkbook Balance	$

Important Information About Your Balance Plus* Line of Credit
Please send Balance Plus billing inquiries to Customer Service Department, P.O. Box 7760, Van Nuys, CA 91409.

1. Finance charges are imposed on extensions of credit beginning on the day funds are advanced to your checking account. We compute finance charges in the following manner:
   a. We determine the ending balance of your Balance Plus Account for each day of the billing period by starting with the day's beginning balance (the previous day's ending balance), adding new advances posted that day and subtracting payments and credits posted that day.
   b. We then multiply each day's ending balance by the daily periodic rate shown on your statement.
   c. We arrive at the FINANCE CHARGE shown on your statement by adding together the daily finance charges for each day of the billing period. We calculate the "New Balance" shown on your statement by adding the total Finance Charge (and any applicable credit life insurance premiums) for the period to the ending balance on the last day of the billing period. The "New Balance" then becomes the beginning balance for the first day of the next statement period.
2. Unless stated otherwise in your agreement, the "Minimum Payment Now Due" will be 5% of the New Balance or $25.00, whichever is greater plus any amount past due. The "Minimum Payment Now Due" must be paid on or before the next statement date. Amounts in excess of your credit limit must be paid immediately. If you have not authorized automatic payments, please enclose a Balance Plus Payment Coupon with your payment.

In Case of Errors or Questions About Your Bill *
If you think your bill is wrong, or if you need more information about a transaction on your bill, write us on a separate sheet at the address shown on your bill as soon as possible. We must hear from you no later than 60 days after we sent you the first bill on which the error or problem appeared. You can telephone us, but doing so will not preserve your rights.
In your letter, give us the following information:
1. Your name and account number.
2. The dollar amount of the suspected error.
3. Describe the error and explain, if you can, why you believe there is an error. If you need more information, describe the item you are unsure about.
You do not have to pay any amount in question while we are investigating, but you are still obligated to pay the parts of your bill that are not in question. While we investigate your question, we cannot report you as delinquent or take any action to collect the amount you question.
• This section applies to non-business accounts.

In Case of Errors or Questions About Your Electronic Fund Transfers **
Telephone or write your local branch of account (the telephone number and address are shown on the front page of this statement) as soon as you can if you think your statement or receipt is wrong or if you need more information about a transfer on the statement or receipt. We must hear from you no later than 60 days after we sent you the FIRST statement on which the error or problem appeared.
(1) Tell us your name and account number.
(2) Describe the error or the transfer you are unsure about and explain as clearly as you can why you believe there is an error or why you need more information.
(3) Tell us the dollar amount of the suspected error.
We will investigate your complaint and will correct any error promptly. If we take more than 10 business days to do this, we will recredit your account for the amount you think is in error, so that you will have use of the money during the time it takes us to complete our investigation.
** These procedures apply to certain consumer transactions as described in the Bank's Preauthorized Transfer, Day & Night Teller, Day & Night Telephone Banking or other electronic fund transfer agreements. Please refer to your particular EFT Agreement for further details.

Pre-authorized Credits
If you have arranged to have direct deposits (e.g. Social Security) made to your consumer account at least once every 60 days from the same person or company, you can call your local branch of account (the telephone number is on the front of this statement) to find out whether the deposit has been made.

First Interstate Bank of California
Formerly United California Bank

Member FDIC

rived at in Step five should agree with the final figure arrived at in the checkbook. If they do the task has been completed.

If balances do not agree. If the checkbook and bank statement balances do not agree, you must determine the source of the error. There are some errors commonly committed in reconciling bank statements; knowing what they are can help you locate the possible source of your error. First, look at the previous month's statement and crosscheck to see if all the oustanding checks noted have been processed. If they have not, be sure that you have included them in the current list and total outstanding. Second, check your mathematical calculations for the outstanding checks, deposits not credited, bank statement reconciliation, and the figures carried forward on the check stubs. Third, review your figures to be sure that you have not transposed any numbers, and finally, be certain that all checks have been recorded in each check stub or in the check register. A shortcut method involves subtracting the lesser number from the greater number of the nonreconciling balances and quickly reviewing the checks, deposits, service charges, and debit and credit memos involved. However, this method will not help you locate mathematical errors or transposed numbers.

Other Bank Services

Banks supply customer services other than checking and savings accounts, including the following:
- Safe deposit boxes;
- Loans;
- Financial planning; and
- Retirement funds.

Medical practices may need some or all of the services available through a bank. Safe deposit boxes, available in various sizes, are used to store valuable documents such as deeds, insurance policies, and wills. An application must be submitted to the bank to obtain a box. Once the box is acquired, the physician-owner is given a set of keys for the box and the bank retains a set for the vault slot. Both keys are needed to gain access to the box. Renters must sign a form, in the presence of a bank employee, each time they want access to the box. These measures are for the protection of the renter and the bank. You may be asked to keep a record of the contents of the box and should periodically review the list with your employer to be certain that the list is current.

The remaining bank services, loans, financial planning, and retirement funds are primarily the physician's responsibility. Your involvement will be minimal and may only involve retrieving tax or employee records. Any paperwork involved will be completed by the physician and bank employees.

BOOKKEEPING
Why Financial Records are Kept

Financial records provide a method of monitoring the status and changes in a medical practice as in any business, and the records that are generated on a daily basis provide the foundation for all subsequent accounting records. These records involve patient relations through the billing system, provide proof of all transactions, provide the information for financial planning, and provide the data for tax purposes.

Information Available from Records

Financial records provide information about four general areas: accounts receivable, gross income, accounts payable, and business expenses by category.

Accounts receivable records contain the dollar value of services rendered daily, which are subsequently consolidated into monthly and annual totals. If the physician wishes, the data can also be developed by the type of service provided to determine the more profitable portions of the practice.

Gross income reflects the total dollars collected from practice business. The largest percentage will be from patient services, either through direct payments or from accounts referred to collection agencies. Other sources of recorded business income include fees for services to professional organizations, reimbursement for expenses related to professional meetings and services, and income for complying with subpoenas and requests for medical reports.

Accounts payable details the funds expended on all goods and services necessary to maintain the practice. These business-related expenses are usually subclassified by category. Be aware of the various categories to indicate the appropriate assignment on checks when preparing them for payment. Most accounts payable can be categorized in one of the following headings:
- Automobile;
- Dues and subscriptions;
- Employee benefits and relations;
- Insurance;
- Janitorial services;
- Laundry;

- Licenses;
- Medical-surgical supplies;
- Office supplies;
- Petty cash;
- Professional meetings;
- Public relations;
- Rent;
- Taxes; and
- Telephone.

Record-Keeping Responsibilities and Methods

As an administrative medical assistant you may be responsible for the basics of accounts receivable and accounts payable. You may also wish to work with the office bookkeeper or accountant to learn the skills involved in posting and balancing the journals and ledgers that will be discussed later. Depending on the size of the practice and the volume of patients, the bookkeeping records may be kept by hand or by computer. Familiarize yourself with the basics of each method and use any opportunity during your externship or career to gain experience. The additional skill will strengthen your position in the health care team.

Develop consistent work habits

The careful attention you pay to details in all aspects of your work also applies to the bookkeeping functions. Time required to assure accurate posting of entries is much less than that required to locate and correct errors. Printing letters and numbers correctly will also decrease the possibility of errors. Any entries in financial records must be made in ink, since they are permanent legal records. When totaling columns, you may note the amounts in pencil until they are double-checked, and you are assured that they balance. Then you may superimpose the verified totals in ink. If errors are noted after an entry has been made, they are corrected in the same manner as a medical record; you should strike through the error with a single line, without obliterating the entry, and insert the correct information.

Regardless of the type of bookkeeping system used, the following rules apply:

- Fees and payments should be posted promptly.
- Checks should be endorsed with a restrictive endorsement stamp as they are received.
- Duplicate receipts should be prepared for all cash payments.
- Deposits should be prepared daily.

- All statements for accounts payable should be checked against invoices for accuracy and due date.
- All financial transactions should be conducted by check.
- A petty cash fund should be established, including a voucher system to account for expenditures.

Bookkeeping Systems

There are three basic types of bookkeeping systems: single-entry, one-write or pegboard, and double-entry. The system selected will depend on the size of the practice and usually involves the opinion of the physician-owner's accountant.

Single-entry bookkeeping

A bookkeeping system is identified as a single-entry system if each dollar amount charged for services, received as income, or paid out for services is recorded in only one place in the accounting records. It is a simple, easily learned, and relatively inexpensive method of keeping records that provides the data necessary for accounting and tax purposes. It does not, however, include a built-in check system to verify all totals. It relies instead on double checks of column totals and the use of calculator tapes to check each entry by hand. The records used in a single-entry system include the following:

- General or fees journal—the log or accumulated day sheets used to enter charges for services and fees paid.
- Accounts receivable journal—the total amount due or currently outstanding for all services provided to all patients. The pegboard day sheet provides a space on each sheet to record this daily, and computer systems produce the information for you automatically. Other billing systems require that you determine the totals by adding up balances due from active accounts receivable cards or statements.
- Accounts payable ledger—the checkbook is the simplest form this record can take, with the stubs and bank statements providing the necessary data. Write-it-once systems automatically produce a ledger sheet that is subsequently stored in an accounting binder, and voucher checks are recorded on a similar ledger sheet purchased for the purpose. Ancillary records in this area include payroll records and a petty cash fund.

One-write pegboard bookkeeping

The one-write system previously discussed under billing systems serves to generate the journal entry at the same time the charge slip and receipt are produced for the patient and the ledger card for the office. The system includes instructions for simple checking techniques and provides space on each day sheet to verify the totals of each column. Any mathematical or entry errors are identified quickly. This method is very feasible for many practices, because the system is easy to learn and maintain. Physician-owners recognize the advantage of daily access to accounts receivable information and the potential control advantages for account collection.

Double-entry bookkeeping

Double-entry bookkeeping systems are more sophisticated than other bookkeeping systems in that they are used by accountants to verify results and provide a built-in mechanism for the rapid identification of entry and computing errors. The fundamental principle of a double-entry system is that each entry to a debit account has a corresponding entry to a credit account and is based on the equation

$$\text{Assets} = \text{Liabilities} + \text{Owner's equity}$$

Any entry on the asset side must have a comparable entry in a liability account, an equity account, or in a combination of liability and equity entries equal to the asset entry. Entries from the daily journals that record services and disbursements are transferred to the appropriate accounts in the general ledger. Entries are totaled for each calendar month, and the correctness of the data is verified if the total of the debit columns equals the totals of the credit columns. The next step is the transfer of monthly totals to the accounts ledger, which contains a separate page for each source of income and each category of disbursements. Verification of accuracy is again possible, because the debit and credit accounts must be equal.

Status Reports

Periodically, reports will be produced by the accountant to demonstrate the financial status of the practice. Data that you have entered in the daily journals and compiled in the ledgers will be used to develop the status reports. You can expect the following reports to be prepared on a monthly, quarterly, semiannual, or annual basis.

An *income statement* summarizes the funds received for professional services and the expenses paid, by category, to maintain the practice. The income received is termed *gross income,* and the funds that remain after all expenses have been paid is *net income.*

A *trial balance* is a method of determining whether or not the accounting records are balanced in a way similar to that discussed under double-entry systems. For the trial balance, the accounts are simply listed by name with their totals placed in the appropriate credit or debit column. The grand total of one column equals that of the other. Any errors are traced and corrected before the trial balance is prepared.

The *balance sheet* is prepared to reflect the condition of the practice as of the specific date of the report, since the variables change on a daily basis. The components of this report are the three elements of the double-entry equation.

If the status reports are produced periodically throughout the year, the information can be easily consolidated into an annual report. Annual reports can then be used for the completion of tax reports, analysis of insurance needs, loan applications, and planning.

Payroll Records

Payroll records are considered separately because of the legal directives involved in maintaining and reporting the information. Employers are responsible for withholding income taxes from gross salaries, depositing the taxes with federal and state agencies, submitting quarterly and annual reports on taxes withheld, and providing reports needed by employees to file their annual tax reports.

Basic documents and data

When establishing a medical practice, each employer must apply for a federal and state employer's tax number that must be used on all forms and correspondence submitted to government agencies. Employees are identified, for tax purposes, by their Social Security numbers.

The first step in establishing a payroll record for each employee is the completion of a W-4 form (Figure 15.9). This form supplies the employer and accountant with the information needed to determine the amount to withhold from the gross income of each employee. The data submitted on the employee's W-4 form are used to determine both federal and state withholding taxes. The factors that influence the amount withheld for state and federal taxes are the employee's marital status, the

Figure 15.9
W-4 form.

1989 Form W-4

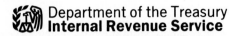 **Department of the Treasury
Internal Revenue Service**

Purpose. Complete Form W-4 so that your employer can withhold the correct amount of Federal income tax from your pay.

Exemption From Withholding. Read line 6 of the certificate below to see if you can claim exempt status. If exempt, only complete the certificate; but do not complete lines 4 and 5. No Federal income tax will be withheld from your pay.

Basic Instructions. Employees who are not exempt should complete the Personal Allowances Worksheet. Additional worksheets are provided on page 2 for employees to adjust their withholding allowances based on itemized deductions, adjustments to income, or two-earner/two-job situations. Complete all worksheets that apply to your situation. The worksheets will help you figure the number of withholding allowances you are

entitled to claim. However, you may claim fewer allowances than this.

Head of Household. Generally, you may claim head of household filing status on your tax return only if you are unmarried and pay more than 50% of the costs of keeping up a home for yourself and your dependent(s) or other qualifying individuals.

Nonwage Income. If you have a large amount of nonwage income, such as interest or dividends, you should consider making estimated tax payments using Form 1040-ES. Otherwise, you may find that you owe additional tax at the end of the year.

Two-Earner/Two-Jobs. If you have a working spouse or more than one job, figure the total number of allowances you are entitled to claim on all jobs using worksheets from only one Form

W-4. This total should be divided among all jobs. Your withholding will usually be most accurate when all allowances are claimed on the W-4 filed for the highest paying job and zero allowances are claimed for the others.

Advance Earned Income Credit. If you are eligible for this credit, you can receive it added to your paycheck throughout the year. For details, obtain Form W-5 from your employer.

Check Your Withholding. After your W-4 takes effect, you can use **Publication 919,** Is My Withholding Correct for 1989?, to see how the dollar amount you are having withheld compares to your estimated total annual tax. Call 1-800-424-3676 (in Hawaii and Alaska, check your local telephone directory) to obtain this publication.

Personal Allowances Worksheet

A Enter "1" for **yourself** if no one else can claim you as a dependent . . . . **A** _____

B Enter "1" if: { **1.** You are single and have only one job; or
2. You are married, have only one job, and your spouse does not work; or
3. Your wages from a second job or your spouse's wages (or the total of both) are $2,500 or less. } . . . . . . **B** _____

C Enter "1" for your **spouse.** But, you may choose to enter "0" if you are married and have either a working spouse or more than one job (this may help you avoid having too little tax withheld) . . . . **C** _____

D Enter number of **dependents** (other than your spouse or yourself) whom you will claim on your tax return . . . . . . **D** _____

E Enter "1" if you will file as a **head of household** on your tax return (see conditions under "Head of Household," above) . . **E** _____

F Enter "1" if you have at least $1,500 of **child or dependent care expenses** for which you plan to claim a credit . . . **F** _____

G Add lines A through F and enter total here . . . . ▶ **G** _____

For accuracy, do all worksheets that apply. {
● If you plan to **itemize or claim adjustments to income** and want to reduce your withholding, turn to the Deductions and Adjustments Worksheet on page 2.
● If you are **single** and have **more than one job** and your combined earnings from all jobs exceed $25,000 OR if you are **married** and have a **working spouse or more than one job,** and the combined earnings from all jobs exceed $40,000, then turn to the Two-Earner/Two-Job Worksheet on page 2 if you want to avoid having too little tax withheld.
● If **neither** of the above situations applies to you, **stop here** and enter the number from line G on line 4 of Form W-4 below. }

- - - - - - - - - - Cut here and give the certificate to your employer. Keep the top portion for your records. - - - - - - - - - -

Form **W-4**
Department of the Treasury
Internal Revenue Service

Employee's Withholding Allowance Certificate
▶ **For Privacy Act and Paperwork Reduction Act Notice, see reverse.**

OMB No. 1545-0010
1989

1 Type or print your first name and middle initial	Last name	**2** Your social security number

Home address (number and street or rural route)	**3** Marital Status	☐ Single ☐ Married ☐ Married, but withhold at higher Single rate. **Note:** If married, but legally separated, or spouse is a nonresident alien, check the Single box.
City or town, state, and ZIP code		

4 Total number of allowances you are claiming (from line G above or from the Worksheets on back if they apply) . . . **4** _____

5 Additional amount, if any, you want deducted from each pay . . . . **5** $ _____

6 I claim exemption from withholding and I certify that I meet **ALL** of the following conditions for exemption:
- Last year I had a right to a refund of **ALL** Federal income tax withheld because I had **NO** tax liability; **AND**
- This year I expect a refund of **ALL** Federal income tax withheld because I expect to have **NO** tax liability; **AND**
- This year if my income exceeds $500 and includes nonwage income, another person cannot claim me as a dependent.

If you meet all of the above conditions, enter the year effective and "EXEMPT" here . . . . . . ▶ **6** | 19

7 Are you a full-time student? (**Note:** Full-time students are not automatically exempt.) . . . . **7** ☐Yes ☐No

Under penalties of perjury, I certify that I am entitled to the number of withholding allowances claimed on this certificate or entitled to claim exempt status.

Employee's signature ▶ _____   Date ▶ _____ , 198_

8 Employer's name and address (**Employer:** Complete 8 and 10 **only if sending to IRS**)	**9** Office code (optional)	**10** Employer identification number

Figure 15.9, cont'd
W-4 form.

Form W-4 (1989)   Page **2**

Deductions and Adjustments Worksheet

Note: *Use this worksheet only if you plan to itemize deductions or claim adjustments to income on your 1989 tax return.*

1	Enter an estimate of your 1989 itemized deductions. These include: qualifying home mortgage interest, 20% of personal interest, charitable contributions, state and local taxes (but not sales taxes), medical expenses in excess of 7.5% of your income, and miscellaneous deductions (most miscellaneous deductions are now deductible only in excess of 2% of your income)	**1** $
2	Enter: $\begin{cases} \$5,200 \text{ if married filing jointly or qualifying widow(er)} \\ \$4,550 \text{ if head of household} \\ \$3,100 \text{ if single} \\ \$2,600 \text{ if married filing separately} \end{cases}$	**2** $
3	**Subtract** line 2 from line 1. If line 2 is greater than line 1, enter zero	**3** $
4	Enter an estimate of your 1989 adjustments to income. These include alimony paid and deductible IRA contributions . .	**4** $
5	**Add** lines 3 and 4 and enter the total	**5** $
6	Enter an estimate of your 1989 nonwage income (such as dividends or interest income)	**6** $
7	**Subtract** line 6 from line 5. Enter the result, but not less than zero	**7** $
8	**Divide** the amount on line 7 by $2,000 and enter the result here. Drop any fraction	**8**
9	Enter the number from Personal Allowances Worksheet, line G, on page 1	**9**
10	**Add** lines 8 and 9 and enter the total here. If you plan to use the Two-Earner/Two-Job Worksheet, also enter the total on line 1, below. Otherwise, **stop here** and enter this total on Form W-4, line 4 on page 1	**10**

Two-Earner/Two-Job Worksheet

Note: *Use this worksheet only if the instructions at line G on page 1 direct you here.*

1	Enter the number from line G on page 1 (or from line 10 above if you used the Deductions and Adjustments Worksheet) .	**1**
2	Find the number in **Table 1** below that applies to the **LOWEST** paying job and enter it here	**2**
3	If line 1 is **GREATER THAN OR EQUAL TO** line 2, subtract line 2 from line 1. Enter the result here (if zero, enter "0") and on Form W-4, line 4, on page 1. **DO NOT** use the rest of this worksheet . .	**3**

Note: *If line 1 is **LESS THAN** line 2, enter "0" on Form W-4, line 4, on page 1. Complete lines 4–9 to calculate the additional dollar withholding necessary to avoid a year-end tax bill.*

4	Enter the number from line 2 of this worksheet	**4**
5	Enter the number from line 1 of this worksheet	**5**
6	**Subtract** line 5 from line 4	**6**
7	Find the amount in **Table 2** below that applies to the **HIGHEST** paying job and enter it here	**7** $
8	**Multiply** line 7 by line 6 and enter the result here. This is the additional annual withholding amount needed	**8** $
9	Divide line 8 by the number of pay periods each year. (For example, divide by 26 if you are paid every other week.) Enter the result here and on Form W-4, line 5, page 1. This is the additional amount to be withheld from each paycheck . . .	**9** $

Table 1: Two-Earner/Two-Job Worksheet

Married Filing Jointly		All Others	
If wages from **LOWEST** paying job are—	Enter on line 2 above	If wages from **LOWEST** paying job are—	Enter on line 2 above
0 - $4,000 . . .	0	0 - $4,000 . . .	0
4,001 - 8,000 . . .	1	4,001 - 8,000 . . .	1
8,001 - 18,000 . . .	2	8,001 - 13,000 . . .	2
18,001 - 21,000 . . .	3	13,001 - 15,000 . . .	3
21,001 - 23,000 . . .	4	15,001 - 19,000 . . .	4
23,001 - 25,000 . . .	5	19,001 and over . . .	5
25,001 - 27,000 . . .	6		
27,001 - 32,000 . . .	7		
32,001 - 38,000 . . .	8		
38,001 - 42,000 . . .	9		
42,001 and over . . .	10		

Table 2: Two-Earner/Two-Job Worksheet

Married Filing Jointly		All Others	
If wages from **HIGHEST** paying job are—	Enter on line 7 above	If wages from **HIGHEST** paying job are—	Enter on line 7 above
0 - $40,000 . . .	$300	0 - $23,000 . . .	$300
40,001 - 84,000 . . .	560	23,001 - 50,000 . . .	560
84,001 and over . . .	660	50,001 and over . . .	660

Privacy Act and Paperwork Reduction Act Notice.—We ask for this information to carry out the Internal Revenue laws of the United States. We may give the information to the Department of Justice for civil or criminal litigation and to cities, states, and the District of Columbia for use in administering their tax laws. You are required to give this information to your employer.

The time needed to complete this form will vary depending on individual circumstances. The estimated average time is: **Recordkeeping** 46 mins., **Learning about the law or the form** 10 mins., **Preparing the form** 70 mins. If you have comments concerning the accuracy of these time estimates or suggestions for making this form more simple, we would be happy to hear from you. You can write to the **Internal Revenue Service,** Washington, DC 20224, Attention: IRS Reports Clearance Officer, TR:FP; or the **Office of Management and Budget,** Paperwork Reduction Project, Washington, DC 20503.

☆U.S. GPO: 1988—205-056

number of allowances claimed, and the pay periods established by office policy. Employees may elect one allowance for themselves and one for each dependent. If they do not complete all appropriate information as requested, the employer will withhold taxes at the rate specified for an (unmarried) individual with no allowances. W-4 forms can be obtained from the federal Internal Revenue Service regional office on written request.

Payroll accounting

Payroll accounting involves keeping a record of the gross salary; taxes withheld, including federal income tax, Social Security (FICA) tax, state income tax, state disability insurance if applicable, and net income. If the write-it-once check system is used, the task is accomplished by stating the net amount on the check and the gross amount and various amounts withheld in the appropriate columns to the right of the check. Other check-writing systems involve the transfer of data to the appropriate ledger accounts. Many offices prefer to maintain a separate payroll book that includes space for all necessary tax data and room to record time off for vacations, holidays, or illness.

Be aware that many payroll services are available for a nominal fee. These services will write checks, make federal withholding deposits, produce monthly payroll records, and produce quarterly tax returns, and W-2 forms. Some of these services are available to a practice with only two employees. These services have proven to be cost-effective and reduce staff time significantly.

Employee taxes withheld

Federal income tax. Employers are required by law to withhold and process federal taxes for each employee. *The Federal Employer's Tax Guide,*Circular E, is supplied to every employer with a federal identification number and includes tables for all possible combinations of variables (Figure 15.10).

FICA tax. Several taxes, commonly known as Social Security tax, are covered under the Federal Insurance Contributions Act (FICA). The amount to withhold from an employee's gross income can also be determined from tables in Circular E and is calculated on a percentage of the gross salary up to an annual maximum income. FICA is different from income tax in that every dollar contributed by an employee is matched by a dollar from the employer, and the funds are used for individuals who are retired or unable to work.

State income tax. Some states have set up a mechanism similar to that of the federal govern-ment that allows employees to withhold a portion of each paycheck for deposit on estimated annual taxes due by employees. Tables to assist employers to determine the appropriate amount are supplied by the state tax board.

State disability insurance. Some states have established funds to protect individuals temporarily unable to work because of illness or injury. The employee contribution is usually very limited, because the risk of needing the service is spread over large numbers of contributors.

Unemployment insurance. Unemployment insurance is available in each state for individuals who have lost their jobs through unavoidable circumstances. The contributions and contributors to this fund vary state to state; you will need to determine the law for your state. The possibilities include contributions only by the employer, by both employer and employee, or by employers with more than three employees. There is also federal unemployment insurance, which is a supplementary fund developed by employer contributions and intended for use after state funds have been exhausted.

Depositing taxes withheld. Employers are required to deposit federal taxes they withhold to a Federal Reserve bank or authorized commercial bank on a monthly or quarterly basis. Tax deposit form 501 is sent to each registered employer before the beginning of each quarter and must be submitted with the deposit. The amount of the deposit equals the total accumulated federal income taxes and FICA taxes withheld from employees and the matching FICA employer contribution.

Deposits to state tax boards are usually done on a quarterly basis directly to the state agency and accompanied by a quarterly report that describes the required payroll information. The funds submitted include state income tax, disability insurance fees, and, where applicable, unemployment insurance.

Required reports. For tax purposes the calendar year is divided into quarters, and the mandatory quarterly reports must be submitted on or before the last day of the month that follows the end of the quarter. For example, forms for the first quarter (January, February, March) must be mailed on or before April 30. Federal and state agencies send the necessary forms during the last month of each quarter.

Annual reports involve the preparation of the W-2 forms and a gederal unemployment insurance form. The W-2 forms are six-part forms supplied by the federal government. Three copies of the W-2 form are given to employees. Employees need the

Figure 15.10
Sample of federal tax table.

MARRIED Persons–MONTHLY Payroll Period
(For Wages Paid After December 1988)

And the wages are–		And the number of withholding allowances claimed is–										
At least	But less than	0	1	2	3	4	5	6	7	8	9	10
		The amount of income tax to be withheld shall be–										
$0	$270	$0	$0	$0	$0	$0	$0	$0	$0	$0	$0	$0
270	280	1	0	0	0	0	0	0	0	0	0	0
280	290	3	0	0	0	0	0	0	0	0	0	0
290	300	4	0	0	0	0	0	0	0	0	0	0
300	320	7	0	0	0	0	0	0	0	0	0	0
320	340	10	0	0	0	0	0	0	0	0	0	0
340	360	13	0	0	0	0	0	0	0	0	0	0
360	380	16	0	0	0	0	0	0	0	0	0	0
380	400	19	0	0	0	0	0	0	0	0	0	0
400	420	22	0	0	0	0	0	0	0	0	0	0
420	440	25	0	0	0	0	0	0	0	0	0	0
440	460	28	3	0	0	0	0	0	0	0	0	0
460	480	31	6	0	0	0	0	0	0	0	0	0
480	500	34	9	0	0	0	0	0	0	0	0	0
500	520	37	12	0	0	0	0	0	0	0	0	0
520	540	40	15	0	0	0	0	0	0	0	0	0
540	560	43	18	0	0	0	0	0	0	0	0	0
560	580	46	21	0	0	0	0	0	0	0	0	0
580	600	49	24	0	0	0	0	0	0	0	0	0
600	640	53	28	3	0	0	0	0	0	0	0	0
640	680	59	34	9	0	0	0	0	0	0	0	0
680	720	65	40	15	0	0	0	0	0	0	0	0
720	760	71	46	21	0	0	0	0	0	0	0	0
760	800	77	52	27	2	0	0	0	0	0	0	0
800	840	83	58	33	8	0	0	0	0	0	0	0
840	880	89	64	39	14	0	0	0	0	0	0	0
880	920	95	70	45	20	0	0	0	0	0	0	0
920	960	101	76	51	26	1	0	0	0	0	0	0
960	1,000	107	82	57	32	7	0	0	0	0	0	0
1,000	1,040	113	88	63	38	13	0	0	0	0	0	0
1,040	1,080	119	94	69	44	19	0	0	0	0	0	0
1,080	1,120	125	100	75	50	25	0	0	0	0	0	0
1,120	1,160	131	106	81	56	31	6	0	0	0	0	0
1,160	1,200	137	112	87	62	37	12	0	0	0	0	0
1,200	1,240	143	118	93	68	43	18	0	0	0	0	0
1,240	1,280	149	124	99	74	49	24	0	0	0	0	0
1,280	1,320	155	130	105	80	55	30	5	0	0	0	0
1,320	1,360	161	136	111	86	61	36	11	0	0	0	0
1,360	1,400	167	142	117	92	67	42	17	0	0	0	0
1,400	1,440	173	148	123	98	73	48	23	0	0	0	0
1,440	1,480	179	154	129	104	79	54	29	4	0	0	0
1,480	1,520	185	160	135	110	85	60	35	10	0	0	0
1,520	1,560	191	166	141	116	91	66	41	16	0	0	0
1,560	1,600	197	172	147	122	97	72	47	22	0	0	0
1,600	1,640	203	178	153	128	103	78	53	28	3	0	0
1,640	1,680	209	184	159	134	109	84	59	34	9	0	0
1,680	1,720	215	190	165	140	115	90	65	40	15	0	0
1,720	1,760	221	196	171	146	121	96	71	46	21	0	0
1,760	1,800	227	202	177	152	127	102	77	52	27	2	0
1,800	1,840	233	208	183	158	133	108	83	58	33	8	0
1,840	1,880	239	214	189	164	139	114	89	64	39	14	0
1,880	1,920	245	220	195	170	145	120	95	70	45	20	0
1,920	1,960	251	226	201	176	151	126	101	76	51	26	1
1,960	2,000	257	232	207	182	157	132	107	82	57	32	7
2,000	2,040	263	238	213	188	163	138	113	88	63	38	13
2,040	2,080	269	244	219	194	169	144	119	94	69	44	19
2,080	2,120	275	250	225	200	175	150	125	100	75	50	25
2,120	2,160	281	256	231	206	181	156	131	106	81	56	31
2,160	2,200	287	262	237	212	187	162	137	112	87	62	37
2,200	2,240	293	268	243	218	193	168	143	118	93	68	43
2,240	2,280	299	274	249	224	199	174	149	124	99	74	49
2,280	2,320	305	280	255	230	205	180	155	130	105	80	55
2,320	2,360	311	286	261	236	211	186	161	136	111	86	61
2,360	2,400	317	292	267	242	217	192	167	142	117	92	67
2,400	2,440	323	298	273	248	223	198	173	148	123	98	73
2,440	2,480	329	304	279	254	229	204	179	154	129	104	79
2,480	2,520	335	310	285	260	235	210	185	160	135	110	85
2,520	2,560	341	316	291	266	241	216	191	166	141	116	91
2,560	2,600	347	322	297	272	247	222	197	172	147	122	97
2,600	2,640	353	328	303	278	253	228	203	178	153	128	103

copies to file their personal state and federal taxes. Another copy is given to employees to retain for their records. Employers must send one copy of the W-2 form to the federal government and one to the state and retain one copy for office records. The federal unemployment tax is submitted with a check for the employer's contribution to the fund.

Employer's personal income taxes

Because of their complexity, the employer's tax reports are usually prepared by an accountant. Tax payments are made on a quarterly basis according to an estimate of the total amount due by the end of the year. The final payment for the previous year must be submitted with the annual reports by April 15 of the present year and represent any amount due over the estimated payments already made.

Computer Services

As record keeping and reporting requirements become more complex, many physician-owners and their accountants will begin to use computers. Computer services and computer programs are available for all accounting functions and can be expected as routine support services in the near future. Computers offer some basic advantages, including the following:

- They save time.
- They have built-in proofing mechanisms for the work they produce.
- They can generate all needed forms.

Some disadvantages can be cited with regard to computer services and equipment, but most of them relate to a lack of understanding of the use or potential of the system. Some basic study and research should eliminate the problems related to computers, including the following:

- Fear of the equipment;
- Selection of inappropriate equipment and programs; and
- Improper use of reports.

Record Retention

Opinions vary on the length of time financial records should be retained. Some feel five years is the maximum necessary for bank statements and tax records; others feel they should be kept indefinately. Currently, the popular opinion is toward indefinite retention of all financial records with anything older than three years being transferred to inactive status.

Conclusion

The management of banking and bookkeeping systems involves a responsibility that can affect all other aspects of a medical practice. Receiving and disbursing funds and the records for reporting these activities require attention to detail, and the fulfillment of your responsibility to these functions will put you in a position of great value.

Review Questions

1. Name the basic bank functions that you will encounter as an administrative medical assistant.
2. List and explain the 10 parts of a check.
3. List and briefly describe in your own words the six types of checks other than the basic bank check.
4. Describe four possible problems associated with checks received for accounts receivable.
5. List and describe the three most common check endorsements.
6. Complete a sample deposit slip for the following receipts:
   Cash: $14.83 ($2.83 in coins)
   Checks:

ABA Number	Amount
11-35/1210	$ 42.00
11-1/1010	$160.00
1-2/1412	$ 17.80
11-35/1200	$682.49
14-3/6060	$ 31.27
12-1/181	$ 92.00

7. Describe the steps you would take on receiving a check back from the bank marked *NSF*.
8. Describe the method of preparing a voucher check for payment of a bill, including materials needed and processing of supporting documents.

9. What is the difference between an invoice and a statement? How are they associated with one another?

10. The five final steps in reconciling a bank statement are as follows:
    a. Note the _____ statement balance.
    b. Add the _____.
    c. Determine the _____.
    d. Subtract the _____.
    e. Compare the final total with the _____.

11. List and describe the four general areas of financial records.

12. List the seven basic rules of an efficient bookkeeping system.

13. What is the difference between a single-entry and double-entry system?

14. Name and describe the three reports prepared to demonstrate the financial status of a practice.

15. List and describe the basic federal and state employee income taxes withheld from paychecks. How are the taxes determined? Which taxes are paid by the employer?

Chapter 16

Facilities and Equipment

- Fundamentals of facilities management
- Physical resources
- Capital equipment
- Expendable equipment and supplies

Objectives

On completion of Chapter 16 the medical assistant student should be able to:

1 Define the terms listed in the vocabulary.

2 Develop a system for managing facilities and equipment founded on the four basic considerations of patient comfort, accessiblility, safety, and security.

3 Define the four distinct internal areas of an office.

4 Describe the importance of space arrangement, color, traffic patterns, and maintenance in a facility.

5 Compare and contrast capital and expendable equipment.

6 Describe an efficient ordering system.

7 Discuss the principles of receiving and storing supplies.

Vocabulary

bottleneck An obstructed area that impedes or slows production or progress.

electrical ground A mechanism to return an electrical current back into the source of the electricity; used to avoid shocking individuals who come into contact with the electrical equipment.

esthetic Beautiful; pleasing to the senses.

monitor To check or keep track of progress or the use of goods.

overload An excessive demand for electrical current.

supplier One who provides materials or provisions.

All of the functions discussed in the previous chapters and those to be covered in Part III of this book are performed within the confines of the medical office or agency. The facilities and equipment of the office or agency provide the structural support for the services provided. Facilities must be organized and maintained for maximum efficiency, and the equipment required to fulfill the various assisting responsibilities must be acquired and monitored.

FUNDAMENTALS OF FACILITIES MANAGEMENT
Assignment of Responsibility

The general responsibility for the management of facilities and equipment is usually assigned to the administrative medical assistant or office manager. Specific duties should be detailed in the office policy manual. In small and moderate-sized practices, the job description for one employee may include the entire responsibility for this management system. Managers of large practices or agencies may

Figure 16.1
Frequently used medical supplies
accessible in treatment room.

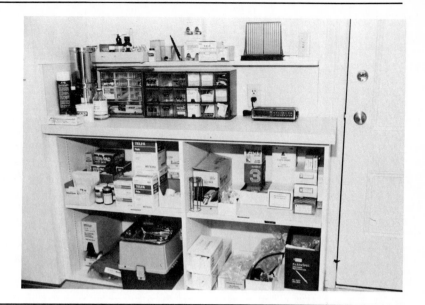

find that the responsibility for facilities and equipment must be divided, usually by administrative and clinical areas, and that job descriptions must be written to reflect the division of duties.

Areas of Consideration

As a system for managing the facilities and equipment is developed, there are four basic factors that must always be considered:
- Patient comfort;
- Accessibility of equipment and supplies;
- Safety; and
- Security.

The comfort of patients during the time they are in the facility is the primary concern of all personnel and involves both psychological as well as physical comfort. You will need to develop methods of conveying a sense of privacy and dignity that will be reassuring to patients.

Accessibility to equipment and supplies is important to personnel as well as patients. Maintaining adequate supplies in convenient locations saves time that can be spent addressing patients' needs. It also eliminates unnecessary, fatiguing movement expended searching for items to accomplish assigned tasks (Figure 16.1).

Monitoring the premises and equipment for safety is the responsibility of all personnel and is for the benefit of patients and employees. Areas of concern include the placement of furniture, ripples in carpets, slippery floors caused by excess wax or spills, frayed or improperly grounded electrical

Figure 16.2
Overloaded electrical outlet.
From Sorrentino S: Mosby's textbook for nursing assistants, St Louis, 1984, The CV Mosby Co.

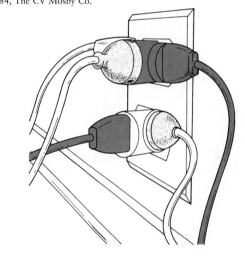

cords, overloading of electrical outlets (Figure 16.2), or improperly labeled or stored fluids and chemicals. These potential problem areas and others unique to your facility require constant monitoring, and you should develop the habit of periodically evaluating the premises from the perspective of someone entering for the first time. The other important safety consideration involves the predetermined course of action to be taken in the event of an emergency involving the facility. An evacuation plan should be developed and practiced in the

Figure 16.3
Fire extinguisher.
From Sorrentino S: Mosby's textbook for nursing assistants, St Louis, 1984, The CV Mosby Co.

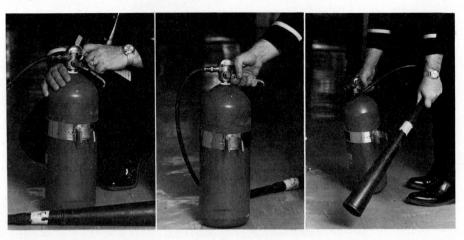

event that a fire occurs. A fire extinguisher should be accessible (Figure 16.3). Each employee should be assigned specific areas of responsibility, with notification of the fire department and attention to patients having the highest priority. If time allows, you will also want to consider closing all filing cabinets to protect records, removing financial records, and notifying the answering service to monitor incoming calls. Plans should also be developed for events common in your geographical area, such as earthquakes, hurricanes, and tornadoes.

A security system is the final area that must be developed to protect the office and contents during and after work hours. While the office is open, a signaling method to indicate when someone enters the reception room will be needed, most commonly a bell that is activated when the door is opened or when an individual passes through a light beam. The door between the reception area and the work areas should remain locked to prevent the entry of unknown individuals. Special attention is required for the protection of medications, expecially narcotics, kept on the premises. After office hours, the office can be protected by checking all windows and doors to be sure thay are securely locked. Office buildings usually have a burglar alarm for additional security (Figure 9.2). Freestanding private offices should have their own alarm systems.

PHYSICAL RESOURCES

Management of a facililty begins with the physical layout of the office, the choices made regarding furnishings and colors, evaluation of traffic patterns, and general maintenance.

Delineation of Space

The internal office space can be thought of as four distinct areas, which are designated as follows:
- Public area;
- Control area;
- Medical area; and
- Storage area.

Activity and maintenance of one area affects the others, but each area will be discussed separately.

Public area

The public area of an office or agency is the reception room and the access entrances to it. Most offices have a single reception area, and it should be evaluated and planned to meet the needs of many individuals (Figure 9.3). Seating should be adequate, with a minimum of three to four chairs provided per physician in the practice. Some large practices with available space can decentralize the waiting area to accommodate special needs, such as a play area for children or an isolation room for infectious cases.

Control area

The space from which personnel can monitor the activity to and from all other areas is the control area, generally known as the administrative offices (Figure 9.2). When working in this area, you will be responsible for reception, registration, appointments, medical records, and telephone activity.

Figure 16.4
Examination–minor surgery room.

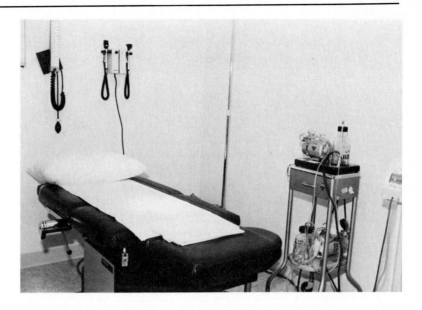

Figure 16.5
Physician's office–consultation room.

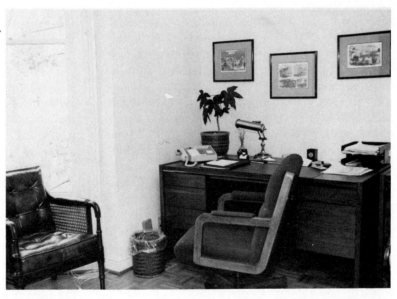

Since all patients and visitors must pass through and stop at this area between the reception and medical areas, it must be organized for efficiency and security. A great deal of activity takes place in the control area, and access to records, funds, and prescription pads requires particular attention.

Medical area

The medical area of the facility includes the rooms reserved and furnished for the examination and treatment of patients (Figure 16.4) and the physician's office or consultation room for patient interviews and postexamination discussions (Figure 16.5). In the examination-treatment rooms, partic-

ular attention must be paid to privacy for patients. Windows should be appropriately covered, and examining tables should not be placed opposite the door, in case it must be opened after an examination has begun. Sound control should be checked to assure confidentiality. Light sources and equipment should be placed for easy access to save time during the course of the examination or treatment.

Storage area

Extra supplies and equipment require storage space that does not intrude on the other areas of the office. Supplies and equipment must also remain readily available to personnel who need to replace items used in the course of daily activities. This area should be spacious enough to receive supplies as they arrive and hold them until invoices can be checked against the items delivered. Visitors and sales personnel should not be permitted in this area.

Arrangement of Space

Furnishings, particularly in the public area and consultation room, should be selected and arranged for utility and aesthetics. Chairs of varying height and firmness should be provided to accommodate the needs and comforts of patients. The arrangement of furniture is particularly important in small areas to give the illusion of more space. Attention should also be given to lighting for safety and reading comfort.

Colors

The colors selected for the walls, carpet, and furnishings should not only be functional but cheerful and soothing. The use of art work throughout the office (may be loaned, leased, or rented from a local artist, museum, or gallery) is particularly pleasing. This can be a diversion for those who are waiting and also lessens the impersonal appearance of the medical environment. The assistant and the physician should see that current publications and/or magazines are available, not only in the reception area, but in the examination and treatment rooms as well. Another positive aspect is the use of music in the examination rooms. Music should not normally be piped into the reception area since it adds to the overall noise.

Traffic Patterns

The corridors through which patients travel to gain access to the various areas of an office should be evaluated to be certain that privacy and confidentiality are provided. Attention should also be directed at timing movement so that bottlenecks do not occur in any one area. This is most likely to occur at the reception window or in the control area where several people may arrive at one time. Staggering patients at the reception and appointment desk will enhance privacy and confidentiality.

Maintenance

The major portion of the maintenance functions will be carried out by a janitorial service that has a written or spoken agreement with the employer or office manager. One employee should be assigned to monitor the efficiency of the service and communicate the needs of the office to the service personnel. You may wish to restrict some areas within the office from the janitorial service, such as areas containing sterile equipment, confidential information, or personal work areas. Responsibility for maintaining the restricted areas must then be assigned to office staff, usually divided along administrative and clinical lines.

CAPITAL EQUIPMENT

Capital equipment is the term applied to items that are considered major and involve funds above a dollar value predetermined by the employer and the accountant. Although the determination of the amount that represents a capital expenditure will vary, it is often placed at or near $500. Items are classified as capital when they are purchased. The accounting differences are handled by the office accountant.

Types of Capital Equipment

Items that are categorized as general capital equipment include the office furnishings, artwork, automobiles purchased by the practice, carpeting, and so forth. Remodeling of the premises is also considered a capital expenditure and is often referred to as a leasehold improvement for an office rented in a medical building. Administrative capital equipment denotes items needed to fulfill the administrative office duties. Typewriters, word processors, copy machines, and computer terminals and printers all fall into this category. In the clinical area, the capital purchases will include the examination room furnishings, particularly the tables, which can be very expensive. Examination and treatment items include major equipment used by specialists such as ophthalmologists, neurologists, radiologists, and gynecologists. Other specialists, such as internists and otorhinolaryngologists, require little capital equipment and more expendable equipment, which will be discussed later. Regardless of the specialty, most offices also maintain equipment used to sterilize clinical supplies, prepare laboratory specimens, or perform some laboratory studies. Most also have a refrigerator to store perishable supplies.

Care and Maintenance of Capital Equipment

All equipment, capital or otherwise, should be handled carefully and used properly to preserve it in the best operating condition for the longest period of time possible. Before using any piece of equipment, thoroughly read the operating instructions and understand the functions that it is capable of performing. If you have any doubt, seek the help of another employee familiar with the equipment or an employee of the firm from which the equipment was purchased.

Equipment that is used extensively and has many moving parts or functions capable of breaking down can be covered by a maintenance contract. Typewriters, computers, and copy machines commonly fall into this category. A maintenance contract is a sort of insurance policy purchased to cover parts and labor charges incurred when a piece of equipment breaks or malfunctions. Maintenance contracts are renewed annually and should be reviewed to determine if the predicted cost of service calls exceeds the cost of the contract. This is more likely to be the case as the equipment ages.

Your responsibility for the office equipment includes using it properly, following maintenance instructions, and acquiring appropriate service when necessary. Because capital equipment is expensive, it is unlikely that you will have comparable back-up items in the event of equipment failure. Therefore it is in your best interest to maintain the equipment properly and seek professional services at the first sign of a problem. This should help reduce the amount of time that you must be without the equipment that has failed.

EXPENDABLE EQUIPMENT AND SUPPLIES

Expendable equipment and supplies include items that you expect to use up within a short period of time and are relatively inexpensive, especially when considered at unit cost.

Expendable administrative equipment and supplies include the following:

- Paper goods—stationery, typing paper, photocopy paper, insurance forms, chart folders, labels, medical record forms, laboratory and radiology request forms, and appointment books.
- Writing utensils—pens, pencils, color highlighters, correcting tape or fluid.
- Typewriter and copy supplies—ribbons, cleaning fluids, copy ink or toners.
- Accounting supplies—statements, ledger cards, accounting forms, adding machine tapes, receipt books or forms, and day sheets.

In the clinical area, expendable items include the following:

- Linens—pillow cases, towels, drapes, laboratory coats, gowns that are used once and laundered.
- Paper supplies—examining-table paper, disposable gowns, drapes, paper towels, wraps and bags for equipment sterilization.
- Examination equipment—ear and nose speculum covers, disposable vaginal specula, disposable proctoscopes and sigmoidoscopes, lubricant, catheters, tongue blades, cotton-tipped applicators.
- Treatment equipment—needles, syringes, cautery tips, suture material, dressings, elastic bandages, tape, and cast materials.

Ordering Systems

Since expendable supplies and equipment must be replaced relatively often, you will need to develop a system to keep an adequate supply on hand.

First, determine a reorder point for the various items. This is the point in time that takes into consideration the amount of supplies remaining against the amount of time needed to order replacement supplies and have them delivered. The object is never to reach the point at which all supplies are depleted before replacements arrive.

Second, develop a method of noting ordering needs. The responsibility may be delegated to one employee or divided according to administrative and clinical areas. A supply ordering notebook can be maintained and divided by type of supply or ordering source. As supplies are placed in the storage area, the boxes can be numbered. The box that indicates the reorder point can be marked in a manner recognized by all personnel. The person who removes the reorder-point item is responsible for noting this in the reorder book.

Third, the person or persons responsible for ordering supplies should be aware of the time required to place the order and the anticipated delivery time. Orders need to be placed far enough in advance of actual need. A copy of the order form should be retained to check against the order when it arrives or to check on the order if it does not arrive within the expected time.

Fourth, there are some basic considerations that should be kept in mind when ordering supplies. A unit-cost saving can usually be realized by ordering in large quantities rather than by single item. For example, if *one* box of 100 syringes is ordered at a cost of $10, then each syringe cost 10¢. The same supplier might reduce the cost per box to $8 if you purchase *five* boxes at one time, which will reduce your unit cost to 8¢ per syringe. Aside from cost, also consider available storage space and the expiration date of some items when you order in quantity. The storage problem could interfere with safety and efficiency, and ordering items that will be outdated before they can be used will be a waste of money rather than a savings.

Suppliers

You will need several suppliers to maintain an office, since administrative and clinical items are usually not available from a single source. Local suppliers provide the convenience of quick delivery and personalized service, while mail-order firms may provide a saving in cost. The preference of the employer and the service capability demonstrated is usually the final deciding factor in selecting a supplier.

Receiving

A single location should be designated as the receiving area within the medical office. All deliveries should be deposited in this location and held until they can be checked for completeness. One person should be assigned the responsibility of receiving and signing for deliveries. The subsequent duties can be divided between administrative and clinical areas, with one person from each area being responsible for checking invoices or packing slips against the items delivered and distributing the goods to the proper storage area.

Storage of Supplies

As supplies are placed in the storage area, the pre-existing supplies should be rotated to a position in which they will be used first. Items that have just arrived should be placed for subsequent use. Storage areas should be arranged so that the most commonly used items are within the closest reach. Conversely, infrequently used items can be stored in less accessible sites. Special consideration must be given to the storage of drugs, particularly narcotics. The law requires that narcotics be locked up and that each item be currently accounted for as either in storage or dispensed.

Conclusion

The orderly management of the office facilities and equipment provides an atmosphere of comfort for patients and efficiency for employees. Evaluating each unique situation, planning for the needs of the various areas within the facility, and maintaining the system in a consistent manner will enhance public image and provide a pleasant working environment.

Review Questions

1. Describe your responsibilities to patients regarding comfort, safety and security, and to co-workers regarding equipment accessibility.
2. List and describe the four areas of internal office space.
3. Describe capital equipment and give three examples of capital items.
4. Define expendable equipment and supplies and give four examples each of expendable administrative and clinical equipment.
5. Describe the reorder point and give an example.
6. Develop an efficient possible plan for reordering expendable supplies.
7. How should supplies be stored?

SUGGESTED READING

Cotton H: Medical practice management, ed 2, Oradell, NJ, 1977, Medical Economics Books.

Part Three

Clinical Theory and Technique

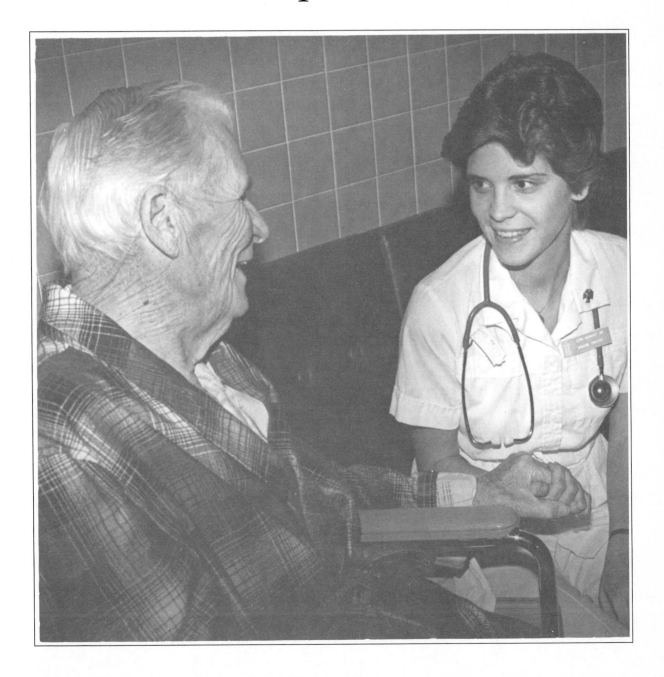

Chapter 17

Physical Measurements: Vital Signs, Height, and Weight

- Vital signs
- Temperature
- Pulse

- Respiration
- Blood pressure
- Physical measurements of height and weight

Objectives

On completion of Chapter 17 the medical assistant student should be able to:

1 Define the terms *vital signs, temperature, pulse, apical heartbeat, respiration rate,* and *blood pressure,* listing the normal average values for each and listing the equipment used to take these measurements.

2 Recall and state the *general* instructions for taking temperature, pulse, respirations, and blood pressure measurements.

3 When given the results of 25 patients' vital signs measurements, state which fall within normal ranges and which do not. State the reasons for the answers given.

4 List two situations in which taking a rectal temperature, two situations in which taking an axillary temperature, and five situations in which taking an oral temperature should be avoided.

5 List 10 situations that will cause variations in a person's pulse rate.

6 List and locate pulsations on the seven major arteries on the body at which the pulse rate can be obtained with relative ease.

7 List five situations that would increase a person's respiratory rate, five that would increase blood pressure, and five that would cause a decrease in each of these measurements.

8 Describe what is meant by the rate, rhythm, and volume of the pulse rate and the rate, rhythm, and depth of respirations.

9 Demonstrate the correct methods for measuring a person's vital signs.

10 Demonstrate the correct method for measuring a person's height and weight, and state six reasons for taking these measurements.

11 Convert temperature readings taken in degrees Fahrenheit to degrees Centigrade and vice versa.

12 Convert weight readings taken in pounds to kilograms and vice versa.

13 Demonstrate the proper methods for caring for stethoscopes, sphygmomanometers, and thermometers after use.

Vocabulary

Among the medical assistant's most routine clinical duties are the taking and recording of the patient's physical measurements, which include vital signs, height, and weight. It is therefore necessary for the medical assistant to know and understand these measurements and be able to correctly obtain and record the values for each. This chapter discusses these six measurements along with procedures and related vocabulary.

It is assumed that the medical assistant student has studied or is currently studying anatomy and physiology. Therefore detailed explanations of how the vital signs are produced by the body will not be included here.

VITAL SIGNS

Vital signs are measureable, concrete indicators that pertain to and are essential for life. The four vital signs are temperature, pulse, respiration (TPR), and blood pressure (BP). These signs are routinely measured in each physical examination. The purpose of obtaining a patient's vital signs is to provide the physician with information that will help accomplish the following:

- Determine the patient's condition by comparing his body temperature, pulse, respiration, and blood pressure with normal values
- Determine a diagnosis, the course, and the prognosis of the patient's condition
- Designate the treatment that will be instituted

TEMPERATURE

Body temperature, the degree of body heat, is a result of the balance maintained between heat produced and heat lost by the body. This is regulated by a center located in a portion of the brain, the hypothalamus, that initiates the various mechanisms to increase or decrease heat loss.

Heat is produced by oxidation of foods in all body cells, especially those in the skeletal muscles and liver. The blood and blood vessels distribute it to other parts of the body. Eighty-five percent of the body heat is lost through the skin by radiation, convection, and evaporation of perspiration. The remainder is lost through the respiratory tract and mouth and through feces and urine.

A variation from the normal range of a patient's temperature may be the first warning of an illness or a change in the patient's condition. As such, it is an important part of the diagnosis and treatment plan for a patient.

Normal Temperature Readings

Body temperature is measured by a thermometer placed under the tongue in the mouth, in the rectum, or in the axilla, because large blood vessels are near the surface at these points. The normal temperature values for these three sites, based on a statistical average, are as follows:

- Oral—98.6° F (Fahrenheit) or 37° C (centigrade or Celsius)
- Rectal—99.6° F or 37.6° C
- Axillary—97.6° F or 36.4° C

Accurate rectal temperatures will register approximately 1° F or 0.6° C higher than accurate oral temperatures. Accurate axillary temperatures will register approximately 1° F or 0.6° C lower than accurate oral temperatures. The rectal temperature is considered to be the most reliable and accurate reading. The mucous membrane lining of the rectum, with which the thermometer comes into contact, is not exposed to the air, and the conditions do not vary as do those of the mouth or axilla.

Variations in Body Temperature

Normal body temperature varies from person to person and at different times in each person.

- The daily average oral temperature of a healthy person may vary from 97.6° to 99° F (36.4° to 37.3° C).
- The lowest body temperature occurs in the early morning (2 AM to 6 AM).
- The highest body temperature occurs in the evening (5 PM to 8 PM).
- In a woman, body temperature may increase *slightly* during the menstrual cycle at the time of ovulation.
- Body temperature is slightly higher during and immediately after eating, exercise, or emotional excitement.
- Body temperature may vary more and is generally higher in an infant or young child than in an adult.

Abnormal temperatures occur when the body's temperature-regulating system is upset by disease or other physical disturbances.

- Body temperature will *decrease* in some illnesses, or if a patient faints, collapses, or hemorrhages, or if the patient is in a fasting state, is dehydrated, or has sustained a central nervous system (CNS) injury. Subnormal temperatures, below 96° F (35.6° C), may occur in cases of collapse.
- Body temperature will *increase* in an infectious process or may increase following a chill. Shivering (chills) is one way the body increases heat production by the muscular activity that occurs; this activity releases heat.

Increases in body temperature are also produced by the following:

- Activity
- Emotions
- Environmental changes
- Age (the aged and infants show 1° F higher)
- Reactions to certain drugs
- The amount and type of food eaten (an increase in metabolic rate increases heat production in the body)

Fever usually accompanies infection and many other disease processes. Fever is present when the oral temperature is 100° F (38.8° C) or higher. Temperatures of 104° F (40° C) or higher are common in serious illnesses.

Vocabulary

constant fever High fever with a variation not exceeding 1° or 2° F (0.6° or 1.2° C) between morning and evening temperatures.

crisis Sudden drop of a high temperature to normal or below; generally occurs within 24 hours.

fever Pyrexia, or elevation of body temperature above normal; 98.6° F (Fahrenheit) or 37° C (centigrade or Celsius) registered orally. Some classify it as follows:

Low:	99° to 101° F (37.2° to 38.3° C)
Moderate:	101° to 103° F (38.3° to 39.5° C)
High:	103° to 105° F (39.5° to 40.6° C)

intermittent fever Variations with alternate rises and falls, with the lowest often dropping below 98.6° F (37° C). An intermittent fever reaches the normal line at intervals during the course of an illness, for example, AM 98° F, PM 100° F; AM 98.6° F, PM 101° F.

lysis Gradual decline of a fever.

onset Beginning of a fever.

remittent fever Variations in temperature but always above 98.6° F (37° C); a persistent fever that has a daytime variation of 2° F (1.2° C) or more, for example, AM 100° F, PM 103° F; AM 99° F, PM 102.4° F.

Thermometers

A thermometer calibrated in Fahrenheit or centigrade (Celsius) degrees is the instrument used to measure body temperature. Various models made of glass or special disposable materials are available. Newer models are electronic. All good thermometers must pass a rigid inspection for proper calibration according to the standards set by the U.S. National Bureau of Standards.

The commonly used glass thermometers vary in shape. The rounded, short bulb is used when taking rectal temperatures as it is held better by the rectal muscles. It may also be used when taking an axillary temperature. The slender bulb is considered more effective for oral temperatures. There are also rounded, short bulb thermometers for both oral and rectal use. These are usually color coded for ease of identification; that is, the oral thermometers have a blue identification mark at the end, and rectal thermometers have a red mark. All register the same temperature, although the "normal" temperature arrow will be on the 98.6° F (37° C) mark for the oral thermometer and may be on the 99.6° F (37.6° C) mark for the rectal thermometer (Figure 17.1).

Safe and easy-to-use battery-operated electronic thermometers are rapid (within 10 to 30 seconds) and accurately calibrated to within two tenths of a degree. They have disposable covers and interchangeable color-coded probes for both oral and rectal use. The temperature is registered on a dial or on a digital display on the equipment (Figure 17.2).

How to read a glass thermometer

When reading a thermometer, hold it between your thumb and index finger at the end away from the bulb. Rotate the thermometer until you see the center (silver) line of mercury toward the bulb. Follow this line up until it ends. Sometimes you can see this line better by changing the direction of the light source. Fahrenheit thermometers are marked off in degrees, with intermediate marks at two tenths of a degree. Centigrade thermometers are marked off in degrees, with intermediate marks at one tenth of a degree. Centigrade readings can be converted to Fahrenheit readings and Fahrenheit degrees converted to centigrade degrees by using

Figure 17.1
A, Three types of thermometers. The slender bulb is best for oral temperatures; the rounded bulb, shown in both Fahrenheit and Centigrade degrees, is best for rectal temperatures and may also be used for axillary temperatures. **B,** One type of disposable thermometer. The last dot to turn dark indicates the temperature reading.

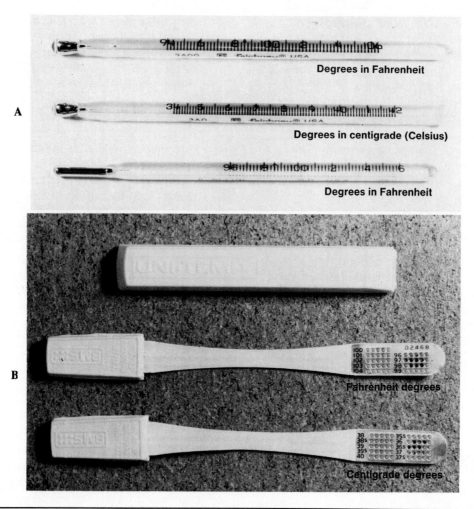

the following formulas. Since the metric system is to be used more frequently, you should know how to convert Fahrenheit degrees to centigrade degrees. The formula for this is $C° = (F° - 32) \times 5/9$. If the Fahrenheit temperature is 98.6°, then the equation is as follows:

$$C° = (98.6° - 32) \times 5/9$$
$$C° = 66.6° \times 5/9$$
$$C° = 33\,3/9$$
$$C° = 37°$$

To convert centigrade to Fahrenheit degrees, the formula is $F° = (C° \times 9/5) + 32$.

Text continued on p. 266.

Figure 17.2
Mark X Electronic Thermometry System, using the latest in electronics and microprocessor technology, is lightweight (about 10 ounces) and is easy to use, maintain, and clean. The 15-second timer can be used for measuring pulse and respiratory rates. Temperature is measured in 30-45 seconds.
Courtesy Electromedics, Inc., Englewood, Colo.

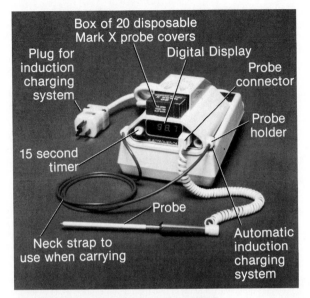

NOTE: The Mark X displays the following letter indications when appropriate:

P = Low battery power, return to charger for a minimum of 4 hours.

H or L = Defective probe, replace with a good probe.

E = Tissue contact lost, eject the probe cover, return the probe to the storage well—repeat all steps for taking patient's temperature.

OPERATING INSTRUCTIONS

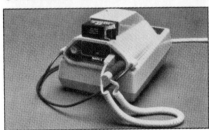

1 Remove the Mark X from the charger base. Select °F or °C (select switch is located on the back of the Mark X).

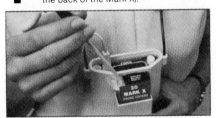

2 Removing the probe from the storage well turns the temperature display, returning the probe to the well shuts off the display. Holding **ONLY** the red or blue collar of the probe, **FIRMLY** insert the probe tip into the probe cover. (Use only HPC-360 probe covers.)

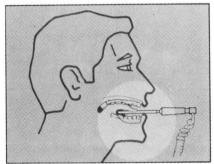

3 For oral temperatures (use blue probe) – Taking 4 to 5 seconds, **SLOWLY** insert the covered probe tip under the patient's tongue into the sublingual pocket.

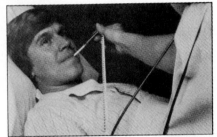

4 Hold probe ensuring good tissue contact until audible tone is heard, record temperature.

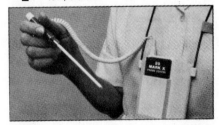

5 DISCARD the probe cover by holding the red or blue collar of the probe between the thumb and fingers while pushing on the white top of the probe with the index finger. Return the probe to the storage well to turn off the dispaly. Also, **ALWAYS** return the Mark X to its charger base when the Mark X is not in use.

Taking Axillary Temperatures – The patients arm should be down against the body 3 minutes prior to **SLOWLY** inserting the covered probe into the axilla. Hold the probe parallel to the trunk of the body until the audible tone is heard.

Taking Rectal Temperatures – Using the (red) rectal probe with probe cover, **SLOWLY** insert probe to depth in accordance with established practice. Slightly tilt probe after insertion, hold the covered probe until the audible tone is heard. Luberication may be used on the tip of the probe cover.

Taking Pulses – Find patient's pulse, push white button on left side of the Mark X front. Count pulses until tone is heard 15 seconds later. Timer may also be used for respiration or I.V. rate. (For best results: **Do Not Use The Timer During** the same moments when taking temperatures.)

Continued.

CARE AND PRECAUTIONS

GENERAL CARE AND PRECAUTIONS
- Read complete instructions before using system
- Keep the unit clean and follow established procedures in your office or clinic on clinical usage and cleaning
- Place unit on the charger base when not in use
- Do not use in the presence of flammable anesthetics
- Do not use acetone or similar products to clean unit as the surface could be damaged
- Please review all information in the manufacturer's manual before using the Mark X system

MARK X THERMOMETER
- Always place unit on charger base when not in use to insure that the batteries are fully charged
- Do not steam sterilize
- Read service instructions before attempting repairs or calibrations. Check the calibration of the unit periodically. This can be accomplished by using the calibration plug and verifying that the readout of the Mark X is the temperature indicated on the calibration plug. Should the unit require calibration, there are internal adjustments for fast service
- Do not reuse probe covers and use only Electromedics probe covers
- Replace components with like specification items

CHARGER BASE
Electrical shock hazard. Do not open case. Refer servicing to qualified personnel.
- Connect to properly grounded outlet
- Do not steam sterilize
- Always perform a current leakage test after any repairs

DESCRIPTION OF FRONT AND REAR PANELS

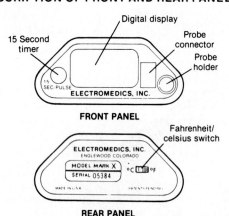

FRONT PANEL

REAR PANEL

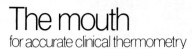

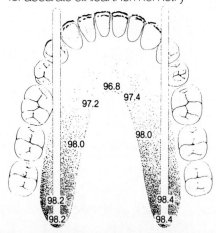

The placement of the thermometer probe tip is important for accurate temperature taking since there may be significant differences in temperature over small distances in the mouth.

The diagram shows the hot spots where maximum temperatures are found. These important heat pockets lie at the junction of the base of the tongue and the floor of the mouth on either side of the frenum. If the probe tip is not placed in the heat pocket, temperature readings can vary significantly.

HELPFUL HINTS
THINGS IN GENERAL

The Mark X probes are cleanable. The blue and red sliders on the probes can be removed to allow for cleaning. If you will hold the probe above the slider and pull the slider while turning at the same time, the slider will pull off the probe shaft. You can clean the probe shaft and the slider with any of the cold wipe agents or they may be gas sterilized.

Hold the probe for the patient. Avoid allowing the patient to hold the probe. It is possible that the patient may move the probe out of the sublingual pocket, which would give an incorrect reading of the temperature.

When taking a rectal temperature, have the patient and supplies ready before removing the probe from the probe well and activating the unit. Pre-lube the rectal probe, ready the patient, remove the oral probe, plug the rectal probe into the Mark X, and then follow established procedures for taking the rectal temperature.

IF GETTING INACCURATE TEMPERATURES

Generally, inaccuracy with electronic thermometers is due to placement in the mouth. The map of the mouth shows the different temperature zones. If one is not careful to place the probe in the sublingual pocket, different temperatures will be experienced.

With electronic thermometers being very accurate in measurement, it is possible to vary a tenth or two tenths of a degree. Most of the glass thermometers do not have the ability to read this area as accurately as the electronic units do, so it may lead you to believe you have an accuracy problem. If your thermometers are within the published accuracy specifications and you are getting higher or lower readings, you should suspect measurement technique.

It is recommended that the patient not take anything orally for at least 15 minutes before taking the temperature. It is recommended that you wait for 15 minutes after an enema before taking a rectal temperature. These procedures will allow the tissue to return to the natural temperature and the measurement will be more accurate.

In some cases, you will have performed all of the proper techniques and have different temperature indications. The manufacturer recommends that you check the unit with the calibration key. This will indicate the electronic function and accuracy. You may want to change probes with another unit and see if you have the same readings. It may be helpful to ask the patient if they have taken anything orally or if they have been chewing gum or eating candy before you attempt to measure the temperature.

IF GETTING LOW TEMPERATURES

Low temperatures may be caused by several things. The most common is what is called "The Draw Down Effect." "Draw Down" is the sudden lowering of tissue temperature because of its contact with a probe at a lower temperature. The "Draw Down" occurs within the first few seconds, while recovery may take several minutes. This "Draw Down" effect results from thermal energy flowing from the skin tissue to the probe, until both the probe and the skin tissue are at the same temperature. Recovery then occurs as both tissue and probe temperatures increase to body temperature.

Measurements of "Draw Down" for various probes show that for an initial probe temperature of 75°F and tissue temperature of 98.6°F, the average recovery time of temperature in the local tissue is at least 3 minutes. To avoid the effect of "Draw Down", simply take 4–5 seconds to slowly insert the probe along the gum line. This process will warm the cold probe and not lower the temperature of the sublingual pocket at the base of the tongue.

The second possibility is the failure to insert the probe into the sublingual pocket. As the map of the mouth shows, there are many areas of varying temperatures located in the mouth. The most accurate for this purpose is the sublingual pocket located at the base of the tongue and close to the blood supply from deep within the body. If you are not in the pocket or if you press into the pocket and restrict the blood flow, you may well experience low temperature readings.

The third possibility is the natural temperature variations of humans. It has been found that people have a natural low temperature in the morning hours and a higher temperature in the evenings. If you have applied proper technique and you are experiencing what appears to be low temperature, you may be reading the natural temperature of that person. You may want to check the patient with another unit after about 5 minutes.

Table 17.1
Comparison of centigrade and Fahrenheit readings

C	F	C	F	C	F	C	F
34.0— 93.2		36.0 — 96.8		38.0—100.4		39.8—103.6	
34.1— 93.4		36.1 — 97.0		38.1—100.6		39.9—103.8	
34.2— 93.6		36.2 — 97.2		38.2—100.8		40.0—104.0	
34.3— 93.7		36.3 — 97.3		38.3—100.9		40.1—104.2	
34.4— 93.9		36.4 — 97.5		38.4—101.1		40.2—104.4	
34.5— 94.1		36.5 — 97.7		38.5—101.3		40.3—104.5	
34.6— 94.3		36.6 — 97.9		38.6—101.5		40.4—104.7	
34.7— 94.5		36.7 — 98.1		38.7—101.7		40.5—104.9	
34.8— 94.6		36.8 — 98.2		38.8—101.8		40.6—105.1	
34.9— 94.8		36.9 — 98.4		38.9—102.0		40.7—105.3	
35.0— 95.0		37.0*— 98.6*		39.0—102.2		40.8—105.4	
35.1— 95.2		37.1 — 98.8		39.1—102.4		40.9—105.6	
35.2— 95.4		37.2 — 98.9		39.2—102.6		41.0—105.8	
35.3— 95.5		37.3 — 99.1		39.3—102.7		41.1—106.0	
35.4— 95.7		37.4 — 99.3		39.4—102.9		41.5—106.7	
35.5— 95.9		37.5 — 99.5		39.5—103.1		42.0—107.6	
35.6— 96.1		37.6 — 99.7		39.6—103.3		42.5—108.5	
35.7— 96.3		37.7 — 99.9		39.7—103.5			
35.8— 96.4		37.8 —100.0					
35.9— 96.6		37.9 —100.2					

*Normal oral temperature.

Methods and Procedures for Taking a Temperature

Following these guidelines determines the correct method of use.
1. *Oral* temperatures should *never* be taken on the following:
   a. Children who are not old enough to know how to hold the thermometer in the mouth (4 years old and under).
   b. Patients with a nasal obstruction, dyspnea, coughing, weakness, a sore mouth, mouth diseases, or oral surgery.
   c. Patients receiving oxygen.
   d. Uncooperative, delirious, unconscious, or intoxicated patients.
2. *Axillary* temperatures should *never* be taken on the following:
   a. Thin patients who cannot make the hollow under the arm airtight.
   b. Perspiring patients whose axilla cannot be kept dry for the required 5 to 10 minutes.
3. *Rectal* temperatures should *never* be taken on the following:
   a. Rectal surgery patients.
   b. Children or other patients whose body movement cannot be controlled for the required 4 to 5 minutes.

Equipment

Thermometer:
Oral—Glass thermometers may be stored in a small container of 70% alcohol solution or other disinfectant solution, with a small pad of cotton in the bottom, and labeled *clean oral thermometers.*
Rectal—Glass thermometers may be stored in a small container of alcohol solution or other disinfectant solution, with a small pad of cotton in the bottom and labeled *clean rectal thermometers.*
Box of tissues or small cotton squares
Container for waste
Containers labeled "soiled oral thermometers" or "soiled rectal thermometers" for the ones used

Continued.

Methods and Procedures for Taking a Temperature—cont'd

Equipment—cont'd

Water-soluble lubricant if a rectal temperature is to be taken, such as K-Y jelly, Vaseline, mineral oil, or baby oil

Disposable rubber gloves for taking a rectal or infant's temperature

General instructions

1. Handle the thermometer with great care, as it is a very delicate instrument.
2. Keep rectal thermometers separate from oral thermometers.
3. Wash your hands before and after handling a thermometer or taking a patient's temperature.
4. Read the thermometer with great care to ensure accuracy.
5. Record the reading and indicate if it was other than oral. This notation must be made because of the differences in temperatures when taken in either the axilla or rectum.

Care of glass thermometers after each use

1. Shake mercury down to below 96° F or 36° C.
2. Wash with soap and cold water, then rinse with cold running water.
3. Place in a disinfectant solution, such as 70% alcohol if it is to be used continuously; then rinse with cold, running water and dry with a small piece of cotton before the next use.
4. If the thermometer is not to be reused within 24 hours, follow steps 1 and 2, then dry it and place it in a container that has cotton in the bottom to provide protection for the bulb. Before the next use, the thermometer must soak for at least 10 minutes in a disinfectant solution then be rinsed in cold running water and dried with a small piece of cotton.

Oral temperature

The thermometer is to be placed in the mouth under the tongue. The lips should be closed.

Procedure	*Rationale*
1. Identify and evaluate the patient. 2. Wash your hands. 3. Assemble equipment.	Defer reading for 15 to 20 minutes if the patient has just finished eating, drinking, or smoking. Patients should not be left alone unless they are absolutely responsible. This is a precaution to observe to avoid any accident or false reading.
4. Instruct the patient to assume a sitting position and explain the procedure.	Complete explanations help gain the patient's cooperation and help the patient relax. Provide for the patient's comfort and safety.
5. Remove clean thermometer from the container. 6. Rinse with cold running water, and wipe dry from the stem downward to the bulb with a tissue or cotton square. Discard cotton square.	
7. With a firm hold on the end of the thermometer, shake it down to 96° F (35.5° C) or lower.	This is done by giving the wrist several quick snaps. Be careful to avoid contact with nearby objects.
8. Place the thermometer well under the patient's tongue. 9. Instruct the patient to keep lips closed, breathe through the nose, and not touch the thermometer with the teeth. 10. Leave the thermometer in place for 3 minutes. 11. The pulse and respirations may be taken while the thermometer is registering.	
12. Remove the thermometer and wipe it from the top toward the bulb.	Never place pressure on the mercury bulb end of the thermometer.
13. Read the thermometer. Hold it horizontally and rotate it slowly until you see the point at which the mercury column stops. 14. Record the reading at once.	Charting example: January 26, 19_____, 9 AM Oral temp 98.8° F *or* Temp 98.8° F J. Sublett, CMA

15. Shake the mercury down to 96° F (35.5° C) or below and place the thermometer in the container for used oral thermometers, or into a container of cool soap solution.
16. If retaking a questionable temperature, the medical assistant should do the following:
    - Check that the thermometer is shaken down to 96° F (35.5° C) or below
      or
    - Use another thermometer
      or
    - Use another method, either rectal or axillary.
17. Wash your hands.

If the temperature is found to be remarkably high or low and there is no apparent reason for this, take it again.

Axillary temperature

The thermometer is to be placed in the axilla (armpit).

Procedure	*Rationale*
1. Perform steps 1 through 7 as for oral temperature technique, using a rounded, short bulb thermometer.	
2. Blot the axillary region dry with tissue or a cotton square.	Avoid rubbing, as friction increases the blood supply in the area, thus increasing the temperature of the skin.
3. Place the bulb end of the thermometer in the hollow of the axillary region with the end of the thermometer slanting toward the patient's chest.	Ensure that the thermometer is in direct contact with the skin surface, not touching clothing or exposed to the air.
4. Have the patient cross the arm over the chest. It may be more comfortable to hold the opposite shoulder.	This prevents as little air as possible coming in contact with the thermometer. When the patient is unable to put his hand on the opposite shoulder, place it there gently and hold it with your own hand or hold the patient's arm close to his side. When taking a child's temperature by axilla, hold the thermometer in place for the entire time.
5. Leave the thermometer in place for 5 to 10 minutes.	This ensures accurate registration of the temperature.
6. The pulse and respirations may be taken while the thermometer is registering.	
7. Remove and wipe the thermometer from the top toward the bulb, and read it.	Never place pressure on the bulb end of the thermometer.
8. Record reading at once.	Charting example: January 30, 19_____,11 AM Axillary temp 97.6° F *or* Temp 97.6° F A M. Kubiak, CMA
9. Shake the mercury down to 96° F (35.5° C) or below and place the thermometer in the container for used thermometers.	
10. Wash your hands.	

Rectal temperature

The thermometer is to be carefully inserted approximately 1 inch into the rectum.

Procedure	*Rationale*
1. Perform steps 1 through 7 as for oral temperature, using a rectal thermometer.	*Never* use an oral thermometer for a rectal temperature.
2. Have the patient turn on the side with the upper leg flexed if possible.	Do not expose patient unnecessarily.
3. Don disposable rubber gloves.	
4. Apply lubricant to the thermometer.	Lubricant allows for easier insertion of the thermometer.
5. Separate buttocks so that anus is exposed.	
6. Gently insert thermometer approximately 1 inch into anal canal and instruct the patient to remain still.	Forceful insertion beyond 1 inch may cause damage to the tissues involved. Movement could cause the thermometer to go further into the rectum and possibly cause tissue damage, or the thermometer could slip out of the rectum.
7. *Hold* thermometer in place for 4 to 5 minutes.	*Never leave the patient alone when taking a rectal temperature.*
8. You may take pulse and respirations while the thermometer is registering.	

Continued.

Methods and Procedures for Taking a Temperature—cont'd

Rectal temperature—cont'd

Procedure

9. Remove the thermometer, wipe from stem to bulb, and read accurately.
10. Record the reading at once.

11. Shake the mercury down to below 96° F (35.5° C).
12. Place the thermometer in the container for used rectal thermometers.
13. Remove gloves and wash your hands.

Taking an infant's temperature

1. Don disposable rubber gloves.
2. Lay the infant on the stomach on a firm surface.
3. With your left hand, spread the cheeks of the buttocks so that you can see the rectum.
4. With your right hand, insert the lubricated bulb end of the rectal thermometer into the rectum approximately 1 inch.
5. Place your right hand on the infant's buttocks, hold the buttocks firmly, and pinch the thermometer firmly between your fingers.
6. Place your other hand in the small of the infant's back, and with your arm straight, lean on the infant slightly. This will help hold the infant still (Figure 17.3).

Figure 17.3
Position for holding thermometer and infant while taking rectal temperature.

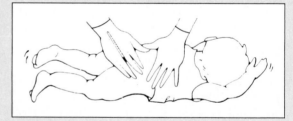

7. Leave the thermometer in place for 5 minutes.
8. Remove the thermometer and place it out of reach of the infant.
9. Support the infant.
10. Wipe the thermometer with a tissue, read the temperature registered, and record it promptly.
11. Remove gloves and wash your hands.

Rationale

Never place pressure on the bulb end of the thermometer. Be certain all fecal material is removed.

Charting example:
    January 31, 19_____, 10 AM
    Rectal temp 99.6° F
    or
    Temp 99.6° F Ⓡ
        Josh Burns, CMA

Remember to keep used rectal thermometers in a separate container.

PULSE

The pulse is the beat of the heart as felt through the walls of the arteries. It is the palpable distention or pulsation of the arteries produced by the wave of blood that travels along the arteries with each contraction of the left ventricle of the heart.

The pulse can also be described as a throbbing caused by the alternate expansion and recoil of an artery.

Characteristics of the Pulse

When you are taking a pulse, the four important characteristics to note are the rate, rhythm, volume of the pulse, and the condition of the arterial wall. These characteristics depend on the size and the elasticity of the artery, the strength of contraction of the heart, and the tissues surrounding the artery. The physician will sometimes spend several minutes examining a patient's pulses to obtain information that may reveal abnormalities of the circulation or the heart.

The *rate* (frequency) of the pulse means the number of pulsations (beats) in a given minute. Normal (average) rates are outlined in the following section. Abnormal rates are those above or below the range of norms, and could be described as bradycardia (slow) or tachycardia (rapid).

Figure 17.4
Common arteries for determining pulse rates.

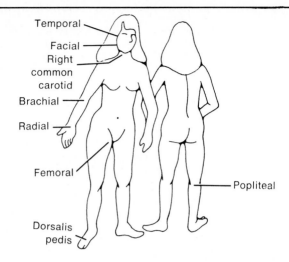

The *rhythm* of the pulse pertains to the time interval between each pulse. Normal rhythm is described as regular; that is, intervals between pulsations are of equal length. Abnormal rhythm may be described as irregular, arrhythmic, bigeminal, skipping beats, or intermittent. Skipping an occasional beat occurs in all normal individuals especially during exercise or after ingesting certain stimulants such as coffee. Most of these irregularities go unnoticed but at times may concern a patient sufficiently to seek medical advice. When there are frequent beats skipped or if the beats are highly irregular, the physician should be alerted, because this could be an important sign of heart disease. In such cases, it is sometimes useful to count the radial pulse rate for 1 minute and then to record the apical rate by listening over the heart (see p. 269). If the apical rate is greater, the difference is referred to as the pulse deficit. The pulse deficit is important in the examination of the patient with atrial fibrillation, one of the more common causes of a very irregular pulse.

A pulse may vary in intensity in association with irregularities of rhythm. A pulse that varies only in intensity but is otherwise perfectly regular is often a manifestation of heart disease. The *volume* of the pulse pertains to the strength of the pulsations and may be described as full, strong, bounding, weak, feeble, thready, febrile, hard, or soft. It depends on the force of the heartbeat and the condition of the arterial walls.

The *force* of the pulse is an indication of the general condition of the heart and the circulatory system. This intensity may vary from being a weak and feeble beat as seen in shock, to being a strong and bounding throb as seen after exercise.

The *condition of the arterial wall* pertains to the texture of the artery that one feels through the skin surface when palpating the pulse. A normal arterial wall is described as soft and elastic; abnormal conditions include hard, ropy, knotty, and wiry.

Common arteries and body locations for determining pulse rate (Figure 17.4)

radial Over the inner aspect of the wrist area, on the thumb side. This site is the one most frequently used and accessible in most cases.
facial Along the lower margin of the mandible.
common carotid At right and left sides of the neck, at the anterior edge of the sternocleidomastoid muscle.
brachial Over the inner aspect at the bend of the elbow.
temporal At the temple, on the side of the forehead.
femoral The anterior side of the hip bone, in the groin region.
popliteal At the back of the knee.
dorsalis pedis On the upper surface of the foot between ankle and toes.

Normal pulse rates (average number of pulsations [beats] in 1 minute)

At birth	130-160 beats per minute
Infants	110-130 beats per minute
Children from 1 to 7 years	80-120 beats per minute
Children over 7 years	80-90 beats per minute
Adults	60-80 beats per minute

Variations in Pulse Rate

Individual pulse rates *normally vary* as a result of a person's sex, age, body size, posture, activity level, health status, functions of the nervous system, and

Procedure for Taking a Radial Pulse

Equipment

Watch with a second hand
Paper or graphic sheet to record pulse
Pen

General instructions

1. Have the patient assume a comfortable position either sitting or lying down, with the arm supported.
2. Do not take a pulse rate immediately after the patient has been emotionally upset or after exertion, unless so ordered.
3. Never use your thumb to take a pulse, because its own pulse is likely to be confused with the one being taken.
4. Always count any unusual pulse for a full minute, and repeat if uncertain.

Procedure	*Rationale*
1. Identify the patient and explain the procedure.	Explanations help gain the cooperation and relaxation of the patient.
2. Wash your hands.	
3. Position the patient with the arm supported and at rest.	
4. Taking a firm hold of the patient's wrist, place your first three fingers on the patient's wristbone just over the radial artery, with sufficient pressure to feel the pulsations distinctly. (Pulse rates at other locations previously noted are taken in similar fashion.)	A firm hold will inspire the patient's confidence. Excessive pressure prevents the pulse from being felt. *Never* use your thumb to take a pulse, because your thumb's pulse can be confused with the patient's.
5. Count the pulse for 60 seconds.	This will give the total beats per minute.
6. Note the rate, rhythm, volume, and condition of the arterial wall.	Always report any deviations from normal. If deviations are noted, always count the pulse rate for 1 full minute, and repeat if uncertain.
7. Write the pulse rate down immediately.	Do not trust it to memory
8. Record accurately on the patient's chart.	Charting example:

        January 15, 19_____, 2 PM, Pulse 78
          or
        Radial pulse, right arm—78
        Regular and strong pulsations
          Rae Evans, CMA

the volume and chemical composition of the blood.

In general, the pulse rate is faster in women (70 to 80 beats per minute) than in men (60 to 70 beats per minute) and usually higher in short people than in tall people. Infants' and children's pulse rates are also more rapid than an adult's. When one is sitting, the rate is more rapid (for example, 70 beats per minute) than when lying down (for example, 66 beats per minute), and increases when standing, walking, or running (for example, 80, 86, and 90 beats per minute respectively). During sleep or rest, the pulse rate may be as low as 45 to 50 beats per minute. In athletes it is not unusual to obtain resting rates as low as 45 to 50 beats per minute. The following list indicates some of the common causes of increases or decreases in the pulse.

Increase	Decrease
Fear or excitement	Mental depression
Physical activity, exercise	Certain types of heart disease
Fever	

Increase	Decrease
Certain types of heart disease	Chronic illness
Hyperthyroidism	Hypothyroidism
Shock	Certain brain injuries that cause pressure
Pain	Certain drugs, such as digitalis
Certain drugs	
Many infections	

Pulse variation vocabulary

abdominal pulse Abdominal aorta pulse.

acrotism (ak′ro-tizm) Apparent absence of pulse.

alternating pulse Alternating weak and strong pulsations.

arrhythmia (ă-rith′mĭ-ă) Irregularities in pulse or rhythm.

bigeminal (bī-jĕm′ĭn-al) **pulse** Two regular beats followed by a longer pause. It has the same significance as an irregular pulse.

bradycardia (brad-ĭ-kar′dĭ-ă) Slow heart action; extremely slow pulse, generally below 60 beats per minute.

febrile (feb′rile) **pulse** A full, bounding pulse at the onset of a fever, becoming feeble and weak when the fever subsides.

formicant (for′mi-kant′) **pulse** A small, feeble pulse.

intermittent pulse A pulse in which occasional beats are skipped.

irregular pulse A pulse with variation in force and frequency; an excess of tea, coffee, tobacco, or exercise may cause this.

pulse deficit The apical rate is greater than the radial pulse rate. The difference between the two is noted as the pulse deficit.

pulse pressure The difference between the systolic and the diastolic blood pressure.

EXAMPLE: If BP is 120/80

$$120 = \text{systolic pressure}$$
$$\underline{-80} = \text{diastolic pressure}$$
$$40 = \text{pulse pressure}$$

A pulse pressure consistently over 50 points or under 30 points is considered abnormal.

regular pulse The rhythm of the pulse rate is regular.

slow pulse A pulse between 40 and 60 beats per minute, often found among the aged and among athletes at rest.

tachycardia (tăk″y-kar′dĭ-ă) A pulse of 170 or more beats per minute; abnormal rapidity of heart action.

thready pulse A pulse that is very fine and scarcely perceptible, as seen in syncope (fainting).

unequal pulse A pulse in which some beats are strong and others are weak; pulse in which rates are different in symmetrical arteries.

venous pulse A pulse in a vein, especially one of the large veins near the heart such as the internal or external jugular. Venous pulse is undulating and scarcely palpable.

Apical Heartbeat Rate

The apical rate is the rate per minute of the heartbeat as determined by auscultation or feeling the apex of the heart. This is the most accurate pulse site. An apical pulse is taken on all children under 2 years of age and on patients with possible heart problems regardless of age. The normal range is 70 to 90 beats per minute; the average rate is 80 beats per minute.

To count the apical beat, place the chestpiece of a stethoscope over the apex of the heart and count the number of heart beats in 1 minute.

The apex of the heart is located in the left fifth intercostal space on the midclavicular line, that is, between the fifth and sixth ribs on a line with the midpoint of the left clavicle. This position is usually just below the nipple.

When recording the results, you must indicate that it was the apical rate that was taken. On completion, wipe the ear-pieces and diaphragm of the stethoscope with an alcohol sponge and return it to the proper storage area.

RESPIRATION

Respiration is the act of breathing, consisting of one inspiration or inhalation, in which air is taken into the lungs, and one expiration or exhalation, in which the lungs expel carbon dioxide. More specifically, respiration is the taking in of oxygen (O_2) and its use in the tissues, and the giving off of carbon dioxide (CO_2). For this reason, respiration may be classified as external and internal. External respiration is the interchange of gases that takes place in the lungs between the alveoli and blood; internal respiration is the interchange of gases that takes place in the tissues between the body cells and blood.

The autonomic control of breathing is controlled by the respiratory center in the medulla oblongata in the lower portion of the brainstem. A buildup of carbon dioxide in the blood stimulates respirations to occur automatically.

In the human body a relationship exists between the body temperature, pulse, and respiratory rates. The usual ratio of respiration to the pulse is one to four (1:4). Respiration and pulse ordinarily rise proportionally to each degree rise in temperature because of the increased metabolism in the tissue cells and the need for more rapid heat dissipation.

Characteristics of Respirations

When you are taking the respiratory rate of a patient, the three important characteristics to note are the rate, rhythm, and depth.

The *rate* of respirations refers to the number of respirations per minute and is best described as normal, below or above normal, or rapid or slow. In adults normal rates are between 14 and 20 per minute; subnormal rates are 12 per minute and below and should be considered a serious symptom; above-normal rates are between 34 and 35 per minute; rapid rates are between 36 and 50 per minute. Any rate above 40 should also be considered a serious symptom. Dangerously rapid rates are those that are 60 per minute and above. Usually rapid respirations are also shallow. They are seen in some diseases of the lungs. Deep respirations are characteristically slow, dependent on oxygen exchange, and common in conditions affecting brain pressure and in some forms of coma.

Procedure for Taking the Respiratory Rate

Equipment

A watch with a second hand
Paper or graphic sheet to record respiration rate
Pen

General instructions

1. Have the patient assume a comfortable position.
2. Do not take the respiratory rate immediately after the patient has been emotionally upset or after exertion, unless so ordered.
3. Count any unusual respiratory rate for an additional minute.

Procedure

1. Wash your hands.
2. Do *not* explain procedure to the patient.

3. Place your fingers on the patient's wrist as though counting the pulse.
4. Count each breathing cycle (inhalation and exhalation) as one breath by watching the rise and fall of the chest or upper abdomen.

5. Count for 1 full minute.
6. Record rate on paper immediately
7. Record on patient's chart.
   - Note any abnormality if present.
   - Note any pain associated with breathing.
   - Note the position the patient assumes, as in some cases it may be significant. Examples include when the patient can breathe easier when sitting up, or when lying on one side or the other.

Rationale

The rate of respiration should be counted and its depth, rate, and rhythm studied without the patient's knowledge. The consciousness of being watched will cause involuntary change in the rate of respiration. A patient can control respirations if he wishes to.

When these movements are scarcely perceptible, place the patient's hand, with your fingers remaining on the wrist, gently but firmly on the patient's chest, and count in this manner.
Do not trust it to memory.

Charting example:
January 15, 19_____, 2 PM
Respirations 22 and regular.
    L. Quarry, CMA

The *rhythm* may be described as regular or irregular. Regular breathing or respiration is characterized by inhalations and exhalations that are the same in depth and rate, whereas in irregular breathing, the inhalations and exhalations may vary in the amount of air inhaled and exhaled and in the rate of respirations per minute.

The *depth* of respirations depends on the amount of air inhaled and exhaled and is best described as either shallow or deep. In shallow respirations, small amounts of air are inhaled; these respirations are often rapid. In deep respirations, larger amounts of air are inhaled, as in a "deep breath."

Normal Respiratory Rates

At birth—30 to 60 respirations/minute
Infants—30 to 38 respirations/minute
Children—20 to 26 respirations/minute
Adults—14 to 20 respirations/minute

Variations in the Respiratory Rate

Certain situations, both in health or in diseased states, will cause variations in the normal respiratory rates. Some of these are listed here:

Increased respiratory rate

Excitement
Nervousness
Any strong emotion
Increased muscular activity, such as running or exercising
Certain drugs, such as ephedrine
Diseases of the lungs
Diseases of the circulatory system
Fever
Pain
Shock
Hemorrhage
Gas poisoning
High altitudes
Obstruction of the air passages
An increase in the carbon dioxide levels in arterial blood, which in turn stimulates the respiratory center

Decreased respiratory rate

Sleep

Certain drugs, such as morphine

Certain diseases of the kidneys in which there is a coma

Diseases and injuries that cause pressure on the brain tissue; for example, a stroke or skull fracture

Decrease of the carbon dioxide level in arterial blood (causes the respiratory centers to be depressed, causing decreased respiration rates)

Respiration and respiratory rate vocabulary

abdominal respirations The inspiration and expiration of air by the lungs accomplished primarily by the abdominal muscles and diaphragm.

accelerated respirations More than 25 respirations per minute, after 15 years of age.

apnea (ap-ne′ah) Cessation or absence of breathing.

artificial respiration Artificial methods to restore respiration in cases of suspended breathing.

Biot respiration Irregularly alternating periods of apnea and hypernea; occurs in meningitis and disorders of the brain.

Cheyne-Stokes (chān-stōks) **respiration** Respirations gradually increasing in rapidity and volume, until they reach a climax, then gradually subsiding and ceasing entirely for 5 to 50 seconds, when they begin again. These are often a sign of impending death. Cheyne-Stokes respirations *may* be observed in normal persons (especially the aged) during sleep or during visits to higher altitudes.

diaphragmatic respiration Performed mainly by the diaphragm.

dyspnea (disp-ne′ah) Labored or difficult breathing.

eupnea (ūp-ne′ah) Easy or normal respiration.

forced respiration Voluntary hyperpnea.

hyperpnea (hi″perp-ne′ah) Increase in rate and depth of breathing.

hyperventilation Increase of air in the lungs above the normal amount; abnormally prolonged and deep breathing, usually associated with acute anxiety or emotional tensions.

hypoxia (hi-pok′se-ah) Reduced amounts of oxygen to the body tissues.

labored breathing Dyspnea or difficult breathing; respiration that involves active participation of accessory inspiratory and expiratory muscles.

orthopnea (or″thop-ne′ah) Severe dyspnea in which breathing is possible only when the patient sits or stands in an erect position.

rales (rahls) An abnormal bubbling sound heard on auscultation of the chest; often classified as either moist or crackling and dry.

stertorous (stĕr′to-rŭs) Characterized by a deep snoring sound with each inspiration.

BLOOD PRESSURE

Blood pressure (BP) is the pressure of the blood against the walls of the blood vessels. The pressure results from the pumping action of the heart muscle. This pressure inside the arteries varies with the contracting and the relaxing phases of the heart beat cycle. Systole is the phase in which the heart contracts, forcing blood through the arteries, and diastole is the phase in which the heart relaxes between contractions. Thus when you are measuring a person's blood pressure there are two readings that you will need to take: systolic pressure and diastolic pressure (systole and diastole).

Systolic pressure is measured in the number of millimeters of mercury (mm Hg), representing the force with which blood is pushing against the artery walls when the ventricles of the heart are in a state of contraction. During systole, blood is forced out of the heart into the aorta and pulmonary artery, and the pressure within the arteries is the highest.

Diastolic pressure is the number in millimeters of mercury that represents the force of the blood in the arterial system when the ventricles of the heart are in the state of relaxation. During diastole the two ventricles of the heart are dilated by blood flowing into them, and the pressure within the arteries is at its lowest point.

These measurements provide the physician with valuable information about a patient's cardiovascular system. Systolic pressure provides information about the force of the left ventricular contraction, and the diastolic pressure provides information about the resistance of the blood vessels.

Clinically, diastolic pressure is more important than systolic pressure because diastolic pressure indicates the strain or pressure to which the blood vessel walls are constantly subjected. Since diastolic pressure rises or falls with the peripheral resistance, it also reflects the condition of the peripheral vessels. For example, if a patient's arteries are sclerosed, both the peripheral resistance and the diastolic pressure will increase.

Blood pressure is recorded and discussed as the systolic pressure over the diastolic pressure. A typical blood pressure is expressed as: 120/80 (mm Hg) *or* 120 over 80. The numerical difference between these two readings (in this case, 40 points) is called the *pulse pressure*, which may indicate the tone of the arterial walls. A normal pulse pressure is about 40; if consistently over 50 points or under 30 points it is considered abnormal. You may see an increase in pulse pressure in arteriosclerosis mainly because of an increase in the systolic pressure, or in aortic valve insufficiency, the result of both a rise in systolic and a fall in diastolic pressure.

Factors that Determine Blood Pressure

A number of factors, acting in dynamic equilibrium and integrated through the central nervous system, determine the arterial blood pressure. They include the following:

- *The pumping action of the heart and cardiac output*—how hard the heart pumps the blood, or the force of the heartbeat; how much blood it pumps and how efficiently it does the job.
- *The volume of blood within the blood vessels*—how much blood the heart pumps into the arterial system.
- *The peripheral resistance of blood vessels to the flow of blood*—the size of the lumen, the central core of the arteries, directly influences the resistance to the arteries, directly influences the resistance to the blood flow. When the lumen is narrow, the blood pressure will be higher; with a larger lumen, the blood pressure will be lower.
- *The elasticity of the walls of the main arteries*—The main arteries leading from the heart have walls with strong elastic fibers capable of expanding and absorbing the pulsations generated by the heart. At each pulsation, the arteries expand and absorb the momentary increase in blood pressure. As the heart relaxes in preparation for another beat, the aortic valves close to prevent blood from flowing back to the heart chambers, and the artery walls spring back, forcing the blood through the body between contractions. In this way the arteries act as dampers on the pulsations and thus provide a steady flow of blood through the blood vessels. This elasticity of the arterial walls lessens with age, and because the arterial wall is resistant, the blood pressure will then be higher.
- *The blood's viscosity, or thickness*—Blood pressure increases as the viscosity of blood increases. Polycythemia, an increase in red blood cells, will cause this.

The exact contribution of each factor is not known, but it is generally thought that the peripheral resistance and cardiac output have the greatest influence on blood pressure.

Normal Readings and Values for Blood Pressure

At birth the systolic pressure is about 80 mm Hg. *At age 10* (young people), systolic blood pressure varies normally from 100 to 120 mm Hg and diastolic 60 to 80 mm Hg. In *adults* the average BP is 120/80. The *average ranges* are 90 to 140 mm Hg for systolic pressure and 60 to 90 mm Hg for diastolic pressure. In *older people* (around 60 years) the systolic blood pressure normally varies from 140 to about 170 mm Hg, and diastolic varies from 92 to 100 mm Hg, the result of a loss of resilience in the vascular tree and physiological changes of aging.

Abnormal Readings

In children around age 10, upper limits of normal are 140/100, with systolic pressure greater than 140 mm Hg generally recognized as being abnormal. In adults, a systolic pressure consistently above 150 mm Hg and a diastolic pressure consistently above 90 mm Hg are generally recognized as being abnormal. *Hypertension* is systolic pressure over 160 mm Hg or diastolic pressure over 90 mm Hg. If the blood pressure is consistently above this level, it could, if not treated, damage the heart, eyes, kidneys, and even the arteries. Diagnosis of hypertension is never based on only one reading. It is based on at least three consecutive daily or weekly blood pressure readings.

Hypotension is systolic pressure consistently under 90 with the diastolic pressure in proportion. In the absence of other signs or symptoms, hypotension is generally innocent. An extremely low blood pressure is occasionally a symptom of a serious condition, such as shock, and may be associated with Addison's disease (underfunctioning of the adrenal glands).

A pulse pressure constantly greater than 50 mm Hg or less than 30 mm Hg is considered abnormal.

Variations in Normal Blood Pressure

The blood pressure can vary between the sexes (with women usually having a lower pressure than men), between different age groups, and even between individuals of the same age and sex. At birth it is the lowest, then continues to increase with age, reaching its peak in advancing age as a rule. Variations are also seen at different times of the day, and the pressure may change with the kind of activity a person is engaged in. When one is standing or sitting, blood pressure is higher than when one is lying down.

The pressure is normally lowest just before awakening in the morning. There are many other situations that will produce changes in the blood pressure. The following lists indicate some of the common causes of an increase or decrease in a person's pressure.

Increased or elevated

Exercise

Stress, anxiety, excitement

Increased arterial blood volume

Conditions in which blood vessels become more rigid and lose some of their elasticity, as seen in old age

Increased peripheral resistance, resulting from vasoconstriction or narrowing of peripheral blood vessels

Endocrine disorders, such as hyperthyroidism and acromegaly

Increased weight

Renal disease and diseases of the liver and heart

In the right arm, it is about 3 to 4 mm Hg higher than in the left arm

Certain drug therapy

Increased intracranial pressure

Decreased or lowered

Weak heart

Massive heart attack

Decreased arterial blood volume (such as in hemorrhage)

Shock and collapse

Dehydration

Adrenal insufficiency

Drug treatment

Disorders of the nervous system

Hypothyroidism

Sleep

Infections, fevers

Cancer

Anemia

Neurasthenia

Approaching death

Blood pressure vocabulary

hypertension (hi'per-ten'shun)   High blood pressure; a condition in which a patient has a higher blood pressure than normal for his age; for example, systolic pressure consistently above 160 mm Hg and a diastolic pressure above 90 mm Hg.

hypotension (hi-po-ten'shun)   A decrease of systolic and diastolic blood pressure to below normal; for example, below 90/50 is considered low blood pressure.

benign (be-nīn) **hypertension**   Hypertension of slow onset that is usually without symptoms.

essential hypertension (idiopathic or primary hypertension)   Hypertension that develops in the absence of kidney disease. Its cause is unknown. About 85% to 90% of the cases of hypertension are in this category.

malignant (mah-lig'nant) **hypertension**   Hypertension that differs from other types in that it is a rapidly developing hypertension and may prove fatal if not treated immediately after symptoms develop, before

damage is done to the blood vessels. This type occurs most often in persons in their 20s or 30s.

orthostatic (or''tho-stat'ik) **blood pressure**   Blood pressure measured when the patient is in an erect, standing position.

orthostatic hypotension   Hypotension occurring when a patient assumes an erect position.

postural hypotension   Hypotension occurring upon suddenly rising from a recumbent position or when standing still for a long period of time.

renal hypertension   Hypertension resulting from kidney disease.

secondary hypertension   Hypertension that is traceable to known causes such as pheochromocytoma (tumor of the adrenal gland), hardening of the arteries, kidney disease, or obstructions to kidney blood flow. Approximately 10% to 15% of the cases of hypertension are secondary. Patients with *secondary hypertension* can often be cured *if* the underlying cause can be eliminated.

Instruments for Measuring Blood Pressure

Blood pressure is measured with two instruments, a sphygmomanometer (sfig''mo-mah-nom'ĕ-ter) and a stethoscope (steth'o-skōp). Various models of each and combination kits are available (Figure 17.5). Two common types of sphygmomanometers (*sphygmo,* pulse; *manos,* slight; *meter,* to measure) are available for general use: the mercury manometer, which uses a column of mercury to measure the blood pressure, and the aneroid (*a,* not; *neroid,* liquid) manometer, which uses compressed air.

Each type has advantages and disadvantages. The mercury manometer offers total reliability, because once it is calibrated at the factory, accuracy is assured. However, it may only be used when the column of mercury is in a vertical position, and it is more fragile and larger than the aneroid type. The aneroid manometer, on the other hand, needs periodic adjustment and calibration against a mercury manometer. However, it is smaller, thus offering more convenience and easier portability. Each manometer has four basic parts (Figure 17.6).

Pressure indicators

Pressure indicators are the scales used to read the blood pressure. The mercury manometer has a glass tube with numbers on the side to indicate the height of the column of mercury in millimeters. When the cuff is inflated, mercury is forced up into the tube; as the cuff is deflated, the column of mercury will fall. At certain points the level of the column of mercury is noted to provide the blood pressure reading. In the aneroid manometer, an inter-

Figure 17.5

Various types of sphygmomanometers. **A,** Desk mercury sphygmomanometer. **B,** Acoustic sphygmomanometer. Wrap cuff around arm in usual way. Make sure microphone is over brachial artery. With cuff in place, raise pressure to approximately 30 mm Hg beyond expected systolic pressure. Watch digital countdown, as pressure automatically releases. Systolic then diastolic pressure is displayed, as the sphygmomanometer responds to appropriate sounds. When both systolic and diastolic readings are displayed, a touch of a button also lets you read the pulse rate. **C,** Wall mercury sphygmomanometer.

A and B courtesy Sybron Corporation, Medical Products Division, Rochester, NY.

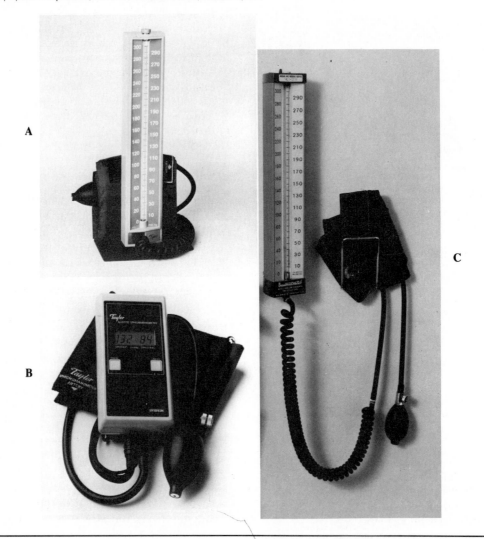

nal gear rotates in response to inflation and deflation of the cuff, which in turn moves a needle across a calibrated dial to provide the blood pressure reading.

Cuff

The compression cuff is a rectangular inflatable rubber bag covered with a nonstretch material.

This is wrapped around the patient's arm and secured with Velcro or clasps. On older models, the end of the cuff is tucked under one of the turns wrapped around the arm. Various sizes of cuffs are available to ensure a proper fit. Small cuffs are available to use on children or very thin people; larger cuffs are available to use on obese people or when taking a pressure reading on the leg (Table 17.2).

Figure 17.6
Four basic parts of a
sphygmomanometer.
Courtesy Sybron Corporation,
Medical Products Division,
Rochester, NY.

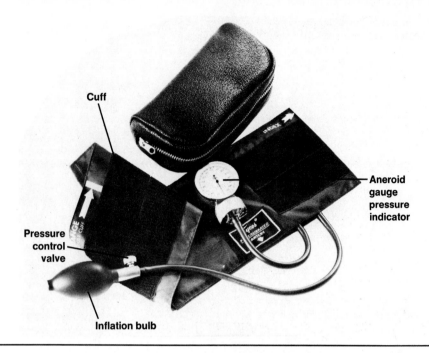

Table 17.2
Recommended widths of compression cuffs

Age	Width of inflatable bladder
Newborn infants	2.5 cm (1 inch)
Children (1 to 4 years old)	6 cm (2.3 inches)
Children (4 to 8 years old)	9 cm (3.5 inches)
Adults	13 cm (5.1 inches)
Obese adults	20 cm (8 inches)

Inflation bulb

The inflation bulb is used to pump air into the cuff through a rubber tube.

Pressure control valve

A valve on the inflation bulb is regulated with a thumbscrew to allow the air in the cuff to escape at different rates as it is opened and closed.

• • •

The second instrument used to measure blood pressure is the stethoscope, a basic diagnostic instrument that amplifies sounds produced by the blood pressure, the heart, and other internal body sounds. The key parts of the stethoscope are shown in Figure 17.7.

chestpiece Has one, two, or three "heads" consisting of bell-shaped or various diaphragm-type sensors that "pick up" body sounds.

diaphragm A waferlike sound sensor whose shape and the pressure applied to it determine which sound frequencies, low to high, are picked up.

tubing Tapered, flexible rubber or plastic tubing through which sound travels from the chestpiece to the binaurals.

binaurals Rigid metal tubes that connect the tubing to the earpieces.

earpieces The tips of the stethoscope to be positioned in the examiner's ear.

spring The external spring that holds the binaurals so that the earpieces are firmly positioned in the ear.

Figure 17.7
Key parts of stethoscope.
Courtesy Sybron Corporation, Medical Products Division, Rochester, NY.

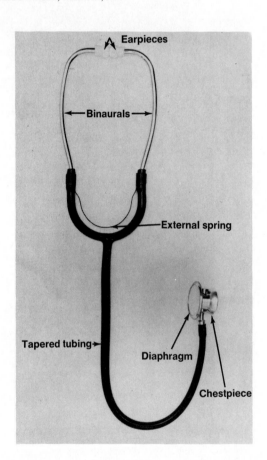

Procedure for Measuring Blood Pressure

Equipment

Sphygmomanometer
Stethoscope
70% isopropyl alcohol
Cotton balls or alcohol sponges
Paper and pencil

Auscultation method

Auscultation (aws''kul-ta'shun) indicates that you will be listening for sounds representing the pressure inside the arteries. The artery most frequently used is the brachial artery at the antecubital space opposite the elbow. Other locations that may be used are the popliteal artery behind the knee, or less commonly, the pedal artery on the foot.

General instructions

1. Before taking the patient's blood pressure, ask if he or she has been or is currently under treatment for high blood pressure. Anyone under treatment should be encouraged to continue, especially if blood pressure is normal at the time of screening, and should be urged to report an elevated blood pressure to the physician. The potential dangers of discontinuing antihypertensive treatment and the desirability of achieving satisfactory control of blood pressure must be strongly emphasized.
2. Arrangements should ensure as much confidentiality as possible during the recording of the blood pressure.
3. Be sure the patient is relaxed and in a comfortable position. Depending on the physician's orders, the patient may be sitting, standing, or lying.
4. If possible, take all subsequent observations with the patient in the same position and using the same arm.
5. Take readings as quickly as possible, as prolonged pressure affects the accuracy of the readings and is unpleasant for the patient.
6. On all new patients, blood pressure should be taken on both arms. If a discrepancy exists, the arm with the higher pressure is used in future recordings. This discrepancy is to be recorded on the chart.
7. Blood pressure is taken routinely on the following patients, the frequency being determined by their condition:
   - Patients receiving a complete physical examination;
   - Patients on hypertensive drugs;
   - Patients with a history of heart, kidney, or hypertensive disease;
   - New admissions to the hospital;
   - Pregnant patients;
   - Postpartum patients;
   - Preoperative patients;
   - Postoperative patients;
   - Patients in shock or those who are hemorrhaging; and
   - All patients with neurological disorders.

   It is suggested to routinely take the blood pressure on *all* patients as a preventive health measure.
8. Check the sphygmomanometer regularly for loss of mercury and for leaks in the tubing, compression bag, and bulb.
9. Before and after each use of the stethoscope, clean the earpieces and the bell or diaphragm with a cotton ball soaked in alcohol or with an alcohol sponge.
10. Handle these instruments gently, as misuse will adversely affect their proper functioning.

Taking blood pressure reading on the arm

Procedure	*Rationale*
1. Wash hands and obtain equipment.	
2. Identify patient and explain the procedure.	Explanations enhance the patient's confidence and relaxation.
3. Position the patient in a comfortable position with the arm extended and supported.	Patient may be sitting, standing, or lying down, depending on the physician's orders.

Continued.

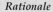

Procedure for Measuring Blood Pressure—cont'd

Procedure

4. Place a mercury sphygmomanometer on a level surface, in a position in which the scale can be easily read.
5. Expose the patient's arm well above the elbow.

6. Apply the cuff of the sphygmomanometer over the brachial artery (see Figure 17.4) 1 to 2 inches above the antecubital space and wrap the remainder of the cuff around the arm so that each turn covers the previous one (Figure 17.8). On older model cuffs, tuck the end under one of the turns; some cuffs will have clasps or hooks to fasten, and the newer models, with Velcro closures, will adhere to the last turn on the cuff.

Rationale

Having the mercury manometer at your eye level enables you to take a more accurate reading.

Clothing should be adjusted to avoid constriction and to prevent rustling of garments.

The cuff should be applied snugly and neatly. Arm may be flexed slightly after the cuff is applied. Use a child's or infant's cuff for small children or on extremely thin patients and the larger cuff on obese patients (Table 17.2)

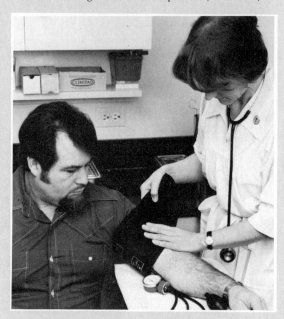

Figure 17.8
Applying cuff of sphygmomanometer above antecubital space of left arm.

7. Locate the strongest pulsation of the brachial artery in the antecubitial space by palpating with your fingers at the bend of the elbow (Figure 17.9).

Figure 17.9
Location of strongest pulsation in antecubital space.

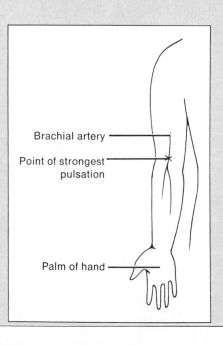

Brachial artery —

Point of strongest — ✕
pulsation

Palm of hand —

Procedure for Measuring Blood Pressure—cont'd

Procedure	*Rationale*
8. Adjust the earpieces of the stethoscope in your ears, place the bell or diaphragm of the stethoscope over the artery pulsation felt, and hold in place (Figure 17.10).	The bell or diaphragm should always be placed below, not under, the cuff and directly over the strongest pulsation felt of the brachial artery.
9. With your free hand, close the air valve on the hand bulb by turning the thumbscrew in a clockwise direction. Pump air into the cuff of the manometer rapidly until the level of mercury is about 180 to 200 mm Hg or about 20 mm Hg above the palpated systolic pressure. (The procedure for taking a blood pressure by palpation is explained on p. 280.)	Blood is cut off when the cuff is inflated. To identify the true systolic pressure, air must be pumped into the cuff rapidly and then the cuff deflated slowly. Inflating the cuff slowly or sending the mercury to a higher level than necessary is very uncomfortable for the patient. To avoid missing the true systolic reading, pressure can initially be taken by the palpation method and then waiting 15 to 30 seconds before the pressure reading is taken by the auscultation method.

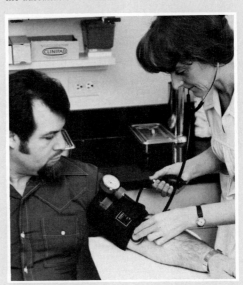

Figure 17.10
Adjusting stethoscope for taking blood pressure.

10. Turn the thumbscrew counterclockwise to open the air valve slowly. Allow for a slow release of air in the cuff so that the pressure falls only 2 to 3 mm Hg at a time (Figure 17.11).	Rapid deflation of the cuff will cause you to miss the exact reading.

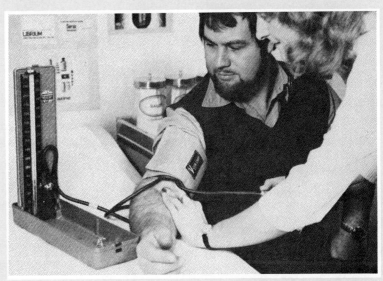

Figure 17.11
Mercury column descending as air is released from the cuff.

Continued.

Procedure for Measuring Blood Pressure—cont'd

Procedure	*Rationale*
11. Listen carefully and read the exact point on the mercury column (or spring gauge if using an aneroid manometer) at which the first distinct sound is heard. Keep this number in mind; this represents the *systolic pressure*.	This sound is caused by an initial spurt of blood into the collapsed artery as deflation of the cuff occurs.
12. Continue to allow the air to escape, thereby letting the cuff deflate slowly. The sounds will get louder, then dull and soft, then fade away (Figure 17.11).	
13. Read the scale when the sound becomes dull or muffled. Keep this number in mind; it represents the *diastolic pressure*.	The level of mercury at the point where the sound changes from loud to dull or muffled is the *diastolic pressure,* representing the pressure in the arteries during diastole of the heart.
14. Continue to deflate the cuff until the sound disappears. Keep this number in mind, as many physicians request that both numbers be reported for diastolic readings.	
15. Open the valve completely to release all the air from the cuff.	The blood in the veins in the lower arm will not be able to return to the heart if all the air in the cuff is not released. It is harmful for blood to become congested in the veins.
16. If there is any doubt of an accurate reading, wait 15 seconds, then repeat steps 7 through 15. Do not repeat more than twice on the same arm, because the reading will be inaccurate because of blood stasis (blood trapped in the arm).	Between readings the cuff must be completely deflated. Failure to do so will produce erroneously high readings.
17. Write blood pressure down on paper as a mathematical fraction. Depending on your employer's preference, you may inform the patient of the numerical value of the blood pressure.	Do not trust it to memory. Record systolic reading over diastolic reading as a mathematical fraction. For example, $^{120}/_{80}$ *or* $^{120}/_{80}$-60 (60 indicating where the sounds disappear).
18. Remove the cuff from the patient's arm.	
19. See that the patient is comfortable.	
20. Return equipment to designated area and prepare for storage according to type of apparatus used. Cleanse earpieces and diaphragm of stethoscope with alcohol sponge.	
21. Record blood pressure on the patient's chart.	Charting example: October 1, 19_____, 2 PM BP $^{118}/_{86}$ rt arm *or* $^{118}/_{86}$-70 Ann Banks, CMA
22. Notify the physician if you have obtained a relatively higher or lower reading than previously recorded.	Further evaluation or only periodic measurement may be needed. Because an initial high reading may reflect only a transient increase, which could be due to anxiety or excitement, the blood pressure should be measured on different days and after the patient has been able to relax for a time.

Palpation method for measuring blood pressure

The palpation method is an alternative way to measure blood pressure. When the blood pressure is inaudible by stethoscope you may use this method, but *only* when the physician directs you to use it, because it is generally thought to be an inaccurate method.

The procedure is similar to the auscultation method except that you use your fingers rather than a stethoscope.

1. Place your fingers over the patient's brachial artery.

2. Pump cuff to 200 mm Hg, or at least 10 to 20 mm Hg after pulsation in the artery has ceased.

3. Release the air valve slowly.

4. The *systolic pressure* is read the moment you feel the first pulsation in the artery.

5. The pulse will increase in force and tension and then gradually become softer; it is at this point of change that the *diastolic pressure* is recorded. (Some feel that this is not an accurate diastolic reading, and therefore do not obtain a diastolic reading for BP taken by the palpation method.)

Procedures for Measuring Height and Weight

Equipment

A weight scale with height measuring bar

Procedure	*Rationale*
1. Wash your hands.	
2. Identify the patient and explain the procedure.	
3. Place a clean paper towel on the scale foot stand.	This is just one form of expected clean technique. Use a clean towel for each patient.
4. Balance the scale.	Unbalanced scales will result in an inaccurate weight measurement.
5. Have the patient remove shoes and any jacket or heavy outer sweater. In some offices or agencies the patient may be weighed in a patient gown.	The removal of heavy outer clothing provides a more accurate reading.
6. Direct and/or assist the patient onto the scale. NOTE: You may raise the height bar above the patient's estimated height and have it in position before the patient steps onto the scale to avoid moving and manipulating it later.	
7. Ask all patients their usual weight, then move the 50-pound weight to the 50-, 100-, 150-, 200-, or 250-pound mark, ensuring that the weight is resting securely in the weight indicator groove (Figure 17.12)	Unless the weight is secured correctly in the groove provided, the patient's weight measurement will be off by many pounds.

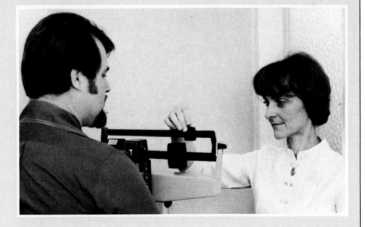

Figure 17.12
Obtaining patient's weight.

8. Gradually move the upper weight across the individual pound register until the arm at the right end of the balance bar rests in a position in the center of the metal frame, not touching either edge of this frame.	
9. Read the weight accurately to the nearest fraction of a pound. NOTE: Pediatric scales will measure weights in pounds and ounces.	
10. Return the weights to zero.	
11. Record the weight on the patient's chart.	When charting, you must indicate if the patient was wearing street clothes or a patient gown.
12. To measure the height, have the patient remain on the scale, standing erect and looking straight ahead.	The patient must be standing very straight to obtain the correct height measurement.
13. If height bar was not raised previously (see step 6), do so now; raise it over the patient's head and extend the hinged arm.	

6. Chart and indicate that the blood pressure was obtained by palpation on the brachial artery.

Continued.

Procedures for Measuring Height and Weight—cont'd

14. Carefully lower the height bar until it touches the top of the patient's head lightly (Figure 17.13)

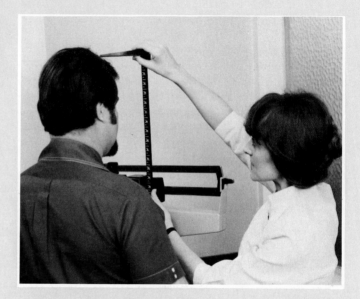

Figure 17.13
Measuring patient's height.

15. Read the height measurement.

The number (in inches) indicating the patient's height is the last digit or fraction visible at the point where the movable part of the bar enters its stationary holder.

16. Assist the patient off the scale if necessary and return the height bar to the resting position.
17. Record the height accurately in feet and inches. Use accepted abbreviations.

Charting Example:
October 27, 19_____, 4 PM
Ht. 5'2"
Wt. 112 lb. in
    street clothes,
    [without] shoes.
        Annie Fox, CMA

PHYSICAL MEASUREMENTS OF HEIGHT AND WEIGHT

The two other important physical or clinical measurements to obtain are the height and weight of the patient. It is common practice to take these measurements as part of a physical examination, because they may provide relevant information for diagnosing, treating, preventing, or evaluating a condition. Height and weight are also measured to determine a child's growth pattern. In addition, the patient's weight is used as a guide for determining the dosage for certain drugs. There are recommended standards set for the average weight that individuals should be for their height, but it is important to remember that these are only ranges, not absolute standards, with latitude for body types.

Overweight as well as underweight can have serious implications when determining the health status of an individual. Frequently complications of overweight include hypertension (high blood pressure), heart disease, and diabetes mellitus. Underweight may indicate malnourishment or metabolic disorders. Either may be the result of psychological problems.

Table 17.3
Conversion table: pounds to kilograms*

Pounds	Kilograms	Pounds	Kilograms	Pounds	Kilograms
1	0.45	100	45.36	205	92.99
2.2	1.00	105	47.63	210	95.26
5	2.27	110	49.90	215	97.52
10	4.54	115	52.12	220	99.79
15	6.80	120	54.43	225	102.06
20	9.07	125	56.70	230	104.33
25	11.34	130	58.91	235	106.60
30	13.61	135	61.24	240	108.86
35	15.88	140	63.50	245	111.13
40	18.14	145	65.77	250	113.40
45	20.41	150	68.04	255	115.67
50	22.68	155	70.31	260	117.94
55	24.95	160	72.58	265	120.20
60	27.22	165	74.84	270	122.47
65	29.48	170	77.11	275	124.74
70	31.75	175	79.38	280	127.01
75	34.02	180	81.65	285	129.28
80	36.29	185	83.92	290	131.54
85	38.56	190	86.18	295	133.81
90	40.82	195	88.45	300	136.08
95	43.09	200	90.72		

*To convert:
Pounds to kilograms: multiply number of pounds by 0.45 (0.4536)
Kilograms to pounds: multiply number of kilograms by 2.2 (2.204)

Table 17.4
Desirable weights—ages 25 to 59 based on lowest mortality*

Men					Women†			
Height (in shoes with 1-inch heels)		Small frame	Medium frame	Large frame	Height (in shoes with 1-inch heels)		Small frame	Medium frame	Large frame
Feet	Inches				Feet	Inches			
5	2	128-134	131-141	138-150	4	10	102-111	109-121	118-131
5	3	130-136	133-143	140-153	4	11	103-113	111-123	120-134
5	4	132-138	135-145	142-156	5	0	104-115	113-126	122-137
5	5	134-140	137-148	144-160	5	1	106-118	115-129	125-140
5	6	136-142	139-151	146-164	5	2	108-121	118-132	128-143
5	7	138-145	142-154	149-168	5	3	111-124	121-135	131-147
5	8	140-148	145-157	152-172	5	4	114-127	124-138	134-151
5	9	142-151	148-160	155-176	5	5	117-130	127-141	137-155
5	10	144-154	151-163	158-180	5	6	120-133	130-144	140-159
5	11	146-157	154-166	161-184	5	7	123-136	133-147	143-163
6	0	149-160	157-170	164-188	5	8	126-139	136-150	146-167
6	1	152-164	160-174	168-192	5	9	129-142	139-153	149-170
6	2	155-168	164-178	172-197	5	10	132-145	142-156	152-173
6	3	158-172	167-182	176-202	5	11	135-148	145-159	155-176
6	4	162-176	171-187	181-207	6	0	138-151	148-162	158-179

Courtesy Metropolitan Life Insurance Co.
*Weights in pounds according to frame (in indoor clothing) weighing 5 pounds for men and 3 pounds for women.
†For women between 18 and 25, subtract 1 pound for each year under 25.

Many patients are very self-conscious of their weight; therefore, it is advisable to have the scales located in an area that ensures patient privacy. Also to reduce embarrassment, you may have the patient stand with the back to the numbers on the scale. It is important in this procedure, as in all procedures, that you maintain a neutral facial expression to avoid communicating your impressions to the patient.

Be alert, and note any unusual weight gains or losses in established patients and comments regarding changes by new patients, either of which may be an important diagnostic aid.

Some scales are calibrated in kilograms and others in pounds. When you wish to convert a weight, use the following formulas. To convert kilograms to pounds (kg to lb):

1 kilogram = 2.2 pounds
Multiply the number of kilograms by 2.2
EXAMPLE: If a patient weighs 60 kilograms, multiply 60 by 2.2

$$60 \times 2.2 = 132 \text{ pounds}$$

To convert pounds to kilograms (lb to kg):

1 pound = 0.45 kilograms
Multiply the number of pounds by 0.45
EXAMPLE: If a patient weighs 132 pounds, multiply 132 by 0.45.

$$132 \times 0.45 = 59.40 \text{ or } 59\tfrac{2}{5} \text{ kilograms}$$

See Table 17.3 for the conversion of pounds to kilograms and Table 17.4 for the average heights and weights for adults.

Conclusion

You have now completed the unit on physical measurements, the most basic clinical procedures that you may be required to perform. When you have practiced these procedures and feel competent in performing them, arrange with your instructor to take a performance test. You will be expected to demonstrate accurately your ability to prepare for and take the vital signs and height and weight measurements on individuals assigned to you by your instructor.

Review Questions

1. List three purposes for taking a patient's vital signs.
2. For the following situations, indicate if you would normally see an increase or a decrease in each of the following: (1) temperature, (2) pulse rate, (3) respiratory rate, and (4) blood pressure.
   a. a patient who faints
   b. a patient who has a severe infection in her throat
   c. a patient who is hemorrhaging
   d. a patient who has just jogged for 2 miles
   e. a patient who has a brainstem injury
   f. a patient who becomes extremely excited or upset
   g. a patient who is sleeping
   h. children as compared with adults
3. List the normal average readings for the following:
   a. oral temperature in adults
   b. axillary temperature in adults
   c. rectal temperature in adults
   d. pulse rate in adults
   e. respiratory rate in adults
   f. blood pressure in adults
4. Convert the following temperatures to centigrade degrees:
   a. 98.6° F   c. 100.4° F
   b. 97.8° F   d. 99.6° F
5. Convert the following temperatures to Fahrenheit degrees:
   a. 39.5° C   c. 38.2° C
   b. 36.0° C   d. 37.2° C
6. List and describe the location of the seven most common arteries where a pulse may be felt.
7. If a patient has an extremely sore mouth, how would you take the temperature?
8. You have just taken a patient's respiratory rate and found it to be 10 respirations per minute. Would you consider this a normal and adequate rate, or as a serious symptom of some physiological change in the body?
9. What action is taking place in the heart during systole? During diastole?
10. Convert the following body weights to measurements in pounds.
    a. 52 kg   c. 47 kg
    b. 68.5 kg   d. 56 kg

Chapter 18

Health History and Physical Examinations

- History and physical examination
- Problem-oriented medical record (POMR)

Objectives

On completion of Chapter 18 the medical assistant student should be able to:

1 Define and pronounce the vocabulary terms listed in this chapter and the medical abbreviations listed in Appendix B.

2 List the eight major components of a patient's medical history/record, and describe the information that is recorded in each.

3 List and define the six parts of the patient's medical history.

4 List eight reasons why information gathered during a history and physical examination is valuable to the physician.

5 List and describe six methods of examination employed by the physician when performing a physical examination on a patient, giving an example of when or how each is used.

6 List the essential parts of a physical examination.

7 Differentiate between information obtained in the review of systems and that obtained during the physical examination.

8 Help take and record a brief medical history or statement of the patient's chief complaint.

9 Discuss the steps taken by a physician when making a diagnosis.

10 List five forms of treatment.

11 List three reasons for diagnostic studies.

Vocabulary

health The state of mental, physical, and social well-being of an individual.

positive findings Evidence of disease or body dysfunction.

prodrome An early symptom indicating the onset of a disease, such as an achy feeling before having the flu.

prognosis A statement made by the physician indicating the probable or anticipated outcome of the disease process in a patient; usually stated simply as *good, fair, poor,* or *guarded.*

sign Sometimes called a *physical sign;* any objective evidence (apparent to the observer) representing disease or body dysfunction. Signs may be observed by others or revealed when the physician performs a physical examination; examples include swollen ankles, a distended rigid abdomen, elevated blood pressure, and decreased sensation.

symptom   Sometimes called a *subjective symptom;* any subjective evidence of disease or body dysfunction; a change in the physical or mental state of the body that is perceptible or apparent only to the individual experiencing the change; examples include anorexia, nausea, headache, pain, itching, and dizziness.

syndrome   A combination of symptoms resulting from one cause or commonly occurring together to present a distinct clinical picture; an example is the dumping syndrome, which consists of nausea, weakness, varying degrees of syncope, sweating, palpitation, and sometimes diarrhea and a feeling of warmth. This may occur immediately after eating in patients who have had a partial gastrectomy.

symmetry   Correspondence in form, size, and arrangement of parts on opposite sides of the body.

To provide a basis for decision making and planning for the care of a patient, information of varied types must be gathered, compiled, and maintained in an orderly and confidential manner. Lack of needed information and confidentiality may jeopardize appropriate patient care. Thus there is the need for the patient's confidential medical record, which is a compilation of information concerning the patient, the care provided, progress, and results obtained. When a physician sees the patient for the first time, identifying information (such as name and address) and all the information necessary for diagnosing the case, prescribing treatment, and planning future care are obtained. Every diagnostic workup has six major components: the history, the physical examination, the summary of positive findings, the interpretation of completed diagnostic studies, the examiner's impression based on all the information gathered, and the care plans including suggested further study.

On subsequent visits the progress or status of the patient's condition is recorded as progress notes. Eventually, when the patient is discharged or the condition has been resolved, the date of discharge and status of the patient at that time are recorded as the discharge summary.

This compilation of information is kept together and called the patient's medical record. These confidential records and reports are arranged in a file folder, binder, or other special type of folder, which is generally referred to as the patient's chart or file.

The medical assistant plays a very important role in obtaining and maintaining data on patients. This responsibility will vary with the preference and specialty of the physician. In some instances the medical assistant is expected to relieve the physician of much of the data collection. In this case, the medical assistant obtains identifying information from the patient, measures the patient's height, weight, temperature, pulse rate, respiration rate, and blood pressure and takes the medical history. In other situations, the medical assistant may only be required to obtain the identifying information from the patient. In addition to recording data, the medical assistant is responsible for preparing the examination room for the examination of the patient, preparing the equipment and supplies needed, preparing the patient both physically and mentally, and assisting the patient, assisting the physician, collecting specimens as requested, and organizing the results of diagnostic studies in the patient's record (See also Chapter 13).

This chapter discusses the components and related information of a patient's medical record, related vocabulary, and the problem-oriented medical record. Chapter 19 presents vocabulary, procedures, and techniques used when preparing for and assisting with various types of physical examinations.

HISTORY AND PHYSICAL EXAMINATION

The history and general physical examination are extremely valuable diagnostic tools used by a physician to gather information about the physiological and sometimes psychological condition of a patient. Many people now recognize the value of a regular physical examination as a measure to prevent or treat disease in the early stages. Most authorities recommend that everyone have at least one a year.

Information gathered from a history and general or special physical examination can be used by the physician to determine the following:

- The individual's level of health
- The body's level of physiological functioning
- A tentative diagnosis of a condition or disease
- A confirmed diagnosis of a condition or disease
- The need for additional special examinations or testing
- The type of treatment to be prescribed
- An evaluation of the effectiveness of the prescribed treatment
- Preventive measures to be used

Preventive techniques include educating patients on healthful living habits, administering vaccinations to prevent communicable diseases, using screening procedures such as blood pressure checks and Pap smears, and treating conditions in the early stages to avoid more serious diseases.

The order followed by physicians when taking a history and performing a physical examination may vary somewhat, but the end result is the same, since the same basic areas are covered. One of the two types of forms may be used to record the information obtained. These include a preprinted outline form (Figure 18.1) or a blank sheet of standard-size paper on which the physician writes out all the information gathered. The pre-printed form serves as a reminder so that essential factors will not be overlooked, and it minimizes necessary writing to a narrative record of the abnormal findings.

History

The history is a record of the information provided by the patient. This includes a series of questions and answers regarding the patient.

Problem areas, either physical or emotional, can be revealed by history taking—not only areas of current problems but also those that may become problems and thus call for preventive care and advice.

Components of history

Chief complaint. The chief complaint is a brief statement, made by the patient, describing the nature of the illness and duration of symptoms that led the patient to consult the physician. Chief complaint is abbreviated CC.

History of present illness. The history of present illness includes the present illness discussed in detail, the health status of the patient until the onset of the present illness, then the onset of symptoms, the character, duration of each, and any other pertinent facts or relation to other events, such as shortness of breath after exertion. History of present illness is abbreviated HPI (or PI, present illness).

Past history. The past history is a summary of all prior illnesses, allergies, drug sensitivities, childhood diseases, surgical procedures, hospital admissions, and serious injuries and disabilities, including the date of each. For women, the number of pregnancies, live births, and abortions if any are also recorded. Past history is abbreviated PH.

Family history. The family history is the health status and age of immediate relatives; if deceased, the date, age at death, and cause are noted. Diseases among relatives that are thought to have a hereditary or familial tendency or cases in which contact may play a role are also recorded. Examples would be cardiovascular, renal, endocrine, metabolic, mental, or infectious diseases, neoplasms or carcinoma, and allergies. Family history is abbreviated FH.

Social and occupational history. The social and occupational history (may also be referred to as personal history and patient profile) includes information relating to where the patient has lived, occupation(s), and environment. This includes statements about the patient's life-style and habits, any of which may have a bearing on the development of disease, and the patient's general health status and perception of his health. These factors may include the following:

- Use of tobacco, alcohol, drugs, coffee, tea, and so on
- Diet, sleep, exercise, hobbies, and interests
- Marital history, children, home life; religious convictions; occupation and employment
- Sexual preferences, problems, and attitudes
- Ways of reacting to stress
- Defense mechanisms
- Resources for support and assistance
- Cultural, educational, and environmental factors that may be related to health status

Review of systems. Review of systems is the last category in the history. The purpose of this systematic review is to reveal subjective symptoms that either the patient forgot to discuss or, at the time, seemed relatively unimportant to the patient. An analysis of the subjective findings, as related by the patient when questioned by the physician, will generally give a clue to the diagnosis and will indicate the nature and extent of the physical examination required. Review of systems is abbreviated ROS.

• • •

The following are the major headings in the order in which they appear in the patient's ROS and the items that are usually reviewed by the physician. The physician will question the patient as to the usual or unusual presence or condition of, and/or occurrence of any of these.

The physician will ask if there has been or is a history of the following conditions and whether as well as what kinds of medications are currently being used for any of the following*:

Text continued on p. 292.

---

*See Appendix C for definitions and pronunciation keys for many of the terms listed.

Figure 18.1
Preprinted forms used for patient history and physical examination. **A,** Form used
for internal medicine.
Courtesy of Histacount Corp Melville, NY.

**A
front**

INTERNAL MEDICINE

CASE NO.   PATIENT'S NAME

ADDRESS _____ DATE _____

TEL. NO. _____ REFERRED BY _____ OCCUPATION _____ DOB ___ SEX ___ S.M.W.D.

INSURANCE _____

CHIEF COMPLAINT: _____

PRESENT AILMENT: _____

PAST HISTORY (INCLUDING SURGERY) _____

FAMILY HISTORY: _____

CASE NO.

PATIENT'S NAME

SYSTEMS REVIEW

HEAD: Headache · Dizziness Fainting	
EYE · EAR NOSE · THROAT:	
RESPIRATORY: Hemoptysis · Cough · Sputum Chest Pain · Night Sweats Chill · Rhinitis · Sinusitis Epistaxis · Post Nasal Discharge	
HEART: Dyspnea · Orthopnea Cyanosis · Pallor · Pain Location · Radiation	
GASTRO-INTESTINAL: Pain · Relation To Food Radiation · Relieved By Med.? Dysphagia · Nausea Anorexia · Flatulence Constipation · Diarrhea Hemorrhoids · Melena · Wt. Loss or Gain	
GENITO-URINARY: Polyuria · Oliguria · Anuria Hematuria · Dysuria · Colic Pain · Frequency · Chills Urgency · Backache	
NEURO-MUSC. SKELETAL:	
VASCULAR:	
HEMATOLOGICAL: Bleeding · Anemia	

HISTACOUNT®   FORM NO. 6951   HISTACOUNT CORPORATION, MELVILLE, L. I., N. Y. 11747

Figure 18.1, cont'd

CASE No._____   PATIENT'S NAME_____

SYSTEMS REVIEW

ENDOCRINE

VENEREAL DISEASE

ALLERGIES

CENTRAL NERVOUS SYSTEM

MENSTRUAL:
Onset · Periodicity · Type
Duration · Pain · L.M.P.

MARITAL:
Miscarriages · Abortions
Children · Sterility · Sexual

HABITS:
Tobacco · Alcohol · Drugs
Diet · Cathartics · Etc.

REMARKS:

PHYSICAL EXAMINATION: TEMP. _____ PULSE _____ RESP. _____ B.P. _____ HT. _____ WT. _____

GENERAL APPEARANCE _____

SKIN _____ MUCOUS MEMBRANE _____

EYES: VISION _____ PUPIL _____ FUNDUS _____

EARS: _____

NOSE: _____

THROAT: _____ PHARYNX _____ TONSILS _____

NECK: _____

CHEST: _____ BREASTS _____

HEART: _____

LUNGS: _____

ABDOMEN: _____

GENITALIA: _____

RECTUM: _____

VAGINA: _____

EXTREMITIES: _____

LYMPH NODES: NECK _____ AXILLA _____ INGUINAL _____ ABDOMINAL _____

REFLEXES: _____

REMARKS: _____

LABORATORY FINDINGS:

(Urine · Blood · Smears · Chemistry · X-Ray
Pregnancy Tests · Stool Occult Blood · VDRL
Tine · Etc.)

Date	

DIAGNOSIS: _____

TREATMENT: _____

DATE			SUBSEQUENT VISITS AND FINDINGS	ACCOUNT RECORD		
MO.	DAY	YR.		CHARGE	PAID	BALANCE

A back

CASE No.

PATIENT'S NAME

Continued.

Figure 18.1, cont'd
B, Patient questionnaire.

**B
front**

PATIENT QUESTIONNAIRE

PATIENT'S NAME _____   BIRTH DATE _____ SEX _____   S. M. W. D.

ADDRESS _____   TEL. NO. _____

INSURANCE _____   REFERRED BY _____   OCCUPATION _____

INSTRUCTIONS: PUT ☑ IN THOSE BOXES APPLICABLE TO YOU AND IN THE "YES" OR "NO" SPACE. IF LINES ARE PROVIDED WRITE IN YOUR ANSWER.

FAMILY HISTORY

	FATHER	MOTHER	BROTHER				SISTER				SPOUSE	CHILDREN					
			1	2	3	4	1	2	3	4		1	2	3	4	5	6
AGE (IF LIVING)																	
HEALTH (G) GOOD (B) BAD																	
CANCER																	
TUBERCULOSIS																	
DIABETES																	
HEART TROUBLE																	
HIGH BLOOD PRESSURE																	
STROKE																	
EPILEPSY																	
NERVOUS BREAKDOWN																	
ASTHMA, HIVES, HAYFEVER																	
BLOOD DISEASE																	
AGE (AT DEATH)																	
CAUSE OF DEATH																	

PERSONAL HISTORY

HAVE YOU EVER HAD...	NO	YES	HAVE YOU EVER HAD...	NO	YES	HAVE YOU EVER HAD...	NO	YES
☐ SCARLET FEVER ☐ SCARLATINA			☐ GONORRHEA ☐ SYPHILIS			ANY ☐ BROKEN ☐ CRACKED BONES		
DIPHTHERIA			ANEMIA			RECURRENT DISLOCATIONS		
SMALLPOX			JAUNDICE			☐ CONCUSSION ☐ HEAD INJURY		
PNEUMONIA			EPILEPSY			EVER BEEN KNOCKED UNCONSCIOUS		
PLEURISY			MIGRAINE HEADACHES			☐ FOOD ☐ CHEMICAL ☐ DRUG POISONING		
UNDULANT FEVER			TUBERCULOSIS			EXPLAIN		
☐ RHEUMATIC FEVER ☐ HEART DISEASE			DIABETES					
ST. VITUS DANCE			CANCER					
☐ ARTHRITIS ☐ RHEUMATISM			☐ HIGH ☐ LOW BLOOD PRESSURE			ANY OTHER DISEASE		
ANY ☐ BONE ☐ JOINT DISEASE			NERVOUS BREAKDOWN			EXPLAIN		
☐ NEURITIS ☐ NEURALGIA			☐ HAY FEVER ☐ ASTHMA					
☐ BURSITIS ☐ SCIATICA ☐ LUMBAGO			☐ HIVES ☐ ECZEMA					
☐ POLIO ☐ MENINGITIS			FREQUENT ☐ COLDS ☐ SORE THROAT			WEIGHT: NOW ONE YR. AGO		
BRIGHT'S DISEASE			FREQUENT ☐ INFECTIONS ☐ BOILS			MAXIMUM WHEN		

ALLERGIES

ARE YOU ALLERGIC TO...	NO	YES	ARE YOU ALLERGIC TO...	NO	YES	ARE YOU ALLERGIC TO...	NO	YES
☐ PENICILLIN ☐ SULFA DRUGS			ANY OTHER DRUGS			ANY FOODS		
☐ ASPIRIN ☐ CODEINE ☐ MORPHINE			EXPLAIN			EXPLAIN		
☐ MYCINS ☐ OTHER ANTIBIOTICS								
☐ TETANUS ☐ ANTITOXIN ☐ SERUMS			ADHESIVE TAPE			☐ NAIL POLISH ☐ OTHER COSMETICS		

SURGERY

HAVE YOU HAD REMOVED...	NO	YES	HAVE YOU HAD REMOVED...	NO	YES	HAVE YOU	NO	YES
TONSILS			☐ OVARY ☐ OVARIES			HAD HERNIA REPAIRED		
APPENDIX			HEMORRHOIDS			HAD ANY OTHER OPERATIONS		
GALL BLADDER			EVER HAVE A TRANSFUSION...			BEEN HOSPITALIZED FOR ANY ILLNESS		
UTERUS			☐ BLOOD ☐ PLASMA			EXPLAIN		

X-RAYS

EVER HAVE X-RAYS OF...	NO	YES	DATE	DISEASE PRESENT
CHEST				
☐ STOMACH ☐ COLON				
GALL BLADDER				
EXTREMITIES				
BACK				
OTHER				

FORM NO. 405

HISTACOUNT CORPORATION, MELVILLE, N. Y. 11746

Figure 18.1, cont'd

SYSTEMS

DO YOU NOW HAVE OR HAVE YOU EVER HAD . . .	NO	YES	DO YOU NOW HAVE OR HAVE YOU EVER HAD . . .	NO	YES
ANY ☐EYE DISEASE ☐EYE INJURY ☐IMPAIRED SIGHT			KIDNEY ☐DISEASE ☐STONES		
ANY ☐EAR DISEASE ☐EAR INJURY ☐IMPAIRED HEARING			BLADDER DISEASE		
ANY TROUBLE WITH ☐NOSE ☐SINUSES ☐MOUTH ☐THROAT			BLOOD IN URINE		
FAINTING SPELLS			☐ALBUMIN ☐SUGAR ☐PUS ☐ETC. IN URINE		
CONVULSIONS			DIFFICULTY IN URINATION		
PARALYSIS			NARROWED URINARY STREAM		
DIZZINESS			ABNORMAL THIRST		
HEADACHES: ☐FREQUENT ☐SEVERE			PROSTATE TROUBLE		
ENLARGED GLANDS			☐STOMACH TROUBLE ☐ULCER		
THYROID: ☐OVERACTIVE ☐UNDERACTIVE ☐ENLARGED			INDIGESTION		
ENLARGED GOITER			☐GAS ☐BELCHING		
SKIN DISEASE			APPENDICITIS		
COUGH: ☐FREQUENT ☐CHRONIC			☐LIVER DISEASE ☐GALL BLADDER DISEASE		
☐CHEST PAIN ☐ANGINA PECTORIS			☐COLITIS ☐OTHER BOWEL DISEASE		
SPITTING UP BLOOD			☐HEMORRHOIDS ☐RECTAL BLEEDING		
NIGHT SWEATS			BLACK TARRY STOOLS		
SHORTNESS OF BREATH ☐EXERTION ☐AT NIGHT			☐CONSTIPATION ☐DIARRHEA		
☐PALPITATION ☐FLUTTERING HEART			☐PARASITES ☐WORMS		
SWELLING OF ☐HANDS ☐FEET ☐ANKLES			☐ANY CHANGE IN APPETITE ☐EATING HABITS		
VARICOSE VEINS			☐ANY CHANGE IN BOWEL ACTION ☐STOOLS		
EXTREME ☐TIREDNESS ☐WEAKNESS			EXPLAIN		

IMMUNIZATION - EKG

HAVE YOU HAD . . .	NO	YES	HAVE YOU HAD . . .	NO	YES
SMALLPOX VACCINATION (WITHIN LAST 7 YEARS)			POLIO SHOTS (WITHIN LAST 2 YEARS)		
TETANUS SHOT (NOT ANTITOXIN)			AN ELECTROCARDIOGRAM WHEN		

B back

HABITS

DO YOU . . .	NO	YES	DO YOU USE . . .	NEVER	OCC.	FREQ.	DAILY
EXERCISE ADEQUATELY			LAXATIVES				
HOW?			VITAMINS				
AWAKEN RESTED			SEDATIVES				
SLEEP WELL			TRANQUILIZERS				
AVERAGE 8 HOURS SLEEP (PER NIGHT)			SLEEPING PILLS, ETC.				
HAVE REGULAR BOWEL MOVEMENTS			ASPIRINS, ETC.				
SEX - ENTIRELY SATISFACTORY			CORTISONE				
LIKE YOUR WORK (HOURS PER DAY) ☐INDOORS ☐OUTDOORS			ALCOHOLIC BEVERAGE				
WATCH TELEVISION (HOURS PER DAY)			COFFEE (CUPS PER DAY)				
READ (HOURS PER DAY)			TOBACCO: ☐CIGARETTES (PKS PER DAY)				
HAVE A VACATION (WEEKS PER YEAR)			☐CIGARS ☐PIPE ☐CHEWING TOBACCO				
HAVE YOU EVER BEEN TREATED FOR ALCOHOLISM			☐SNUFF				
HAVE YOU EVER BEEN TREATED FOR DRUG ABUSE			APPETITE DEPRESSANTS				
RECREATION: DO YOU PARTICIPATE IN SPORTS OR HAVE HOBBIES WHICH GIVE YOU RELAXATION AT LEAST 3 HOURS A WEEK.			THYROID MEDICATION: ☐NO ☐YES, IN PAST ☐NONE NOW NOW ON GR. DAILY HAVE YOU EVER TAKEN . . . ☐INSULIN ☐TABLETS FOR DIABETES ☐HORMONE SHOTS ☐TABLETS ☐NO				

WOMEN ONLY

MENSTRUAL HISTORY . . .				NO	YES
AGE AT ONSET			ARE YOU REGULAR: ☐HEAVY ☐MEDIUM ☐LIGHT		
USUAL DURATION OF PERIOD DAYS			DO YOU HAVE ☐TENSON ☐DEPRESSION BEFORE PERIOD		
CYCLE (START TO START) DAYS			DO YOU HAVE ☐CRAMPS ☐PAIN WITH PERIOD		
DATE OF LAST PERIOD			DO YOU HAVE HOT FLASHES		

PREGNANCIES . . .	NO	YES		NO	YES
CHILDREN BORN ALIVE (HOW MANY)			STILL BORN (HOW MANY)		
CESAREAN SECTIONS (HOW MANY)			MISCARRIAGES (HOW MANY)		
PREMATURES (HOW MANY)			ANY COMPLICATIONS		

EMOTIONS

ARE YOU OFTEN . . .	NO	YES	ARE YOU OFTEN . . .	NO	YES
DEPRESSED			JUMPY		
ANXIOUS			JITTERY		
IRRITABLE			IS CONCENTRATION DIFFICULT		

Review of Systems—cont'd.

GENERAL—Chills, fever, sweats, weight gain or loss, fatigue, weakness, nightmares, insomnia, nervousness, loss of memory.

HEAD—Headaches, trauma, sinus pain, fainting.

EYES—Vision, pain, burning, eyestrain, redness, photophobia, diplopia, blurred vision, excessive tearing, discharge, any eye diseases, prescription glasses, date of last eye examination.

EARS—Hearing loss, pain, discharge, tinnitus, dizziness, mastoiditis, trauma, noise exposure, vertigo.

NOSE—Smell, head colds, discharge, postnasal drip, epistaxis, pain, obstruction, trauma, allergies.

MOUTH—Taste, dryness or excessive salivation, condition of lips, tongue, gums, teeth, dentures.

THROAT—Redness, sore throat, tonsillitis, hoarseness, laryngitis, voice changes, speech defects, dysphagia.

NECK—Pain, tenderness, swelling, limitation of motion, trauma.

RESPIRATORY—Chest pain, cough, expectoration, hemoptysis, asthma, wheezing, dyspnea, orthopnea, hyperventilation, night sweats, recurrent respiratory tract infections.

CARDIOVASCULAR (CV)—Chest pain, hypertension, palpitation, tachycardia, bradycardia, peripheral edema, varicosities, cyanosis, dizziness, syncope.

GASTROINTESTINAL (GI)—Appetite, anorexia, bulimia, abdominal pain, nausea, vomiting, hematemesis, food intolerance, indigestion, dysphagia, diarrhea, constipation, laxatives, color and form of stools, melena, jaundice, distention, flatus, colic, hemorrhoids, rectal pain, presence of blood, pus, or mucus, pruritus ani, hernia or masses.

GENITOURINARY (GU)—Dysuria, oliguria, polyuria, frequency, hesitancy, nocturia, incontinence, enuresis, urgency, retention, hematuria, pyuria, glycosuria, abnormal color or odor, pain, renal colic, stones, pruritus, discharge, sexually transmitted disease(s), sexual habits, potency, prostate disease, testicular masses, history of urinary tract infections.

FEMALE REPRODUCTIVE—Leukorrhea, discharge, itching, pain, dyspareunia, date and results of last Pap smear, breast self-examination routine.

MENSES (MENSTRUAL PERIODS)—Age at onset, regularity, amount, duration, date of last menstrual period, premenstrual tension, dysmenorrhea, amenorrhea, irregular bleeding, spotting, menopause (age of onset), postmenopausal bleeding, menopausal symptoms.

OBSTETRICAL HISTORY—Number of pregnancies, live births and living children, complications during pregnancy and labor, abortions if any.

BIRTH CONTROL—Method if used.

METABOLIC—Change in weight and appetite.

ENDOCRINE—Excessive thirst, goiter, hair distribution, falling hair, change in skin texture or color, temperature intolerance, speech, voice, growth changes, sexual vigor and abnormalities, symptoms of diabetes, hormone therapy.

BLOOD—Bruising or bleeding tendencies, blood disorders.

SKIN—Allergies, rash, pruritus, moles, sores or ulcers, color change (redness, jaundice, cyanosis, pallor), infections, dryness, sweating, alopecia, past dermatitis.

MUSCULOSKELETAL (MS)—Muscle or joint pain, swelling, stiffness, limitation of movement, spasm, tetany, weakness, numbness, coldness, deformities, atrophy, dislocations, fractures, discoloration, varicosities, cramping, edema, thrombophlebitis.

NEUROLOGICAL—Headaches, vertigo, fainting, sense of balance, nervousness, sleeping irregularities, tremor, convulsions, loss of consciousness, memory, paralysis, paresthesia, pain.

PSYCHIATRIC—Personality type, emotional stability, previous mental illness.

Physical Examination

After the history is completed, the physician will proceed with the physical examination, often referred to as a physical or a PE. This differs from the history in that it involves a thorough examination of the patient from head to toe for anatomical and physiological functioning.

The key to a physical examination is systematic thoroughness. Generally, a physician will formulate a logical, methodical approach by examining each body system or part, beginning with the head and working down. The information obtained in the history or the chief complaint as stated by the patient will help determine the extent of the examination to be performed. Sometimes a limited or a specific examination of one body part or system may be indicated.

Methods of physical examinations

Various methods of physical examinations are used by the physician to learn about the patient's condition. The standard methods follow (Figure 18.2).

Figure 18.2
Methods of physical examinations. **A,** Inspection. **B,** Palpation. **C,** Percussion. **D,** Auscultation.

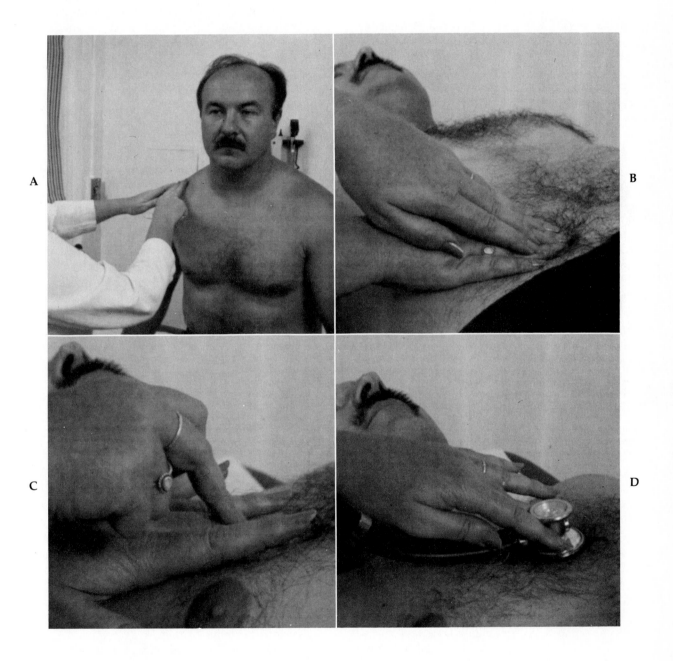

Inspection. Inspection is the <u>visual observation</u> of the body as a whole and of its individual parts. The physician will observe the patient's general appearance, color of the skin, size and shape of the body as a whole and the individual parts. The physician will also note any rashes, scars, trauma, deformities, swelling, injuries, and nervousness.

In the detailed examination, the physician will use the otoscope to look into the ears and the ophthalmoscope to inspect the eyes. A tongue blade will be of help when inspecting the mouth and throat.

Palpation. Palpation is performed by applying the tips of the fingers, the whole hand, or both hands to the body part. Pressure may be slight or forcible, continuous or intermittent. The physician feels, touches, and sometimes manipulates the external surface of the various parts of the body to determine the physical characteristics of tissues or organs, and also to note if pain or tenderness is present.

Also involved are the physician's senses of temperature, vibration, position, and kinesthesia as the examination is in progress. Some of the organs and parts of the body examined by this method are the breast, chest, abdomen, liver, kidney, bladder, and lymph nodes. In conjunction with external palpation, internal palpation may be done on the uterus, ovaries, and rectum.

Percussion. In medical diagnosis, percussion is done by tapping the body lightly but sharply with the fingers. The physician places one or two fingers of one hand on the part of the body to be examined and then strikes those fingers with the index or middle finger of the other hand.

The purpose of percussion is to determine the density, size, and position of the underlying organs and also to determine the presence of pus or fluid in a cavity. The differing densities of the various parts of the body give off different sounds when struck by the examiner's fingers. The more hollow the part struck, the more drumlike the sound. The sounds that are emitted help the physician make a diagnosis. A solid mass in a hollow organ can be noted because of a change from the normal density. Also, the borders of certain organs such as the heart can be mapped out by comparing the density in the organ with surrounding tissues.

Percussion is most commonly used on the chest and back for examination of the heart and lungs, but may also be done on the abdomen, bladder, or bones.

A physician may also use an instrument, the percussion hammer, to check a patient's reflexes by striking the tendon just below the knee and also at the elbow or ankle with this instrument. Failure of the desired reflex gives the physician more information for a diagnosis.

Auscultation. Auscultation is the process of listening to sounds produced in some of the body cavities as the organs perform their functions. A stethoscope is usually used in this method, but it can also be done by placing one's ear directly over a bared or thinly covered body surface. It is used chiefly on the chest to listen to the heart and lungs and also on the abdomen to diagnose an abdominal aneurysm or listen to fetal heart sounds or peristaltic waves. Listening to the sounds produced in these body cavities helps determine the physical condition of the organs.

Mensuration. Mensuration is the process of measuring. Clinical measurements include weight, height, temperature, pulse, respirations, and blood pressure. Head circumference is also measured in young children. When recorded and compared with previous measurements, these are extremely important guides for some diagnoses. Chest measurement may also be done to ascertain the amount of expansion and retraction of the two sides, accompanying inspiration and expiration. This is important when diagnosing or treating chest conditions such as emphysema, in which there is often a loss of elasticity of the lung.

Smell. Smell is a much less frequently used method, but it is still a relevant method for detecting a disease process. Odors from the breath, sputum, urine, feces, vomitus, or pus can provide valuable information to help the physician make a diagnosis.

Essentials of a thorough physical examination

A complete physical examination report should cover the following as the physician observes, tests, and measures each for normal or abnormal structure and function.

general inspection General appearance, nutritional status, apparent age, color, sex, height, weight, attitude, communication.

vital signs Temperature, pulse, respiration, blood pressure.

skin Color, texture, turgor, warmth, hair distribution, pigmentation, rashes, scars, lesions, moles, warts.

head Position, proportion to rest of body, distribution of hair, masses, evidence of trauma.

face Symmetry, size, appearance, facial expression, tenderness.

eyes Visual fields, visual acuity, eyeball movement, conjunctiva, sclera, cornea, iris, pupils, eyelids, ptosis, tearing, discharges.

ears Hearing, ear canals, tympanic membranes, cerumen, discharge.

nose Size, shape, color, deformity, septum, airways, mucosa, discharge, bleeding.

mouth Breath, lips, gums, teeth, tongue, mucosa.

throat Tonsils, pharynx, larynx.

neck Suppleness, thyroid gland, lymph nodes, vessels, carotid pulses, position of trachea, tenderness, stiffness, masses.

breasts Size, contour, symmetry, nipples, masses, discharge, tenderness.

chest Shape, symmetry, expansion, lesions.

lungs Rate and quality of respiration, breath sounds, cough, sputum, friction rubs, resonance, fremitus.

heart Rate, rhythm, point of maximum impulse (PMI), sounds, murmurs, dullness, thrills, gallop.

arteries Pulses, vessel walls, bruits.

veins Pulsation, dilation, filling.

lymph nodes Enlargement.

abdomen Contour; appearance; liver, kidneys, and spleen (LKS); bladder; scars; peristalsis; tenderness; rigidity; spasm; masses; fluid; hernia.

female genitalia External appearance, Bartholin and Skene glands, discharge, masses; vaginal— bimanual examination of uterus and adnexa, tenderness, masses, Pap smear if required.

male genitalia Penis, scrotum, scars, lesions, discharge, tenderness, masses, atrophy, enlargement.

rectal Sphincter tone, prostate gland, seminal vesicles, fissure, fistula, hemorrhoids, masses, discharge, feces.

back and spine Posture, curvature, balance, mobility, gait, tenderness, masses, costovertebral tenderness.

extremities Proportion to trunk, range of motion, color, pulses, edema, swelling, deformity, tenderness, ulcers, varicosities.

fingernails Contour, color.

neurological status Consciousness, cranial nerves, reflexes, coordination, gait, balance, muscle tone and strength, tactile, pain—deep and superficial, discriminatory sensation.

mental status Orientation to time, place, and person; appearance; behavior; mood and thought content.

See Appendixes B and C for additional vocabulary used by the physician when recording physical findings, terms used to describe pain, commonly used medical abbreviations, and an example of a patient's case history.

Other tests that a physician may have performed as part of the physical examination include a routine urinalysis (UA), a complete blood count (CBC), a chest x-ray film, and an electrocardiogram (ECG or EKG). Physical examinations will vary according to the needs or complaints of a patient. Frequently a patient may have a complaint or situation that can be handled in a few minutes or that requires a special type of examination such as a sigmoidoscopy. Other patients may require a complete physical examination. In this case, all of the preceding information will be obtained.

Special examinations

Certain types of examinations are more specific and restricted. These are local or special examinations, which are confined to specific parts and organs or special functions of the body. They are extensive and detailed and performed to establish complete information of a complex nature. Frequently they are done to examine the interior of body cavities and passages. Some of the local or special examinations are vaginal and obstetrical examinations, proctoscopy, sigmoidoscopy, cystoscopy, bronchoscopy, and skin tests. Other specialized examinations include ultrasound, roentgenological, neurological, ophthalmological, and cardiac studies.

Summary of Positive Findings

Based on the subjective findings as related by the patient and the objective findings as found by the physician during the physical examination, the physician will sometimes outline a brief summarization of all of the positive findings of the case.

Diagnostic Data

The physician arrives at a diagnosis by employing and reviewing multiple factors and information obtained on the patient's condition, that is, the physician uses various studies to arrive at a diagnosis.

Three reasons for diagnostic studies are as follows:

- To determine (diagnose) the condition from which the patient is suffering so that treatment may be initiated if feasible.
- To discover disease in its early stage before the patient experiences any signs or symptoms. This is called screening. Screening for disease often permits the cure of the disease, because treatment can be started in the early stages of the disease process (for example, cancer), or early treatment can delay the progression of the disease (for example, hypertension).
- To evaluate past or ongoing treatment received by the patient.

As the field of medical science continues to expand, newer, more accurate, and more sophisticated techniques are made available to help physicians diagnose disease processes. Diagnostic procedures and studies include but are not limited to physical examinations, surgical intervention, and laboratory studies. Laboratory data may include a set of routine laboratory examinations that were performed at the time of the patient's physical examination with the results recorded if the tests have been completed. Other procedures used in diagnosing and treating disease processes may involve the specialized areas of radiology (roentgenology), nuclear medicine, special skin tests, physical medicine, physiotherapy, and electrocardiography. These areas of health care and treatment will be elaborated on in later chapters of this book.

Impression

Once all this information has been gathered, the physician will indicate an impression of the patient's condition. This may include any or all of the following:

Diagnosis:

Primary diagnosis—a statement that indicates the cause of the patient's current, most important problem/condition.

Secondary diagnosis—a statement that indicates a problem/condition that is less important or urgent than the patient's primary diagnosis.

Tentative or provisional diagnosis: A probable diagnosis. This reflects the physician's impression of the patient's condition, but it is made before any further tests have been completed and a final diagnosis has been reached.

Differential diagnosis: A possible diagnosis. A statement based on comparison of signs and symptoms of two or more similar diseases to determine from which the patient is suffering. Thus, by a process of elimination, the provisional diagnosis may be made.

Rule out (R/O): A statement that indicates those conditions that the physician believes might be causing the patient's problem/condition. Each condition will be investigated thoroughly and ruled out as a diagnosis, if and when negative testing results are obtained. Again by a process of elimination a diagnosis may be reached. (The current trend is discouraging the use of this term for purposes of more definitive record keeping. In place of *rule out,* the term *possible diagnosis* is used by some.)

Problem list: This is used in the most recent system of recording called the Problem-Oriented System (POS). A problem is any situation, disease, or condition for which the patient needs help or any questions that requires a solution. In the problem list, each problem drawn from the data base is numbered, dated, and listed in order of occurrence. (Data base refers to all of the preceeding parts of the medical record as discussed.) Problems may be stated in terms of the following:

- Diagnosis
- Symptom or physical findings
- Physiological findings
- Abnormal laboratory results
- Social or personal problems
- Environmental problems
- Behavior factors
- Patient education

Additional explanations of the problem-oriented system and the problem-oriented record will be discussed at the end of this chapter.

Prognosis: A statement of the probable or anticipated outcome of the patient's condition.

Care Plans and Suggested Further Study

The next part of the medical case record will include the physician's clearly stated plans, which may include one or a combination of the following forms of treatment: drug therapy, physical therapy, diet therapy, surgery, and psychotherapy. In addition, hospitalization will be noted if required. For all of these treatments patient education should be included. The medical assistant, as a member of the health care team, may be required to do part of the patient teaching. All treatments prescribed and medications ordered are entered on the record in detail.

Suggested further studies will list the laboratory tests, x-ray studies, or any other special tests that the physician deems necessary for the treatment and care of the patient. Instructions for follow-up visits will be stated. Also included may be a statement that the patient has been referred to another physician for consultation or treatment when this is advisable.

After the completion of any special test or consultation, a report is made, which is then incorporated into the patient's medical record.

Progress Notes

After each future visit, the physician's observations, the status of the patient's condition, and the patient's own report, if it is relevant, are added to the medical record. Any change in treatment or medication is recorded. This is called the progress report or progress note, and each entry must be dated and signed. In a hospital, progress notes are also written by other health care providers, for example, physical therapists.

Discharge Summary

If the patient is discharged, the date and final statement about the patient's health and condition at that time are recorded on the medical record. These may be written at the end of the progress notes or on a separate form.

If death occurs, a statement describing the cause of death is recorded, and the history is marked *deceased.*

Hospital discharge summaries contain more detailed information. A copy of the patient's hospital discharge summary should be obtained from the hospital for the patient's permanent office record. This summary will be of some importance to the physician for providing continuity of care to the patient on return to the office for follow-up care or future checkups. Other uses of this form may include research, statistical, insurance, and legal purposes.

PROBLEM-ORIENTED MEDICAL RECORD (POMR)

Over the past few years, the problem-oriented medical record has gained great momentum and support from health care providers in a variety of settings. Pioneered by Lawrence L. Weed, MD, of the University of Vermont College of Medicine, the problem-oriented medical record provides a systematic way of recording data pertinent to patient care. Its purpose is to obtain and record in an organized manner all the knowledge needed to accurately diagnose, treat, and provide complete follow-up care for a patient's condition disease, or situation. This record consists of four basic parts, which are as follows:

- Data base
- Problem list
- Plans
- Progress notes

The *data base* provides the data necessary to identify and solve the problem(s). It consists of the patient's medical history, the physical examination, and known laboratory data, all of which were previously described.

The *problem list* results from the information obtained in the data base. All the problems identified are titled, numbered, and dated in order of occurrence. This information is usually placed on the front page of the patient's chart to provide a quick diagnostic profile of the patient. The problems may be stated in various terms as outlined on p. 298.

At subsequent visits any new problems are noted as they arise, dated, and numbered consecutively. As problems are resolved, the fact is noted with the date it occurred. The number of a resolved problem is not used again for another problem.

The problem list can be adapted in various ways to accommodate short-term or temporary problems that are seen frequently in the physician's office or clinic. One recommendation is the use of two problem lists: one for short-term or temporary problems, the other for long-term or permanent problems. When a short-term problem persists beyond a reasonable time, or recurs frequently, it is added to the long-term or permanent list and removed from the short-term list.

Another recommendation is to use only one problem list, but not to record quickly resolved temporary problems here. The temporary problems are simply indicated as such in the progress notes and are not numbered.

The *plans* state what will be done to start to solve the problem(s). They are made for each titled and numbered problem. A plan for a problem may be classified as follows:

- Diagnostic, that is, evaluative studies, such as laboratory tests and x-ray films, consultations requested, and interviews with the patient's family, all of which help acquire additional information.
- Therapeutic, that is, medical, surgical, diet, psychological, and/or physical treatment used to meet the goals of the physician when providing health care.
- Educative, that is, what the patient is told about the therapy and condition, what instructional material, if any, was given to the patient, and what the expectations from the patient are as a partner in the care and treatment plan.

The *progress notes* are added to the record as the plan(s) are carried out. Each progress note is dated and titled and numbered relating to the problem under discussion. Each problem is evaluated for current status, noting new findings or thoughts, changes in treatment plans, or resolution of the problem.

Each progress note should contain four parts and be recorded according to the following format.

Number and Title of the Problem

S *Subjective findings*—Statements made by the patient; how the patient feels; other information from the patient's family.

O *Objective findings*—What is observed or measured by the examiner; specific things done for/on the patient; results of laboratory, x-ray, and other diagnostic reports.

A *Assessment*—Evaluation and interpretation of the patient's status (the S plus O). Assessment may be what the examiner thinks is happening, reasons for changing management of the problem, or significance of the findings; it may be expressed as an impression or as a diagnosis

P *Plan*—diagnostic, therapeutic, and/or educative methods that will be used

After the data base has been completed and evaluated, the POMR may appear as follows.

Problem List

Nov. 4, 19____

   Problem No. 1: Hypertension, essential arterial
   Problem No. 2: Obesity, exogenous
   Problem No. 3: Upper abdominal pain—Resolved 11/7/____

Plan

Nov. 4, 19____

   Problem No. 1: Aldactazide 50 mg, 1 tab bid; recheck patient in 1 week
   Problem No. 2: 1200-calorie diet; multivitamin × 1 daily; suggested to patient to join a Weight Watchers club
   Problem No. 3: UGI series; oral cholecystogram

Progress Notes

Nov. 4, 19____

   Problem No. 1: Hypertension, essential arterial
      S —patient states that fatigue and headaches decreasing some
      O —BP ↓ 20 points to 160/84
      A —positive effects from the medication
      P —continue medication for 2 weeks, then to be checked
   Problem No. 2: Obesity
      S —patient has joined a Weight Watchers club, but states she hates dieting
      O —wt. ↓ 4 lb to 176
      A —dieting effective
      P —continue 1,200-calorie diet and multivitamin × 1 daily
   Problem No. 3: Upper abdominal pain
      S —patient states that the abdominal pain is less severe but persists
      O —UGI and GB series—negative; no abdominal distention
      A —deferred until all results complete
      P —abdominal ultrasound

Nov. 11, 19____

   Problem No. 1: Hypertension
      S —patient states that headaches have stopped, but still remains fatigued
      O —BP 140/84
      A —medication effective
      P —reduce Aldactazide to 1 tab daily

Problem No. 2: Obesity

S —patient states is now adjusting to the diet much better

O —wt. ↓ 2 lbs. to 174

A —weight loss will benefit problem No. 1

P —continue 1,200-calorie diet

Problem No. 3: Upper abdominal pain

S —patient states pain has subsided— 11/7/____

O —x-ray results and ultrasound reports negative

A —temporary condition, resolved 11/7/____

P —patient to report if pain recurs and advised that x-ray studies and ultrasound were negative

As you can see, the POMR is an orderly method of providing a chronological profile of a patient that helps the physician and other health care providers conduct total patient care. This system provides a quick current reference of the patient's medical case record, including problem management. It greatly reduces the possibility of an oversight, especially for patients receiving long-term care or those with multiple problems.

Conclusion

You have now completed the chapter on health history and physical examinations. You will be expected to discuss the parts and the importance of a patient's health history and other components that make up a medical record. In addition, you should be able to describe the methods used by a physician when performing a physical examination. When you are familiar with the contents of this chapter, arrange with your instructor to take a performance test.

Review Questions

1. Information gathered on a history and physical examination is used for varied purposes. List four of these purposes.

2. List and define the six parts of a patient's history.

3. The following information has been obtained from physicians' notes. For each statement, indicate the correct component of the patient's record in which this information would be recorded. Choose your answers from the following headings: chief complaint; history of present illness; past history; family history; social or occupational history; review of systems; physical examination; and impression.

   a. The patient is a 25-year-old white obese female who was in good health until approximately 10 PM last evening.

   b. There is no history of past operations.

   c. Neck: thyroid is not enlarged.

   d. Head: there is no history of headaches, sinus pain, or trauma.

   e. The arteries are full, soft, and readily compressible.

   f. "I have a lump in my left breast."

   g. Patient had measles and chickenpox when she was a child.

   h. R/O diabetes.

   i. There is decreased muscle tone in all four extremities.

   j. Patient's father has a history of hypertension for 5 years.

   k. GU system: There is no history of dysuria, hematuria, frequency, or nocturia.

   l. The patient denies the use of alcohol, tobacco, and drugs of any kinds.

4. Define the following methods of examination, and state one body part or system that is examined in each method.

   a. Inspection

   b. Percussion

   c. Palpation

   d. Auscultation

   e. Mensuration

5. Describe the difference between the ROS and the PE.
6. List five forms of treatment that may be used for the care of a patient.
7. List three reasons why diagnostic studies are important for patient care.
8. State the purpose of the problem-oriented medical record.
9. List and explain the four parts of the problem-oriented medical record.

SUGGESTED READINGS

Collen MF: Periodic health examination, Primary Care 3:197, 1976.

Malasanos L et al: Health assessment, ed 2, St Louis, 1981, The CV Mosby Co.

Weed LL: Medical records, medical education, and patient care, Cleveland, 1971, The Press of Case Western Reserve University.

Chapter 19

Assisting with Physical Examinations

- Preparing for and assisting with physical examinations

Objectives

On completion of Chapter 19 the medical assistant student should be able to:

1 Define and pronounce the vocabulary terms listed.

2 Summarize the medical assistant's responsibilities in assisting the physician during an examination of a patient.

3 List, identify, and state the function of each instrument commonly used during a complete physical examination, including the following: rectal and vaginal examinations; a proctosigmoidoscopy; a neurological examination; an ear examination; and an eye examination.

4 State two purposes for positioning a patient and three purposes for draping a patient for physical examinations.

5 State the purpose of and discuss the following special examinations: neurological; ear; eye; obstetrical; and breast self-examination.

6 Discuss the American Cancer Society's guidelines for examinations for the early detection of cancer in people without symptoms.

7 Prepare a patient for a physical examination by providing clear, simple instructions and explanations that are easy to understand.

8 Position and drape a patient in the positions outlined in this chapter.

9 Select, identify, and prepare for use equipment and supplies required for the following: a complete physical examination that is to include a rectal examination and a pelvic examination with Pap smear; and a proctosigmoidoscopy.

10 Demonstrate correct assisting techniques during physical examinations.

11 Assist the patient before, during, and after physical examinations.

12 Record the procedures and results (when applicable) of physical examinations.

13 Measure the patient's distance visual acuity using the Snellen eye chart.

Vocabulary

bimanual (bi-man′u-al) With both hands, as bimanual palpation.

bronchoscopy (bron-kos′ko-pĭ) The internal inspection of the tracheobronchial tree with the use of a bronchoscope; used for diagnostic or treatment purposes. For diagnosis, the physician will inspect the interior of the bronchi and may obtain a sample of secretions or a biopsy of tissue; for treatment, foreign bodies or mucus plugs that may be causing an obstruction to the air passages can be located and removed.

cystoscopy (sis-tos′kop-ĭ) The internal examination of the bladder with a cystoscope. Samples of urine for diagnostic purposes can be obtained by passing a catheter through the cystoscope into the bladder or beyond, up into the ureters and kidneys. Also, radiopaque dyes may be injected through the cystoscope into the bladder or up into the ureters when taking x-ray films of the urinary tract.

digital (dij'it-al) Denoting the use of a finger to insert into a body cavity, such as the rectum, for palpating the tissue.

endoscopy (en-dos'ko-pĭ) The visual examination of internal cavities of the body with an endoscope, for example, a proctoscope, bronchoscope, cystoscope, gastroscope, and laryngoscope.

gastroscopy (gas'tros'ko-pĭ) The internal inspection of the stomach with a gastroscope.

oral examination An examination pertaining to the mouth

Papanicolaou smear or test (pap"ah-nik"o-la'oo) A smear examined microscopically to detect cancer cells from body excretions (urine and feces), secretions (vaginal fluids, sputum or prostatic fluid), or tissue scrapings (as obtained from the stomach or uterus); most commonly done on a cervical scraping to detect abnormal or cancerous cells in the mucus of the uterus and cervix. This test is often referred to as a Pap smear or test.

pelvic examination An examination of the external and internal female reproductive organs.

roentgenological (rĕnt-gĕn-ŏl'ŏj-i-cal) Pertaining to an examination with the use of x-ray films (radiographs).

Instruments used for physical examinations (Figure 19.1)

anoscope (an'no-skōp) A speculum or endoscope inserted into the anal canal for direct visual examination.

applicator A slender rod of glass or wood with a pledget of cotton on one end used to apply medicine or to take a culture from the body.

biopsy (bi'op-se) forceps Two-pronged instruments of varying sizes and shapes used to remove tissue from the body for examination.

bronchoscope (brong'ko-skōp) An endoscope designed specifically for passage through the trachea to allow visual examination of the interior of the tracheobronchial tree.

cystoscope (sist'o-skōp) A hollow metal tube instrument (endoscope) designed specifically for passing through the urethra into the urinary bladder to permit internal inspection. The bladder interior is illuminated by an electric bulb at the end of the cystoscope. Special lenses and mirrors allow the bladder mucosa to be examined for calculi (stones), inflammation, or tumors.

endoscope (en'do-skōp) A specially designed instrument made of metal, rubber, or glass that is used for direct visual examination of hollow organs or body cavities. All endoscopes have similar working elements, even though the design will vary according to its specific use. The viewing part (scope) is a hollow tube fitted with a lens system that allows viewing in a variety of directions. Each endoscope has a light source, power cord, and power source; examples include bronchoscope, cystoscope, proctoscope, and sigmoidoscope.

insufflator (in'suf-fla-tor) An instrument, device, or bag used for blowing air, powder, or gas into a cavity.

laryngeal (lar-in'je-al) mirror An instrument used to view the pharynx and larynx consisting of a small rounded mirror attached to the end of a slender (metal or chrome plate) handle.

laryngoscope (lar-in'go-skōp) An endoscope used to examine the larynx. It is equipped with mirrors and a light for illumination of the larynx.

nasal speculum (n'azl spēk'ū-lŭm) A short, funnellike instrument used to examine the nasal cavity.

ophthalmoscope (ŏf-thăl'mō-skōp) An instrument used for examining the interior parts of the eye. It contains a perforated mirror and lens. When the ophthalmoscope is turned on and brought close to the eye, it sends a narrow, bright beam of light through the lens of the eye. By looking through the lens of the instrument, the physician is then able to examine the interior parts of the eye to detect any possible disorders.

otoscope (ōt'ō-skōp) An instrument used to examine the external ear canal and eardrum.

percussion (pŭr-kŭsh'ŭn) hammer A small

hammer with a triangular-shaped rubber head used for percussion.

proctoscope (prŏk′tō-skōp) A specially designed tubular endoscope that is passed through the anus to permit internal inspection of the lower part of the large intestine.

sigmoidoscope (sĭg-moy′dō-skōp) A tubular endoscope used to examine the interior of the sigmoid colon.

speculum (spĕk′ū-lŭm) An instrument used for distending or opening a body cavity or orifice to allow visual inspection; a bivalve speculum is one having two parts or valves.

Sims vaginal speculum A form of bivalve speculum used in the examination of the vagina and cervix.

stethoscope An instrument used in auscultation to amplify the sounds produced by the lungs, heart, intestines, and other internal organs; also used when taking a blood pressure reading (see pp. 275-276).

tongue blade A flat, thin, smooth piece of wood or metal with rounded ends approximately 6 inches long; also called a tongue depressor. It is used for pressing tissue down to permit a better view when examining the mouth and throat. In addition, it may be used for application of ointments to the skin.

tonometer (to-nome e-ter) An instrument used to measure tension or pressure, especially intraocular pressure.

tuning fork A steel, two-pronged, forklike instrument used for testing hearing; the prongs give off a musical note when struck.

PREPARING FOR AND ASSISTING WITH PHYSICAL EXAMINATIONS

The physical examination is done in an examination or treatment room, whereas the history is commonly obtained from the patient in the physician's private office.

This chapter covers positioning the patient for an examination and preparing for and assisting with the common examinations performed by a physician. It outlines *one* way in which examinations are conducted and lists *one* group of instruments and equipment for each. The physician(s) or agency for whom you work may use other methods and equipment; therefore you must be able and willing to adapt to individual needs as required.

General instructions and responsibilities for medical assistants when assisting with examinations are given before the procedures. These instructions should be followed in every procedure that requires your assistance. Keep them in mind as you are preparing for all examinations, as they are not repeated before each individual procedure.

Commonly, during any of the examinations that are outlined in this chapter, various types of specimens may be obtained. Detailed information for collecting and labeling specimens will be covered in Chapter 22.

Cleansing and sterilization techniques to be used in the care of used, nondisposable equipment will be discussed in Chapter 20. It is suggested that you refer to these chapters for this specific information.

General Instructions and Responsibilities for the Medical Assistant

1. Always wash your hands thoroughly before setting up the required equipment for an examination and assisting the physician.
2. Prepare the patient, the examination room, and the equipment and instruments required by the physician for the examination according to office or agency policy.
3. Make certain that electrical and battery-operated equipment and all other lights are in working condition.
4. Place the equipment for the examination so that it is conveniently located for the physician's use.
5. Check to make sure that the examination room is comfortably warm, well aired, and spotlessly clean.
6. Cover the examination table with a clean cover, either a cotton or muslin sheet, crepe paper, or a covered rubber sheet on the lower part of the table. A towel may be placed over a pillow at the end of the table.
7. Assist the patient as required. Have a sturdy step stool for the patient to use when getting on and off the examining table. Offer support; guard against falling. Never leave a confused patient or a child alone on the examining table because of the danger of falling.
8. Assist the physician as required. You must learn the physician's methods and preferences for each examination.

Text continued on p. 308.

Figure 19.1
Instruments used for physical examinations.
Line drawings courtesy Miltex Instrument Co, Div of Miltenberg, Inc, Lake Success, NY.

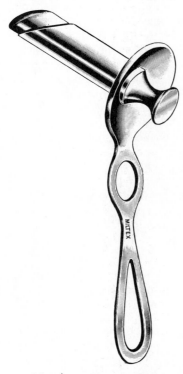

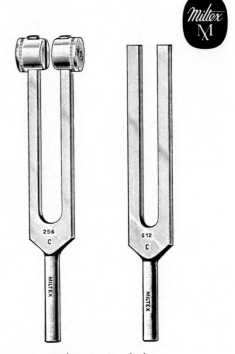

Hirschman anoscope

Miltex tuning forks

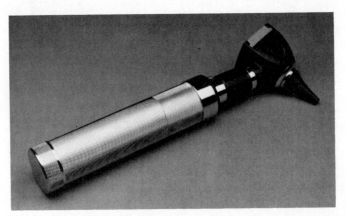

Otoscope

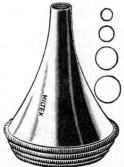

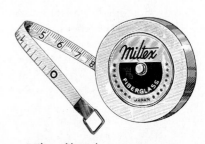

Boucheron and Toynbee ear specula to be used with an otoscope

Miltex fiberglass tape measure

Figure 19.1,
—cont'd

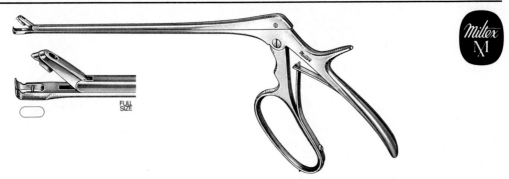

Tischler cervical biopsy punch forceps

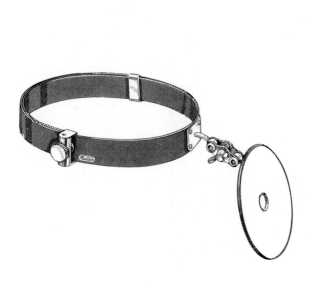

Frankel head band and mirror set

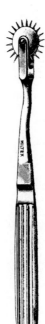

Wartenberg neurological
pin wheel

Laryngeal mirror

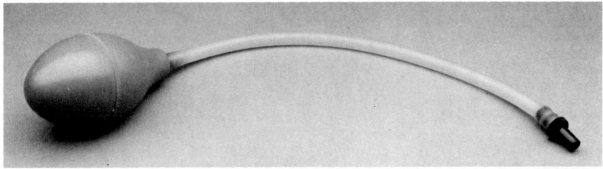

Insufflator   *Continued.*

Figure 19.1—cont'd

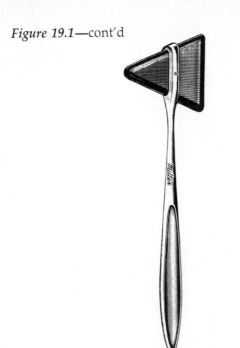

Taylor percussion hammer

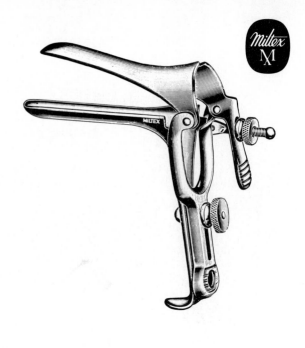

Graves vaginal speculum

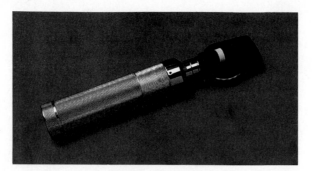

Ophthalmoscope

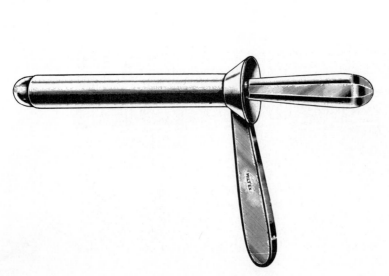

Kelly proctoscope

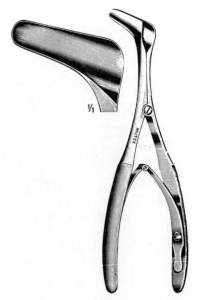

Sonnenschein nasal speculum

Figure 19.1—cont'd

Schiotz tonometers

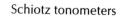

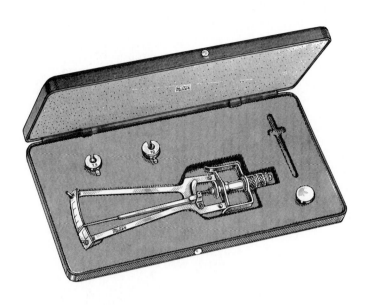

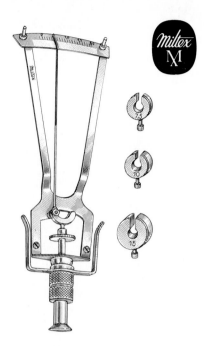

Original model with 3 weights (5.5, 7.5, and 10 g), plunger, footplate, and test block

Improved model with 4 weights (5.5, 7.5, 10, and 15 g), mirror insert on scale reduces error of parallax

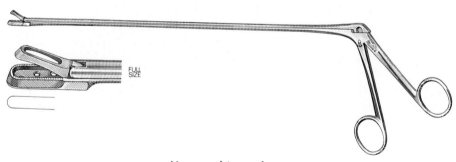

FULL SIZE

Yeoman biopsy forceps

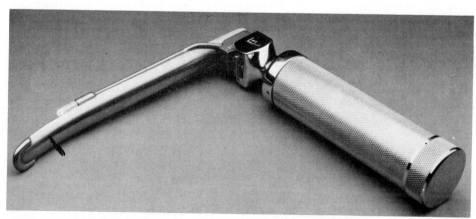

Laryngoscope

9. Never expose the patient unnecessarily. Only those parts of the body being examined are to be exposed.

10. A female assistant should remain in the room if the patient is female and the physician is male. This may not only help the anxious patient to feel more relaxed but also protect the physician from unwarranted lawsuits. There can be no false allegations if the witness observes the entire examination.

11. Observe the patient for various types of reactions. A change in facial expression may indicate that the patient is apprehensive or experiencing pain. Note any unusual weakness, change in breathing pattern, change in skin color, or fainting. Your observations may provide the physician with important information that will help make a diagnosis and provide treatment for the patient.

12. Inform the patient of any special instructions. When the physician has completed the examination, inform the patient that he is free to leave after getting dressed, or if required, to check at the front desk to schedule a future appointment or laboratory or x-ray examination. Often the physician requests that certain tests be run or specimens be gathered. Some offices and agencies have a printed sheet that the physician uses to check each test that is to be performed on the patient. The medical assistant should make the proper arrangements, notify the technologist, or collect the specimens requested before the patient leaves.

13. Handle specimens obtained according to office or agency policy.

14. On completion of the examination, carry out your responsibilities for the disposal, cleansing, disinfecting, or sterilizing of the used equipment and the treatment room to prevent the spread of microorganisms.

15. Record findings from the examination accurately and completely. Use correct medical abbreviations, when applicable, in recording all information. Most physicians will record all the necessary information on the patient's chart, so frequently this will not be one of the medical assistant's responsibilities. The policy regarding this will vary and will be established by the physician or agency for whom you work. If it is your responsibility the following items are usually to be included:
    - Date, time, and type of examination and the findings/results, when applicable.
    - Name of the examiner.
    - If specimens were obtained, the type, how

they were handled, the test(s) to be performed.
- Any pertinent observations that you have made that will help describe the patient's general condition. Be specific in the type of information you record; for example, "Patient complained of slight nausea and a transient pain in the right lower abdominal quadrant."
- Future directions given to the patient.
- Your signature.

Positioning the Patient for Physical Examinations

A physical examination is facilitated by the use of an examining table and proper gowning, positioning, and draping of the patient. The purposes of positioning a patient are as follows:
- To allow for better visibility and accessibility for the physician during the examination of the patient
- To provide support for the patient when being examined

The purposes of gowning and draping the patient are as follows:
- To avoid unnecessary exposure of the patient's body during an examination, thereby protecting the patient's modesty
- To contribute to the patient's feeling of being cared for, which helps the patient relax
- To provide some comfort and warmth and avoid chilling

The principle of gowning and draping is that only the part of the body that is being examined should be exposed, other than the head, arms, and sometimes the legs, and only when the physician is about to begin the examination.

There are different positions used for various types of examinations. In all positions the patient must be well supported, as most positions are uncomfortable and difficult to maintain for any length of time. The position chosen will depend on the type of examination or procedure to be performed, and on the patient's age, sex, and physical condition. The various positions used most frequently in a general or special physical examination follow. The medical assistant must explain what is required and why it is necessary in order to gain full cooperation from the patient.

Equipment
- Examination table
- Patient gown, either cotton or disposable paper
- Paper or sheets to cover the table

Figure 19.2
Dorsal recumbent position.

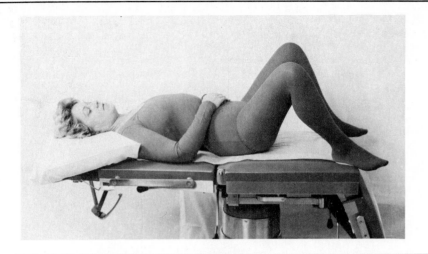

Figure 19.3
Lithotomy position.

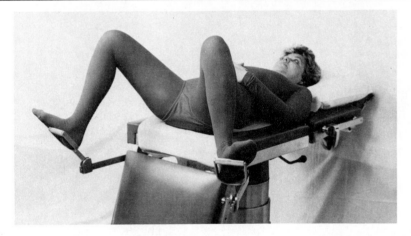

- Small towel, cloth or paper
- Small pillow
- Drape sheet; two drape sheets are needed for the jackknife and Trendelenburg positions
- Stirrups on the examining table for the lithotomy position
- A binder to support the patient on the table when placed in the Trendelenburg position

Dorsal recumbent and lithotomy positions

In the lithotomy position the patient's feet are placed in stirrups that are raised approximately 12 inches from table level, although the stirrups on some examining tables cannot be elevated. These positions are used almost exclusively for pelvic, bladder, and rectal examinations (Figures 19.2 and 19.3).

- The patient lies on the back with the legs separated and flexed.
- The feet are supported in stirrups, or the soles of the feet are flat on the table.
- The buttocks are brought to the edge of the examining table.
- The arms are placed either at the side or crossed over the chest or under the head.

Jackknife or proctological position

In the jackknife or proctological position the patient lies on the abdomen with both the head and legs lowered, so that the buttocks are elevated. Arms are placed along the side of the head. This position is used for rectal examinations and occasionally for surgery. A special examining table that can be adjusted to facilitate this position is required (Figure 19.4).

Knee-chest position

In the knee-chest position the patient rests on the knees and chest, with the head turned to one side. Arms may be placed under the head to help support the patient. Buttocks extend up in the air, and the back is straight. This position is used for the

Figure 19.4
The Ritter Procto Table raises, lowers, and tilts at the touch of a toe on the foot control.
Courtesy Sybron Corp, Medical Products Division, Rochester, NY.

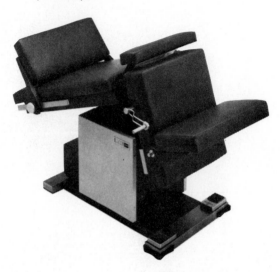

Procto

Figure 19.5
Knee-chest position.

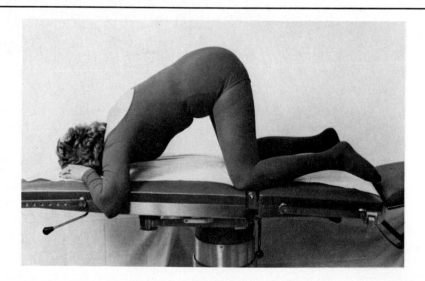

rectal examinations and sometimes for vaginal and prostatic examinations (Figure 19.5).

Sims or left lateral position

In the Sims or left lateral position the patient lies on the left side and chest, with the left leg slightly flexed and the right leg sharply flexed on the abdomen. The left arm is drawn behind the body with the body inclining forward. The right arm is positioned forward according to the patient's comfort. The buttocks are brought up to the long edge of the table. This position is used frequently for rectal examinations and when giving enemas. The vagina and abdomen can also be examined in this position, and it may be used when the lithotomy position is too difficult to maintain (Figure 19.6).

Trendelenburg position

In the Trendelenburg (trĕn-dĕl′ĕn-burg) position the patient lies on the back with the head lower than the rest of the body. The body is elevated at an angle of about 45°, and the knees are flexed over the lower section of the examining table,

Figure 19.6
Sim's or left lateral position.

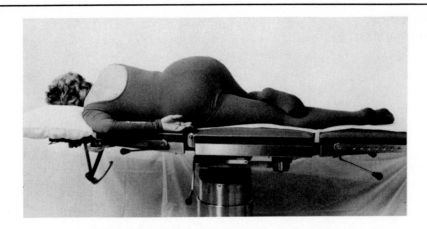

Figure 19.7
Trendelenburg positions.

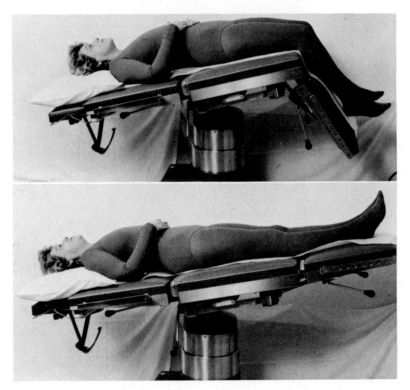

which is lowered. The patient should be well supported to prevent slipping.

This position is not used routinely for an office examination, but often is used in the operating and x-ray rooms. It displaces the intestines into the upper abdomen.

An alternate form of the Trendelenburg position is one in which the patient's body is placed on an incline with the feet elevated at an angle of 45° and the head lowered. One may use this position to prevent shock or when the patient is in a state of shock or has low blood pressure. It is also used for some abdominal surgery. Some physicians will have the patient positioned in the Sims position along with this form of the Trendelenburg position for rectal examinations (Figure 19.7).

Supine position

In the supine position the patient lies flat on the back, arms placed at the side, and head elevated

Figure 19.8
Prone position.

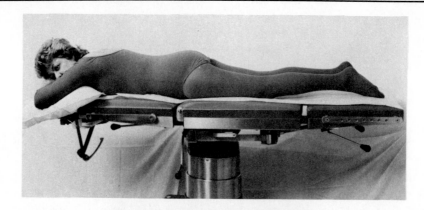

Figure 19.9
Fowler's (sitting) position.

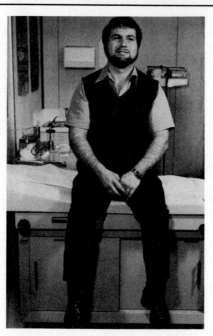

slightly on a pillow. This position is used for examinations of the abdomen, breasts, some surgical and x-ray procedures, and on occasion for examination of the chest.

Prone position

In the prone position the patient lies flat on the abdomen, arms flexed under the head, which is turned to one side. It may be used in examinations of the back in musculoskeletal and neurological examinations, and for some surgical procedures (Figure 19.8).

Fowler's position

In the Fowler's position the patient sits up. This position is used for examining the head, ears, eyes, nose and throat, neck, chest, and breasts (Figure 19.9).

Semi-Fowler's position

In the semi-Fowler's position the patient lies in a supine position, with the head of the table or bed raised 18 to 20 inches above the level of the feet. This may be used rather than the supine or Fowler positions when the comfort and physical condition of the patient require it, such as a patient with dyspnea (Figure 19.10).

Erect or standing position

In the erect or standing position the patient stands erect with arms down at the sides and feet facing forward. This position is used for part of a neurological and musculoskeletal examination and also during some x-ray procedures (Figure 19.11).

Text continued on p. 327.

Figure 19.10
Semi-Fowler's position.

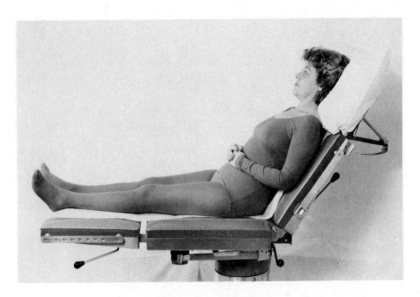

Figure 19.11
Standing position.

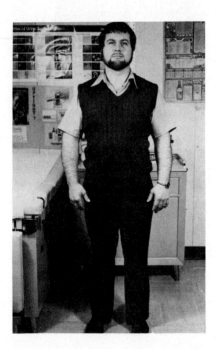

Procedure for a Complete Physical Examination

Equipment

The exact amount and type of equipment to be assembled for physical examination will depend on the following:
- Purpose of the examination;
- Type and extent of the examination;
- Preferences of the physician; and
- Condition of the patient.

In some physicians' offices and agencies, the equipment required for examinations will be kept on a special tray ready for use and in a central location. In others it may be necessary for you to assemble all the equipment that will be needed.

Although there are differences among physicians and agencies the following list includes items that are commonly used and should be available, ready for use (Figure 19.12).

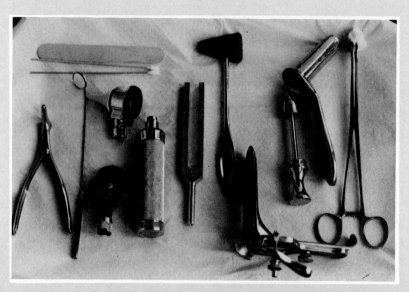

Figure 19.12
Instruments and supplies commonly used for a physical examination. *Left to right:* Nasal speculum, laryngeal mirror, otoscope (top) and ophthalmoscope (bottom) attachments with battery-operated handle, tuning fork, percussion hammer, vaginal speculum, anoscope, and sponge stick (forceps) with sponge. *Top left corner:* Tongue blade, cotton tip applicators.

Examination table covered with a clean sheet
Patient gown, either cloth or paper
Draping material, drape sheet, small towel
Watch with a second hand
Stethoscope
Thermometer
Sphygmomanometer
Scale with height measure rod
Tape measure
Tuning fork
Percussion or reflex hammer
Tongue blades
Laryngeal mirror
Head mirror
Flashlight and/or gooseneck lamp

Otoscope
Ophthalmoscope
Nasal speculum
Safety pin
Tissues
Cotton balls
Alcohol or prepackaged alcohol swabs
Urine specimen bottle
Laboratory request form
X-ray request form
Emesis basin or waste container used for soiled equipment and/or waste
  Additional equipment is required for a visual acuity test and vaginal and rectal examinations. This will vary with the purpose of the examination, the condition of the patient, and the physician's preference.
Visual acuity test: A Snellen eye chart is used most commonly to measure distance visual acuity.
Vaginal examination:
  Vaginal speculum
  Sterile rubber gloves
  Lubricant, such as K-Y jelly
  Uterine sponge or uterine dressing forceps
  Sponges
  Two glass slides for smears; *or* one glass slide and one sterile culture tube with applicator
  Cotton-tipped applicators or wooden cervical spatulas
  Fixative spray *or* cytology jar with solution
  Plastic container for slides if using fixative spray
  Laboratory request form
Rectal examination:
  Rectal glove or sterile rubber gloves or rubber finger cot
  Lubricant, such as K-Y jelly
  Rectal speculum, proctoscope, or anoscope—depending on the extent of the examination
  Tissues
  Sponge forceps
  Sponges
  Cotton-tipped applicators

Procedure	*Rationale*
1. Wash your hands.	
2. Assemble and prepare the necessary equipment for the physician.	Equipment is to be arranged on a table or tray covered with a clean towel.
3. Identify the patient, and explain the procedure.	An explanation allows the patient to understand what will be done, that is, what will occur, how it may feel, and how he can help in the examination. It also provides some reassurance for the patient.
4. Have the patient void to empty the bladder.	Instruct the patient how to collect a urine specimen if one is required (see pp. 419-420). When the bladder is full, it is difficult for the physician to palpate the abdomen adequately. It is also very uncomfortable for the patient to have a full bladder while being examined.

5. Take the following physical measurements and record accurately:
  TPR
  BP
  Height
  Weight
	This will vary with your job requirements. At times the physician may wish to do these tests rather than have you do them. Height and weight should be taken after the patient removes shoes and heavy outer clothing.

6. Instruct the patient to disrobe completely and put on a patient gown with the opening in the front.	Gown donned with opening in the front permits access to the chest for examination while the shoulders and back are still covered.
7. Have the patient sit on the edge of the examining table with a towel under the buttocks. Place a drape sheet over the patient's lap.	

Continued.

Procedure for a Complete Physical Examination—cont'd

Procedure

8. Call the physician when the patient is ready and when you have all necessary recordings completed and equipment assembled. The patient's chart should be given to the physician before the examination begins.
9. Assist the physician as required.

10. While the patient is in a sitting position, the physician will examine the head, ears, eyes, nose, mouth, and throat; the neck and axillae; the chest, breasts, and heart; the neuromuscular reflexes and sensations, such as the pinprick; as well as a general observation of skin and body symmetry.

11. When handling or accepting a tongue blade from the physician, hold it in the center. Break it at the center after use (without touching the end used) and then discard in the emesis basin or waste container.
12. Warm the laryngeal mirror by placing the mirrored end under warm running water or in a glass of warm water.
13. After step 10 is completed, the patient is to assume a supine position. Help the patient attain this position if necessary.
14. Place the drape sheet to cover the patient from shoulders to feet. It can be moved down when the physician is ready to examine the breasts and abdomen. When the physician examines the breasts, fold the sheet down to the patient's waist, and open the patient's gown.
    When the abdomen is being examined, the patient's gown can be used to cover the breasts, and you are to fold the drape sheet down to the pubic hair line.

Rationale

A female assistant should remain in the room if the patient is female and the physician is male and/or if the physician requires assistance in performing the examination (see p. 305).

Depending on the physician's preference, you may have to be ready to hand up the instruments as needed. The physician will proceed with the examination from head to toe, examining the body systems and parts as described previously under the physical examination in Chapter 17.

Equipment:
   Tuning fork
   Otoscope
   Ophthalmoscope
   Nasal speculum
   Tongue blade
   Flashlight
   Head mirror
   Laryngeal mirror
   Stethoscope
   Safety pin
   Percussion hammer

By handling the tongue blade this way you avoid contamination to the patient and also to yourself.

It must be warmed to prevent fogging. Be sure to dry it before it is used.

Give reassurance and support as needed. Often just placing your hand on the patient's shoulder or arm gives the patient a feeling of support and of being cared for.

When the patient is in this position, the physician will palpate breasts, liver, spleen, and other abdominal organs. The groin will be checked for a possible hernia.

The physician may use a stethoscope to listen to abdominal sounds as part of the examination of the abdomen.

Procedure

15. For a vaginal and rectal examination, help the patient assume the correct position. Assist the physician as required.

16. Observe the patient for any unusual reactions, such as a feeling of weakness or pain, facial grimace, change in color.

17. When the examination has been completed, the patient may sit up.

18. Check with the patient if there are any questions to be answered.

19. Inform the patient of any special instructions (see No. 12, p. 308).

20. If necessary, help the patient dress; otherwise leave the room so that the patient may have some privacy.

21. On returning to the examining room, assemble all used equipment and supplies to be disposed of properly.

22. Replace clean equipment as needed.

23. Clean the examination table and put on a fresh cover.

24. If smears or cultures were obtained, send them to the laboratory or place them in a refrigerator or a cool dark place until you can transfer them to the laboratory.

25. Wash your hands.

26. Do any recording required of you completely and accurately (see no. 15, p. 308). Use accepted medical abbreviations when recording.

Rationale

Positions and procedures for these examinations are discussed next. Vaginal and rectal examinations are included in the complete physical examination of a female patient. For the male patient, the physician will examine the genitals, the rectum, and prostate gland.

It may be advisable to allow the patient to remain in the supine position for a few minutes before getting up.

Frequently a patient may have questions, but does not feel free to ask or may feel that there is not time to do so.

Frequently patients are left in the room after the examination not knowing if they are to talk further to the physician or are free to leave. Do not let this happen.

Remove all linens and place in the soiled laundry. Place disposable equipment in a covered waste container. Take instruments to your cleanup area. Depending on the instrument and its requirements, you may rinse it with cool water, or wash or soak it in soap and water until you are ready to prepare it for sterilization or disinfection (see Chapter 20). Others, such as the tuning fork, may be wiped off and then replaced in the usual storage area.

Make sure that specimens are properly labeled and that you have completely filled out the appropriate laboratory request form.

Charting example:

Jan. 27, 19_____ 1 PM

Complete physical examination done by Dr. Short. Patient referred to lab for a CBC (complete blood count) and UA (urinalysis) and to the x-ray department for a chest x-ray film. Patient to return in 1 week to discuss the results of these tests with the doctor.

Ann O'Reilly, CMA

Pelvic Examination and Papanicolaou Smear

Pelvic (vaginal) examinations and Papanicolaou (Pap) smears are essential for the adult female. Most general practitioners and internists as well as gynecologists and obstetricians will perform them routinely. These examinations, done to diagnose abnormalities of the female reproductive system, include inspection of the vulva, vagina, and cervix, and a bimanual palpation of the uterus, fallopian tubes, and ovaries. The physician notes the size, shape, position, and consistency of the uterus and whether any masses are present in the uterus, fallopian tubes, or ovaries. The purpose of the Pap smear is to detect precancerous conditions, any unusual cell growth, or cancer of the cervix or uterus. The value of the test is that it can detect potential problems early so that they can be treated.

Instruct the patient not to put any creams or foams in the vagina, not to douche, and not to have sexual intercourse for 24 hours (some suggest 48 hours) before having a Pap smear taken. Any of these circumstances will interfere with the specimen obtained and make the test invalid. Also, a Pap smear must not be taken during the patient's menstrual period because the red blood cells will interfere with obtaining accurate findings.

The smear will be examined in the laboratory by a pathologist who will report the findings as one of the following five classifications:

Class I Normal. Only normal cells are seen.

Class II Possibly abnormal. Some atypical cells are seen. These may be due to inflammation of the vagina or cervix.

Class III Abnormal. Mild dysplasia.

Class IV Abnormal. Severe dysplasia, suspicious cells.

Class V Abnormal. Carcinoma cells are seen.

When the Pap smear is abnormal it does not mean that the patient has cancer unless the findings are in Class V. Abnormal findings indicate the need for further diagnostic studies.

Frequently a physician will first do a colposcopy. In this examination an instrument called a colposcope magnifies and focuses an intense light on the cervix. This allows the physician to observe the cervical anatomy in greater detail. If the colposcopy reveals an inflammatory process, a vaginal cream may be all that is needed for treatment. If the colposcopy reveals areas of abnormal tissues, the physician may use one or more diagnostic and therapeutic procedures, which include a biopsy, cryosurgery, endocervical curettage, and possibly a cone biopsy or more extensive surgery (see also pp. 302 and 440).

Equipment (Figure 19.13)

Examination table (stirrups if available) covered with a clean sheet or paper
Patient gown
Drape sheet
Small towel
Small pillow
Gooseneck lamp
Vaginal speculum
Lubricant, such as K-Y jelly
Sterile rubber gloves
Uterine sponge or uterine dressing forceps
Sponges or cotton balls
Two glass slides for smears *or* one glass slide and one sterile culture tube with applicator.
Two cotton-tipped applicators or wooden cervical spatulas
Fixative spray, such as Cyto-Fix, Spray-cyte; *or* cytology jar with solution, for example, 95% isopropyl alcohol solution is preferred, although formalin 10% may be used.
Plastic container for slides when using the fixative spray
Tissues
Laboratory request form

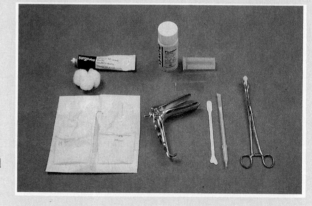

Figure 19.13
Equipment for a pelvic examination and Pap smear.

Procedure

1. Wash your hands.
2. Assemble and prepare the necessary instruments and equipment. Prepare the room.
3. Identify the patient. Explain the procedure, and reassure the patient.

4. Have the patient empty her bladder.

5. You may be required to take the patient's pulse and blood pressure.

6. Provide a patient gown, and have the patient remove all clothing from the waist down.
7. Position the patient on the table in a dorsal-recumbent or lithotomy position and drape. Remember to do the following:
   - Place the stirrups far enough out so that the knees are apart.
   - Avoid exposing the patient unnecessarily.
   - Make sure that there is a small towel under the buttocks.
8. Call the physician.
   NOTE: You may call the physician into the room and then have the patient assume the required position.
9. Assist the physician as required.
   - Lower the foot of the examining table (if it is a table that splits), or push the foot piece in on newer model tables.
   - Pull back the drape sheet exposing *only* the perineal region.
10. Be prepared to hand the physician the various instruments and materials that may be needed. Some physicians will request that you put some K-Y jelly out on a gauze sponge; others will squeeze it out when they are ready to lubricate the rubber gloves and vaginal speculum. Direct the light on the area being examined.
11. If a smear is to be obtained, mark the patient's name on the slides and the cytology jar *or* on the container where they will be placed after using a fixative spray. Label the slides No. 1 and No. 2.
12. You may instruct the patient to breathe deeply through the mouth.
13. The *physician* will begin the examination. If a Pap smear is to be obtained, the *physician* will do the following:
    a. Insert a dry speculum into the vagina.
    b. Open the speculum so that the cervix can be seen clearly.
    c. Insert a cotton-tipped applicator or wooden vaginal spatula and draw it across the cervix to obtain a specimen, which is then smeared evenly and moderately thin across the No. 1 glass slide.

Rationale

Make sure the lamp is working and that there is a clean paper or sheet on the table.
An explanation gives the patient some understanding of the need for the examination and what to expect, that is, what will occur, how it may feel.
Explain to the patient how to collect a specimen if a urinalysis is to be done.
This is usually done if the woman is taking birth control pills; also frequently done routinely in many offices as a screening process for high BP.
Shoes may be left on if the heels will fit into the stirrups.

This will vary with the physician's preference and the patient's condition. The Sims position may also be used for a vaginal examination of an elderly woman.

Remain in the room if necessary (refer to No. 10, p. 308).

If you do not have to assist the physician with the instruments and materials, give your attention to the patient. You may stand by the patient on one side and offer support and reassurance. Frequently support can be given just by having your hand placed gently on the patient's arm or shoulder.
The vaginal speculum may be warmed by running warm water over it. Alternatives used in some offices and agencies are to keep the instruments on a heating pad or in a warming pan. Other agencies use plastic disposable specula; warming these specula is not necessary.

Paper clips should be attached to the ends of the slides to prevent them from sticking together if they are to be placed in a cytology jar with the isopropyl alcohol or formalin solution.

This helps relax muscles.

NOTE: (a) If a smear is *not* to be obtained, the speculum would be lubricated for easier insertion into the vagina. Steps (c) through (e) would then be omitted.

Continued.

Pelvic Examination and Papanicolaou Smear—cont'd

Procedure

d. Insert another applicator or spatula and draw it across the posterior fornices or pools of the vaginal canal to obtain a second specimen, which is then smeared evenly and moderately across the No. 2 glass slide. If the material is spread too thickly, it will be difficult for the laboratory worker to visualize individual cells.

e. Place these two slides immediately (within 4 seconds to prevent drying and death of cells) into the cytology jar with solution, or spray them thoroughly with the cytological fixative spray and place them in the designated container after the fixative has dried thoroughly (drying takes about 5 to 10 minutes).

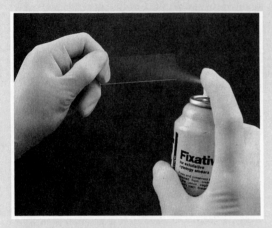

Figure 19.14
Spraying smear with a cytologic fixative spray.

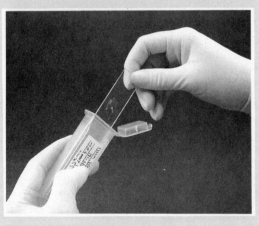

Figure 19.15
Placing slides in container for transport to a laboratory.

Rationale

NOTE: Frequently an endocervical smear is more desirable than one obtained from the posterior vaginal pool. In this case, the physician would insert an applicator into the cervical os, rotating it completely around the os until the cotton is saturated. A smear is then prepared with this specimen.

NOTE: The *medical assistant* may be required to hold the slide while the physician smears the specimen on the slide and then spray the slide with the cytological fixative spray. When spraying the slides, hold the nozzle of the can at least 5 to 6 inches away from the slide and spray lightly from left to right and then from right to left (Fig. 19.14). Allow the slides to dry thoroughly before placing them in the designated container for transport to an outside laboratory (Fig. 19.15). To avoid contaminating yourself, it is suggested that you wear disposable rubber gloves when handling these slides.

NOTE: These slides will be sent with a properly labeled laboratory request form to the laboratory for cytological examination. Enter on the request form the following information:

- Date
- Physician's name and address
- Patient's name and age
- Source of specimen
- Tests(s) requested

Also enter all of the following that apply:

- Date of last menstrual period (LMP)
- Hormone treatment (which includes birth control pills)
- Postmenopausal
- Postpartum
- Pregnant
- Previous surgery
- X-ray treatment
- Previous normal
- Previous abnormal and date

NOTE: Rather than making two smears, many agencies and physicians will obtain one endocervical smear for cytology studies and one culture for gonorrhea screening. This is done more frequently now, as often patients will have an infection without any signs or symptoms. This has been found to be a very beneficial screening process that enables early treatment of asymptomatic infections.

Procedure

    f. Remove the speculum, and place in an area designated for used equipment.

    g. Apply lubricant to the gloved index finger of the dominant hand.

    h. Insert the gloved, lubricated finger into the vagina to palpate internally for any abnormalities such as displacement or growths of the uterus, cervix, ovaries, and fallopian tubes. Place the other hand on the patient's abdomen and apply pressure so that the movable abdominal organs may be felt more easily during this bimanual examination.

14. When the physician has completed the examination, wipe off the excess lubricant or discharge from the patient's perineal region.

15. Remove small towel from under the patient's buttocks.

16. Raise or pull out the foot of the examining table.

17. Help the patient remove her feet from the stirrups and place her legs down on the table.

18. The patient may now slide up toward the head of the table and then sit up.

19. Remove drape sheet.

20. If necessary, help the patient get up and get dressed. Provide extra tissue and a sanitary pad and belt if required.

21. Inform the patient of any special instructions, if she is free to leave after she is dressed, or if the physician wishes to speak to her further. Ask the patient if she has any questions (see No. 12, p. 308).

22. Leave the patient to dress in privacy if your assistance is not required.

23. Return to the examining room to assemble all used equipment and supplies to be disposed of properly.

24. Replace clean equipment as needed.

25. Clean the examination table, and put on a fresh cover.

26. If smears or cultures were taken, send them to the laboratory with request form, or place in a cool, dark place until you can transfer them to the laboratory.

27. Wash your hands.

28. Do any recording required of you completely and accurately (see No. 15, p. 308).

Rationale

You may use tissues or the small towel that was placed under the patient's buttocks.

This varies with the type of examining table used.

If you are helping the patient lower her legs, lift and move both legs together to avoid any undue strain to the pelvic area.

Frequently it is desirable or advisable to allow the patient to rest for a few minutes before getting up.

Always provide for the patient's safety, comfort, and well-being.

Provide accurate and complete information, or refer the patient's questions to the physician if you cannot answer them. Part of patient care includes patient education and providing information and answers as necessary.

Remove any linens, and place in the soiled laundry. Place disposable equipment in a covered waste container.

Take instruments to your cleanup area wearing disposable rubber gloves: rinse with cool water. These may be soaked in soap and water until you are ready to prepare them for sterilization (see Chapter 20).

It is very important that all the required information appears on the cytology lab request, including notation of cervical and vaginal smears (see No. 13 (e), under NOTE, p. 320).

Charting example:
Jan. 27, 19_____, 2 PM
Pelvic exam done by Dr. Short, Pap smear sent to laboratory for cytology studies. Patient had no specific complaints and left office in good spirits.
Sandi Wilcox, CMA

Rectal Examination

The rectal examination is used to detect polyps, early cancer, lesions, inflammatory conditions, and hemorrhoids. In addition, examination of the rectum can show how far the uterus is displaced and if there are any masses in the rectum or pelvic region in a female and the size, any enlargement, and texture of the prostate gland in a male. A more extensive examination of the interior surfaces of the rectum is done by proctoscopy.

Equipment (Figure 19.16)

Examination table
Sheet or paper to cover the table
Patient gown
Drape sheet
Small pillow
Small towel
Tissues
Rubber glove or finger cot
Lubricant (K-Y jelly)
Sponge forceps
Sponges
Rectal speculum and/or anoscope
Cotton-tipped applicators

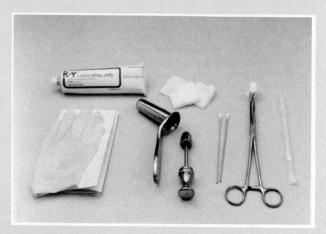

Figure 19.16
Equipment for a rectal examination including a Culturette (far right) to obtain a culture.

Procedure	*Rationale*
1. Wash your hands.	
2. Identify the patient and explain the procedure.	An explanation gives the patient some understanding of the need for the examination and provides some reassurance.
3. Have the patient empty the bladder.	Explain to the patient how to collect a specimen if a urinalysis is to be done (see Chapter 22).
4. Provide a patient gown; have the patient remove all clothing from the waist down and put the gown on with the opening in the back.	
5. Assemble the necessary instruments and equipment.	This will vary somewhat depending on the extent of the examination to be done and the physician's preference. Frequently only the glove and lubricant will be necessary.
6. Position the patient on the examination table in a Sims, jackknife, or knee-chest position.	This will vary according to the physician's preference. Refer to p. 309 for positioning techniques.
7. Drape the patient.	NOTE: You may call the physician and then position the patient. By doing this, you prevent the patient from having to be in an uncomfortable position for an excessive period of time.
8. Call the physician.	
9. When the examination is ready to begin, pull the drape sheet back, exposing only the rectal area.	Avoid exposing the patient unnecessarily.
10. Assist the physician as required.	A female assistant should remain in the room if the patient is female and the physician is male, even if she does not have to assist during the examination (see No. 10, p. 308).

Procedure

11. Be prepared to hand the physician the various instruments and equipment. Some physicians will request that you put some K-Y jelly out on a piece of gauze; others will get it themselves to lubricate the gloved finger and anoscope if used. If a light is used, direct it on the part to be examined (the rectal region).

12. The *physician* will begin the examination by inserting a gloved, lubricated finger into the rectum, then palpating the rectum internally to determine if there are any hemorrhoids, polyps or other obstructions, growths, or enlargements. This will be done gently, as it is often painful for the patient. If the anoscope is used, it will be lubricated, then the physician will insert it into the anal canal gently, and remove the obturator. If there is any bleeding or discharge, the physician may insert the sponge forceps and sponge through the anoscope to swab the area dry. This will allow better viewing of the internal surfaces. A good light will be needed so that the physician can view the internal lining of the anal canal. If a culture is to be taken, the physician will put a cotton-tipped applicator through the anoscope and swab the area. The cotton-tipped applicator will then be placed in a sterile culture tube, often one that has a special broth solution in it, so that the culture will not dry out.

13. When the physician has completed the examination, wipe the patient's anal region for any excess lubricant or discharge.

14. Help the patient, if required, assume a supine position.

15. Remove the drape sheet.

16. If required, assist the patient to a standing position and in getting dressed. Provide extra tissues to the patient, if required, for additional cleansing of the anal region.

17. Tell the patient of any special instructions, if the patient is free to leave after getting dressed, or if the physician wishes to speak further to the patient in the office. Inquire if the patient has any questions, (see No. 12, p. 308).

18. If your assistance is not required, leave the patient to dress in private.

19. On returning to the examining room, assemble all used equipment and supplies to be disposed of properly.

20. Replace clean equipment as needed.

21. Clean the examination table and put on a fresh cover.

22. If smears or cultures were obtained, send them to the laboratory or place them in a refrigerator or a cool, dark place until you can transfer them to the laboratory.

23. Wash your hands.

24. Do any recording required of you completely and accurately (see No. 15, p. 308).

Rationale

If you do not have to assist the physician, give your attention to the patient. Provide support and observe for any unusual reaction, such as a feeling of weakness, a change in skin color, or facial grimace, which may be an indication of pain.

You may use tissues, or the small towel under the patients buttocks, which is then removed.

Frequently it is desirable to allow the patient to remain lying down for a few minutes.

Always provide for the comfort and welfare of the patient at the conclusion of an examination.

Always provide complete and accurate information.
Refer the patient's questions to the physician if you cannot answer them completely and accurately.
Never leave a patient in the examining room wondering if the office visit and examination are completed.

Remove any linens and place in soiled laundry. Place disposable equipment in a covered waste container.
Take instruments to your cleanup area wearing disposable rubber gloves; rinse with cool water. These may be soaked in soap and water until you are ready to prepare them for sterilization (see Chapter 20).

Make sure that specimens are properly labeled and that you have completely filled out the appropriate laboratory request form.

Charting example:
Jan. 27, 19_____, 3PM
Rectal exam done by Dr. Short. No specimens were obtained. Patient complained of a sharp, continuous pain in the anal region when leaving the office and stated will call the doctor if it continues.
Betty Fox, CMA

Endoscopic Examinations: Proctoscopy and Sigmoidoscopy

The purpose of a proctoscopy (prŏk-tŏs′kō-pĭ) and sigmoidoscopy (sig′moi-dos′ko-pe) is to examine the rectum and lower sigmoid colon for possible lesions, tumors, ulcers, polyps, inflammatory conditions, strictures, varicosities, and hemorrhages. Carcinoma will appear as a nodular, often cauliflower-like growth with superficial ulceration. Polyps are recognized easily by their pedicle. In doubtful cases, a biopsy of the growth will be done.

If found early and treated properly, 75% to 80% of all cases of cancer of the rectum and lower bowel can be cured. Most cases occur in individuals 55 to 75 years of age. Bowel cancers tend to grow slowly and are possible to detect at the most curable stage, before symptoms appear. Anyone with a personal or family history of rectal or colon cancer, of polyps in the rectum or colon, or of ulcerative colitis should be examined carefully.

The American Cancer Society recommends that individuals have the following:
- An annual digital rectal examination after the age of 40;
- An annual stool test for occult (hidden) blood after the age of 50 (see Chapter 22);
- A proctosigmoidoscopy examination every 3 to 5 years after the age of 50 (*following* two initial negative examinations that were performed one year apart).

Many physicians also recommend that a sigmoidoscopy be included as part of the annual physical examination for men over the age of 40 because of the relatively high incidence of cancer of the rectum and sigmoid colon in this age group.

A proctosigmoidoscopy takes approximately 10 to 15 minutes and requires special preparation of the patient beforehand.

Check with your physician or agency for specific instructions. It is the medical assistant's responsibility to check that the patient is prepared before the examination begins. Generally the preparation includes:
- A laxative the evening before (type and amount as prescribed by the physician);
- Only liquids for breakfast;
- Tap water or saline enemas until the return is clear, usually 1 hour before the examination.

NOTE: Enemas are usually avoided for patients who have colitis, bleeding from the rectum, or Crohn's disease.

Equipment (Figure 19.17)

Examination table covered with a clean sheet
Patient gown
Drape towel
Drape sheet
Small towel
Small pillow
Place and assemble the following equipment
    from the contents of the rectal diagnostic set
    on a clean drape towel (Figure 19.17):
    Sigmoidoscope with obturator
    Proctoscope with obturator (depending on the
      physician's request)
    Transilluminators (light source)
    Rheostat
    Extension cord
    Insufflator with bulb attachment
    Suction tip for suction machine
    Biopsy forceps (sterile)
    Metal sponge holder

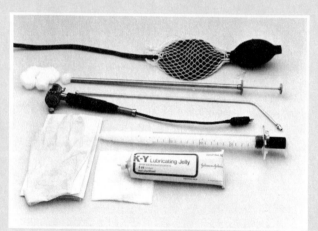

Figure 19.17

Equipment for sigmoidoscopy. *Top to bottom:* Insufflator with bulb attachment, metal sponge holder, suction tip, light source, sigmoidoscope with obturator, disposable gloves, sponges and lubricating jelly. Biopsy forceps may be added when required.

When these have been assembled, add the following:

Rubber gloves
Doctor's gown
Rectal dressing forceps
Cotton-ball sponges
4 × 4 inch gauze
Tissues
Lubricant (K-Y jelly)
Specimen bottle with preservative if biopsy is to be taken
Laboratory request form
Kidney basin
Suction machine

Procedure	Rationale
1. Wash your hands.	
2. Assemble and prepare the necessary equipment and supplies on a clean drape towel.	Disposable scopes may be used instead of the metal ones.
3. Test the suction apparatus and the light on the scopes to make sure that they are working properly.	
4. Identify the patient, and explain the procedure carefully.	This provides the patient with some understanding of the need for the examination and what to expect, that is, what will occur and how it may feel; and it also enables the patient to cooperate more readily and to feel somewhat reassured.
5. Have the patient empty the bladder.	Explain to the patient how to collect a specimen if a urinalysis is to be done. (Refer to Chapter 21 for specimen collection procedure).
6. Have the patient remove all clothing from the waist down and put on the patient gown.	Patient gown should have the opening in the back.
7. Position the patient.	
a. Knee-chest position Many examining rooms have a special proctoscopic table that is tilted in a way that supports the patient in the knee-chest position (see Figures 19.4 and 19.5). Draping remains the same.	This is often preferred as it allows the abdominal contents to fall away from the pelvis, making it easier and less painful for the patient to be examined. NOTE: This is an uncomfortable position and usually cannot be tolerated for a long period.
b. Sims or left lateral position. Position of the patient may vary with the physician's preference.	This may be more comfortable for the patient, depending on age, weight, and condition.
8. Drape the patient completely.	
9. Call the physician into the room.	NOTE: You may call the physician into the room and then position the patient, as this would avoid the necessity of having the patient in an uncomfortable position for an excessive period of time.
10. When the physician is ready to begin the examination, pull the drape sheet back to expose only the anal area.	Avoid exposing the patient unnecessarily.
11. Assist the physician as required. Be prepared to hand the physician the various instruments and equipment.	A female assistant should always remain in the room if the patient is female and the physician is male. (See No. 10, p. 308). If not assisting the physician, give your full attention to the patient. Provide support and reassurance. Observe the patient for any unusual reaction.
12. The physician will begin the examination.	*Method of examination:*
a. Put a generous amount of lubricant on 4 × 4 inch gauze square, and place on the towel with the equipment. Use this for lubricating the instruments and the physician's gloved finger when the examination begins.	The physician will first do a manual rectal examination. A liberal amount of lubricant is applied to the gloved index finger for easier insertion into the anal canal.
b. Warm the metal scopes by placing them in warm water or by rubbing them with your hand. Avoid additional discomfort for the patient that a cold instrument would cause.	This will vary with office or agency preference. Disposable scopes do not need to be warmed.
c. Hand the physician the scope. Attach the inflation bulb to the scope.	The physician or you then lubricates the distal end of the scope with the obturator in place.

Continued.

Endoscopic Examinations: Proctoscopy and Sigmoidoscopy—cont'd

Procedure	Rationale
d. To help the patient relax the anal sphincter for easier insertion of the scope, instruct the patient to bear down slightly, as though having a bowel movement at the time when the physician inserts the scope. Also, instruct the patient to take deep breaths through the mouth, as this also helps relax the anus and rectum.	If right-handed, the physician will separate the buttocks with the left hand, and then slowly and gently insert the scope about 3 cm to 4 cm. Force is *never* used when inserting the scope, as injury to the bowel must be avoided. The obturator is removed and can be placed in the kidney basin.
e. Attach the light source to the scope and adjust the light to the proper intensity. NOTE: You may turn off the lights in the room when the physician begins the visual examination through the scope. This allows for better inspection.	The physician will visually inspect the bowel as he or she advances the scope to its full length. Complete inspection and observation of the bowel will be performed.
f. Observe the patient throughout the procedure for fatigue, weakness, or fainting.	Next, the physician pumps the inflator bulb attachment slowly to inject a small amount of air into the bowel. Although this is quite painful for the patient, it is necessary for proper inspection of the bowel. NOTE: This step is omitted in cases of ulcerative colitis or diverticulitis, because of the fragility of the bowel.
g. Turn on the suction machine if it is to be used.	When there is bleeding or loose discharge in the bowel, the physician may place a long metal sponge holder with a sponge through the scope, to swab the area clean, or the suction tip may be used.
h. You may hand the biopsy forceps to the physician.	A biopsy forcep will be placed through the scope if a biopsy is required.
i. Have ready a labeled specimen jar.	When a specimen is obtained, it should be placed immediately into a labeled specimen jar.
j. Continue to offer reassurance and support to the patient. Frequently, just placing your hand on the patient's shoulder, arm, or hand gives the patient a feeling of being cared for as an individual.	On completing the examination, the physician will remove the scope slowly, which may then be placed in the kidney basin.
13. At the completion of the examination, take tissues and wipe the anal area for any lubricant and/or body discharge.	Provide for the patient's comfort.
14. Help the patient assume a supine position.	Frequently, it is desirable to allow the patient to rest for a few minutes before getting up, as he may feel faint.
15. Remove the drape sheet.	
16. When required, help the patient get up and get dressed. Provide the patient with extra tissues to cleanse the anal region more completely.	Always provide for the safety and comfort of the patient.
17. Inform the patient of any special instructions. Inquire if the patient has any questions (see No. 12, p. 308).	Provide complete and accurate information. Never leave a patient alone in a room after an examination without an understanding of what is to be done after getting dressed.
18. If your assistance is not required, leave the patient to dress in privacy.	
19. If specimens were obtained, send them to the laboratory.	Be sure that all specimens are properly labeled and sent to the laboratory with the correct requisition form.
20. Return to the examining room to assemble all used equipment and supplies.	Remove linens and place in soiled laundry. Disposable equipment should be removed and placed in a covered waste container. Take the instruments to your cleanup area. Wearing disposable rubber gloves, rinse thoroughly with running water. You may then soak the instruments in soap and water until you are ready to prepare them for sterilization. NOTE: Do not soak the light attachment for the scope; cleanse it thoroughly with an alcohol sponge.
21. Wash the examination table with a disinfectant solution, and cover with a clean sheet of paper.	Prepare the examination room for the next patient.
22. Replace clean equipment as needed.	
23. Wash your hands.	
24. Do any recording required of you completely and accurately (see No. 15, p. 308).	Charting example: Jan. 29, 19_____, 1:15 PM Sigmoidoscopy done by Dr. Short. Tissue biopsy sent with requisition to laboratory. Gary Greaves, CMA

Figure 19.18
Evaluation for sensation and superficial pain using the sharp point of a safety pin.

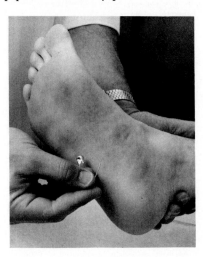

Figure 19.19
Alternate use of the dull end of the pin for evaluation of sensation and pain.

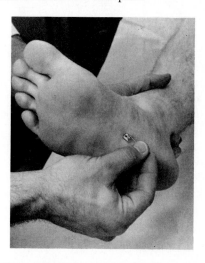

OTHER SPECIAL EXAMINATIONS

Numerous other special or more specific examinations may be performed to gain pertinent information about a body part or system.

Neurological examination

The neurological examination tests for adequate functioning of the cranial nerves, the motor and sensory systems, and the superficial and deep tendon reflexes.

Equipment and supplies
- Pins and cotton to test the senses of touch, sensation, and pain on the external surfaces of the body (Figures 19.18, 19.19, 19.20)
- Tuning fork to test hearing
- Ophthalmoscope to examine the interior of the eye
- Flashlight to test pupil reactions and equality
- Tongue depressor to test the gag and corneal reflexes and pharyngeal sensation
- Percussion hammer to test superficial and deep tendon reflexes
- Test tubes with hot and cold water to test the skin for heat and cold sensation
- Bottles of sweet, bitter, salty, and sour solutions to test the sense of taste
- Bottles of substances that have common familiar odors to test the sense of smell

The physician also observes the patient's level of consciousness, behavior, and the higher functions of speech and writing. Coordination, balance, gait, muscle tone, and strength will be noted for adequate functioning of the motor system. The senses

Figure 19.20
Test of light touch sensation using cotton applied to stimulate the sensory nerve endings.

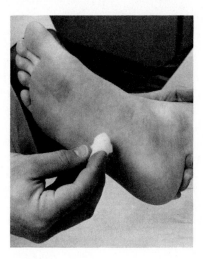

of touch, pain—deep and superficial—and temperature and discriminatory sensations are noted in the examination of the sensory system.

Hearing examination

To detect impaired hearing, the physician will use an otoscope to inspect the external ear canal and the eardrum and a tuning fork to test for hearing acuity.

The tuning fork is used to determine the distance at which the patient can hear a certain sound (air conduction test) and for bone conduction tests. In the bone conduction test, the vibrating end of the tuning fork is placed on the patient's skull. This test is valuable in distinguishing between perceptive and transmission deafness.

A more accurate test to gauge and record hearing is done with the use of an audiometer, a delicate instrument consisting of complex parts. For audiometry the patient is placed in a soundproof room and puts on earphones. Timing circuits, sound wave generators, and other complex pieces of equipment are used to measure the patient's acuity of hearing for the various frequencies of sound waves. Results are plotted on a graph called an audiogram. No special preparation of the patient is required for this test. Physicians, audiometric technicians, or other specially trained individuals will perform this test.

Eye examinations

External eye examinations

Distance visual acuity. Visual acuity means acuteness or clearness of vision. This may be measured on patients having complete physical examinations but more specifically is measured on patients having a specific visual complaint. Visual acuity is also measured on some patients because of employment requirements or for meeting the requirements established by the Department of Motor Vehicles for obtaining specific types of drivers' licenses, such as a chauffeur's or truck driver's license. The visual acuity test is also performed in schools and on preschool-aged children as a means of vision screening. Imperfect refractive powers of the eye such as myopia (nearsightedness), hyperopia (farsightedness), and astigmatism (another refractive error of the eye resulting from irregularities in the curvature of the cornea and/or surfaces of the lens of the eye) can be detected by using the Snellen eye chart to measure distance visual acuity. The Snellen eye chart consists of varied-sized block letters arranged in rows in gradually decreasing sizes. Another chart used for preschoolers, individuals unable to speak English, slow learners, and those unable to read is the "E" chart, which consists of the letter *E* arranged in different directions in decreasing sizes (Figure 19.21). Charts with pictures of common objects, such as a house and a truck, are available to use when testing preschoolers, although some children are unable to identify the objects because of a lack of knowledge rather than a defect in visual acuity. On the Snellen chart there are two standardized numbers to the side of each row of letters; these numbers, shown one on top of the

other, indicate the degree of visual acuity measured from a distance of 20 feet, the standard testing distance. The top number is 20, indicating the number of feet between the chart and the person taking the test; the bottom number indicates the distance in feet from which the normal eye can read the row of letters. The large letter on the top of the chart can be read by the normal eye at a distance of 200 feet. This is indicated as 20/200. In each of the succeeding rows, from top to bottom, the size of the letters decreases to where the normal eye can read the row of letters at distances of 100, 70, 50, 40, 30, 25, 20, 15, 13, and 10 feet. The row marked 20/20 indicates normal visual acuity and is expressed as 20/20 vision. A measurement of visual acuity of less than 20/20 vision is an indication of a refractive error or some other eye disorder. When the letters on the row marked 20/50 are read, the person is said to have 20/50 vision, and so on. This means that the person can read at only 20 feet what the normal eye can read at 50 feet. The larger the bottom number of the row read, the poorer the vision is. A reading of 20/15 indicates above-average distance vision (Figure 19.21, *A* and *B*). This test is to be given in a well-lighted room with the person taking the test standing or sitting 20 feet away from the chart, with the chart placed at eye level to the person. Each eye is to be tested separately, with and without glasses or contact lenses. However, reading glasses should not be worn during the test, as they tend to blur distance vision. The results must be recorded indicating the reading for each eye without and with glasses or contact lenses. Both eyes are not usually tested together, because the stronger eye will usually compensate for the weaker eye.

Patients who are unable to see even the largest numbers on the Snellen chart (top line 20/200) are given additional tests to determine if they can see enough to count fingers (this is recorded as C.F.), perceive hand movements (H.M.), perceive light (L.P.), or perceive light with projection (L.P.cP.). N.L.P. is used to record "no light projection." An ophthalmologist considers patients to be blind when they cannot even perceive light. Legal blindness is defined as vision of 20/200 or less in both eyes when wearing correction glasses.

There are also electric testing devices on the market, such as the Titmus II Vision Tester, which is the product of advances in computer-designed optics (Figure 19.22). This compact instrument, using eight test slides, can screen patients of all ages (preschool through adults) for *all* common vision problems—problems that the standard wall chart

Figure 19.21
A, Snellen eye chart consisting of varied-sized letters arranged in rows in gradually decreasing sizes. **B,** Snellen "Big E" eye chart consisting of the letter "E" arranged in different directions in decreasing sizes.

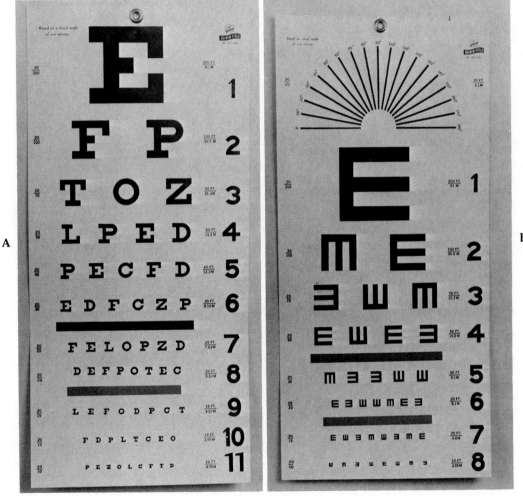

Figure 19.22
Titmus II Vision Tester.
Courtesy Titmus Optical, Inc, Petersburg, Va.

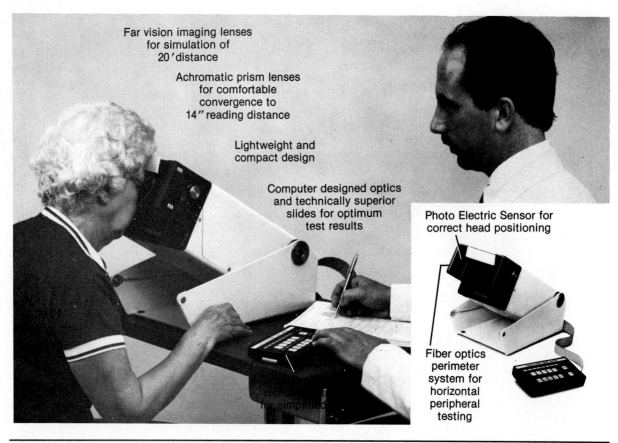

misses. The Titmus II Vision Tester measures acuity (both far and near), hyperopia, binocularity, muscle balance, color perception, depth perception, and, with the optional equipment, peripheral vision and intermediate vision, all within five minutes. The standard wall chart measures only distance vision. The fiber optics perimeter system determines if peripheral vision is adequate, a basic requirement for employees who operate machinery and mobile equipment. The intermediate distance feature tests the intermediate distance (20-40 inches) viewing capabilities important to machine workers and to the increasing number of video display terminal operators. Because of its extremely compact and lightweight design, the Titmus II Vision Tester can be used virtually anywhere. It is especially convenient when performing vision screening tests on large groups or in small areas where space is less than 20 feet. Only five square feet of space is required for using this instrument. Patients of all ages and statures can be easily screened because of the unit's balanced height adjustment. The

unit's face mask, in addition to eliminating outside light, is designed to accommodate all sizes and types of eyeglasses. A training manual, complete with an instructional cassette supplied as standard equipment, provides correct testing techniques that are easy to learn. The Titmus II Vision Tester is a complete system for all vision screening in each individual office situation.

Visual fields. The patient will be asked to look directly at a central point, then the extent of peripheral and side vision is spot checked with an instrument called a perimeter. A target screen method may also be used. The patient is asked to focus on a small target that is moved to different points on a screen. The patient has a visual field defect in the areas in which the target cannot be seen.

Color vision. The patient will be asked to identify colored figures and numbers on a color plate from a standardized distance, usually 75 cm.

Refraction. The physician will instill atropine drops (or any mydriatic, a drug used to dilate the

Measuring Distance Visual Acuity Using the Snellen Chart

Equipment

Snellen eye chart   Pen
Opaque card or eye cover   Paper

Procedure

1. Wash your hands.
2. Prepare the room; determine a distance 20 feet from the point at which the chart will be posted to the point at which the patient will be positioned.
3. Assemble supplies and equipment.
4. Identify the patient and explain the procedure. Do not allow time for the patient to study and memorize the chart before the examination begins.
5. Position the patient comfortably, either standing or sitting, 20 feet from the location of the chart.
6. Position the center of the Snellen eye chart at eye level to the patient.
7. Provide the patient with the opaque card or eye cover. Instruct the patient to cover the left eye with the card, and to keep the left eye open at all times.
8. Instruct the patient to use the right eye and to verbally identify the letters as you point to each row. Start at row 20/70 (or a row several rows above the 20/20 row). (Figure 19.23).

Rationale

When this test is used frequently, this distance can be permanently marked to save time.

Explanations help the patient to feel comfortable and more relaxed, in addition to gaining the patient's confidence as you proceed with the examination.
Twenty feet is the standard testing distance.

To position the chart correctly, the patient must first be positioned.
The right eye (OD) is traditionally tested first. The hand or fingers are not to be used to cover the eye not being tested.
The patient is to read as many letters as possible in the rows as you point to them. Starting with row 20/70, which has larger letters than those on row 20/20, allows the patient to gain confidence in identifying the letters.

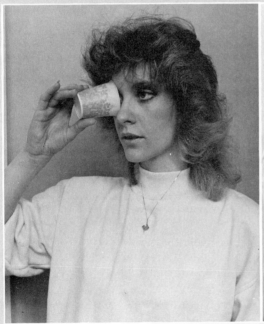
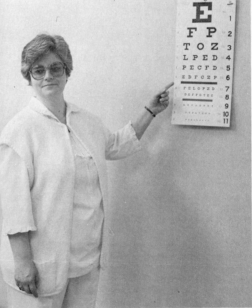

Figure 19.23
Using the Snellen chart for distance visual acuity testing.

9. As the patient identifies the letters in the first row that you point to, proceed down the chart until the patient has identified as many rows of letters as possible. If the patient is unable to identify row 20/70, proceed up the chart having the patient identify the rows of letters until the smallest row of letters is identified.

To obtain the correct visual acuity measurement, the patient is to identify the smallest letters possible.

Continued.

Measuring Distance Visual Acuity Using the Snellen Chart—cont'd

Procedure	Rationale
10. Provide instructions to the patient during the test, such as what line to read and not to squint. Observe the patient for any unusual reactions, such as tearing in the eyes, blinking, squinting, or leaning forward to read the chart.	These reactions may indicate that the patient is experiencing difficulty with the test and must be recorded.
11. Continue testing until the smallest line of letters that the patient can read is reached, or until a letter is misread.	
12. Record the results of visual acuity of the right eye on a piece of paper.	It is important to write the results down when determined so that errors are avoided when charting the results on the patient's record.
13. Instruct the patient to cover the right eye with the opaque card or eye cover and keep the eye open (Figure 19.23).	
14. Measure the visual acuity of the left eye (OS) using the method described in steps 8 through 12.	
15. Give further instructions to the patient as required.	
16. Replace equipment and leave the room neat and clean.	

17. Record the results for each eye on the patient's chart using proper medical abbreviations. When one or two letters are missed or misread in a row, the results are recorded with a minus sign and the number of letters missed or misread next to the bottom number. That is, if the patient identified the rows of letters down to row 20/25 and could not read two letters in this row, you would record this result as 20/25-2. Record as sc (without correction) when the patient isn't wearing glasses or contact lenses, and cc (with correction) when the patient is wearing glasses or contact lenses.	Charting example:
	  Oct. 31, 19_____, 5 PM
	  Snellen chart eye test given. Results without glasses:
	    OD20/20
	    OS 20/15-2
	      H. McMullen, CMA

eyes) into the eye. With the use of these drops, the lens of the eye is unable to accommodate, thus allowing the physician to determine eye function when the lens is at rest.

Internal eye examinations

Ophthalmoscopic examination. With the use of the ophthalmoscope, the physician examines the anterior chamber, the lens, the vitreous body, and the retina of the eye. When using the ophthalmoscope, the physician may want the room darkened, as this causes the pupils to dilate and thus aids the examination. Visualization of the retina with the ophthalmoscope is known as funduscopic examination.

Tonometry. After the instillation of a local anesthetic into the eye, a tonometer is gently rested on the eyeball to measure the tension of the eyeball and intraocular pressure. This is an important test to determine the presence of an eye condition termed *glaucoma,* in which the pressure within the eyeball is increased. Glaucoma is the most common cause of blindness in adults. A normal tonometry reading is 11 to 22 mm Hg. A reading of 24 to 32 mm Hg suggests glaucoma.

Obstetrical examinations

After pregnancy has been confirmed, monitoring both the physical well-being of mother and fetus and the progress of the pregnancy is highly recommended and considered vital by some. The initial physical examination of the pregnant woman will include the following:

- Weight—the ideal weight gain during pregnancy is considered by most to be 22 to 26 pounds. Excessive weight gain or loss is an important symptom and requires further follow-up.
- Blood pressure—any rise in blood pressure is cause for concern.
- Urinalysis—a complete urinalysis, then on subsequent visits the urine will be tested for sugar and albumin. Glucose levels are normally lower during pregnancy; any sign of albumin in the urine must be reported immediately, as this is considered an early warning sign of toxemia.
- Blood tests—these include a complete blood count (CBC), blood typing and cross-matching, and an automated reagent test (ART) to

test for syphilis. If the ART results are positive, a venereal disease research laboratory (VDRL) or fluorescent treponemal antibody (FTA) test will be performed to confirm the first positive results. A rubella titer to determine if the patient has immunity to rubella (German measles) is also done.

- Patient history—family history, past medical history, personal history of the present pregnancy, that is, date of last menstrual period (LMP), symptoms, and estimated date of birth.
- Physical examination—have the patient empty her bladder before the examination. Palpation and auscultation of the abdomen are done to determine the size and position of the fetus and to listen to the fetal heart rate. During a pelvic examination, an estimation of pelvic measurement is made to determine a difficult delivery in cases of cephalopelvic disproportion. A vaginal examination will be done to check the birth canal for any abnormalities, obtain further pelvic measurements, obtain a Pap smear and usually a culture for gonorrhea.

On subsequent visits the weight, blood pressure, urine testing for sugar and albumin, CBC (when deemed necessary), and auscultation and palpation of the abdomen are continually monitored. The vaginal examination is done only periodically to check the progress of the pregnancy.

All visits should also include educating the mother in healthful living habits and various aspects of her pregnancy, as education is an integral part of antepartum care.

Figure 19.24
How to examine your breast.
Courtesy California Div, Inc, of the American Cancer Society.

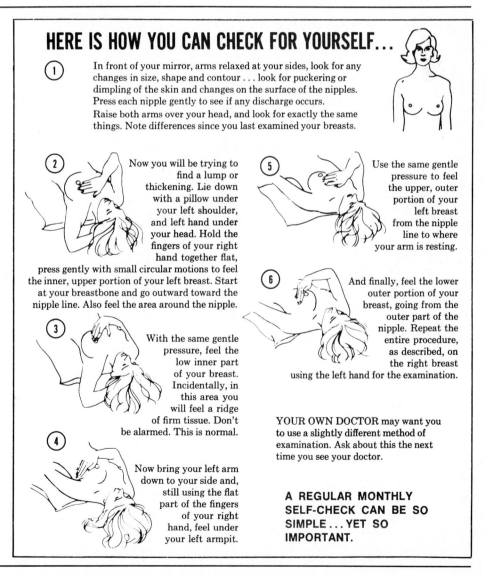

HERE IS HOW YOU CAN CHECK FOR YOURSELF...

① In front of your mirror, arms relaxed at your sides, look for any changes in size, shape and contour . . . look for puckering or dimpling of the skin and changes on the surface of the nipples. Press each nipple gently to see if any discharge occurs.
Raise both arms over your head, and look for exactly the same things. Note differences since you last examined your breasts.

② Now you will be trying to find a lump or thickening. Lie down with a pillow under your left shoulder, and left hand under your head. Hold the fingers of your right hand together flat, press gently with small circular motions to feel the inner, upper portion of your left breast. Start at your breastbone and go outward toward the nipple line. Also feel the area around the nipple.

③ With the same gentle pressure, feel the low inner part of your breast. Incidentally, in this area you will feel a ridge of firm tissue. Don't be alarmed. This is normal.

④ Now bring your left arm down to your side and, still using the flat part of the fingers of your right hand, feel under your left armpit.

⑤ Use the same gentle pressure to feel the upper, outer portion of your left breast from the nipple line to where your arm is resting.

⑥ And finally, feel the lower outer portion of your breast, going from the outer part of the nipple. Repeat the entire procedure, as described, on the right breast using the left hand for the examination.

YOUR OWN DOCTOR may want you to use a slightly different method of examination. Ask about this the next time you see your doctor.

A REGULAR MONTHLY SELF-CHECK CAN BE SO SIMPLE . . . YET SO IMPORTANT.

Figure 19.25
Cancer-related checkups.
Courtesy American Cancer Society,
New York, NY.

GUIDELINES
For the early detection of cancer in people without symptoms
TALK WITH YOUR DOCTOR
Ask how these guidelines relate to you.

AGE 20-40	AGE 40 & OVER
CANCER-RELATED CHECKUP EVERY 3 YEARS	**CANCER-RELATED CHECKUP EVERY 3 YEARS**
Should include the procedures listed below plus health counseling (such as tips on quitting tobacco use) and examinations for cancers of the thyroid, testes, prostate, mouth, ovaries, skin and lymph nodes. Some people are at higher risk for certain cancers and may need to have tests more frequently.	Should include the procedures listed below plus health counseling (such as tips on quitting tobacco use) and examinations for cancers of the thyroid, testes, prostate, mouth, ovaries, skin and lymph nodes. Some people are at higher risk for certain cancers and may need to have tests more frequently.

AGE 20-40

BREAST
- Exam by doctor every 3 years
- Self-exam every month
- One baseline breast x-ray between ages 35-39.
  > Higher Risk for Breast Cancer: Personal or family history of breast cancer, never had children, first child after 30

UTERUS
- Pelvic exam every 3 years

Cervix
- All women who are, or have been sexually active, or have reached age 18 years, have an annual Pap test and pelvic examination. After three or more consecutive satisfactory normal annual examinations, the Pap test may be performed less frequently at the discretion of her physician.
  > Higher Risk for Cervical Cancer: Early age at first intercourse, multiple sex partners

Remember, these guidelines are not rules and only apply to people without symptoms. If you have any of the Seven Warning Signals listed on the back, see your doctor or go to your clinic without delay.

AGE 40 & OVER

BREAST
- Exam by doctor every year
- Self-exam every month
- Breast x-ray every year after 50; between ages 40-49, 1 every 1-2 years as recommended.
  > Higher Risk for Breast Cancer: Personal or family history of breast cancer, never had children, first child after 30

UTERUS
- Pelvic exam every 3 years

Cervix
- All women who are, or have been sexually active, or have reached age 18 years, have an annual Pap test and pelvic examination. After three or more consecutive satisfactory normal annual examinations, the Pap test may be performed less frequently at the discretion of her physician.
  > Higher Risk for Cervical Cancer: Early age at first intercourse, multiple sex partners

Endometrium
- Endometrium tissue sample at menopause if at risk
  > Higher Risk for Endometrial Cancer: Infertility, obesity, failure of ovulation, abnormal uterine bleeding, estrogen therapy

COLON & RECTUM
- Digital rectal exam every year
- Stool slide test every year after 50
- Procto exam—**after 2 initial negative tests 1 year apart**—every 3 to 5 years after 50
  > Higher Risk for Colorectal Cancer: Personal or family history of colon or rectal cancer, personal or family history of polyps in the colon or rectum, ulcerative colitis

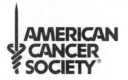

AMERICAN CANCER SOCIETY®

Breast self-examination

Generally, the physician will examine the patient's breasts at each physical examination. During the time that individuals are unattended by a physician, they should examine their own breasts to detect any abnormality, which can be brought to the physician's attention immediately. The following information is supplied to the public for their general information by the American Cancer Society.

Why you should examine your breasts monthly. Most breast cancers are first discovered by women themselves. Since breast cancers found early and treated promptly have excellent chances for cure, learning how to examine your breasts properly can help save your life. Use the simple 6 step breast self-examination (BSE) procedure shown in Figure 19.24.

For the best time to examine your breasts. Follow the same procedure once a month about a week after your period, when breasts are usually not tender or swollen. After menopause, check breasts on the first day of each month. After hysterectomy, check your doctor or clinic for an appropriate time of the month. Doing BSE will give you monthly peace of mind and seeing your doctor once a year will reassure you there is nothing wrong.

What you should do if you find a lump or thickening. If a lump or dimple or discharge is discovered during BSE, it is important to see your doctor as soon as possible. Don't be frightened. Most breast lumps or changes are not cancer, but only your doctor can make the diagnosis.

Know cancer's warning signals!

C Change in bowel or bladder habits
A A sore that does not heal
U Unusual bleeding or discharge
T Thickening or lump in breast or elsewhere
I Indigestion or difficulty in swallowing
O Obvious change in wart or mole
N Nagging cough or hoarseness
   IF YOU HAVE A WARNING SIGNAL, SEE YOUR DOCTOR.

The medical assistant should see that the office or clinic has literature for women on this subject in addition to the information given in Figure 19.25. (See also "Mammography" in Chapter 27.)

Conclusion

You have now completed the chapter on assisting with physical examinations. After you have practiced the procedures and are ready to demonstrate your skills and knowledge attained, arrange with your instructor to take a performance test. You will be expected to demonstrate accurately your ability in preparing for and assisting with the procedures and examinations discussed in this chapter and to measure a patient's distance visual acuity. In addition, you will be expected to identify by name the equipment and instruments used for each examination if and when you are questioned by your instructor.

Review Questions

1. List and summarize the medical assistant's general responsibilities when assisting the physician with a complete physical examination.
2. Indicate what body part or system is examined with the following instruments:
   a. Otoscope
   b. Laryngeal mirror
   c. Ophthalmoscope
   d. Anoscope
   e. Tuning fork
   f. Bronchoscope
   g. Cystoscope
   h. Percussion hammer
   i. Stethoscope
3. In what position is the patient placed for the following:
   a. A vaginal or pelvic examination?
   b. A rectal examination and proctosigmoidoscopy?
   c. A chest examination?
   d. An examination of the ears and eyes?
4. List the purpose(s) and the common instruments required for the following examinations:
   a. General physical examination
   b. Vaginal examination
   c. Pap smear or test
   d. Rectal examination
   e. Proctosigmoidoscopy
5. If a physician suspects a growth in the sigmoid colon that is considered doubtful as to being benign or malignant, what procedure will the physician usually perform?
6. You have a 50-year-old obese patient who cannot tolerate the jackknife position for a sigmoidoscopy. Name an alternate position that may be used for this examination.
7. Explain why it is important for a female assistant to remain in the room when a female patient is being examined by a male physician.
8. Explain why it is important that you check battery-operated and electrical equipment before an examination.
9. What is a Snellen chart, and how is it used?
10. When is the best time of the month for a woman to examine her breasts for any unusual lump or thickening? Explain how a woman performs a breast self-examination.

SUGGESTED READINGS

Hirsh R: Can your examining rooms pass this test? Med Econ June 13, 1977, p 191.

Hirsh R: Can your office soundproofing pass this test? Med Econ June 27, 1977, p 131.

Oppenheim M: Suppose you were getting that physical exam, Med Econ June 13, 1977, p 249.

Chapter 20

Infection Control: Practices of Medical Asepsis and Sterilization

- Basic concepts and goals
- Infectious process and causative agents
- The body's defenses against disease and infection
- Infection control
- Methods to control microscopic agents

Objectives

On completion of Chapter 20 the medical assistant student should be able to:

1 Define and pronounce the terms presented in the vocabulary and throughout the chapter.

2 List the five classifications of microorganisms that are capable of causing a disease process, giving examples of diseases caused by each.

3 List the six factors that are essential for the development of an infectious process, discussing briefly components of each.

4 List and describe the body's natural defense mechanisms used to control or prevent disease and infection.

5 Discuss and compare the various types of immunity.

6 List the classical signs and symptoms of inflammation and briefly describe the inflammatory process.

7 Differentiate between medical and surgical asepsis; list and describe procedures used to accomplish each and medical situations in which each is employed.

8 Differentiate between sanitization, disinfection, and sterilization; describe and demonstrate the procedures employed by these methods when working with contaminated instruments, syringes and needles, rubber goods, and other equipment, selecting the most effective method for controlling microscopic agents.

9 Describe and demonstrate how items are to be wrapped, positioned, and removed from a sterilizer for sterilization to be effective, and how items are to be positioned and removed from a boiler.

10 Demonstrate how to wash hands, wrists, and forearms, explaining the reasons for the actions taken.

11 Given packs that have been removed from an autoclave, determine if sterilization has been effective and then store each for use at a later date.

12 Discuss the causes of inefficient sterilization of supplies.

13 Discuss and apply the principles of the universal blood and body substance precautions.

Vocabulary

antiseptic (an′tĭ-sep′tik) A substance capable of inhibiting the growth or action of microorganisms without necessarily killing them; generally safe for use on body tissues.

asepsis (ā-sep′sis) The absence of all microorganisms causing disease; absence of contaminated matter.

bactericide (bak-tēr′ĭ-sīd) A substance capable of destroying bacteria but not spores.

bacteriostatic (bak-te″re-o-stat′ik) A substance that inhibits the growth of bacteria.

contaminated, contamination (kon-tam″ĭ-na′shun) The act of making unclean, soiling, or staining, especially the introduction of disease germs or infectious material into or on normally sterile objects.

decontaminate To remove infectious agents from body surfaces or from inanimate surfaces or articles. Decontamination is the process which renders an item safe for handling.

disinfectant (dis″in-fek′tant) A substance capable of destroying pathogens, but usually not spores; generally not intended for use on body tissue, because it is too strong.

fungicide (fun′jĭ-sīd) A substance that destroys fungi.

germicide (jer′mĭ-sīd) A substance that is capable of destroying pathogens.

immunization (im″u-nĭ-za′shun) The process of rendering a person immune (protected from or not susceptible to a disease) or of becoming immune; frequently called vaccination or inoculation. A process by which a person is artificially prepared to resist infection by a specific pathogen.

incubation (in″ku-ba′shun) period The interval of time between the invasion of a pathogen into the body and the appearance of the first symptoms of disease.

infection (in-fek′shun) A condition caused by the multiplication of pathogenic microorganisms that have invaded the body of a susceptible host.

acute rapid onset, severe symptoms, and usually subsides within a relatively short period of time.

chronic develops slowly, milder symptoms, and lasts for a long period of time.

latent dormant or concealed; pathogen is ever-present in the host, but symptoms are present only intermittently, often in response to a stimulus. At other times the pathogen is dormant.

localized restricted to a certain area.

generalized systemic; involving the whole body.

medical microbiology The study and identification of pathogens, and the development of effective methods for their control or elimination.

necrosis (ne-kro′-sis) The death of a cell or group of cells because of injury or disease.

normal flora Microorganisms that normally reside in various body locations such as in the vagina, intestine, urethra, upper respiratory tract, and on the skin. These microorganisms are nonpathogenic and do not cause any harm (they may become pathogenic and cause harm if they are introduced into a body area in which they do not normally reside).

pathogenic (păth″ō-jĕn′ĭk) Productive of disease.

pathogenic microorganism A microorganism that produces disease in the body.

reservoir (rez′er-vwar) The source in which pathogenic microorganisms grow and from which they leave to spread and cause disease.

resistance (re-zis′tans) The ability of the body to resist disease or infection with its own defense mechanisms.

sepsis (sep′sis) A morbid state or condition resulting from the presence of pathogenic microorganisms.

spore (spōr) A reproductive cell, usually unicellular, produced by plants and some protozoa and possessing thick walls to withstand unfavorable environmental conditions. Bacterial spores are very resistant to heat and must undergo prolonged exposure to very high temperatures to be destroyed.

sterile (ster′il) Free from all microorganisms.

toxin (tok′sin) A poisonous substance produced by pathogenic bacteria and some animals and plants. The toxins produced by bacteria include toxic enzymes, exotoxins, and endotoxins. Toxins in the body cause antitoxins to form, which provide a means for establishing immunity to certain diseases.

vaccination (vak″sĭ-na′shun) The introduction of weakened or dead microorganisms (inoculation) into the body to stimulate

the production of antibodies and immunity to a specific disease.

virulence (vir′u-lens) The degree of ability of a pathogen to produce disease.

BASIC CONCEPTS AND GOALS

Since the early days of civilization there has been concern with the control of disease and the spread of infection. The history of medicine documents the wealth of knowledge attained by numerous individuals on the anatomy and physiology of the human body, certain diseases, and many therapeutic agents. Not until the last half of the nineteenth century was a connection between disease and pathogenic microorganisms established through the work of Louis Pasteur and Robert Koch. Among things documented, Pasteur discovered important properties of bacteria, and Koch was credited with establishing the germ theory of disease. Koch's theory states that to prove an organism is actually the specific pathogen causing the disease, one must establish a causal relationship between the microbe and the disease.

Microorganisms (microbes) are defined as minute living creatures that are too small to be seen by the naked eye. The classifications or divisions of microscopic life include viruses, rickettsiae, bacteria, fungi, and parasites. Microorganisms in each of these divisions that cause disease are termed *pathogens*. It is important to keep in mind that many members of these microscopic divisions are either beneficial or harmless to humans or animals. The term *medical microbiology* implies the study of pathogens and involves identification and development of effective methods of control or elimination.

Pathogenic microorganisms are everywhere around us. They are easily spread directly from person to person or indirectly by animate and inanimate vehicles to humans. Disease or infection transpires when pathogens invade a susceptible host. Although we have antibiotics for use in the treatment of many infectious processes, the best method available for infection control is to prevent the spread of disease-producing microorganisms. It is our responsibility as health professionals to take an active, conscientious role in the process of infection control. Lack of knowledge as to how pathogens spread or how to control the process is frequently the cause of major outbreaks of infection or disease. The goals of infection control are to prevent the spread of pathogenic microorganisms, to attain a state of asepsis (absence of pathogens), and to educate the public in ways that they too can

help. Asepsis, or aseptic technique, is divided into two categories: medical asepsis and surgical asepsis. It is important to distinguish between these two methods.

The rest of this chapter discusses disease-producing organisms, how they are spread, the body's own defense mechanisms, infection control precautions, and medical and surgical asepsis with techniques and sterilization procedures used to prevent transmission of pathogens. Surgical asepsis (aseptic technique) is discussed in greater length in Chapter 21.

INFECTIOUS PROCESS AND CAUSATIVE AGENTS

Six factors are essential for the development of the infectious process. The mere presence of a pathogenic organism is not enough to promote infection. There must be a sequential connection between the following factors:

1. A cause or an etiological (e-tē-o-loj′ik-ăl) agent (pathogen);
2. A source or a reservoir of the etiological agent;
3. A means of escape of the etiological agent from the reservoir (portals of exit);
4. A means of transmission of the etiological agent from the reservoir to the new host;
5. A means of entry of the etiological agent into the new susceptible host (portals of entry);
6. A susceptible host.

Cause or Etiological Agent

Infection begins with the invasion of the body by a pathogen that is the causative agent of the disease in question. The pathogenic organisms must be present in a sufficiently high concentration and be adequately capable of causing disease. The causative agent or pathogen may be one or more of the following.

Viruses

Viruses (vī′rŭs) are the smallest pathogens and require susceptible host cells for multiplication and activity.

To observe viruses an electron microscope must be used. A phenomenon that characterizes viral in-

Figure 20.1
Classification of bacteria
according to their
morphology.

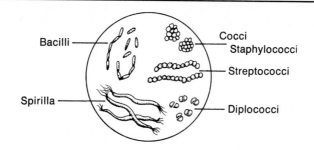

fections as the most insidious is the fact that viruses, as intracellular parasites, can only multiply inside a living cell. Viruses attach themselves to a living cell, inject a compound of protein and a nucleic acid, either DNA (deoxyribonucleic acid) or RNA (ribonucleic acid), and take over the normal cellular metabolism. The cell proceeds to make new cells in addition to new viruses, then bursts, dies, and releases numerous viruses that can then invade other cells. Chemotherapy for viral diseases is extremely difficult, because the viruses surviving an initial dose of a drug have the ability to change their characteristics so that they rapidly become resistant to the drug.

Viruses are also more resistant to chemical disinfection than bacteria, but can be destroyed by heat, as is done when sterilizing equipment in an autoclave.

There is a greater variety of viruses than of any other category of microbial agents of disease. Viruses are the causative agents of flu, poliomyelitis, colds, mumps, measles, rabies, smallpox, chickenpox, as well as hepatitis A, hepatitis B, herpes simplex type 1, and herpes simplex type 2.

Rickettsiae

Rickettsiae (rĭk-ĕt′sē-ă) are also obligate intracellular parasites. They differ from viruses in that they are visible under a conventional microscope by special staining techniques and are also susceptible to antibiotic suppression of replication.

Rickettsiae are the causative organisms for the various "spotted fevers," such as Rocky Mountain spotted fever, and also typhus, Q fever, and trench fever. They are generally tick-borne and therefore are not common in sanitary urban areas.

Bacteria

Bacteria (bak-te′re-ah) can readily multiply outside of living cells. Bacteria are single-celled organisms that can be cultivated on artificial media and then, with appropriate staining techniques, be made readily visible under a microscope. These charac-

teristics make bacteria much simpler to identify than viruses and rickettsiae. There are many varieties, only some of which cause disease; most are nonpathogenic, and many are useful. Bacteria are classified in three groups according to their shape and appearance (morphology) (Figure 20.1).

- Cocci (kok′sē) are spherical bacteria; among the cocci are the following three types:

  Staphylococci (stăf″ĭl-ō-kŏk′sē)—forming grape like clusters of cells, these are the most common pus-producing organisms known to man. They are readily found in pimples, boils, suture abscesses, and osteomyelitis.

  Streptococci (strĕp″tō-kŏk′sē)—forming chains of cells, these are the cause of strep throat, rheumatic heart disease (RHD), scarlet fever, and septicemia (infection in the blood stream).

  Diplococci (dĭp-lō-kok′sē)—forming pairs of cells, different types of diplococci are the causative organisms for gonorrhea, pneumonia, and meningitis.

- Bacilli (bah-sil′i) are rod-shaped bacteria; these organisms cause tuberculosis (TB), typhoid and paratyphoid fever, tetanus (lockjaw), gas gangrene, bacillary dysentery, and diphtheria.

- Spirilla (spi-ril′ah) are spiral organisms; these organisms cause cholera, syphilis, and relapsing fever.

Fungi

Fungi (fun′ji) are the lowest form of infectious agents that bridge the gap between free-living and host-dependent parasites.

Fungi are unicellular or multicellular. They can be grown on artificial media and then identified under the microscope. Fungi appear in the form of molds and mushrooms, as well as in microscopic growth. Disease-producing fungi are seen as the causative agent in some infections of the skin, such as athlete's foot and ringworm.

The fungus *Candida albicans* (Monilia) is responsible for the disease known as thrush (an infection of the mouth and throat) and also some vaginal infections.

Parasites

Parasites (par′ah-sīt) are organisms that live in or on another organism from which they gain their nourishment. Parasites include single-celled and multicelled animals, fungi, and bacteria. Viruses are sometimes considered to be parasitic. Examples include the following:

- Protozoa (pro″to-zo′ah) are single-celled microscopic organisms. Some can be cultivated, fixed, and stained for viewing under a microscope. The most well-known protozoa cause malaria, amebic dysentery, and trichomonas infections of the vagina.
- Metazoal (met″ah-zo′al) parasites are multicellular organisms that cause conditions such as pinworms, hookworms, tapeworms, and trichinosis in pork.
- Ectoparasites (ek″to-par′ah-sīt) can superficially affect the host, like lice and scabies mite, or can invade the integument, such as the larvae of dipterous flies.

Source or Reservoir of Etiological Agent

Areas in which organisms grow and reproduce are called reservoirs and are found mainly in human beings and animals. *Human reservoirs* include the following:

- Overt cases: people who are obviously ill with the disease.
- Subclinical cases: abortive and ambulatory (walking) cases of the disease, for example, "walking" pneumonia.
- Human carriers: people unaware of their condition who circulate freely in their communities until detected and diagnosed, for example, the "Typhoid Marys," or people who are in the convalescent stage of an infection.

Animal reservoirs include mainly domestic animals and rodents. Zoonosis (zo″o-no′sis) is the term given to an animal disease that is transmissible to humans. In this case, the infection is usually derived from the animal and is not further transmitted from human to human. An example is rabies.

Means of Escape of Etiological Agent from Reservoir (Portals of Exit)

Pathogens commonly exit from their reservoir through one or more of the following:

- Respiratory tract in secretions from the nose, nasal sinuses, nasopharynx, larynx, trachea, bronchial tree, and lungs
- Intestinal tract through discharge with the feces
- Urinary tract through discharge or in the urine
- Skin or mucous membranes, or open lesions or discharges on the surface of the body
- Reproductive tract through discharges
- Blood
- Across the placenta

Means of Transmission of Etiological Agent from Reservoir to New Host

The means of transmission is the method by which the pathogen is transmitted from the portal of exit in the reservoir to the portal of entry in the new host. After an infecting organism has escaped from its reservoir, it can cause a new infection only if it finds its way to a new susceptible host. Transmission may occur by either of the following:

- *Direct transmission*—The organism passes from one person to another through inhalation or by actual physical contact, such as sexual contact or direct contact with an open lesion. The organism goes from one host to another without the aid of intermediate objects.
- *Indirect transmission*—The organism is capable of survival for a period of time outside the body and is transferred to the new host by a vehicle, which is either animate or inanimate. Animate vehicles are called vectors and include the various insects that spread infection. Inanimate vehicles are nonliving objects or substances and include water, milk, foods, soil, air, excreta, clothing, instruments, toiletries, or any contaminated article.

Means of Entry of Etiological Agent into New Susceptible Host

The infecting organism enters the new host through a part of the body, which is called the portal of entry. The main portals of entry are as follows:

- Respiratory tract—organisms may be inhaled
- Gastrointestinal tract—organisms may be ingested
- Skin or mucous membranes—organisms may be introduced via cuts, abrasions or open wounds
- Urinary tract—organisms may be introduced through external body orifices
- Reproductive tract—organisms may be introduced through external body orifices

Table 20.1
Factors of infectious process

Disease	Cause/agent	Reservoir/ source	Means of escape from the reservoir	Means of transmission from reservoir to new host	Means of entry into new host	Susceptible host
German measles (rubella)	Virus	Humans	Mouth, na-sopharynx	Water droplets	Mouth	Humans
Pneumonia	Bacteria	Humans	Mouth, na-sopharynx	Droplets, sputum Fomites, such as a pencil (indirect transmission)	Mouth, respira-tory mucosa	Humans

From Zakus SM: Clinical skills and assisting techniques for the medical assistant, ed 2, St Louis, 1988, The CV Mosby Co.

- Blood
- Across the placenta

Although avenues of escape or portals of exit correspond to the portals of entry, the pathogen can escape from one site in the reservoir and enter the new host in another site. An example of this is when the pathogen leaves from the respiratory tract in the reservoir (as through sputum or water droplets) and enters the new host through the skin (as through an open wound when a dressing is being changed).

Susceptible Host

For the infectious process to be completed, the pathogenic organism must enter a host whose resistance is so low that it cannot fight off the invading organism. Even if a pathogen gains entry to the body disease or infection may not develop, since the body possesses certain defense mechanisms to protect itself. These mechanisms may also help destroy invading pathogens. Such defense mechanisms are called resistance, and if they are sufficiently great, they constitute immunity (ĭ-mū′nĭ-tē).

Table 20.1 outlines the six essential factors of the infectious process for two diseases. All infectious diseases can be outlined in this manner.

Stages of an Infectious Process

The stages of an infectious process generally include the following:
1. The invasion and multiplication of the pathogen in the body.
2. The incubation period, which may vary from a few days to months or years.
3. The prodromal period when the first mild signs and symptoms appear. The person is highly contagious during this period.
4. The acute period when signs and symptoms are at the most severe stage.
5. The recovery and convalescent period when signs and symptoms begin to subside and the body heals itself, returning to a state of health.

THE BODY'S DEFENSES AGAINST DISEASE AND INFECTION

The body's resistance level to undesirable microorganisms is influenced by the general health status of the individual and other related circumstances, such as the following:
- Amount of rest, sufficient or insufficient
- Dietary intake of nutritional foods, adequate or inadequate
- How the individual copes with stress
- Age of the individual (the young and aged are most susceptible to infection because of the immaturity of the immune system in the young and the decline of this system in the aged)
- Presence of other disease processes in the body
- Condition of the external environment (such as poor living conditions)
- Influence of genetic traits (for example, people with diabetes mellitus and sickle cell anemia are more prone to some infections than other individuals)

Physical and Chemical Barriers

The body has natural defense mechanisms, either physical or chemical, that act as barriers to the invasion of pathogenic organisms.

Skin

Skin tissue is the largest barrier against infection. As long as it remains intact, the skin serves as a physical barrier to a tremendous number of microorganisms. Chemical barriers of the skin include the acid pH of the skin (which inhibits bacterial infection), sweat, and lysozyme (which functions as an antibacterial enzyme in the skin).

Mucous membrane

Mucous membrane tissue holds in check many microorganisms because of the repelling forces in the secretions that bathe these membranes. The cilia of some mucous membranes serve to keep their surfaces swept clean.

Respiratory tract

The mucosal lining of the respiratory tract is very sensitive and thus readily stimulated by foreign matter. Certain reflexes, such as coughing or sneezing, help remove foreign matter, including microorganisms. The hairs lining the nostrils, along with the moist membranes, serve as a physical barrier. The cilia lining the bronchi beat upward to carry mucus and small, interfering, foreign materials such as dust, bacteria, and soot to the throat. The tortuous passageway from the mouth to the lungs also serves as a barrier.

Gastrointestinal tract

Hydrochloric acid in the stomach has an important bactericidal action, destroying many disease-producing agents. Bile, when in the small intestine, is thought to have a germicidal effect.

Blood and lymphoid tissue

Blood and lymphoid tissue contains and produces cells and antibodies that are able to exert a tremendous influence in protecting the body against disease. White blood cells (leukocytes) are particularly active when pathogenic microorganisms invade the body. In the inflammatory process, some leukocytes surround, engulf, and digest the pathogens. This process is known as phagocytosis (fag"o-si-tō'sis), which is basically the ingestion of the pathogen or "cell-eating." Lymphoid tissue produces antibodies, which are basically protein compounds that help combat infection.

Antigen-Antibody Reaction

Another internal defense mechanism that the body gradually develops against invasion by foreign substances (antigens) is the formation of antibodies.

Antibodies are protein substances produced mainly in the lymph nodes, spleen, bone marrow, and lymphoid tissue in response to invasion by an antigen. Different types of antibodies are produced in response to different antigens, with each antibody being effective only against the specific antigen that stimulates its production. The antibodies can either neutralize the antigens, render them harmless, rupture their cell membranes, or prepare them in a way that makes them more susceptible to destruction by phagocytes (cells that ingest and destroy microorganisms, cells, and cell debris).

The antigen-antibody reaction is the reaction of the body to the invasion of antigens. When antibodies are produced in sufficient quantities, the body becomes immune. Since the body is capable of continuing to produce antibodies for weeks to several years, it is possible for immunity to last for months or years.

Immunity

Immunity, the resistance of the body to pathogenic microorganisms and their toxins, occurs as a result of the antigen-antibody reaction. Specific types of immunity are as follows:
- Active immunity develops when antigens are introduced into the body.
- Passive immunity develops when ready-made antibodies are introduced into the body.
- Natural immunity is an inborn resistance to a disease as a result of antibodies that are normally present in the blood.
- Acquired or induced immunity results from antibodies that are not normally present in the blood.

Both active and passive immunity are produced by natural and acquired means.

Natural immunity

Inherited (active) immunity is acquired by being a member of a race or species. Some races are highly or less susceptible to certain diseases. The longer a race has been exposed to a certain disease, the less susceptible its members become. Humans do not contract many diseases common to lower species of animals, and lower species of animals do not contract most human diseases.

Congenital (passive) immunity is the immunity possessed at birth; antibodies are passed from the mother through the placenta to the fetus. The duration of this immunity may be from 5 to 6 months.

Acquired immunity

Natural active immunity results from being a carrier, recovering from or having a disease, or having an atypical or subclinical case of the disease.

Artificial active immunity is acquired through vaccinations with inactivated (dead) or attenuated (weakened) organisms. Inactivated or dead vaccines include the typhoid, whooping cough, and influenza vaccines, and the Salk vaccine for polio. Attenuated vaccines include vaccines for polio (the Sabin vaccine), smallpox, measles (rubeola), mumps, and German measles (rubella). Toxoids are exotoxins that have been modified to reduce the toxicity. These include the diphtheria and tetanus toxoids.

Artificial passive immunity is obtained by injecting various products, which are usually prepared commercially to produce a high level of antibodies immediately. These products are used to modify, treat, or prevent disease and include gamma globulin and antitoxins.

Gamma globulin, obtained from the blood, is sometimes used for treatment, but is more commonly used for the prevention of viral hepatitis and measles. Antitoxins include the following:

- Diphtheria antitoxin, produced by vaccinating horses and then extracting the gamma globulin fraction of the blood, is used for the immediate prevention and treatment of diphtheria.
- Tetanus antitoxin, obtained by extracting the gamma globulin fraction from the blood of people recently vaccinated with the tetanus toxoid, is used for the immediate prevention and treatment of tetanus.
- Immune sera, either bacterial or viral in origin, are obtained from the gamma globulin fraction of blood from an artificially immunized animal. The rabies immune serum and the pertussis (whooping cough) immune serum are the most commonly used products.

Inflammatory Process

The inflammatory process is a nonspecific defense response of the body to an irritating, invasive, or injurious foreign substance. In other words, it is a process by which the body responds to injury. Acute inflammation is stimulated by necrosis and degeneration of tissue (injuries), invading microorganisms (infection), and antigen-antibody reactions (allergies). The inflammatory process includes dilation of the blood vessels because of increased blood flow, oozing of watery fluids and protein into tissue spaces (exudation) from the dilated blood vessels because of their increased permeability, and infiltration of neutrophils and monocytes (white blood cells) from the blood into the tissue of the injured area to phagocytize (ingest) necrotic tissue and bacteria, if present.

After phagocytosis is complete, the liquified remains diffuse back into the blood vessels or are carried away by the lymphatic vessels that drain into regional lymph nodes. Here the contents are filtered to prevent the spread of foreign substances or bacteria to other parts of the body. By now the process of repair has started at the original site of inflammation. Classical signs and symptoms of inflammation include both local signs and symptoms, which are a result of the changes seen in the blood vessels and the effect on the surrounding tissues, and systemic signs and symptoms. These are as follows:

Local	Systemic
Redness	Leukocytosis (increased
Heat	number of white blood
Swelling	cells in the blood)
Pain	Fever
Limitation of function	Increased pulse rate
in the area	Increased respiration rate

INFECTION CONTROL

To control and prevent the infectious process, the sequential connection between the six factors involved must be broken at the weakest point. Various medical and surgical aseptic practices can break this cycle so that microorganisms cannot spread to and invade a susceptible host.

Medical Asepsis

Medical asepsis refers to the destruction of organisms after they leave the body. Techniques employed to accomplish this include those practices that help reduce the number and transfer of pathogens. We observe many of these practices in everyday living, such as washing the hands after using the bathroom or before handling food, covering the nose and mouth when sneezing or coughing, and using ones' own hair comb, toothbrush, and eating utensils.

Common medical aseptic practices to follow to break the cycle of the infectious process when working with patients include the following:

- Wash your hands before and after handling supplies and equipment and before and after assisting with each patient. The handwashing procedure is discussed in detail in this chapter.

- Handle all specimens as though they contain pathogens.
- Use disposable equipment when available, and dispose of it properly according to office policy. All equipment is considered contaminated after patient use.
- Clean nondisposable equipment before and after patient use.
- Use gloves when handling highly contaminated articles to protect yourself.
- Use clean or sterile equipment and supplies for each patient.
- Avoid contact of used supplies with your uniform to prevent the transfer of pathogens to yourself and to other patients.
- Place damp or wet dressings, bandages, and cottonballs in a waterproof bag when discarding them to prevent the possible spread of infection to the individuals who will handle the garbage.
- Cover any break in your skin as a protective measure against self-infection.
- Discard items that fall on the floor or clean them before using, because all floors are contaminated.
- Use damp cloths for dusting or cleaning to avoid raising dust, which carries airborne microorganisms.
- If you are unsure whether supplies are clean or sterile, do not use them until they have been cleaned or sterilized.

These practices are used during "clean" procedures, which involve parts of the body that are not normally sterile. Specific examples include aseptic procedures used when taking a temperature; obtaining urine, stool, or sputum specimens; obtaining smears or cultures from the throat or vagina; administering oral medications; removing and discarding used supplies; and cleaning a treatment room after use.

UNIVERSAL BLOOD AND BODY SUBSTANCE PRECAUTIONS (BSP)

The following is in accordance with recommendations from the U.S. Public Health Service, Center for Disease Control (CDC).

Vocabulary

aerosol Dispersion of fine particles into the air.

body substance Any fluid or substance produced by the body that may carry infectious agents, for example, blood, urine, sputum, and stool.

body substance precautions (BSP) System that focuses on the cautious handling of potentially infectious body substances through the use of barrier precautions.

detergents Chemicals used for cleaning purposes sometimes in combination with germicides, for example, LpH and Staphene.

universal precautions (Same as body substance precautions) Use of uniform infection control procedures with all patients and all work situations based upon the degree of risk of exposure to body substances, not based on diagnosis.

wastes

infectious waste

- Laboratory wastes, including cultures of etiologic agents that pose a substantial threat to health due to their volume and virulence.
- Pathologic specimens, including human tissues, blood elements, excretions, and secretions that contain etiologic agents, and attendant disposable fomites.
- Surgical specimens, including human parts and tissues removed surgically or at autopsy that, in the opinion of the attending physician, contain etiologic agents and attendant disposable fomites.
- Sharps (needles, sharp disposable instruments, glass slides).

contaminated waste All moist waste, including products that have been in contact with the patient's bodily fluids, or wastes that might attract vermin (for example, tongue blades, diapers, urine cups, moist blood-stained dressings, non-sharp disposable instruments, and food waste).

other wastes Paper materials and other office materials.

Infection control systems are designed to prevent health care workers from transferring infections to patients and prevent health care workers from acquiring infections themselves. Infection precautions previously used were based on diagnosis. Body substance precautions (BSP) improve on the traditional systems because they protect workers during the period before a patient's diagnosis is known. It is not possible to tell by looking which patients are infected. It is not practical to test all patients for all possible infections and not timely, as exposure would occur prior to obtaining the results. Pathologic agents may be present in body substances regardless of whether they are recognized to be present. These agents may be transmitted from clinically healthy individuals.

BSP are designed to be used with all patients, not just the identified infected patient and are based on the knowledge of disease transmission and the prevention of disease transmission. BSP are also based on degree of risk of exposure to blood and other body substances, not on diagnosis. You should determine precautions based on degree of risk.

Precautions with all patients should include routine use of appropriate *barrier precautions* to prevent skin and mucous membrane exposure when contact with blood or other body substances of any patient is anticipated. Since the BSP method considers all patients and laboratory specimens as potentially infected, it provides protection from not only the known infected cases but the unrecognized cases as well, and therefore protects patients and health care workers alike.

Health care workers who have weeping dermatitis or exudative lesions should not take part in direct patient care and should not handle patient-care equipment until the condition is resolved.

Barrier Precautions

The following barrier precautions should be used:

1. *Handwashing.* Body substances that may contain disease microorganisms easily contaminate your hands. Should these microorganisms enter an opening in the body (the mouth, for example), infection may occur. Handwashing is one of the most effective means of infection control. You should wash your hands:

- Before eating or preparing food, drinking, and smoking;
- Before performing clean or sterile invasive procedures;
- Before and after performing a clinical procedure;
- Before and after assisting the physician with a clinical procedure;
- Before and after touching wounds or other drainage;
- After contact with blood or body fluids, mucous membranes, secretions, or excretions, such as saliva, urine, blood, and feces;
- After handling soiled linen or waste;
- After handling devices or equipment soiled with body substances, for example, urine collection containers;
- After removing gloves;
- After using the toilet;
- After blowing your nose or coughing into your hands;
- Between each patient contact.

The most important function of handwashing is to remove infectious organisms. No handwashing product on the market kills all disease-causing organisms. Physical removal, washing soil and organisms down the drain, is the most effective practice. If properly used, any handwashing product approved by your facility, whether antibacterial or not, will achieve this goal. Soap-impregnated towelettes should be used only out in the field where handwashing facilities are not available. They should not be substituted for soap and water in the office or clinic except during an internal disaster. Do not use other chemicals such as alcohol or bleach to wash your hands. They may damage your skin and cause open or chapped areas that are more easily infected.

Your skin may become dry and chapped with frequent handwashing. Use lotion to replace the oils removed by handwashing. Always wash your hands before using lotion. If you use a lotion bottle while your hands are dirty, you are likely to contaminate the lotion container and, thereafter, contaminate your hands each time you touch it. Medicated lotion claims to control this problem have less than satisfactory test data. Use your own bottle of lotion. Leave it in a locker or other location where you will be the sole user. In this way you will be aware if the lotion becomes contaminated. Do not leave "community" lotion bottles in staff bathrooms. (See the procedure for handwashing on p. 351.)

2. *Gloves.* For the care provider, gloves are used to add an additional layer of protection beyond that of intact skin and handwashing. Gloves provide additional safety and should be worn whenever contact with blood or other body fluids or tissue is expected. Both vinyl and latex gloves are suitable for patient care activities. Each has a 95% effectiveness rate. *All gloves* tear with heavy or prolonged use. This needs to be considered and the glove replaced when torn as soon as patient safety permits.

Gloves should be worn for the following procedures:

- When touching blood and body fluids, mucous membranes, or nonintact skin of all patients.
- When handling items or surfaces moist with blood or body fluids and substances.
- When performing venipuncture or other vascular access procedures.
- When working with blood, specimens containing blood, body fluids, excretions, and secretions.
- When cleaning reusable instruments and equipment. Wear heavy rubber gloves over disposable gloves, a plastic apron or gown, and safety glasses, goggles, or personal glasses

when involved in decontamination activities of instruments and equipment.

- When decontaminating areas contaminated with body substances.
- When cleaning up blood spills and other contaminated areas. Wipe up small spills with disposable absorbent towels. If there is broken glass, scoop it up with several paper towels and dispose of it in the red sharps container. Then mop the area with a disinfectant. Large blood spills should also be mopped up with a disinfectant.

Wear *sterile gloves* for all sterile procedures to protect both the patient and yourself.

Wear *nonsterile gloves* for non-sterile patient care procedures where worker protection is needed.

Wear *finger cots* or *gloves* to cover cuts, abrasions, rashes, or minor infections on your hands while working.

If your glove is torn or punctured by a needle stick or other accident, remove the damaged glove, wash your hands, and put on a new glove as promptly as patient safety permits.

If your gloves are contaminated, *do not* touch telephone receivers, other uncontaminated surfaces, or other areas of the same patient's body which may be uncontaminated.

You must change gloves between patients and wash your hands immediately after glove removal.

Always remove gloves when answering the telephone, opening a door or drawer, handling a record book or worksheet, and when performing other clean procedures.

Handwashing remains the most effective infection control procedure. Glove use, as described, is to augment the barrier provided by intact skin against infectious agents. Gloves can transport infectious agents from one person to another or to the mouth as easily as ungloved hands. Therefore these policies are not to be interpreted as replacing the need for handwashing.

3. *Masks and protective eyewear.* Masks and protective eyewear should be worn to prevent exposure of the mucous membranes of your mouth, nose, and eyes during procedures that are likely to generate aerosol droplets, splashes of blood, or other body fluids, and when cleaning equipment that may have disease-producing microorganisms on it. Masks should cover both the nose and mouth and should fit close to the face so that air can be breathed only through the mask. Do not loosen your mask. Over time, your mask will become impregnated with moisture from your breath

and it will become harder to breathe. When this occurs, change the mask—*do not* loosen it. Discard masks after each use or when they become damp as regular, not infectious, waste.

Protective eyewear—personal glasses, goggles, safety glasses, or face shields—should be worn to protect your face from any splashes. Procedures when eyewear might be needed include certain diagnostic procedures, such as endoscopies or any invasive surgical procedure, and when cleaning and decontaminating reusable instruments and equipment. Face shields are best suited for non-patient-care activities such as when sorting laundry. After use, undamaged eyewear must be washed with soap and water and then dried before it is used again.

4. *Gowns and aprons.* A gown or apron should be worn to protect your arms and clothes during all procedures that are likely to generate splashes or soiling from blood or body fluids. Wear a gown when cleaning noncontaminated equipment, when cleaning and decontaminating reusable instruments and equipment, and when performing procedures involving contact with large amounts of patient substances. When performing laboratory procedures you should wear either a long-sleeved gown with a closed front or a long-sleeved laboratory coat that is buttoned shut. Remove the gown or laboratory coat when leaving the laboratory area. Change a gown or laboratory coat immediately if it becomes contaminated with blood or body fluids. You must also change them at appropriate periods to ensure cleanliness. Contaminated gowns and laboratory coats should be placed into a biohazard bag before they are sent to the appropriate laundry as arranged by your facility of employment. If laboratory gowns or coats are contaminated with a microbiological agent due to a laboratory accident, the gown or coat should be sterilized in the steam sterilizer before it is sent to the laundry.

Wear a disposable plastic apron if there is a significant probability that blood or body fluids may be splashed on you. At the completion of the task being performed, the disposable apron, if contaminated, should be discarded in a biohazard container or sterilized in the steam sterilizer before being discarded as ordinary waste. Never store used laboratory wear with street clothes.

5. *Sharps.* Needles, scalpel blades, and any other sharps that can easily puncture the skin must be handled with extreme caution to prevent infection with HIV and hepatitis. Most needle sticks happen when used needles are not handled prop-

erly. Broken skin or mucous membrane contact and a needle stick or other blood-to-blood accident may transmit infection. The following procedures must be followed to prevent any undue infection:

a. Place used disposable needles and syringes, scalpel blades, and other sharp items in a rigid, puncture-resistant disposable container with a lid (needle container) that is easily recognized (for example, a red container) and clearly marked as a biohazard. The container should preferably be made of rigid plastic. Do not use cardboard or paper containers. *Never* put needles or sharps in the trash or linen. This is dangerous to others.

b. Keep the puncture-resistant containers located as close as practical to the area where needles and other sharps will be used. The sharps containers should be located in each treatment room, at each laboratory table, and in any other area where syringes, needles, and slides will be used in the office or clinic.

c. Keep needle containers at a level where the top opening can be seen. Needles should not project from the top of the container.

d. *Never* try to take anything out of a needle box. If a needle will not go in easily, and the box is not full, use a large syringe to dislodge it. Do not push or force items with your hands. If the box is full, arrange to have it replaced.

e. Place the cover on sharps containers to close and seal them when they are three fourths full and dispose of as infectious waste. No additional protective garb is necessary for handling these containers. One suggestion to dispose of the full sharps containers is to place the full container into a brown cardboard box labeled "infectious waste" and lined with plastic sheeting. The location of the box should be in a centralized, authorized area. A contract scavenger company should then pick up the sealed boxes and deliver them to an incineration company on a weekly basis.

f. Pick up improperly discarded needles with extreme caution and dispose of them in the nearest sharps container. Do not attempt to cap the needle. Wash your hands after you dispose of it. Use tongs or forceps to pick up sharps.

g. *Never* purposely bend or break by hand a used needle. *Never* recap a used needle unless absolutely necessary or in approved special circumstances. An example of a special circumstance in which the needle should be recapped is when drawing blood for blood gases. To recap Vacutainer needles, put the cap on the table and slide the needle into it without holding the cap. Then tighten the cap at the needle hub.

h. *Never* remove a used needle from a used disposable syringe. Discard the syringe with the needle in place.

i. *Never* put a used needle into your pocket.

j. Wear gloves if doing laboratory work where a needle needs to be removed from a syringe. Discard the gloves immediately if they become contaminated with blood. It is preferable to use a needle disposal container that has an integral device for removing the needle without touching the needle with your hands.

k. Discard Vacutainer sleeves in the sharps container at the end of each day or when they are soiled with blood.

l. *Reusable sharps:* Place reusable sharps in a suitable puncture-resistant container after use and take them to the decontamination area where they will be cleaned and disinfected or sterilized. When doing this cleaning you should wear protective garb, that is, a gown and/or an apron, gloves, and face protection.

6. *Ventilation devices.* Mouthpieces, resuscitation bags, or other ventilation devices should be available for use in areas where the need for resuscitation is predictable. Use these devices on all patients instead of mouth-to-mouth resuscitation.

7. *Laboratory specimens.* All laboratory specimens should be handled and transported according to the following procedures to control the spread of infection and to protect the health of employees, patients, and the public:

• Laboratory specimens should be contained for transport. Gloves should be used for handling laboratory specimens when contamination of the hands is anticipated. Care must be taken when collecting specimens to avoid contamination of the outside of the container or the laboratory slip.

• Special secure, stiff, and impermeable containers, such as the igloo-type containers, should be used by the messenger service personnel when transporting blood and other body fluids from the office or clinic to a laboratory. Specimens may be placed in test tube racks before being placed into the secure transport container. Some facilities also require that the specimen be placed into a Ziploc or other hand-sealed plastic bag and sealed shut before being placed into the secure transport container for delivery to the laboratory. If the specimen container is too large to fit in a Ziploc, use tape to secure the cap and enclose the entire item in a plastic bag with a twist tie. The laboratory slip should be attached by rubber band or tape to the outside of the bag.

- Specimen mailers must have a metal inner container and a rigid cardboard outer container, complying with CDC regulations (see Figures 22.1 and 22.2).
- Centrifuge all blood or body fluid specimens in carriers with safety domes. Decontaminate the carrier and dome according to the manufacturer's directions. Human tissue, blood, body secretions and excretions, or other specimens and cultures should be autoclaved before they are disposed of by sanitary landfill.
- Put on disposable gloves and dispose of urine specimens into a toilet or utility sink and feces into toilets that empty into a sewer system. Sinks should then be rinsed thoroughly and toilets flushed. (To avoid cross-contamination, this sink should *not* be used for other activities such as preparation of clean supplies or supply of drinking water. Other sinks should be used for routine handwashing.) Dispose of specimen containers and gloves into a closed waste container that is lined with a strong plastic or vinyl bag.
- Wash your hands after handling all specimens and after removing gloves. Hands and other skin surfaces contaminated with blood or other body fluids must be washed immediately and thoroughly. Decontaminate laboratory work surfaces with a disinfectant, such as a 1:10 dilution of sodium hypochlorite (household bleach) or staphene germicide solution when the procedures have been completed or if a specimen is spilled.
- All potentially contaminated materials used in laboratory tests should be decontaminated, preferably by steam sterilization, before disposal or reprocessing. All infectious laboratory waste should be treated by steam sterilization, incineration, or disinfection prior to disposal so as to render the waste harmless. Promptly contact your supervisor when you have had an exposure to blood or other body fluids.

Handling of Equipment, Supplies, and Waste From Patient Care Areas and The Laboratory, and Care of Environmental Surfaces

Waste equipment and supplies should be handled as follows.

Reusable equipment

All used reusable equipment not classified as sharps should be placed as soon as possible, if appropriate, in an Environmental Protection Agency (EPA) approved detergent, such as hemosol or coleo, and transported to the decontamination area. Items that require sterilization or high-level disinfection must first be thoroughly cleaned and decontaminated. Cleaning and decontamination activities should be done by personnel wearing gloves, gown, and face protection. Each facility must develop cleaning and decontamination procedures appropriate to its needs.

Blood pressure equipment, scales, and other reusable room equipment should be decontaminated at the end of each day with a disinfectant solution. Stethoscope earpieces must be cleaned after each use with an alcohol swab. Tonometers must be disinfected with alcohol swabs, rinsed thoroughly in clean water, and then left to air dry or dried with a clean nonlint material after *each* use. Centrifuges should be cleaned with 70% alcohol swabs or disposable cloths soaked in 70% alcohol or LPH solution mixed according to the product's directions after each use when visibly soiled or weekly. Tourniquets can be soaked in a 1:10 5% sodium hypochlorite solution for 15 minutes. Discard blood-stained tourniquets. Goggles and heavy rubber gloves used during decontaminating procedures must be decontaminated after each use with alcohol. Brushes and buckets or basins used for decontamination procedures must be decontaminated after each use with a detergent solution, rinsed, and then placed in areas that are specifically designated for such supplies. This equipment should be sterilized weekly.

Sharps

Sharps containers must be closed when filled and disposed of as infectious waste. No additional protective garb is necessary when handling these containers.

Reusable sharps should be placed in suitable containers for transportation to the decontamination area where they should be cleaned and disinfected and/or sterilized. Employees who do this cleaning must wear protective garb (aprons, gloves, and face protection) (see also "Sharps" on p. 346).

Tissues, body fluids, and cultures

- Patient specimens and their containers should be collected and treated as infectious waste.
- Cultures and their containers should be collected and treated as infectious waste.
- Human tissues or body parts should be treated as infectious waste.
- Large volumes of blood or drainage as from suction machines should be flushed down the sewer or disposed of in their collecting containers as infectious waste.
- Used disposable dialysis equipment should be treated as infectious waste.
- Large volumes of urine, stool, or dialysate should be flushed down the sewer with appropriate precautions to guard against spillage.

While awaiting transport for disposal, infectious waste must be contained at the site of origin in covered or bagged leak-proof waste containers. Infectious waste must be collected in identifiable containers or bags and transported to a separate disposal site. If a can that does not have a working lid must be used, moist trash must be bagged before being placed in an open can. All trash containers must have liners that are thick enough to withstand needed handling and that can be tied shut for disposal. Waste containers should be cleaned weekly with a disinfectant solution.

Other waste

All other waste, such as paper towels and packaging materials, should be placed into the regular waste containers lined with plastic or vinyl liners strong or thick enough to withstand needed handling. For convenience, small items such as contaminated cotton balls may be disposed of in the sharps containers. Other disposable, moist waste generated by clinics or offices should be collected in *covered*, foot-operated cans lined with impervious bags. When removed, the bags should be closed, not emptied, and disposed of as ordinary waste.

Waste container liners must be removed as a single unit and tied shut without turning the container upside down to consolidate waste. Waste containers must be strong enough to resist tears and leaks under normal handling. Final disposal of waste is by approval of the county health officer and includes incineration, autoclaving, sewer system, or sanitary landfill.

Surfaces

- When body fluids are spilled on environmental surfaces, the visible material should be removed, followed by decontamination with an approved disinfectant such as a 1:10 dilution of sodium hypochlorite (household bleach) or Bytech solution. Gloves must be worn for this process.
- Laboratory work surfaces should be decontaminated with a disinfectant, such as a 1:10 dilution of sodium hypochlorite or staphene germicide solution at the completion of work activities or in the event of a specimen spill.
- Regular cleaning of diapering areas is recommended given the potential for the presence of fecal-oral transmitted agents.
- Environmental surfaces in patient care areas should be cleaned with an approved disinfectant weekly and as needed.
- Periodic cleaning of the clinic or office environment is to be considered good housekeeping rather than an infection control concern.
- Materials used for clean-up should be disposed of in the moist infectious waste covered container.
- Covers on examination tables and Mayo stands must be changed after each patient.
- At the end of the day, examination tables, counters, Mayo stands, and other equipment should be decontaminated with a disinfectant solution (for example, LpH solution).
- Supply closets should be dusted and cleaned at least monthly. Use a rag saturated with 70% alcohol to wipe the shelves, then let the shelves air dry. You should leave the door to the room open while doing this procedure to avoid any reaction to fumes.
- Janitorial staff must be taught how to handle and dispose of ordinary, contaminated, and infectious waste.

Uniforms and clothing

Uniforms and clothing that are soiled with body secretions should be cleaned with soap and *cool* water, then washed following normal laundering procedures. Clothing with large amounts of contaminates should be changed as soon as practical.

AIDS (Acquired Immunodeficiency Syndrome) Infection Precautions

In addition to the preceding practices, the following safeguards are recommended for the prevention of the possible transmission of the presumed AIDS infectious agent, human T-cell lymphotropic virus (HTLV-III, HIV, LAV, or ARV), to susceptible individuals, and to provide protection against other infectious agents that may infect patients with AIDS. The precautions described here are designed to protect individuals working with these patients, other patients, and employees.

- Treat all blood and body fluids as potentially infectious.
- Wear rubber gloves when handling potentially infectious body fluids or specimens and when using needles for medications or laboratory procedures.
- All blood specimens from all patients whether known to be infected or not should be handled with caution. All specimens from AIDS patients must be labeled with "H/A (hepatitis/AIDS) Precautions" labels, placed in Ziploc bags, and sealed for transport to prevent spills from broken tubes. A laboratory requisition should also be labeled and attached to the *outside* of the bag.
- Use disposable syringes and needles whenever possible. Dispose of contaminated needles in puncture-resistant containers without bending, breaking, or recapping the needle. The needle box should be as close as possible to the area of use. Handle and dispose of these and all sharp instruments with extraordinary care to prevent accidental injury.
- Carefully dispose of any contaminated dressings, tissues, waste matter, or trash in tear-proof sealed bags and dispose of them as local regulations require.
- Wipe up any spills involving potentially infectious body fluids immediately with a 1:10 solution sodium hydrochlorite (household bleach). Don gloves and use paper towels to wipe up the spill. Place the used towels in an infectious waste container.
- Special precautions such as gowns and masks are needed only in situations involving invasive procedures or procedures that could involve more extensive splashing of blood or body fluids, or in other uncontrollable infection sources.
- Follow general guidelines for sterilization, disinfection, and waste disposal. Use appropriate protective equipment.
- Use pocket masks, resuscitation bags, or other ventilation devices to resuscitate a patient to minimize exposure that may occur during emergency mouth-to-mouth resuscitation. These devices should be kept where the need for resuscitation is likely.
- *Education:* Know the modes of transmission and prevention for these infections.

Handwashing

To prevent the spread of microorganisms, handwashing is one of the very first procedures that all health personnel must learn. *Correct handwashing is the foundation of aseptic technique.* Hands that are not properly cleansed are commonly the cause in spreading infection, as the hands are in constant use when working with or around patients. This procedure must become an automatic part of your work, as its importance *cannot* be overemphasized, and conscientiousness on your part *cannot* be overstressed. The time involved to wash the hands, wrists, and forearms well should be 1 to 2 minutes—2 to 4 minutes if they are highly contaminated. (See also "Barrier Precautions—Handwashing" on p. 345.)

Equipment

Clean paper towels
Sink with running water
Soap

Procedure	*Rationale*
1. Stand in front of the sink, making sure that your clothing does not touch the sink.	Sinks are always considered contaminated.
2. Turn water on; adjust it to a lukewarm temperature and a moderate flow to avoid splashing.	Warm water makes better suds than cold water; hot water may burn or dry the skin.
3. Wet hands and apply soap. Liquid soap is preferred. Germs grow on bar soap and in soap dishes. When using bar soap, keep the bar in your hands throughout the whole procedure.	Apply enough soap to develop a good lather. If you drop the bar of soap, you must repeat the procedure. Only the inside of a bar of soap is sterile when in use; all other objects are considered contaminated.
4. Wash hands (palm, sides, and back), fingers, knuckles, and between each finger, using a vigorous rubbing and circular motion (Figure 20.2).	Friction caused by vigorous rubbing mechanically removes dirt and organisms. You must wash *all* areas on the hands.
5. During the procedure, keep the hands and forearms at elbow level or below.	This prevents water from running down to the elbows, which are areas of less contamination than the hands.
6. Rinse hands well under the running water.	
7. Wash wrists and forearms as high as contamination is likely.	Washing the wrists and forearms after the hands prevents the spread of microorganisms from the hands to these areas.
8. Rinse soap bar off, and drop in the dish without touching the dish.	Soap bars are excellent media for bacteria to grow on; therefore, they must be rinsed after use. The soap dish is considered contaminated and therefore must not be touched.
9. Rinse hands, wrists, and forearms under running water.	Running water rinses away the dirt and organisms that have been loosened during the washing process.
10. Clean nails with an orangewood stick or nail brush at least once a day when starting work and each time hands are very contaminated; then rinse well under running water.	Microorganisms collect and can remain under the nails unless cleansed away.
11. Repeat steps 3 through 10 when the hands are highly contaminated.	A second washing is necessary when the hands are heavily contaminated to ensure that all the microorganisms have been removed.
12. Use a paper towel to turn water faucet off (Figure 20.3).	The faucet is contaminated; using a paper towel allows the hands to remain clean.
13. Take another paper towel to thoroughly dry hands, wrists, and forearms.	Drying the skin completely prevents chapping.
14. Use hand lotion as necessary.	Lotion helps replace the skin's natural oils and prevents chapping. Chapped skin is more difficult to keep clean and more likely to crack. Once the skin is broken, microorganisms can easily enter and cause an infection.

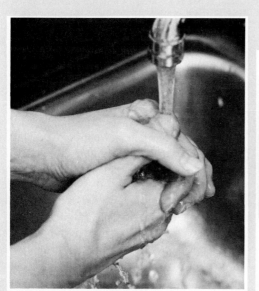

Figure 20.2
Handwashing technique.

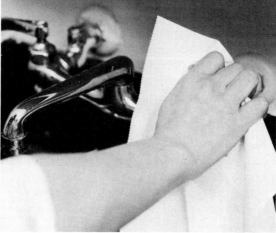

Figure 20.3
Turn water faucet off using a paper towel after washing your hands.

SURGICAL ASEPSIS

Surgical asepsis refers to the destruction of all microorganisms, pathogenic as well as nonpathogenic, before they enter the body. The goal of surgical asepsis is to prevent infection or the introduction of microorganisms into the body.

Practices of surgical asepsis are usually referred to as sterile techniques. These techniques are used in all procedures in which entry into normally sterile body parts occurs, for example, when administering injections and during all surgical procedures. Surgical asepsis or sterile techniques are those practices followed when an area and supplies in that area are made sterile and kept sterile at all times. As an additional example, when changing dressings on a wound, a sterile field, sterile equipment, and sterile technique are maintained to prevent infection from developing.

Measures used to obtain and provide surgical asepsis include absolute sterilization of all instruments and supplies that will come in contact with normally sterile body parts and open wounds, thorough washing of the hands with a detergent or surgical soap, and wearing sterile gloves during sterile procedures other than when administering injections. During surgical procedures, the physician and those directly involved with the procedure also wear a sterile gown, cap, and mask to help prevent contamination.

Methods of sterilization and disinfection are discussed in this chapter. The use of other surgical aseptic or sterile techniques and practices are discussed in Chapter 21.

STERILIZATION

Sterilization is a precise scientific term with a single exact meaning when applied to medical supplies and instruments. We define sterilization as those processes or methods that completely destroy all microorganisms on objects.

Using specific procedures, sterilization is accomplished by subjecting objects to chemical or physical agents that are capable of killing the microorganisms. It must be emphasized that there are no degrees of sterility—objects are either sterile or unsterile.

Sterilization plays a vital role in protecting the health and lives of patients who seek treatment in both physician's offices and hospitals. The use of presterilized disposable equipment has greatly helped reduce the spread of microorganisms and the need for sterilization procedures. Almost all equipment that may be used in a physician's office or clinic is now available in disposable form. Nonetheless there are certain items that are used repeatedly on many patients, such as a stethoscope, in addition to the nondisposable equipment still used by many. Therefore, the microorganisms that contaminate nondisposable supplies must be destroyed by appropriate measures.

The preceding information in this chapter should aid your understanding of the need for and importance of correct sterilization methods.

METHODS TO CONTROL MICROSCOPIC AGENTS

Sanitization, disinfection, and sterilization are the three principal methods used for inhibiting the growth of and for destroying microscopic life. Each represents a different level of decontamination, and though often used jointly, one must not be confused or substituted for the other.

Sanitation, the first step that must always be done before items can be reliably disinfected or sterilized, is a process of cleansing and scrubbing items with agents such as water and soap, detergents, or chemicals.

Disinfection involves methods that destroy *most* infectious microorganisms. However, some resistant and spore-forming bacteria and some viruses, such as the virus of Hepatitis B, are not adequately destroyed by these methods. Agents employed to disinfect items include various types of chemical germicides and boiling water or flowing steam.

Sterilization is the complete destruction of all forms of microscopic life. Methods used to accomplish sterilization include the following:
- Dry heat
- Moderately heated chemical gas mixtures
- Chemical agents
- Steam under pressure (autoclaves)
- Unsaturated chemical vapor (Chemiclaves)

The first three methods are limited to certain applications and require longer exposure periods to sterilize items; therefore they are not often employed. The autoclave, the most commonly used sterilizing method, and the Chemiclave are considered the most efficient, reliable, and practical ways to meet the sterilizing needs in the physician's office or clinic.

Preparation of Materials for Sterilization or Disinfection

The initial step in sterilizing or disinfecting contaminated items is to remove them from the treatment room to the work area that is designated for dirty equipment. Care must be taken to avoid contamination to yourself or injury from any sharp instrument and to prevent dulling any sharp blade or scissors while you are handling instruments. When handling heavily contaminated items or if you have any break in your skin, wear heavy rubber gloves over disposable rubber gloves, a plastic apron or gown, and safety glasses, goggles, or personal glasses when sanitizing supplies. After cleaning all supplies, wash your hands as described previously. (See also "Barrier Precautions," p. 345.)

Sanitizing instruments

Procedure	*Rationale*
1. Bulk rinse the instruments in water containing a blood solvent or low-sudsing detergent or any approved germicide solution.	This first step is to clean all debris, oil, blood, and grease off the instruments.
2. Rinse the instruments in another sink or pan of fresh water.	
3. Scrub each instrument thoroughly with a brush and a warm nonionizing detergent solution (such as Tide or Joy) (Figure 20.4).	Special attention must be given to serrated edges and other areas where blood, oil, or grease, may collect.
4. Using hot water, thoroughly rinse all detergent off the instruments.	Soap solutions are not to be used, as they are alkaline and not compatible with germicides. Any soap residue on an instrument will prevent disinfection.
5. Remove the excess moisture from the instruments by rolling them in a towel.	
6. Check all instruments for working condition, and check to see that they are thoroughly cleaned. Never oil instruments even if they are stiff when using them.	Oil on an instrument may protect a contaminated area from a sterilizing agent.
7. Wrap the instruments for sterilization.	
8. When instruments cannot be cleaned immediately after use, soak them in a solution of water and an effective blood solvent.	

Sanitizing syringes and needles

Disposable syringes and needles have largely replaced the reusable units. However, if you are still using reusable units you must take special care before sterilizing them, because they are a common means of transmitting hepatitis B. **Remember to wear heavy rubber gloves over disposable gloves, a plastic apron or gown, and protective eyewear when cleaning all instruments.**

Procedure	*Rationale*
1. Rinse immediately by filling the syringe with cool tap water and flushing it through the needle (Figure 20.5).	Rinsing immediately prevents coagulation of materials in the syringe and needle.

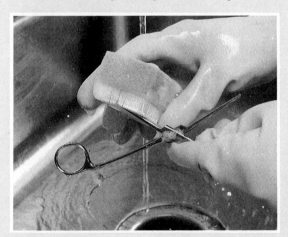

Figure 20.4
Step three for sanitizing instruments.

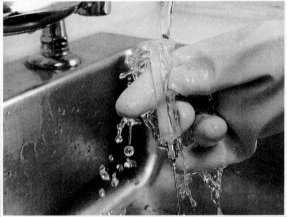

Figure 20.5
Flush cool tap water through syringe and needle after use.

Continued.

Procedure

2. Disassemble the unit.
3. Place the needle in a separate tray; then put into the sterilizer for 30 minutes at 250° F (121° C).
4. Put syringe in water containing a low-sudsing, non-etching detergent, and thoroughly brush the interior of the syringe barrel.
5. Clean the inside of the tip and the plunger.
6. Flush the syringe twice with tap water and once with distilled water.
7. The syringe is now ready to be wrapped and sterilized.
8. Remove needles from sterilizer after the 30 minutes of exposure.
9. Clean the inside of the hub with a cotton-tipped applicator that is soaked with water and blood solvent or detergent solution (Figure 20.6).
10. Pass a stylet in and out of the interior (lumen) of the needle several times.
11. Check the point of the needle.

12. Thoroughly clean the exterior of the needle.
13. Rinse the hub and exterior of the needle well under running tap water (Figure 20.7).
14. Using a syringe, flush tap water through the interior of the needle twice.
15. Rinse both the exterior and the interior with distilled water.
16. The needle is now ready to be wrapped and sterilized.

Rationale

Needles must first be decontaminated so they can be handled safely when cleaned.
All parts of the syringe must be cleaned to remove any foreign matter and contamination.

The needles are now decontaminated.

This removes any foreign matter or tissue left in the needle.
If it is damaged or dull, it must be resharpened and re-cleaned before sterilizing. Use a special whetstone or smooth oil stone (Arkansas stone) for sharpening. Directions for using these are provided by the manufacturer.

Both the exterior and the interior parts of the needle must be rinsed.
Rinsing is repeated with distilled water to ensure that all detergent is removed.

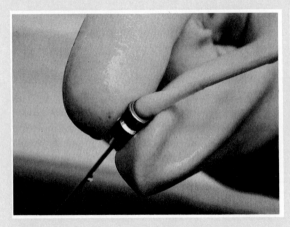

Figure 20.6
Cleaning inside hub of needle.

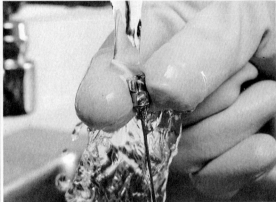

Figure 20.7
Rinse hub and needle exterior well with water.

Sanitizing rubber goods

All rubber goods must also be cleaned and some must be sterilized. Such items as hot water bottles, ice caps, and rubber sheets should be covered with a towel or sheet before being used in patient care. Since they normally do not come in direct contact with the patient, these items are not usually sterilized, but must be thoroughly washed, rinsed, and dried after each usage. Other rubber goods, such as gloves, catheters, and tubing require special care and sterilization. Immediately after use they should be washed in cold water, then washed in warm water and a low-sudsing detergent, rinsed thoroughly, dried, and wrapped for sterilization.

Procedure for cleaning rubber gloves

Procedure

1. Immediately after use, wash in cold water.
2. Wash thoroughly in warm water with a low-sudsing detergent, and rinse.

Rationale

Cold water will remove blood and other soiling.

Procedure	*Rationale*
3. Turn gloves inside out to wash and rinse again with fresh tap water.	Thorough rinsing is necessary to remove all detergent.
4. Fill gloves with water or air and inspect for punctures and unremoved soil.	Water or air will leak out if any puncture hole is present.
5. Dry the gloves; pat with a towel to remove excess moisture, then allow to air dry. When exposed side is dry, turn to expose the inner surface for drying.	
6. The gloves are now ready to be wrapped for sterilization.	

Wrapping instruments and related supplies for sterilization

The next step before sterilizing items that are to be stored for future use is to wrap them in protective coverings, such as clean muslin or special disposable paper or bags. These materials are used because they can be permeated by steam or the chemical vapor from the sterilizer, but not by airborne or surface contaminants during handling and storage.

Items that will be used immediately or those that do not have to be sterile when used (for example, supplies used for "clean" procedures) can be sterilized by placing them in the sterilizer tray with muslin or other material designated by the manufacturer under and over them. When the sterilizing process has been completed, these items are to be removed with sterile transfer forceps and then either used or placed in the proper storage area.

However, those items that are to be kept sterile for future use must be wrapped. Materials and instruments that will be used together may be wrapped together. Hinged instruments, such as hemostats, must be left open when being sterilized for immediate or future use. Also containers with lids are to be sterilized with the lid off; the lid is placed at the side or at the bottom of the container, with the inner surface facing outwards.

The method for wrapping instruments and other supplies, such as dressings, is the same. Figure 20.8 explains and illustrates the method to be used for wrapping these items. Study and practice this procedure of preparation.

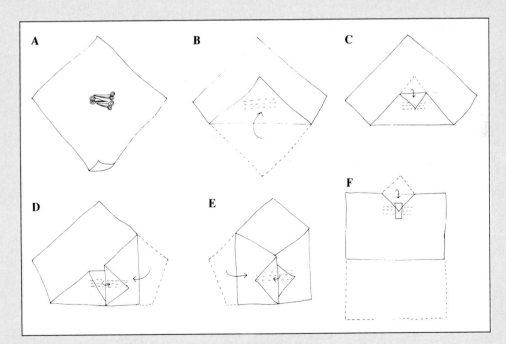

Figure 20.8
Wrapping technique. **A,** Place all instruments in center of wrapper. **B,** Fold the material up from bottom to cover instruments. **C,** Double back a small corner of material folded up over instruments. **D,** Fold right edge over to center, leaving corner doubled back. **E,** Fold left edge over to center, again leaving corner doubled back. **F,** Fold pack up from bottom and secure it with pressure-sensitive tape. Date and label pack according to its contents. Pack must be wrapped firmly enough that it will not fall apart when handled, but loosely enough to allow proper circulation of steam when pack is placed in the autoclave.

Another aid to sterilization has been the introduction of disposable packaging materials. These include paper, pouches, and tubing of paper and plastic. They are convenient for the sterilization and storage of syringes, tubing, and special purpose items.

ATI Steriline bags are made of a special surgical-grade paper that allows rapid steam penetration during sterilization. They also act as a barrier against airborne bacteria during storage.

Each Steriline bag is printed with a temperature and steam-sensitive indicator consisting of an indicator line that changes color during sterilization to show that an item has been processed through the sterilizer (Figure 20.9, *A*).

ATI pouches and tubing offer a clearly labeled package that can be used either for steam or ethylene oxide gas sterilization. They offer advantages similar to those of Steriline bags plus the benefits of content visibility and an easy, peel-open feature. Their use minimizes the risk of damaging expensive items by using the wrong sterilizing method.

A

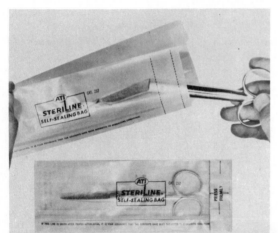

Figure 20.9
A, Disposable bags used for sterilizing instruments, needles, and syringes. Line going across bottom third of bag is sterilization indicator. If line is green after autoclaving, this is assurance that contents have been subjected to sterilizing conditions. **B,** ATI self-seal peel pouches and heat-sealable peel pouches. **C,** ATI instrument protector.
Courtesy Aseptic-Thermo Indicator, North Hollywood, Calif.

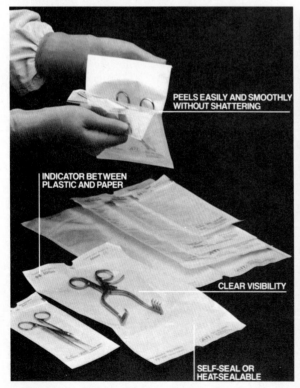

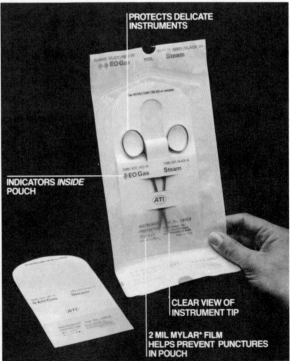

B   **C**

The steam indicator changes color from blue to gray/black during processing in either a gravity displacement or pre-vacuum, high-temperature steam sterilizer. The gas indicator changes color from yellow to rust/red during processing in an ethylene oxide gas sterilizer (Figure 20.9, *B*).

ATI Instrument Protectors are convenient, disposable holders for delicate surgical instruments. They protect instrument tips from being cracked or broken and help prevent the instrument from pen-

etrating the pouch or package in which it is placed. Chemical indicators on each protector verify steam or ethylene oxide (EO) gas processing. To use these holders, first insert the instrument through the slots of the protector until the tip is completely covered by the plastic flap. Open hinged instruments, such as scissors, and fold the antilock flap forward between the handles. For added protection and holding ability, tuck the antilock flap into the top-most slot. Slide the loaded instrument protector into a

---

Wrapping Reusable Syringes and Needles

Syringes are best wrapped in special disposable paper bags that are available for sterilization.

Procedure	Rationale
1. Write the size of the syringe and the date on the outside of the bag.	Size must be indicated for identification. Date must be indicated, because if not used within 21 to 30 days (will vary with office or agency preference), it must be resterilized.
2. Place matching separated syringe and plunger inside the bag.	
3. Fold the top of the bag and seal securely.	
4. When the needle is to be sterilized with the syringe, place the needle in a disposable paper form (Figure 20.10).	The paper form protects the point of the needle, provides a means for sterile handling when putting the needle on the syringe tip for use, and also prevents the needle from piercing the bag.
5. Label the bag with the size of syringe and needle and the date.	
6. Place the needle in the bag with the syringe and plunger; fold the top of the bag and seal.	
7. When the needle is to be sterilized individually, place it in a glass tube with constricted sides, and top the tube with a gauze, cotton, or rubber stopper (Figure 20.11).	The constriction in the tube prevents the sharp needle point from touching the bottom of the tube, thus preventing damage to the point.

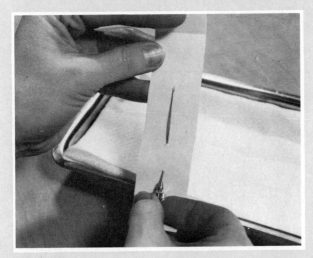

Figure 20.10
Reusable needle placed in paper form for sterilizing with syringe in disposable paper bag.

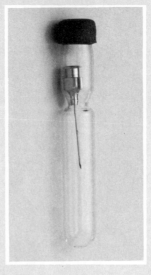

Figure 20.11
Needle in glass tube with constricted neck ready for autoclaving.

sterilization pouch, with the instrument facing the film side. Seal the pouch in the normal manner and sterilize (Figure 20.9, *C*).

Autoclave—Steam Sterilization
Positioning loads in autoclave

Proper positioning of all instruments and materials in the autoclave is extremely important because of the pattern that steam follows as it circulates through the autoclave. *A direction booklet, which must be read carefully, is supplied with every sterilizer.* Usually, when the sterilizing cycle begins, steam will build up at the top of the inside chamber and will move downward from the point of admission. Dry, cool air will be forced downward and out an exhaust drain at the bottom front part of the chamber. All materials must be placed so that steam can flow between the packs and penetrate them. To avoid forming air pockets, you must place containers, tubes, cups, and similar items on their sides so that cool air can drain out in a downward direction and be replaced by steam. If placed upright, air would be trapped in the item, which in turn would prevent steam from contacting all surfaces. The result would be incomplete sterilization.

Syringes wrapped in the disposable paper bags are to be placed horizontally (on their sides) in the sterilizer tray so steam will circulate inside the syringe barrel. Constriction tubes with needles are to placed horizontally so that steam can circulate inside the tube. Place linen and dressing packs in a vertical position.

When sterilizing linen packs and hard items in the same load, place the linen packs on top and the hard items on the bottom to prevent water condensation from dripping down on the linen packs. Items should not rest against plastic utensils so that the plastics will retain their shape even though exposed to very high temperatures.

Above all, *do not* overload the sterilizer chamber regardless of the items being sterilized. Place the articles as loosely as possible inside the chamber. Leave a space between all articles and the surrounding walls in the chamber. Correct positioning and spacing of all materials will allow effective sterilization to occur when the proper temperature, pressure, and time requirements are also met (Figure 20.12).

Exposure times

All loads placed in a sterilizer must be timed carefully after the sterilizer has attained the proper temperature. The length of sterilization time varies with the items and whether wrappers, paper, or fabric are used. Suppliers of such materials will supply correct exposure data to ensure observance of adequate exposure periods.

The *high temperature* attained is the *sterilizing influence* that destroys the microorganisms. The amount of pressure used only makes it possible to develop the high temperature. An accurate thermometer should be used to provide a positive indication that sterilizing conditions have been met in the chamber. Thus the three variables in the sterilizing cycle of an autoclave are *time, temperature,* and *pressure.* Alteration of any one of these means that adjustments are necessary in the others.

Figure 20.12
Instruments in autoclave for sterilization must be well spaced and hinged handles left open.

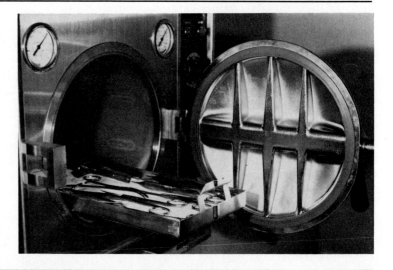

In the autoclave, when steam is in contact with all surfaces of the items, 15 minutes at 250° F (121° C) is adequate time to kill all known microorganisms. However, in practice, longer periods are necessary to achieve this exposure. Recommended exposure times for items placed in an autoclave at 250° F are as follows:

Wrapped surgical instruments	30 minutes
Wrapped syringes and needles	30 minutes
Wrapped rubber goods (excessive exposure will cause heat damage to the rubber)	20 minutes
Wrapped dressings	30 minutes
Wrapped suture materials	30 minutes
Wrapped treatment trays	30 minutes
Unwrapped utensils, glassware, and similar items, when inverted or placed on edge	15 minutes
Unwrapped instruments covered with muslin	20 minutes
Unwrapped and unassembled syringes and needles	15 minutes

Again, methods of wrapping, time of exposure, and the temperature must be scrupulously watched, since the purpose of autoclaving is to sterilize every article completely. Each manufacturer's direction booklet must be read and followed carefully to achieve adequate sterilization.

Sterilization indicators

Numerous commercial devices are used to indicate the effectiveness of the sterilization process. Used correctly, these devices, known as sterilization indicators, are adequate assurance of the sterility of items as long as the wrapper or container has not been torn or handled when moist, as that would contaminate the contents. These indicators work on the principle that specially prepared dyes will change color when exposed to the high temperature and saturated steam in the autoclave for a specific time. Individual disposable indicators in which the color change is to be observed after sterilization include the Sterilometer-Plus and Sterilometers (Figure 20.13). Sterilometer-Plus represents the most precise, complete chemical indicator available. It consists of two indicator bars covered by a clear plastic overlay. The indicator bars contain a special reactive pigment that changes color from purple to green only in the presence of steam, not just heat (the water molecules in the steam actually are part of the color-change reaction, so that the reaction cannot take place without steam present). The clear plastic overlay prevents the indicator areas from coming into contact with items being sterilized.

When the indicator is exposed to steam in a sterilizer, the steam begins to work on the indicator inks. The heat energy and water content of the steam react with the purple pigment in the ink and cause it to turn green. The ink contains other chemicals that carefully control the amount of time necessary for the ink to completely change color, so that the indicator will change only when the conditions necessary for complete sterilization have been met.

The Sterilometer is a disposable tag that is placed in the center of a pack with the nonindicator end extended outside the wrapper. This enables the indicator to be removed without touching the contents of the pack. Sterilization is assured if the

---

Removing Loads from the Autoclave

Procedure	Rationale
1. Exhaust steam pressure from the chamber.	Read and follow precisely the manufacturer's directions for exhausting steam.
2. When the pressure has reached zero and the temperature has decreased to 212° F, (100° C), open the door of the autoclave slightly.	Stand back from the door to avoid steam burns to the face and hands.
3. Allow the contents to dry for approximately 15 minutes before removing them.	Some modern autoclaves automatically provide a sterilization cycle that includes drying, thus eliminating the need for these steps.
4. Regardless of the type of sterilizer you use, all dry wrapped items and unwrapped items that do not have to remain sterile can then be removed with your clean and dry hands.	Do not remove unwrapped metal objects too soon with bare hands, because they retain heat and you could get burned.
5. Remove unwrapped items that are to remain sterile for immediate use with sterile transfer forceps; place items to be used later in sterile storage containers.	

Figure 20.13

A, Sterilometer-Plus sterilization indicators. The color changes from purple to green on the indicator bars point out when the conditions necessary for complete sterilization have been met. **B,** Sterilometer sterilization indicators.

Courtesy Aseptic-Thermo Indicator, North Hollywood, Calif.

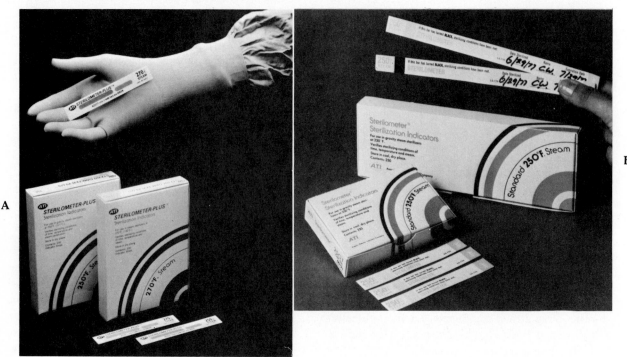

wide bar at the opposite end has changed completely from white to black. If these color change standards do not result, the pack must be resterilized.

Also, specific areas or markings on the outside of commercially prepared packages and on special disposable bags that are available for wrapping instruments, syringes, and needles will change color if sterilization standards have been met (see Figure 20.9). These preceding indicators are superior to the frequently used autoclave tape indicators because the dark diagonal lines that appear on the tape at the end of the sterilization cycle merely indicate that the pack has been exposed to steam and the autoclaving process (Figure 20.14).

There are many other indicators available for various types of sterilization processes. Figure 20.15 illustrates the dry heat sterilization indicator on a pressure-sensitive label, which changes from tan to black when exposed for 5 minutes at 340° F. When any sterilization indicator is used, the manufacturer's directions for use must be followed. Ster-

ilization indicators must be stored in a dry place and away from excessive heat.

Causes of inefficient sterilization

Failure of the indicators to change colors completely indicates a serious lack of steam penetration into the pack. This is a warning that there may be a sterilizer malfunction or an error in the sterilization technique. *Never neglect this warning.* Causes of sterilization failure are numerous, elusive, and often difficult to locate. The problem may require minute examination of every part of the sterilizer and/or complete reexamination of your preparation, wrapping, and loading techniques. Some of the most common problems are as follows:

- Faulty preparation of materials;
- Improper loading of the sterilizer;
- Faulty sterilizer;
- Air in the sterilizer;
- Wet steam.

Figure 20.14
Autoclave indicator tape used to seal and label
packages before sterilization. Dark diagonal lines
appear on the tape after the sterilization cycle to
indicate that the pack has been exposed to steam
and the autoclaving process.
Courtesy Aseptic-Thermo Indicator, North Hollywood, Calif.

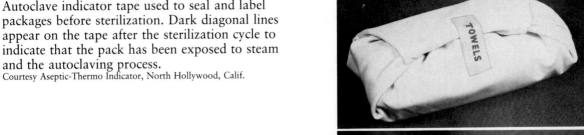

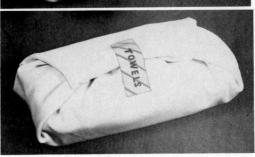

Figure 20.15
Dry heat sterilization indicator labels.
Courtesy Aseptic-Thermo Indicator, North Hollywood, Calif.

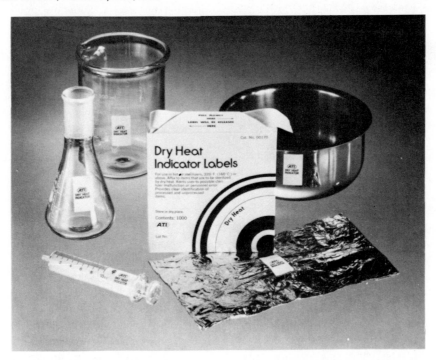

All materials must be sanitized completely beforehand, then wrapped and secured properly as
described previously. You must position the load
correctly in the sterilizer and not overload the
chamber. Timing for adequate exposure times
must begin *after* the sterilizer has attained the
proper temperature. If all of these conditions have
been met satisfactorily, it will be necessary to have
the equipment checked for a defect and repaired as
necessary (see Table 20.2).

Table 20-2
Problems encountered in sterilizing technique

Probable Causes	Corrections
Damp or wet loads	
Clogged strainer in exhaust line; clogged steam trap	Remove strainer; free openings of lint and sediment daily; use trisodium phosphate solution weekly
Placing warm sterilized packs on cold surfaces	Allow packs to cool before removing from sterilizer, or place on surfaces covered with several layers of towels or drapes
Sterilized goods removed too soon from sterilizer following completion of cycle	Allow goods to remain in sterilizer at completion of cycle an additional 15 minutes—door slightly opened ½ inch
Improper loading; tightly loaded packs	Leave space between items; arrange items to present least possible resistance to passage of air and steam through layers of load; position load so water does not collect in utensils; place packs on edge
Pools of water on floor of chamber	Bottom of sterilizer must lean toward exhaust port so condensation can drain
Wet stream	Contact manufacturer in charge of maintenance
Deposits on interior	Weekly cleaning of sterilizer
Corroded instruments	
Poor cleaning; residual protein	Improve cleaning; do not allow protein to dry on instruments; use correct cleaning solution for each instrument
Improper use of instrument milk	Follow procedures for instrument milk
Moisture—not dried properly	Check sterilizer for drying efficiency; packs should air dry in sterilizer; store packs in dry area
Exposure to harsh chemicals	Do not expose instruments to harsh chemicals and abrasives such as steel wool and powder cleaner
Metallic deposits resulting from reaction with sterilizer components	Keep sterilizer free of deposits on chamber walls, shelves, and trays

Storing sterile supplies

Special storage places for each type of supply should be maintained away from areas in which contaminated materials are handled. Storage places must be clean, dry, and dustproof. Sterile items wrapped in cloth or paper can safely be stored for 21 to 30 days. Wrapped items that are placed in sterile plastic duster covers can be stored for 6 months, and items wrapped in plastic teel-packs (special envelopes with one side of transparent plastic and the other side of paper) for 3 months. After these time periods are exhausted, all packs should be reprocessed and resterilized before use. Instruments sterilized unwrapped are to be used immediately and are not to be stored if they are to be sterile when used.

In summary, some points should be remembered when sterilizing items in an autoclave (steam sterilization). All items must be treated as follows:

- Sanitized (cleaned) properly before sterilization.
- Correctly wrapped, sealed, and labeled (for identification) or covered to prevent recontamination. When using cloth or paper wrappers, include a sterilization indicator in or on the pack.
- Positioned correctly in the sterilizer so steam will contact all surfaces.
- Able to fit easily into the chamber—*do not overload.*
- Exposed to saturated steam at 250° F (121° C) for 15 to 30 minutes (varies with the items).
- Allowed to dry before removing from the sterilizer.
- Stored in specific clean, dry, and dustproof places.
- Checked at intervals to determine if the period (date) of sterility has been exhausted.

Figure 20.16
MDT/Harvey Chemiclave 5000 represents the most sophisticated use of the basic principle of unsaturated chemical vapor sterilization.
Courtesy MDT Corp, Gardena, Calif.

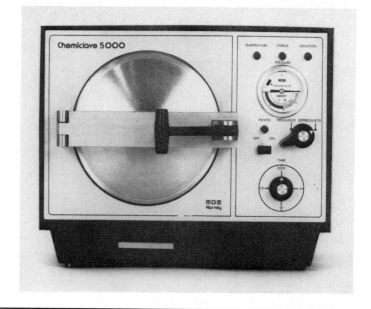

Figure 20.17
Harvey 100/Vibraclean—an ultrasonic cleaner.
Courtesy MDT Corp Gardena, Calif

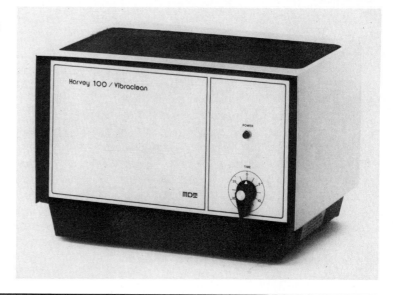

- Reprocessed and resterilized when they are no longer sterile because of wrap damage or date expiration.

Unsaturated Chemical Vapor Sterilization

A practical, efficient, and reliable method of sterilization, the unsaturated chemical vapor sterilizer (now known as the MDT/Harvey Chemiclave, Figure 20.16) depends on pressure, heat, and a specific solution, the Vapo-Sterile Solution, a formulation of proven effective liquid bactericidal chemicals and minimal water. When it is heated and pressurized to 270° F (132° C) and at least 20 pounds per square inch pressure, all living micro-

organisms are consistently killed within 20 minutes.

All items to be sterilized must first be cleaned. To avoid hand scrubbing of instruments and the possibility of transmitting pathogenic microorganisms between patients and medical personnel, an ultrasonic cleaning device, such as the Vibraclean 100 or 200, may be employed for this purpose (Figure 20.17). Once cleansed, instruments must be thoroughly rinsed in cold running water to remove any residue or ultrasonic solution or soap, which would inhibit sterilization or damage the sterilizer, and then towel dried before being placed in the sterilizer. Small, hard-to-dry items should be dipped in a shallow tray of Vapo-Steril solution in lieu of drying. The items are then to be placed in an instrument tray lined with a Harvey chemically pure hard surface tray liner. If storage of sterile instruments is desired, they are to be sterilized in Harvey Sterilization Indicator bags. These bags permit penetration by the chemical vapor, but preclude contamination by air-borne bacteria.

The Chemiclave (the unsaturated chemical vapor sterilizer) uses mechanical principles substantially different from those of other systems. The sterilizer is preheated before the initial use and remains at 270° F (132° C) for immediate use. No further preheating is necessary. Unlike the steam autoclave, in which an unmeasured amount of water is recirculated over the heating element, the unsaturated vapor sterilizer valving system measures a precise amount of solution into the closed, preheated chamber. This solution condenses on the cooler objects in the chamber to begin bactericidal activity. As the objects heat, vaporization of the solution occurs, and unsaturated chemical vapor acts to complete the sterilization cycle. Temperature monitoring is unnecessary, as this sterilizer provides both audible and visual signaling upon completion of the cycle. A thermostatically controlled heating unit maintains the chamber temperature, and a temperature indicator light registers that the heating element is functioning properly. Any failure in the system is immediately evident, as the pressure in the chamber will not be attained, and, unless all operating criteria are met, the pressure switch will not activate the cycle timer.

Cutting edges, even those of carbon steel, and surgical instruments, handpieces, forceps, and similar items vulnerable to dulling, corroding, rusting, or loss of temper in autoclaves or dry heat units are safely and effectively sterilized in a Chemiclave. Many "soft" items may also be safely sterilized in this unit; and since sterilization is achieved in a water-unsaturated environment, materials such as gauze and cotton are dry and ready for immediate use when the cycle is completed. Only low-grade plastic and rubber items, liquids, agars, and items damaged at 270° F (132° C) *should not* be placed in the Chemiclave. As with all sterilizers, the directions for operation from the manufacturer must be followed explicitly to obtain maximum results.

Dry Heat Sterilization

To sterilize items with dry heat, a special combined autoclave–dry heat sterilizer or an individual dry heat sterilizer is required. In essence, the dry heat sterilizer is like an oven.

Before being sterilized, all items must be thoroughly cleaned. Instruments and glass items, such as syringes, should be placed on the tray or wrapped in aluminum foil. Sharp items should be placed on gauze in racks or wrapped in aluminum foil. Rubber goods and dressings must be well dispersed in a container or wrapped in aluminum foil. As for all methods of sterilization, both exposure time and temperature must be considered. Dry heat sterilizers require longer exposure periods and higher temperatures than the autoclave (steam under pressure). The exposure time for dry heat is at least 1 hour at 320° F (160° C). If the items being sterilized cannot tolerate this temperature, reduce the temperature and extend the time proportionately. This method is suggested for instruments that corrode easily, sharp cutting instruments, and glass syringes, because moist heat will dull the cutting edges and the ground-glass portion of the syringe. Needles, powders, oils, ointments, lensed instruments, dressings, rubber goods, and polyethylene tubing can also be sterilized by this method.

Gas Sterilization

Gas sterilizers, using moderately heated mixtures of ethylene oxide gas, are useful for sterilizing heat- and moisture-sensitive items, including rubber and plastic goods, delicate items such as lensed instruments, glass, ophthalmological surgical instruments, catheters, and anesthesia equipment. Items to be sterilized by this method should be cleaned, wrapped, and positioned in the gas chamber using the same steps that were discussed for autoclaving. The temperature in a gas sterilizer is lower (140° F [50° C]); thus the exposure time is extended to suit the temperature, moisture, and gas concentration being used. (Time required is 2 to 6 hours plus additional time for aeration, which can be as long as 5 to 7 days for certain porous materials). Specific instructions for the times and temperatures required are supplied by the manufacturer with the sterilizer and must be followed explicitly.

Chemical Sterilization

Many studies have shown that chemical sterilization (cold sterilization) is difficult to accomplish. Therefore this method is generally limited for items that are heat-sensitive, such as delicate cutting instruments and nonboilable sutures, or used when heat sterilization methods are not available. Chemical solutions are more commonly used for disin-

Procedure for Chemical Sterilization

Procedure

1. Sanitize items as discussed for autoclaving.
2. Pour chemical solution into a designated container with an airtight cover (Figure 20.18).

3. Completely immerse the item into the solution, and close the cover.
4. Leave for required time, which will vary with the chemical used. Exposure time may be from 20 minutes to 3 hours or more.
5. Before using, lift tray out of container, and rinse items in pan of sterile distilled water.
6. Using sterile transfer forceps, remove items from the tray for use.
7. Change the solution in the container every 7 to 14 days or as recommended by the manufacturer.

Rationale

Follow the directions for each chemical accurately. Some may need to be diluted before use, but if diluted too much, the solution will lose its effectiveness.

Correct exposure time is extremely important to ensure sterilization.

Often the solutions used are toxic; therefore, items must be thoroughly rinsed before being used on patients.

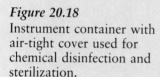

Figure 20.18
Instrument container with air-tight cover used for chemical disinfection and sterilization.

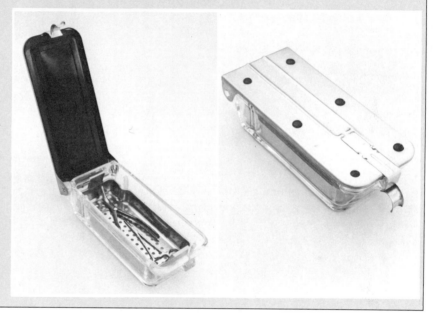

fection rather than for sterilization. Nonetheless, a variety of chemical solutions are on the market for sterilization and disinfection. They are classified as germicidal, bacteriocidal, disinfectants, antiseptics, and so on.

Three chemical solutions that have been recognized as reliable for both sterilization and disinfection procedures are Cidex, Ideal solution, and Formaldehyde Germicide. These solutions are capable of destroying bacteria, including spore-forming types, and viruses and are safe to use on instruments, rubber, and plastic goods. Reliable manufacturers always indicate which microorganisms can be expected to be killed by the chemical solution, items on which the solution can and cannot be used, and specific directions for use.

Disinfection Procedures
Chemical disinfection

Many medical procedures are termed *clean* procedures; this means they do not require the use of strict aseptic (sterile) technique. Instruments and equipment used in clean procedures are in contact only with the patient's skin or shallow body orifices. Since they do not bypass the body's natural defenses, they can be used safely after being disinfected. Examples of such supplies are thermometers, percussion hammers, laryngeal mirrors, blunt instruments not used on open skin surfaces or on sterile materials, such as dressings that will touch an open wound, and also stainless steel goods, such as kidney basins.

When disinfecting such items, thoroughly wash,

Procedure for Disinfection with Boiling Water

Procedure	*Rationale*
1. Fill boiler half full with cold water, preferably distilled water.	Distilled water does not leave sediment on the inside of the boiler as tap water would.
2. Clean items thoroughly.	All soil must be removed before the items are boiled.
3. Place items on the tray in the boiler. Hinges or clamps on instruments must be open; jars and similar containers must be placed on their side (Figure 20.19).	The boiling water must come in contact with all surfaces to provide thorough disinfection of the item.
4. Lower the tray so items are completely immersed in the water.	
5. Close lid of boiler, and turn power switch on.	
6. Once the water is boiling (212° F [100° C]) vigorously, start timing the exposure period.	Recommended exposure time is 15 to 20 minutes. Do not boil for less than 15 minutes.
7. Once the cycle has been completed, stand back or to the side of the boiler, and open the lid to allow steam to escape.	Standing away from or to the side of the boiler prevents a steam burn.
8. Allow the items to cool, then remove and dry thoroughly.	Items can be removed with clean hands, or by using sterile transfer forceps.
9. Store the items in designated area, unless needed for immediate use.	

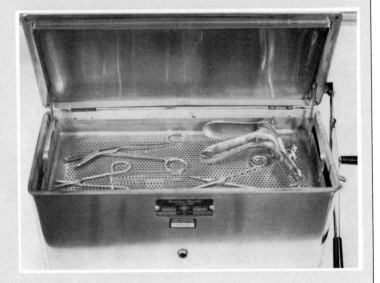

Figure 20.19
Instruments correctly placed in a boiler for disinfecting process.

rinse, and dry, as for sterilization. Then apply a disinfectant or antiseptic solution to the surface of the item or immerse it completely in such a solution (refer to the procedure for chemical sterilization).

Certain items, such as sphygmomanometers, stethoscopes, and ophthalmoscopes may be ruined if washed and immersed in any solution. Disinfect these only by wiping them with gauze or cloth moistened with a disinfectant. Chemical solutions suggested for use include Cidex, Ideal solution, Solucide, 70% to 90% isopropyl alcohol, Deo-Fect, iodophor solutions, Zephiran chloride, Formaldehyde Germicide, and Chlorophenyl.

Boiling water

The other method for disinfection involves the use of boiling water. Formerly considered safe for sterilization, investigations have now shown that many bacterial spores can withstand exposure to boiling water for several hours. Therefore use boiling water only to disinfect items that do not penetrate body tissues.

If you do not have access to an autoclave for sterilizing and must use the boiler, remove items from the boiler with sterile transfer forceps, dry with a sterile towel, and then transfer to a sterile field for use.

When the boiler is used frequently, it must be cleaned regularly to remove any sediment that has gathered on the sides. It may be necessary to scrub the interior surfaces with a stiff brush and cleanser. Follow the specific instructions provided by the manufacturer of the equipment that you use.

The limitations of disinfection procedures must be recognized and must *not* be substituted for ster-

ilization. These procedures can be effective in controlling many forms of microbial life on appropriate items but may not destroy viruses. Also, spore-forming bacteria can withstand boiling water even after several hours exposure.

Conclusion

When using instruments and other equipment, the spread of numerous pathogens can be prevented only by the proper sterilization of reusable items, or by the use of presterilized disposable items, in addition to meticulous aseptic technique.

Because few procedures more directly affect the continued health of the patient you attend, the physician, and yourself, conscientious attention must be given to sterilizing all items at all times. Periodic reexamination of the techniques employed should be done to check their adequacy. The use of disposable equipment is highly recommended to

help control infectious processes and has been found to be most economical in the long run.

On completion of this chapter, practice the procedures until you feel confident with the performance of your skills. Then arrange with your instructor to take a performance test. You will be expected to demonstrate accurately your skill in preparing for and performing all of the procedures outlined in this chapter. In addition, you should be prepared to discuss briefly the infectious process and the methods used for infection control.

Review Questions

1. State three goals of infection control, and explain how you and the general public can play an active role in this.
2. Describe the inflammatory process, listing five local and four systemic signs and symptoms of inflammation.
3. You are given three pieces of equipment; one is to be sanitized, one to be disinfected, and the other to be sterilized. Explain the difference between these three processes, and list methods used to accomplish each effectively.
4. At your place of employment you have an autoclave, a Chemiclave, a dry-heat sterilizer, a gas sterilizer, and chemical solutions. List at least three items that you would sterilize in each of these.
5. If you are busy and cannot clean soiled instruments immediately after use, what should you do?
6. When an instrument is to be boiled for 20 minutes, when do you start to time the exposure period?
7. On checking your storage area of sterile supplies, you find a pack that has been there for 1½ months. What should your next action be regarding this pack?
8. When removing a dry pack from the autoclave, you observe that the sterilization indicator has not changed color. What would you do?
9. Discuss the principles and procedures involved in the "Universal Blood and Body Substance Precautions."

SUGGESTED READINGS

Dubay EC and Grubb RD: Infection: prevention and control, ed 2, St Louis, 1978, The CV Mosby Co.

Perkins J: Principles and methods of sterilization in health sciences, ed 2, Springfield Ill, 1982, Charles C Thomas, Publisher.

Sellars D: A basic understanding of immunology for the medical assistant, Prof Med Assist 10:8, July/Aug 1977.

Chapter 21

Surgical Asepsis and Minor Surgery

- Background of sterile technique
- Principles and practices of surgical asepsis
- Handling sterile supplies
- Minor surgery
- Wounds
- Dressing and bandages

Objectives

On completion of Chapter 21 the medical assistant student should be able to:

1 Define and pronounce the vocabulary terms.

2 State at least 15 principles and practices of aseptic technique.

3 List and differentiate between three types of local anesthesia.

4 State the purpose of suture materials, differentiate between absorbable and nonabsorbable suture material, and given an example of each.

5 Differentiate between an open wound and a closed wound. Give one example of a closed wound and five examples of open wounds.

6 List two goals of wound care.

7 Differentiate between dressings and bandages and know the types and purposes of each. List eight purposes of dressings and four purposes of bandages.

8 Prepare the patient physically and mentally for a minor surgical procedure.

9 Select, assemble, and prepare sterile and nonsterile supplies and equipment needed for a minor surgical procedure using aseptic technique. Identify by name the instruments and supplies selected.

10 Assist the patient and the physician during a minor surgical procedure.

11 Change the patient's dressing, and obtain a wound culture.

12 Identify by name the instruments and supplies used in minor surgical procedures.

13 Apply roller, triangular, and Tubegauz bandages.

Vocabulary

anesthesia (an″es-the′ze-ah) The loss of sensation or feeling.

asepsis (a-sep′sis) The stage of being free from infection or infectious matter.

biopsy (bi′op-se) Removal of tissue from the body for examination.

incisional biopsy Incision into and removal of part of a lesion.

excisional biopsy Removal of an entire small lesion.

aspiration/needle biopsy Removal of material from an internal organ by means of a hollow needle inserted through the body wall and into the affected tissue.

cautery (kaw′ter-ē) A hot instrument used to cut or destroy tissue, causing hemostasis at the time.

don To put on an article, such as gloves or a gown.

ligate (li′gāt) To apply a ligature.

ligature (lig′ah-tūr) A suture; material used to tie off blood vessels to prevent bleeding, or to constrict tissues.

Mayo (mā′ō) stand A stand with a flat metal tray used to hold sterile supplies during an aseptic procedure.

preoperative (pre-op′er-ah-tiv) Pertaining to the time preceding surgery.

postoperative (post-op′er-ah-tiv) Pertaining to the period of time following surgery.

sterile field A work area prepared with sterile drapes (coverings) to hold sterile supplies during a sterile procedure.

sterile setup Specific sterile supplies used in a specific sterile procedure.

suture (soo′cher) Various types and sizes of absorbable and nonabsorbable materials used to close tissue with stitches.

transfer forceps A type of instrument (forcep) that is kept in a chemical disinfectant or germicide and used for transferring or handling sterile supplies and equipment.

This chapter discusses the common practices of and some procedures requiring surgical asepsis (sterile technique). To control the sources and spread of infection when performing and assisting with certain medical procedures, knowledge of and adherence to the correct performance of aseptic practices are essential.

A good preparation for studying this chapter is to review Chapter 20, which discussed concepts of infection control, medical and surgical asepsis, practices of medical asepsis, and disinfection and sterilization of supplies.

BACKGROUND OF STERILE TECHNIQUE

Sterile techniques as we know them today have gradually evolved since the turn of the century. The history of medicine shows evidence of some understanding of asepsis as early as the time of Hippocrates, the father of medicine, in 460 BC. It was Hippocrates who started to use boiled water when irrigating wounds; later Galen (131-210 AD) boiled instruments before using them when caring for wounds. Throughout the centuries up to present times, numerous individuals, too many to mention here, played vital roles in describing diseases and their causes, theories for contagious diseases, how infection was spread by improperly washed hands, the role of bacteria in causing disease, how heat could inhibit the growth of microorganisms, and the germ theory for the causes of disease.

Joseph Lister (1827-1912) introduced the use of chemical to destroy microorganisms in infected wounds (antisepsis) and later procedurs to exclude bacteria from surgical fields (asepsis). Surgery as we know it today was essential Lister's gift to humanity.

In the later years of the nineteenth century, the concepts of vaccinations against disease were introduced. Edward Jenner discovered the value of vaccination against smallpox. This was a discovery that led to further advances, such as Louis Pasteur's principle of inoculation by means of vaccines against viral and bacterial diseases.

Sterilization of items by boiling began around 1880, and the principles and practices of autoclaving (steam under pressure) began around 1886. Rubber gloves were first used to protect the hands from harsh antiseptics. Eventually they were accepted and used as a protective measure to prevent contamination to the patient. Thus sterile technique or aseptic practices—as we know them—evolved.

PRINCIPLES AND PRACTICES OF SURGICAL ASEPSIS

Surgical asepsis, more commonly referred to as *sterile technique* or *aseptic technique,* is the practice used when an area and supplies in that area are to be made and kept sterile. These techniques are used in all procedures in which entry is made into normally sterile body parts, such as when administering an injection, making a surgical incision, or caring for any break in the skin, such as open wounds or skin ulcers. Strict sterile or aseptic technique is required at all times in such procedures, because body tissues can easily become infected. Breaks in technique may lead to infections that the body cannot combat. Even more infections delay recovery and are costly—mentally, physically, and financially, to the patient. It is the responsibility of the medical assistant and the physician to adhere to the following principles and practices at all times when assisting with or performing a sterile procedure.

1. Sterilize all supplies used for sterile procedures either previously or at the time for immediate use.
2. When in doubt about the sterility of an object, consider it nonsterile.
3. When putting on sterile gloves, do not touch the outside of the gloves with bare hands.
4. People who have sterile gloves on must touch only sterile articles; people who are not gloved must touch only nonsterile articles, except when using sterile transfer forceps to move sterile items.
5. If a glove is punctured by a needle or instrument during a sterile procedure, remove the damaged glove, wash your hands, and put on a new glove as promptly as patient safety permits. Remove the needle or instrument from the sterile field.
6. The outer wrappings and the edges of packs that contain sterile items are not sterile, thus are handled and opened by the person who is not wearing sterile gloves.
7. Open sterile packages with the edges of the wrapper directed away from your body to avoid touching your uniform or reaching over a sterile field.
8. Touch only the outside of a sterile wrapper.
9. Once a sterile pack has been opened, use it; if it is not used, rewrap and resterilize it.
10. Avoid sneezing, coughing, or talking directly over a sterile field or object.
11. Do not reach across or above a sterile field or wound. Your clothes and skin are not sterile. If you touch the sterile field or drop debris onto it or into the wound, contamination results. Movements around the area should be kept to a minimum.

12. Avoid spilling solutions on a sterile setup. Any moisture that soaks through a sterile area to a non-sterile one produces a means of transporting bacteria to a sterile area. Thus, the wet areas are considered contaminated and must either be covered with sterile towels or drapes until the top surface is dry or be removed and redraped.
13. Hold sterile objects and gloved hands above waist level or level to the sterile field. Anything below this level is considered unsterile. Keeping objects or hands in sight helps avoid contamination.
14. Since skin cannot be sterilized, any object that touches it is considered contaminated.
15. Have a special receptable or waxed paper or plastic bag to receive contaminated materials.
16. A sterile field should be away from drafts, fans, and windows. Microorganisms can be carried in air current to the patient or the sterile field.
17. Stores sterile packages in dry areas. If they become wet, they must be resterilized or discarded.
18. Hands are the greatest source of contamination; therefore wash frequently using correct technique.
19. Be constantly aware of the need for very clean surroundings.

In summary, keep in mind these five basic rules:
- Know what is sterile.
- Know what is not sterile.
- Keep sterile items separate from nonsterile items.
- Prevent contamination.
- Remedy a contaminated situation immediately.

HANDLING STERILE SUPPLIES

Opening Sterile Packages

Many commercially prepared sterile packages have instructions for opening printed on them. Read these directions carefully before opening the package to avoid contamination of the contents. To open *peel-down packages,* such as those in which syringes and dressing materials are supplied, use the following procedure.

Opening peel-down packages

Procedure

1. Wash your hands..
2. Using both hands, grasp both sides of the extended edges provided.
3. Pull evenly along the sealed edges (Figure 21.1,*A*).
4. Do not touch the inside of the wrapper; place on a flat surface

or

5. Using sterile forceps, remove the contents from the wrapper and transfer to a sterile field or use immediately in a sterile procedure, such as a dressing change (Figure 21.1,*B*).
6. Holding the bottom of the package with the edges folded back, allow a person with sterile gloves on to take the contents.

or

7. If the item is a syringe to be used by you, grasp the plunger end of the syringe with one hand while holding onto the package with your other hand.

Rationale

Pull evenly in a downward motion to avoid tearing.
The inside of the wrapper is sterile and can be used as a sterile field until using the contents.

Keep your fingers away from the contents to avoid contamination.

The bottom part of the plunger does not have to remain sterile, because this is the way in which you take hold of the syringe to remove it from the sterile package.

A   B

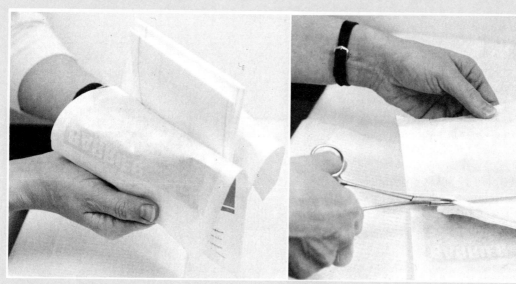

Figure 21.1
A, Technique for opening a peel-down package with sterile contents. **B,** Technique for removing sterile dressing from package.

Continued.

Opening Sterile Packages—cont'd

Opening an envelope wrap

Procedure

1. Wash your hands.
2. Place package on a flat surface so that the folded edges are on top.
3. Remove tape or string fastener, and discard in waste container.
4. Pull out the tucked under corner (if present), and unfold this top flap away from you (Figure 21.2).

Rationale

At this time you should also check the date and sterilization indicator to make sure that the contents are sterile.
Unfolding away from you avoids the necessity of reaching over the sterile field later and causing contamination. Avoid touching the pack with your uniform or person.

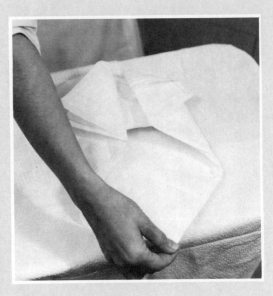

Figure 21.2
Opening sterile pack, step 1: Unfold top flap away from your body.

5. Using both hands, grasp the second layer of folded corners, and open these flaps to the sides of the package (Figure 21.3), or open first one side and then the other.
6. Without reaching over any of the uncovered area, grasp the last fold or fourth corner, and open toward your body (Figure 21.4).

The contents of the package are still covered with the last layer of the wrapper.

Lift this corner up and toward you, dropping it on the surface holding the package. Do not touch the inside of the package nor the contents with bare hands, as this would contaminate everything.

You now have a sterile field that can be used as a sterile work area. Additional sterile items that may be needed for the procedure may be added to this sterile field. To organize the items contained in the package you just opened, use sterile transfer forceps as discussed next (Figure 21.5) or don sterile gloves.

Small packages can be held in the hand and unwrapped in the same fashion. Have someone who is wearing sterile gloves take the item from the opened wrap, or remove it with sterile transfer forceps or very carefully place the item on a sterile field, avoiding contamination to the item and field. Be sure that the wrapper corners do not touch the sterile field.

Figure 21.3
Opening sterile pack, step 2:
Open second layer of flaps to
each side.

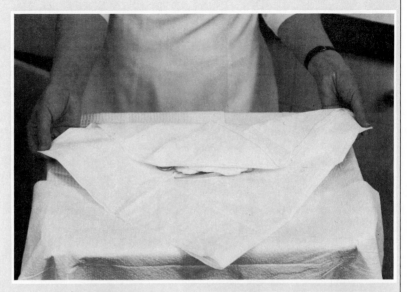

Figure 21.4
Opening sterile pack, step 3:
Open last flap toward your body.

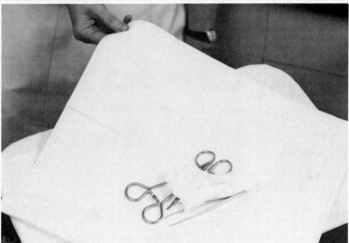

Figure 21.5
Using sterile forceps, arrange
sterile supplies on sterile field
for use.

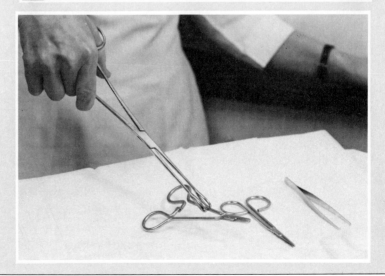

Handling Sterile Transfer Forceps

Sterile transfer forceps are used to transfer or handle sterile equipment to avoid contamination by the hands. The use of these forceps, which are kept in a container with a disinfectant or germicide solution, is being discouraged by many health care practitioners who feel these forceps are very vulnerable to contamination and therefore a cause of further contamination. The more common and recommended practice is to use an individually wrapped sterile forceps for each procedure when needed. Despite the fact that sterile transfer forceps are now not used as often, they remain as standard equipment in many offices and clinics. The following describes how they are to be handled if and when you must use them.

Procedure	*Rationale*
1. Keep only one forceps in the container of clean germicidal solution.	When more than one forceps is kept in the container, the change of contaminating one against the other when removing one is too great.
2. Wash your hands.	
3. When removing from container, keep the prongs together and facing downard; grasp handles and lift vertically without touching any part of the container above the solution line (Figure 21.6).	The container is not sterile above the solution line. Sterile parts are contaminated when touching unsterile parts.
4. You may tap the prongs together gently over the container to remove excess solution.	Excess solution falling on sterile field would contaminate it. You must avoid this.
5. Keep forceps in a downward position when using to prevent any solution on prongs from flowing up to the handle.	The handle is not sterile. Solution that flows to the handle will flow back to the prongs when returned to a downward position, thus contaminating the forceps.
6. Use as required to handle, transfer, or assemble sterile supplies and equipment (Figure 21.5).	
7. Never touch the tip of the forceps to the sterile field when putting supplies on it after a procedure has begun.	After a procedure has begun, the forceps will be contaminated for any other procedure if you touch the present sterile field and must be resterilized before being returned to the container.
8. After use, return the forceps to the container without touching any parts of the container.	Remember that the container is not sterile except inside below the solution level.
9. Sterilize the forceps and container and refill container with fresh germicide solution weekly or more frequently if indicated.	The more frequently these items are resterilized and the solution changed, the more likely this procedure will be safe to use.

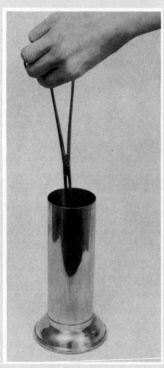

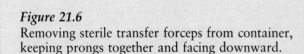

Figure 21.6
Removing sterile transfer forceps from container, keeping prongs together and facing downward.

Pouring Sterile Solutions

When required to pour a sterile solution, you must use aseptic technique to avoid contamination to the solution.

Procedure	*Rationale*
1. Wash your hands.	
2. Obtain the solution and check the label.	Solutions are drugs. All drug labels must be checked three times before using or administering:
	• When removing from storage area
	• Before pouring
	• When replacing container in the storage area
3. Obtain sterile container to be used for the solution, and unwrap.	Follow procedure for unwrapping as described previously.
	NOTE: When using prepackaged sterile trays, a container for the solution may be included in the pack.
4. Remove bottle cap; place on a level surface with the top of the cap resting on the surface or hold it in your hand with the top facing downwards (Figure 21.7).	The inner part of the cap is considered sterile. If you place the cap with top facing up, you have contaminated the inner surface, which then cannot be replaced on the container until it has been sterilized.
5. Hold the bottle with the label in palm of your hand and about 6 inches above the container (or less, when pouring very small amounts of solution), and pour the solution (Figure 21.7).	Holding the bottle this way prevents damage to the label if the solution runs or spills; also undue splashing is avoided. Pour a small amount of solution into a waste container to cleanse the side of the bottle, and then pour from the same area.
6. When pouring a solution on a sponge, pick up the sponge with forceps and pour the solution over the spone. The excess solution will drip into the basin or discard container (Figure 20.8).	
7. Pick the cap up by the sides, and replace it on the bottle securely.	Do not contaminate the inside of the cap, because it is considered sterile and must cover the sterile solution in the bottle.
8. Check the label of the bottle, and replace it in the correct storage area.	

Figure 21.7
Pouring solution into container on sterile field.

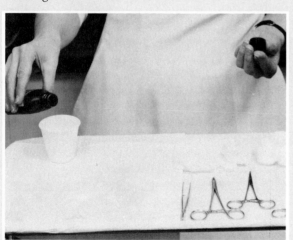

Figure 21.8
Pouring solution onto sterile sponge.

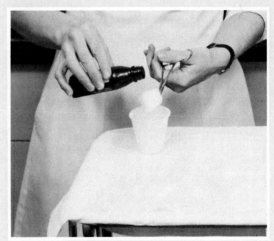

Donning Sterile Gloves

Sterile gloves are worn to protect the patient from infection caused by microorganisms that may be on your hands and to provide a means of safely handling sterile supplies and equipment without contaminating these items. They are also worn to protect the health care worker from possible infection. (See also Chapter 20, page 345.)

Procedure	*Rationale*
1. Wash your hands.	
2. Obtain wrapped gloves, and place on a clean, dry, flat surface with the cuff end toward you.	
3. Open the wrapper by handling only the outside.	The inside part of the wrapper is sterile.
4. Using your left hand, pick up the right-hand glove by grasping the folded edge of the cuff and lifting up and away from the wrapper (Figure 21.9).	The folded edge of the cuff will be against your skin and is contaminated as soon as you touch it. *Do not* touch the outside of the glove with your ungloved hand.
5. Pulling on the edge of the cuff, pull the right glove on.	Keep your fingers away from the rest of the glove.
6. Place fingers of the right gloved hand under the cuff of the left-hand glove (Figure 21.10).	Be sure that your gloved fingers do not touch your skin. The area inside the folded cuff is considered sterile.
7. Lift the glove up and away from the wrapper and pull it onto your left hand.	Be sure that the left thumb does not stray up and touch the right glove. Keep the right gloved fingers under the cuff and straight; keep the right glove thumb bAck to avoid touching skin.
8. Continue pulling the left glove up over your wrist.	The area inside the folded cuff is considered sterile.
9. With the gloved left hand, place fingers under the cuff of the right glove and pull the cuff up over your right wrist (Figure 21.11).	
10. Adjust the fingers of the gloves as necessary.	If, when putting on either glove, the fingers get into the wrong space, you must proceed with the rest of the gloving procedure and then adjust the gloves with gloved hands.
11. If either glove tears during the procedure, remove and discard, then begin the procedure again with a new pair of gloves.	
12. To remove gloves:	
• Grasp the cuff of the right-hand glove with your left hand.	
• Pull the glove down over the hand.	The glove will turn inside out as it comes off.
• Discard in the appropriate place.	
• Repeat using the right hand to remove left glove. Grasp the inside and top of the left-hand glove with your right hand, pull the glove down over the hand, and discoard.	Do not touch the outside of the glove because it is considered contaminated after use.
Reusable gloves must be washed and resterilized; disposable gloves are discarded in the appropriate waste container.	

Figure 21.9
Technique for donning first sterile glove.
Grasp folded edge of cuff, lift up and
away from wrapper, and pull onto right hand.

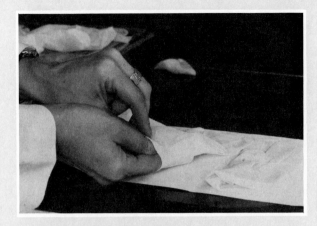

Figure 21.10
Technique for donning second sterile glove.
Place fingers of gloved hand under cuff of
other glove and pull onto left hand.

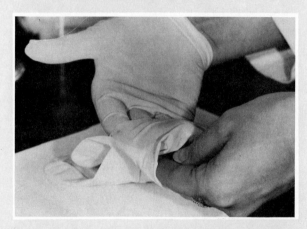

Figure 21.11
Technique for donning sterile gloves.
Adjust cuffs on gloves, avoiding
contamination.

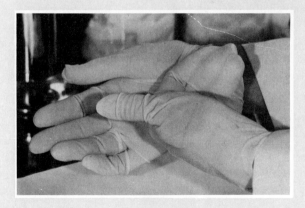

MINOR SURGERY

Only "minor" surgery is performed in the physician's office, although commonly even these procedurs are due in the emergency room or outpatient department of a hospital.

Minor surgical procedures include those that can be done with or without the use of a local anesthetic, such as suturing a laceration; the incision and drainage of an abscess or cyst; incision and removal of foreign bodies in subcutaneous tissues; removal of small growths such as warts, moles, and skin tags; various types of biopsies; cauterization of tissue (such as cauterization of the uterine cervix, or of a wart, mole, or skin tag); and insertion of an intrauterine device (IUD). After minor surgery performed in the office or at the hospital, the patient may come to the physician's office for dressing changes and for removal of sutures as part of the postoperative care. Inspection of the wound is also done at that time to determine the amount of healing that has occurred and to ensure that there is no developing infectious process.

As the physician's assistant, you may be called on to assist with the surgical procedures or to change a dressing for a patient. Assisting in any surgical procedure is a highly responsible job, and strict aseptic techniques must always be used. The nature of the surgery or postoperative care will govern the duties and responsibilities of the medical assistant.

Anesthesia

For minor surgery and very painful treatments, some type of local anesthesia is usually required. Local anesthesia to the absence of feeling or sensation and pain in a limited area of the body without the loss of consciousness. The extent and severity of the procedure will determine the type and amount of anesthetic used, which can be administered by injection or by topical application. Local anesthetics produce their effects in 5 to 15 minutes. These effects may last from 1 to 3 hours, depending on the type and dose administered.

Types of local anesthesia

- Infiltration—The anesthetic solution is injected under the skin to anesthetize the nerve endings and nerve fibers at the site to be worked on. The sensory nerves become insensitive and remain so for several hours, depending on the amount of drug administered. (Rules for the administration of medications and injections as described in Chapter 23 apply here.) Examples of infiltration anesthetics include procaine (Novocaine) 1% to 2% and lidocaine (Xylocaine) 1% to 2%.
- Nerve block or block anesthesia—The anesthetic solution is injected into or adjacent to accessible main nerves, thus desensitizing all the adjacent tissue. Examples of nerve block anesthesia include procaine (Novocaine) 1% to 2% and lidocaine (Xylocaine) 1% to 2%.
- Topical or surface anesthesia—The anesthetic solution is painted or sprayed directly onto the skin or mucous membrane involved to deaden sensation and relieve pain. Examples of topical anesthetics include lidocaine 4% solution, for accessible mucous membranes of oral and nasal cavities, and ethyl chloride spray, for external topical use, because it is too harsh for use on mucous membranes. Before a topical anesthetic is applied the patient's skin must be washed and dried well.

Allergic reactions

Before the administration of a local anesthetic, every patient must be asked if he is allergic to any drug, if he has any cardiac or respiratory problems, and if he has had any type of anesthetic before. This information is very important, as some local anesthetics can cause anaphylactic shock or violent allergic reactions in patients who are allergic to the drug. Frequently skin tests are made beforehand when deemed necessary. An emergency tray with sterile syringes and needles, sterile alcohol sponges, and ampules of a stimulant such as epinephrine (Adrenalin) must be kept within reach when an anesthetic is to be administered in preparation for an emergency if one does arise.

Suture Materials and Needles

The purpose of sutures is to hold the edges of tissues together until healing occurs. When suture materials are needed for a procedure, they can be added to your sterile field. The most commonly used are the sterile prepackaged sutures with or without an attached suture needle (Figure 21.12). The label on these packages indicate the type and size of the suture and needle enclosed. Sutures are prepared from materials that are either absorbable or nonabsorbable. *Absorbable sutures* do not have to be removed when used, as they are absorbed or digested by the body fluids and tissues during and after the healing process, for example, surgical gut (catgut). *Nonabsorbable sutures* used on outer skin surfaces are removed after the wound has healed because body fluids and cells do not absorb or di-

Figure 21.12
Prepackaged sterile suture materials. Cover of package indicates type and size of suture material, and the curved line under the suture label represents the type and size of needle included. Included is a needle holder and a suture needle with attached black suture material.

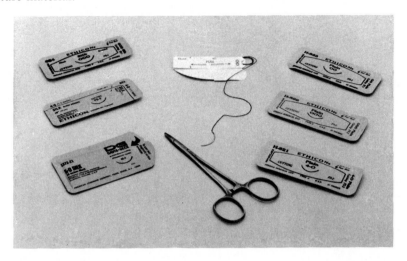

gest them. When used internally, they are not removed and remain as foreign bodies. Usually they become encysted and cause no trouble, for example, cotton, silk, nylon, and wire. The size, or gauge, of most sutures is labeled in terms of 0s. That is, 0, which is the thickest, then 00, 000, and so on, each decreasing in size up to 10-0, which is the thinnest. Sizes 2-0 up to 6-0 are used most frequently; 10-0 silk, is being extremely fine, is used for ophthalmological and vascular procedures. A few types of sutures are designated as 1, 2, 3, 4, and 5 (the thickest); others are designated simply as fine, medium, and coarse. The size of the suture used is determined by the areas and the purpose for which it will be used. Thicker sutures are used when closing large wounds, medium ones on lacerations, and very fine sutures are used on more delicate tissues, such as the eye, or on facial tissues.

Suture needles are either straight or curved and have either a sharp, cutting point or a round, noncutting point. They are supplied in individual packages or in packages with suture materials (Figure 21.12). Some needles have an eye through which you thread the suture material. Other needles come attached to the suture material as one unit. These are called *swaged needles* (Figure 21.13) and their package will be labeled as the type and size of the needle and type, size and length of the suture material.

Sharp cutting needles are used on stable tissues,

such as the skin, where the sharp point is useful in pushing the needle through the tissue. Round, noncutting needles are used on less firm tissues, such as subcutaneous tissues, and on the internal organs of body cavities. Curved needles are held in a needle holder (see Figure 21.13, *D*) when used in order to get in and out of the tissue, as when suturing small skin incisions. Straight needles are held by hand as they are pushed through adjoining tissues when suturing large skin incisions. The size and type of suture needle needed is determined by the area and the purpose for which it will be used.

An alternative to the use of sutures for holding the edges of tissue together is the use of adhesive skin closures. These are sterile nonallergenic tapes that are supplied in a variety of lengths and widths. An example of a commercial adhesive skin closure is Steri-Strips. The edges of the tissue are held together and the Steri-Strips are applied transversely across this area and left in place until the wound has healed.

Instruments Used for Minor Surgery

Surgical instruments are tools or devices designed to perform a specific function, such as cutting, grasping, retracting, or suturing (Figure 21.14). They are usually made of steel and are treated so that they are durable, rust resistant, heat resistant,

Text continued on p. 385.

Figure 21.13

Types of suture needles: **A,** Straight. **B,** Curved with sharp point. **C,** Swaged. **D,**
Swaged needle positioned for use in needle
holder.

A, B, and C, courtesy Miltex Instrument Co.,
Lake Success, NY.

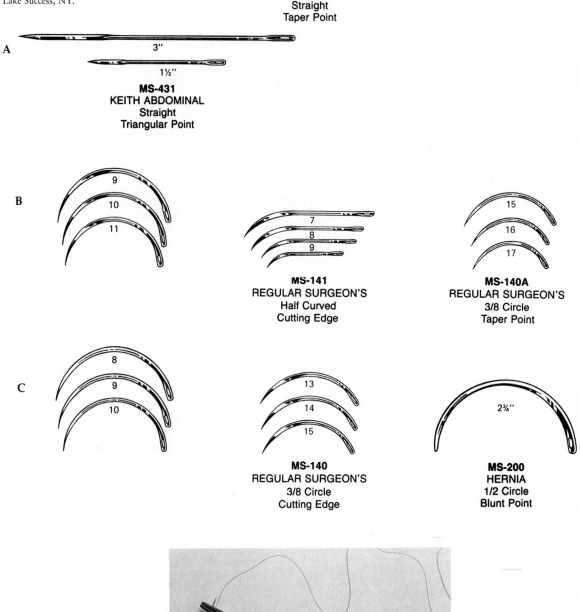

MS-122
FINE INTESTINAL
Straight
Taper Point

A   3″

1½″

MS-431
KEITH ABDOMINAL
Straight
Triangular Point

B   9
10
11

MS-141
REGULAR SURGEON'S
Half Curved
Cutting Edge

7
8
9

MS-140A
REGULAR SURGEON'S
3/8 Circle
Taper Point

15
16
17

C   8
9
10

MS-140
REGULAR SURGEON'S
3/8 Circle
Cutting Edge

13
14
15

MS-200
HERNIA
1/2 Circle
Blunt Point

2¾″

D

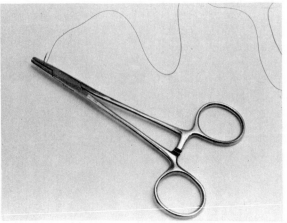

Figure 21.14
Instruments used for minor surgery.
Courtesy Miltex Instrument Co., Lake Success, NY.

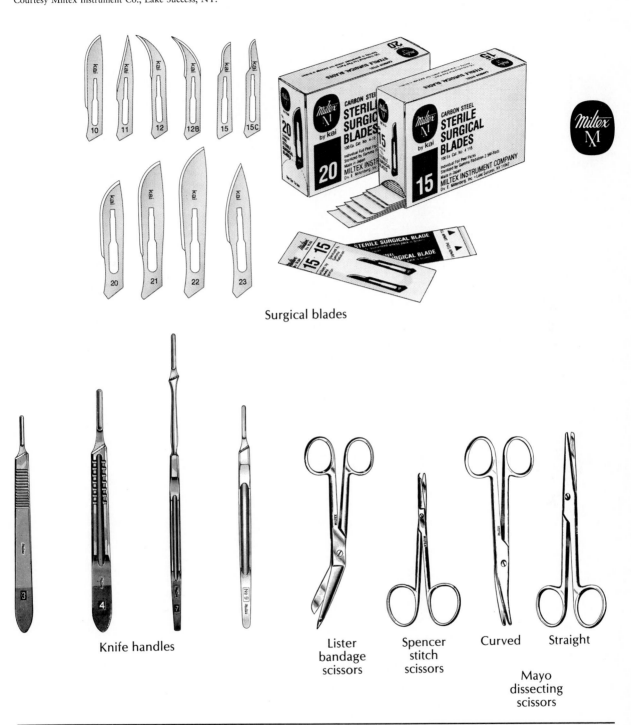

Surgical blades

Knife handles   Lister   Spencer   Curved   Straight
                 bandage   stitch
                 scissors scissors
                                      Mayo
                                      dissecting
                                      scissors

Continued.

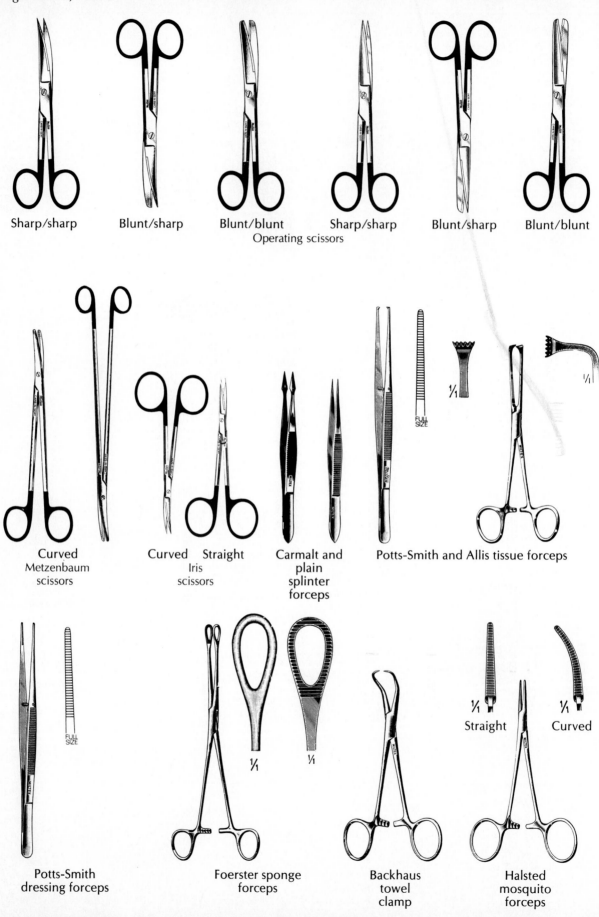

Sharp/sharp   Blunt/sharp   Blunt/blunt   Sharp/sharp   Blunt/sharp   Blunt/blunt

Operating scissors

Curved
Metzenbaum
scissors

Curved   Straight
Iris
scissors

Carmalt and
plain
splinter
forceps

Potts-Smith and Allis tissue forceps

Potts-Smith
dressing forceps

Foerster sponge
forceps

Backhaus
towel
clamp

Halsted
mosquito
forceps

Straight   Curved

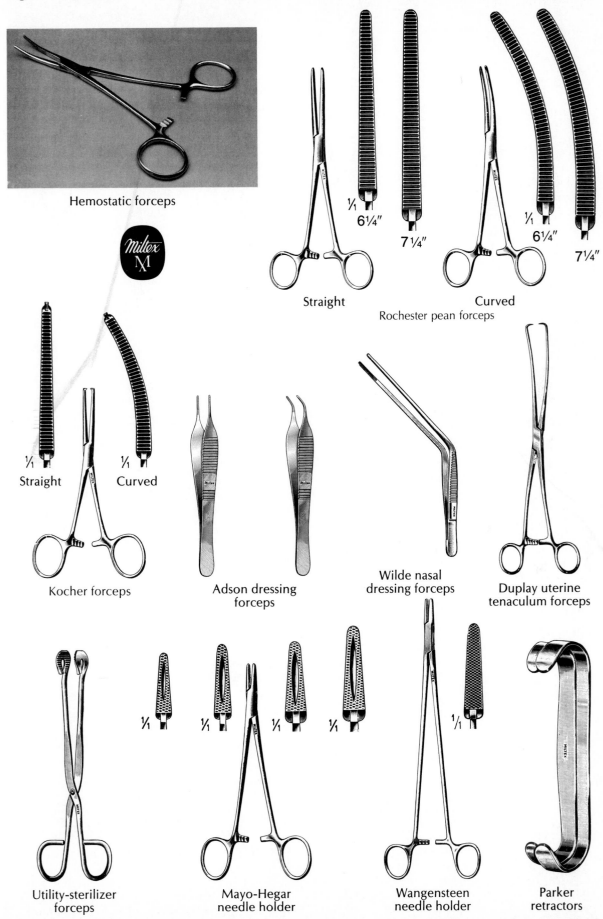

Figure 21.14, cont'd

Hemostatic forceps

⅟₁ 6¼″

7¼″

Straight

⅟₁ 6¼″

7¼″

Curved

Rochester pean forceps

⅟₁ Straight   ⅟₁ Curved

Kocher forceps

Adson dressing
forceps

Wilde nasal
dressing forceps

Duplay uterine
tenaculum forceps

⅟₁   ⅟₁   ⅟₁   ⅟₁   ⅟₁

Utility-sterilizer
forceps

Mayo-Hegar
needle holder

Wangensteen
needle holder

Parker
retractors

Continued.

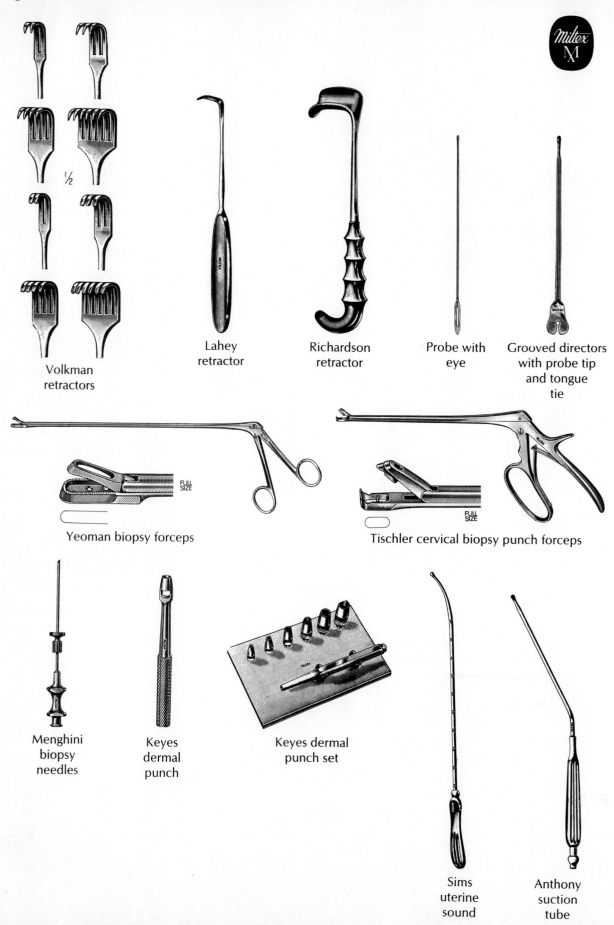

Volkman
retractors

Lahey
retractor

Richardson
retractor

Probe with
eye

Grooved directors
with probe tip
and tongue
tie

Yeoman biopsy forceps

Tischler cervical biopsy punch forceps

Menghini
biopsy
needles

Keyes
dermal
punch

Keyes dermal
punch set

Sims
uterine
sound

Anthony
suction
tube

and stainproof. Proper care of all surgical instruments is essential. You must see that they are used correctly, handled carefully, inspected for any defects, and sterilized and stored correctly. As a medical assistant you should be able to identify a variety of surgical instruments, know how they are used, sterilized, and stored, and be able to select the correct instruments for a variety of minor surgical procedures that may be performed in the physician's office or clinic. Some of the more common surgical instruments will be discussed. Figure 21.14 illustrates many of these instruments. Additional figures in this chapter illustrate tray set-ups for specific procedures with some of these instruments.

Scalpels

Scalpels are used to make incisions into tissues. They are small surgical knives that usually have a convex edge. Scalpel blades are supplied in various sizes and shapes that are designed for making different types of incisions in various tissues. Most scalpels are now disposable and some are supplied with a disposable handle; others are reusable. The no. 3 and no. 7 hands are the most commonly used; the no. 7 handling being the thinner handle.

Scissors

Surgical scissors are used to cut or dissect tissues and to cut sutures. Others are used to cut bandages when they are to be removed. These instruments consist of two opposing cutting blades, which may be straight or curved. The tips on the blades will vary. On some scissors both tips are sharp; on others both tips are blunt; others will have one sharp tip and one blunt tip. *Bandage scissors* have one blunt tip with the other tip having a flat blunt probe on it. These are used to remove bandages and dressings without puncturing the tissues. *Suture scissors,* used to remove sutures, have one blunt tip and a hook on the second tip. When removing sutures the hook goes under the suture. The blunt tip prevents one from puncturing the tissue. Common *dissecting scissors* are the straight or curved Mayo scissors; the short, curved Metzenbaum scissors, which is used on superficial, delicate tissue; and the long, blunt, curved Metzenbaum, which is used on deep, delicate tissue. The tips of dissecting scissors are blunt so that tissue will not be inadvertently punctured. *Operating scissors* have straight blades and may have any one of the combination type of plades (sharp/sharp, blunt/blunt, or sharp/blunt). The type of scissors used in a procedure will vary, depending on its intended function.

Forceps

Forceps are instruments of varied sizes and shapes used for grasping, compressing, or holding tissue or objects. They are two-pronged instruments with either a spring handle or a ring handle with a ratchet closure. The ratchet is a toothed clasp that allows for different degrees of tightness to be applied to the tissue or object on which the instrument is used. The inner surfaces of some forceps have saw-like teeth that are called serrations (Figure 21.17, C). Serrations prevent tissue from slipping out of the forceps jaw. The tips may be either plain-tipped or tooth-tipped. Plain-tipped forceps are used to pick up tissue, dressings, or other sterile objects. A toothed-tipped forceps is especially useful for grasping tissue. The teeth prevent the tissue from slipping out of the grasp of the instrument.

Examples of forceps with a *spring handle* are the thumb, tissue, splinter, and dressing forceps. Examples of forceps with a *ring handle* and ratchet closure are Allis tissue forceps, Foerster sponge forceps, Backhaus towel clamps, and straight or curved hemostatic forceps or hemostats. Hemostats include Halsted mosquito hemostatic forceps, Kelly hemostatic forceps, Rochest-Pean hemostatic forceps, and Ochsner-Kocher hemostatic forceps.

Forceps with a *toothed tip* include standard tissue forceps, Allis tissue forceps, and Ochsner-Kocher hemostatic forceps. *Plain-tipped* forceps include standard thumb forceps, plain splinter forceps (these have sharp points), Adison dressing forceps, and the Halsted mosquito, Kelly, and Rochester-Pean hemostatic forceps.

Sponge forceps are used for holding sponges and have serrated ring-like tips. *Towel clamps,* having two sharp points, are used to hold the edges of sterile drapes or towels together. *Hemostats* are used to compress, hold, or grasp a blood vessel. They are also used by some medical personnel to apply or remove a dressing.

Needle holders

Needle holders have a ring handle, a ratchet closure, and serrated tips. Some needle holders have a groove in the middle of the serrations (see Fig. 21.17, C). These instruments are used to hold a curved needle used for suturing tissues.

Retractors

Retractors are instruments used to hold back the edges of tissues or organs to maintain exposure of the operative area. Examples include a double-ended Richardson retractor and a Volkmann rake retractor.

Probes

Probes are slender, long instruments used for exploring wounds or body cavities or passages. The end of a probe may be straight or curved. The body area being explored will determine the type of probe to be used.

Biopsy instruments

Biopsy instruments are used to obtain a small piece of tissue from the body for examination. There are various sizes and shapes of biopsy forceps. Three common ones that you may see in the office or clinic are the rectal biopsy punch, the cervical biopsy forceps, and a 6 mm biopsy punch used to obtain a small sample of skin.

Instrument Care

Points to keep in mind for the care of instruments include the following:

1. Use the instrument *only* for the intended purpose and in the correct manner. *Handle with care.*
2. Rinse or soak, then sanitize and sterilize instruments as described in Chapter 20 as soon as possible after use.
3. Inspect each instrument for any defect and proper working condition.
4. Never toss instruments around nor pile them on top of each other, as damage could result.
5. Keep sharp and lensed instruments separate from other instruments to prevent damage.
6. Keep ratchet handles open when not in use. This will prolong the usefulness of the treatment.

Preparing the Patient for Minor Surgery

When a patient is to have minor or major surgery, or other major forms of therapy, it is the duty of the physician to explain the nature of the procedure, the alternatives to the procedure, and the risks of the procedure. This allows the patient to give an *informed consent* for the procedure. Informed consent is a *right*—not merely a privilege. By law, the patient's consent is required for these types of treatment.

A consent form must be signed by the patient before the procedure is started. This form gives the physician permission to perform the procedure. If this is not done, numerous legal complications may result. Although it is the physician's responsibility to give the patient an explanation, frequently the medical assistant will have to briefly explain the

procedure once again on the day of surgery while preparing the patient and be ready to answer questions the patient may have. Remember, any surgical procedure is an invasion into body parts not normally interfered with; and although it may be a minor surgical procedure, it often does not appear minor to the patient. Many patients are anxious, nervous, or concerned about what is going to happen. The medical assistant can and must help the patient relax and allay any fears of apprehensions. Having everything ready when the patient arrives is the initial step. The room must be spotlessly clean, well lighted, and at a comfortable temperature. Supplies and equipment required for the procedure should be prepared in advance. Do not have instruments exposed for the patient's view, as these alone may add more apprehension to some patients.

When the patient enters the office, greet and usher her/him into the treatment room. Provide a gown and give directions for the removal of clothing. Attend to the patient's needs for comfort and communication, and give emotion support and reassurance. Once again, a simple explanation of the procedure may be needed. Be willing to answer any questions the patient may have. Always maintain a calm and confident manner to help reassure and relax the patient.

The best of care can be enhanced by evaluating every patient and situation individually. In this way the most suitable environment can be provided for each individual. Also, when deemed necessary, have the patient arrange to have someone accompany her/him to the office or clinic and provide transportation home.

Materials for Office Surgeries

The following are sample lists of equipment used for minor office surgeries that may vary with the individual physician's preferences and the case. Additional supplies and instruments can be added, or deleted, to meet the requirements of the particular situation. Once you learn the physician's preferences, lists can be prepared for each procedure and used as a reference when preparing for minor surgery. In this way, the required instruments and supplies will not be omitted (Figure 21.17). Figure 21.18 shows supplies and instruments used for procedures involving incisions *without* suture closure, and Figure 21.19 shows supplies and instruments used for procedures involving an excision of tissue and closure *with* sutures.

Text continued on p. 388.

Assisting With Minor Surgery

Careful preparation and adherence to aseptic technique are required when preparing for office or clinic surgery. The responsibilities of the medical assistant during minor surgery include preparing the room and supplies; preparing the patient, both physically and mentally; and assisting the physician as needed. An efficient assistant can make the procedure easier for the patient and the physician by giving attention to both. Similar preparatory steps and equipment are used in most minor surgical procedures, although they may vary according to the physician's preferences.

Procedure	*Rationale*
1. Check that the room is spotlessly clean, well ventilated, and well lighted.	
2. Wash your hands.	
3. If electrical or battery-run equipment is to be used, check it for working order.	
4. Assemble and prepare supplies and equipment.	
• Open and place a sterile drape towel on a tray or Mayo stand.	This will be used as a sterile field.
• Place the required supplies and instruments on this sterile field.	Sterile supplies are to be handled with sterile transfer forceps or sterile gloved hands (refer to the section on handling sterile supplies)
• When the required instruments come wrapped in the same package, or in a commercially prepared package, open the wrapper and use it for the sterile field. Then with sterile transfer forceps or gloved hands, organize the instruments for use (see Figures 21.2 to 21.5).	Refer to the previous section on opening sterile packages.
5. Cover this sterile setup with sterile towel until ready to use (Figure 21.15).	Avoid contamination to the sterile setup.
6. Obtain any medications or solutions that will be required during the procedure.	
7. Open outer wrap of the sterile glove pack for the physician.	
8. Prepare the patient.	Refer to the preceding discussion on preparing the patient for minor surgery.
• Explain the procedure.	
• Provide a gown, and instruct what clothing must be removed.	
• Have the patient void if necessary.	

Figure 21.15
A, Using sterile transfer forceps to organize instruments for minor surgery. **B,** Cover sterile setup with a sterile towel until ready to use.

A 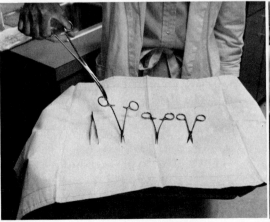   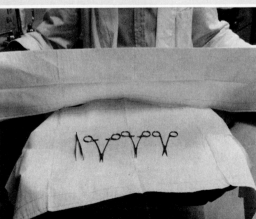 B

Continued.

Assisting With Minor Surgery—cont'd

Procedure	Rationale
• Position the patient according to the type and location of surgery that is to be performed.	The patient must be made comfortable, whether sitting or in a prone or supine position, to avoid any undue tension or movement during the operation.
• If required, wash the operative site with soap and water and then shave the area. • Drape the patient. 9. Summon the physician.	The physician will drape the area with sterile drapes after painting the skin with an antiseptic solution.
10. When the physician has donned the sterile gloves, remove the sterile towel that is covering the tray of instruments.	Standing behind or to the side of the instrument tray, carefully grasp the two distal corners of the towel. Slowly lift the towel off by lifting it towards you. You must not touch anything but the two distal ends of the towel, otherwise you may contaminate the sterile setup.
11. Assist the physician as requested. If additional supplies are needed, you must use aseptic technique when handing them to the physician or placing them on the sterile field.	Refer to the previous section on handling sterile supplies.
12. Offer physical and emotional support to the patient. It may be necessary for you to steady the patient's arm, hand, leg, head, or any body part so that moving or jerking is avoided while the physician is operating. Casually and calmly talk to the patient.	Casual and calm conversation may help to direct attention from any pain or discomfort being experienced and may help the patient relax.
13. Do not stand between the patient and the physician, between the physician and the light source, or too near the sterile setup.	The operative area must not be obstructed. Sterile supplies must not be contaminated.
14. If you actually help the physician and handle the sterile supplies during the procedure, you must again scrub your hands thoroughly before the procedure is to begin, don sterile gloves, and, at times, also don a sterile gown. Then during the procedure, you will be expected to hand the instruments to the physician, and to receive them after use.	When directly assisting the physician with the instruments, you must anticipate the physician's needs. That is, you must know when the physician will need each instrument or other supplies. You must hand an instrument over so that when the physician grasps it, it is ready to use without making adjustments.
15. Hold containers for collecting specimens or drainage or discharge near the work area when needed.	
16. Place soiled instruments in a basin or container when they are no longer needed.	These should be placed out of the patient's view. Avoid contaminating the remaining sterile supplies.
17. Soiled sponges and dressings should be placed in a waxed paper or plastic bag.	Do not allow wet items to sit on a sterile field, because contamination will result.

Materials basic to all procedures

Sterile transfer forceps or individually wrapped sterile forceps
Sterile gloves for the physician
Sterile gloves for the assistant when directly assisting the procedure
NOTE: When using instruments for the following setups that have been soaking in a chemical solution, rinse them in sterile water before using.

Materials for preparing the skin area

Surgical detergent for washing the skin
Sterile sponges (cotton balls and gauze—2 × 2 inch and 4 × 4 inch)

Sterile forceps
Antiseptic solution such as povidone-iodine (Betadine) for disinfecting the skin
Razor and blade (if skin is to be shaved)
Draping materials

Materials to administer local anesthesia

Sterile antiseptic in sterile container, such as povidone-iodine (Betadine) solution
Applicators or cotton balls and a forceps to use when painting the skin. Prepacked sterile povidone-iodine applicators are available and may be used instead
Sterile syringe (3-cc or 5-cc)

Procedure

18. When a biopsy is obtained, immediately place it into the designated jar containing a preservative solution (Figure 21.16).
19. After the surgery, it is often advisable to allow the patient to rest for a short while.

20. Help the patient prepare to leave the office. Do not allow the patient to leave the office without the physician's knowledge. Check with the physician regarding future treatments, medications, and appointments.
21. Provide clear and concise postoperative instructions to the patient, when necessary.

Rationale

When sedation has been administered, *never leave the patient alone on the examining table* unless it has guard rails.

Frequently the physician will give the patient instructions regarding postoperative care to be performed at home by the patient.

When indicated, make sure that the patient knows and understands about the following:
- Compresses
- Elevation of the affected part
- Presence of a drain
- Changing dressing—how often, how it should be done, what to look for (drainage, healing, and so on), and how long to continue
- The possibility of pain and the use of medications ordered for this.

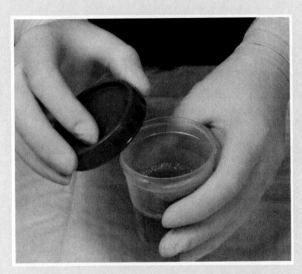

Figure 21.16
Hold container for receiving specimens or discards near work area.

22. When the patient has left, attend to sanitization of the reusable instruments and supplies, dispose of disposables properly, and clean and prepare the room for the next patient. When time permits, clean all instruments for sterilization, sterilize, and return to the proper storage area.
23. Wash your hands.

Sterile needles: 25-gauge, ½-inch, and 23- or 24-gauge, 1½-inch (size and gauge will vary with site to be infiltrated)

Local anesthetic: ampules or vials of lidocaine 1% to 2% or procaine hydrochloride 1% to 2%. For a topical spray anesthetic, ethyl chloride may be used

Sterile gloves (depending on physician's preference and procedure to be performed).

This setup may be prepared individually or added to the sterile setup used for the procedure.

Materials for suturing lacerations

Materials for preparing the skin
Local anesthetic setup

Sterile gloves
Tooth tissue forceps
Hemostat
Needle holder
Suture scissors
Suture material with suture needle
Sterile gauze 2 × 2 inch and 4 × 4 inch (for sponging and dressing wound; larger dressings are needed for lacerations larger than 3 inches)
Adhesive or preferably7 hypoallergenic tape and bandage scissors to cut it
Container for used instruments and sponges

If the wound is infected or abscesses are to be incised, suture material is not needed because infected wounds are usually not sutured.

Figure 21.17
Instruments used for medical-surgical purposes. **A,** Types of scissors. *Left to right:* Straight iris scissors, curved iris scissors, suture scissors, curved Metzenbaum blunt blade scissors, disposable suture scissors, bandage scissors with flat blunt tip to prevent puncturing skin when used. **B,** *Left to right, top:* Punch biopsy forceps, no. 11 scalpel blade and handle; *bottom:* Straight mosquito forceps, curved mosquito forceps, straight Kelly forceps, curved Kelly forceps, tissue forceps (plain tip), tissue forceps (toothed tip), Allis clamp, needle holder. **C,** *Left:* Serrated tip on forceps. *Right:* Serrated tip with groove in the middle seen on some needle holders.

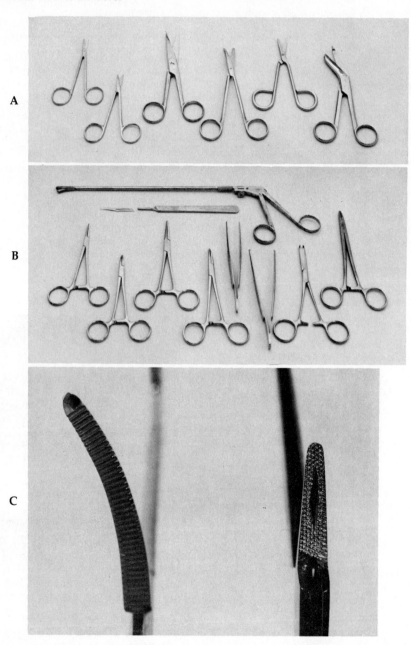

Figure 21.18
Supplies and instruments used for minor surgery involving incisions *without* suture closure. Materials for preparing the skin: container with sponges in surgical detergent and razor with blade. Materials for local anesthesia: vial of local anesthetic medication, 3-cc syringe with needle, alcohol sponge (other antiseptic solutions could be used rather than alcohol sponge). Other supplies and instruments: sterile gloves for surgeon, 4 × 4-inch and 2 × 2-inch sponges, and instruments *(left to right)*, no. 3 scalpel blade handle, scalpel blades *(top to bottom)*, no. 11. no. 10, and no. 15 curved iris scissors, straight mosquito forceps, tissue forcep (plain tip).

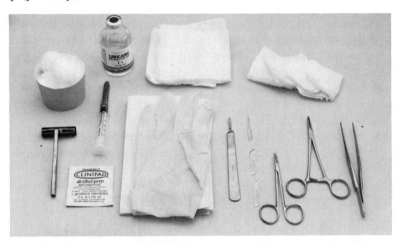

Figure 21.19
Supplies and instruments used for minor surgery when excising tissue and closing the skin *with* suture materials. Left side of picture and along the top includes materials for preparing the skin and administering local anesthesia, sponges, and sterile gloves for the surgeon. Additional supplies and instruments from left to right include: no. 3 scalpel blade handle, no. 10 *(top)* and no. 15 scalpel blades, toothed tissue forceps, curved iris scissors, curved and straight mosquito forceps, straight and curved Kelly forceps, suture scissors, needle holder with mounted curved atraumatic needle with suture material, and container for tissue specimen with preservative solution.

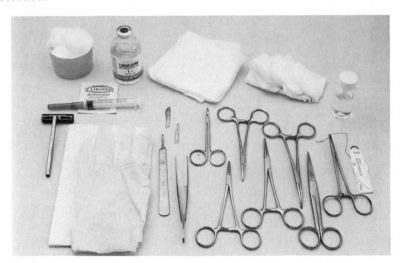

Materials for incision and drainage (I and D) of an abscess or cyst (Figure 21.18)

Materials for preparing the skin
Local anesthetic setup
Sterile gloves
Scalpel handle and blade; usually a no. 11 blade—
   or a no. 15 blade for finer and smaller incisions
Iris (small) sharp scissors to dissect and cut with;
   sometimes larger blunt scissors will also be
   needed
Tissue forceps
Hemostat
Rubber drain to be inserted to provide for drainage
   during healing, when indicated. (Size will vary
   with the size of the incision and area drained. If
   this is sutured to the skin for support, suture material, suture needle, and needle holder are
   needed
Sterile gauze for sponging and dressing the wound
   (2 × 2 inch and 4 × 4 inch)
Adhesive or, preferably, hypoallergenic tape and
   bandage scissors to cut it
Container for used instruments and gauze sponges

Materials for removing foreign bodies in subcutaneous tissues, small growths, and tissue biopsy specimens (Figure 21.19)

Materials for preparing the skin
Local anesthetic setup
Sterile gloves
Mosquito forceps, straight and curved
Kelly forceps, straight and curved
Scalpel handle and blade (no. 10 or no. 15 blade)
   and the electrocautery unit, including a lubri-
   cated lead plate, which is placed under the pa-
   tient for grounding purposes. This plate is not
   needed when the table is grounded. Some tables
   are supplied with an electrical system that is
   grounded to an electrical wall outlet
Iris scissors (small sharp scissors)
Tooth tissue forceps
Suture scissors
Suture material and needle
Needle holder
Sterile gauze for sponging and dressing the wound
   (2 × 2 inch and 4 × 4 inch)
Adhesive or, preferably, hypoallergenic tape and
   bandage scissors to cut it.
Container for used instruments and sponges
Specimen bottle containing a preservative solution
   for a tissue biopsy specimen. Zenker's solution
   or formalin 10% are the preferred solutions used
   to preserve small tissues, warts, and moles
Biopsy forcep is also needed for obtaining a biopsy

from certain body sites, such as the uterine cervix. In this case, dressing materials or tampons
are needed to pack the area after the biopsy has
been obtained, in addition to instruments used in
a pelvic examination (see p. 318).
Laboratory requisition

Materials for a cervical biopsy

Materials for preparing the skin (skin antiseptic so-
   lution)
Sterile gloves
Vaginal speculum
Uterine dressing forceps
Cervical biopsy punch
Coagulant gel or foam
Sponges
Uterine tenaculum
Vaginal packing or tampon
Specimen bottle with preservative solution such as
   10% formalin
Laboratory requisition

Materials for a 6 mm skin biopsy

Materials for preparing the skin (skin antiseptic so-
   lution or an alcohol sponge)
Local anesthetic setup—sterile needle: 25 gauge,
   ⅝ inch *or* 30 gauge, ½ inch; 3 cc syringe; 1%
   lidocaine
Sterile gloves
Scalpel handle and a no. 15 blade
6 mm biopsy punch
Suture set with straight sharp scissors (scissor used
   to remove the top two layers of skin)
Suture material: 5-9 black silk and curved needle
Needle holder
Sterile gauze (2 × 2 and 4 × 4)
Specimen bottle with 10% formalin
Band-Aid (used for the dressing over surgical site)
Laboratory requisition

Materials for an aspiration (needle) biopsy of the breast

Syringe, a no. 18 needle, and a sterile culture tube
   to receive the specimen. Most laboratories prefer
   to receive the specimen in the culture tube, as
   each may use different procedures for fixing,
   staining, and examining the specimen. A Band-
   Aid is usually sufficient for the dressing.
Laboratory requisition when a specimen is sent for
   cytological or histological examination.

Figure 21.20
Supplies and instruments for electrocauterization.

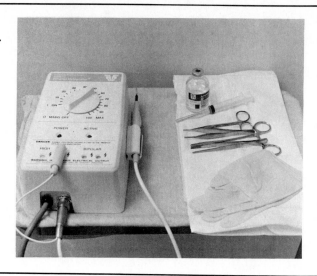

Materials for removing sutures

Suture removal kit that includes suture scissors, plain-tipped tissue forceps, sterile gauze 4 × 4 inch
Antiseptic solution in container (or disposable povidone-iodine applicators)
Sterile applicators or gauze or cotton balls
Container for removed sutures, used instruments, and sponges

Materials for electrocauterization (Figure 21.20)

Materials for skin preparation
Local anesthetic setup (depending on extent and site of area to be cauterized; at times this may not be required)
Sterile gloves
Electrocautery unit
Extension electrode for the cautery and instruments used for a pelvic examination (see p. 318) for cauterization of the uterine cervix
Container for used instruments, sponges
Dressing materials: size and type determined by size and type of area cauterized. A Band-Aid may be applied to a small area to protect it from irritants; frequently dressings are not applied to small, superficial areas

Insertion of an Intrauterine Device (IUD)

An intrauterine device is inserted into the uterus for the purpose of contraception. On January 31, 1986, all IUDs with the exception of the Progestasert were removed from the U.S. market. In 1988 the FDA approved a new copper IUD. Other types are still available outside of the United States.

The physician will insert it usually on the third day of the patient's menstrual period, as at this time the cervix may be dilated somewhat, and it is assumed that the patient is not pregnant. Before the insertion of an IUD, the patient should have had a Pap smear. On occasion, the physician may choose to insert an IUD 5 to 10 days after the patient's menstrual period. The patient is positioned and draped as for a pelvic examination.

Equipment (Figure 21.21)

Surgical soap and water
Alcohol or povidone-iodine
Sterile sponges
Vaginal speculum
Sterile gloves
Sterile single-tooth tenaculum
Sterile uterine sound
Sterile sponge stick
Sterile suture scissors
IUD and inserter

Procedure

The physician will do the following:
1. Introduce the vaginal speculum into the vagina.
2. Perform a pelvic examination.
3. Prepare the cervix with a surgical soap and water, then with alcohol or povidone-iodine.
4. Grasp the cervix with the single-toothed tenaculum.
5. Introduce the uterine sound into the uterus to check for depth.
6. Prepare and insert the IUD.

Figure 21.21
Equipment for the insertion of an intrauterine device. **A,** The Copper-T 380A intrauterine device. **B,** Sterile rubber gloves and vaginal speculum (left), scissors (top), uterine sound and single tooth tenaculum.

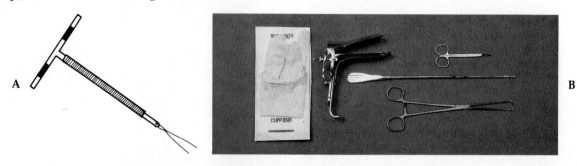

7. Withdraw the IUD inserter.
8. Cut the string attached to the IUD with suture scissors.
9. Perform a digital examination.

The medical assistant should now do the following:

10. Help the patient assume a suppine position for 5 to 10 minutes to prevent the state of shock.
11. Elevate the patient's head 45° to 50° for 5 minutes.
12. Have the patient sit up with legs over the side of the table and maintain this position for a few minutes to ensure that her condition is stable.
13. Give the patient further instructions:
    • If bleeding, fever, or pain occurs, notify the physician;
    • Check for the presence of the IUD string in the vagina once a month after her menstrual period (if she cannot find the string, she should make an appointment to see the physician);
    • A yearly checkup with the physician is necessary;
    • If a Copper 7 IUD was inserted, it must be changed every 2 years, as effectiveness decreases after that time span; then
    • Once dressed, she is free to leave.
14. Ask the patient if she has any questions; answer them adequately, or refer the patient to the physician.

WOUNDS

A wound is a break in the continuity of external or internal soft body parts, caused by physical trauma to the tissues. An *open wound* is one in which the skin and mucous membranes are broken; in a *closed wound,* the skin is not broken, but there is a contusion (bruise) or a hematoma (hēm-a-to′ma), a tumorlike mass of blood.

Types of open wounds include the following (Figure 21.22):

abrasion (ab-rā′zhun) A scrape on the surface of the skin or on a mucous membrane, for example, a skinned knee.
avulsion (ā-vul′shun) A piece of soft tissue that is torn loose or left hanging as a flap.
incision A straight cut caused by a cutting instrument, such as a scalpel (surgical knife) for surgical purposes.
laceration (las″ē-rā′shun) A tear or jagged-edged wound of body tissues.
puncture A small external opening in the skin made by a sharp, pointed object, such as a needle or nail.

Microganisms can invade both open and closed wounds, and an infection can result. Signs and symptoms that indicate the presence of an infection include redness, heat, pain, swelling, and at times, the presence of pus and a throbbing sensation at the wound site. Fever often accompanies infection. As the temperature rises, pulse and respiration rates also rise. An indication that an infection is spreading from a wound caused by needle pricks, splinters, or small cuts is the presence of a red streak running up the extremity from the wound site.

Wounds that are most susceptible to infection are those in which there is not a free flow of blood, those in which there is a crushing of the tissues, and those in which the break in the skin closes or falls back in place, thus preventing entrance of air, as seen in puncture wounds.

Figure 21.22
Types of wounds.

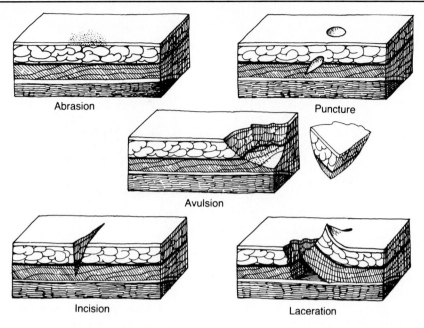

Abrasion

Puncture

Avulsion

Incision

Laceration

Common pathogenic organisms causing a wound infection include the following:

staphylococci (stăf-ĭl-ŏ-kŏk′sĭ) Bacterial that occur in grapelike clusters; gram-positive cocci. Pathogenic species cause suppurative conditions.

streptococci (strĕp″tō-kŏk′sĭ) A type of bacteria occurring in chains; gram-positive cocci.

colon bacillus (Escherichia coli or E. coli) A type of bacteria; a normal inhabitant of the intestinal tract; gram-negative cocci. Pathogenic *E. coli* are responsible for many infections of the urinary tract and for many epidemic diarrheal diseases, especially in infants.

gas bacillus (Clostridium perfringens) A type of bacteria; gram-positive cocci; anaerobic; the most common cause of gas gangrene. (Gas gangrene is a condition often resulting from dirty lacerated wounds in which the muscles and subcutaneous tissue become filled with gas and serosanguineous exudate. It is caused by the species of *Clostrium* that breaks down tissue by gas production and toxins. An exudate is material that has escaped from blood vessels and has been deposited in a body cavity, in tissues, or on the surface of tissues, usually as a result of iflammation).

tetanus bacillus (Clostridium tetani) A type of bacteria; gram-positive cocci, anaerobic, spore-forming rods, the causative organism of tetanus or lockjaw. This organism enters the body through a break in the skin, expecially through puncture wounds. In this case infection is often obvious. Tetanus and gas bacilli are common in puncture wounds because they are anerobic, that is, they grow in the absence of oxygen.

One of the body's natural defense mechanisms against infection or trauma is the inflammatory process. It works to limit damage to the tissue, remove injured cells and repair injured tissues (see also p. 343).

The Healing Process

Wounds heal by first intention or by second intention, depending on damage or loss of tissue. When the edges of wounds can be brought together, as in sutured surgical incisions, or when there is a minimal amount of tissue loss or damage, as in a relatively clean and small cut, they heal by first intention. There will be little inflammation and minimal scarring, if any.

Where the wound edges cannot be approximated because of extensive tissue loss or damage, healing by second intention occurs. This will be seen in open and infected trauma or surgical wounds, such as after the incision and drainage of abscesses, or in major lacerations. Since large amounts of granulation tissue form to fill the gap between the wound edges and to allow epithelial cells to migrate across the wound surfaces from the edges, this healing process is also known as healing by granulation or indirect healing. This is a slower process than healing by first intention; thus it involves a greater risk of infection and usually produces greater scarring.

The healing process normally occurs in three stages.

1. Lag phase: Blood serum and cells form a fibrin network in the wound. A clot is formed that fills the wound and begins to knot the edges together with shreds of fibrin. Dried proteins then form a scab.
2. Fibroplasia: Granulation tissue (fragile, pinkish red tissue) forms as the fibrin network absorbs and epithelial cells start forming from the edges to form a scar.
3. Contraction phase: Small blood vessels are absorbed, fibroblasts (cells from which connective tissue develops) contract, and the scar begins to shrink and changes in color from red to white.

The body's ability to heal after any trauma is affected by the general health status of the individual. Good health helps the body deal successfully with injuries and infections.

Care of Wounds

The goals of wound care are to promote healing and prevent additional injury. There are two schools of thought regarding the care of a wound; that is, some prefer to leave the wound undressed, and others prefer to dress a wound.

Most closed wounds are left undressed, as well as some wounds that have sealed and can be protected from additional injury, irritation, and contamination. Exposure to the air helps keep the wound dry and can promote healing. Open wounds covered with a dressing provide a warm, dark, moist area that is suitable for the growth of microorganisms. Dressing applied incorrectly can interfere with adequate circulation to the area, which will interfere with the healing process; also, if a dressing does not stay in place, it can cause further irritation to the wound and possibly cross-contamination.

Regardless of the method used (dressed or undressed), a wound must be kept clean, have dead tissue removed, and be allowed to drain freely.

When a dressing is changed, it and the wound must be inspected for the amount and character of drainage, if present. The amount is best described as scant, moderate, or large; the character refers to the color, odor, and consistency of the drainage.

Common terms to describe drainage

serous   Consisting of serum.
sanguineous   Consisting of blood or blood in abundance.
serosanguineous   Consisting of blood and serum.
purulent   Consisting of or containing pus.

The condition of the wound, the degree of healing, and the integrity of sutures and drains must also be observed during a dressing change.

DRESSINGS AND BANDAGES

Techniques of applying dressings and bandages vary according to the extent and location of wounds, injuries, or burns, the materials to be used, and the purpose of which they are applied.

Dressings

Dressings are materials of various types placed directly over wounds, open lesions, and burns as the immediate protective covering. When used correctly, dressings serve the following eight basic purposes:

- To protect wounds from additional trauma;
- To help prevent contamination of the wound;
- To absorb drainage;
- To provide pressure for controlling hemorrhage, promoting drainage, and reducing edema;
- To immobilize and support the wound site;
- To ease pain;
- To provide a means of applying and keeping medications on the wound; and
- To provide psychological benefits for the patient by concealing, protecting, and giving support to the wound.

To prevent contamination and the possibility of an infection developing, sterile technique and sterile dressing materials must be used when applying or changing a dressing. The only exception is in emergency situations when the patient has serious bleeding. On those occasions it is more important to stop the bleeding than worrying about contaminating the wound with unsterile materials.

Dressing materials

Various types and sizes of commercial sterile dressings are available. Many are made of gauze, such as folded gauze sponges* available in sizes of 2 × 2 inch, 4 × 4 inch, 3 × 4 inch, and so on; and gauze fluffs, which are loosely foled large gauze squares used to absorb large amounts of drainage or to pack an opening. Some dressings are made from vicose rayon and cellulose materials, such as folded Topper* sponges supplied in 3 × 3 inch, 4 × 3 inch, and 4 × 4 inch sizes; still others are made from a unique, nonwoven, binderless soft

---

*Johnson & Johnson, New Brunswick, NJ.

fabric called Sof-wik,* for example, Sof-wik dressing sponges, available in 4 × 4 inch and 2 × 2 inch sizes. Larger absorbent gauze and dressings made from similar materials are available for dressing large wounds, major burns, or major surgical wounds, for example, Surgipad Combine Dressing* supplied in 5 × 9 inch, 8 × 7½ inch, and 8 × 10 inch sizes; and ABDs.

Other dressing materials have a special covering over the gauze to prevent them from sticking to an open or draining skin area. These are called nonadhering dressings. Examples of these include Band-Aid Surgical Dressing,* which is a complete dressing in a single package, consisting of a nonadherent facing, enclosing an absorbent filler, and backed by Dermical* tape, available with tape 4 × 6 inch, pad 4 × 3 inch; and tape 8 × 6 inch, pad 8 × 3 inch. Telfa† is a gauze dressing having a plasticlike covering on the side that is to be placed over the wound that is also available in various sizes. Steripak is another complete dressing, made of layers of absorbent cellulose and covered with a nonadhering perforated plastic material that is secured to a vented adhesive tape. Steripak is available in 4 × 8 inch, 4 × 4 inch, and 2 × 4½ inch sizes. The Adaptic* nonadhering single-layer dressing, made of a highly porous weave, is used as the immediate covering over a wound under an absorbent secondary dressing; it is available in a foil envelope in sizes 3 × 3 inch, 3 × 8 inch, 3 × 16 inch, and in a bottle in dimensions of ½ inch × 4 yards for a packing strip. Vaseline‡ petrolatum gauze, a fine-mesh absorbent gauze impregnated with white petrolatum is a nonadhering dressing that clings and conforms to the wound. This is used over open or draining wounds to prevent the top dressing from sticking to the wound or disrupting newly formed tissue.

A third type of dressing materials is kept in a package; some are premedicated. These are used for debriding tissue, for treating open or ulcerated wounds, and sometimes for dermatological conditions.

There are also the spray-on dressing materials that, when sprayed over the wound, form a transparent protective film. These are nontoxic and somewhat bacteriostatic and allow for close observation for an incision or wound site. Fluff cotton or cotton balls are never to be used for dressings, because the fibers may get imbedded in the wound and are difficult to remove if they do.

To hold dressings in place securely, various types and sizes of tape are available. The types of tape include hypoallergenic cloth tape, hypoallergenic paper tape, transparent tape, elastic cloth tape, and adhesive tape; sizes range from ½ inch to 3 inches.

When changing or applying an initial dressing, select the dressing materials according to the purposes to be accomplished; in other words, know why the wound is to be dressed. This will enable you to select the proper types and amounts of dressing materials. Any dressing must be large enough to cover the wound completely and extend at least an inch or more beyond.

In addition to caring for patients who have had minor surgery in the office, patients who have had surgery in the hospital may come to the physician's office for a dressing change or wound culture when necessary. The medical assistant may assist the physician with these procedures or perform them alone.

Text continued on p. 402.

---

*Johnson & Johnson, New Brunswick, NJ.
†Kendall Col, Greenwich, Conn.
‡Chesebrough Pond Inc., Greenwich, Conn.

Procedure for Dressing Change with a Wound Culture

When infection is suspected a wound culture is taken to determine the presence and type of microscopic organisms that is causing the infection. Cultures can be obtained from wounds on any part of the body. Soiled dressings are removed and replaced by a clean sterile dressing.

Equipment (Figure 21.23)

To obtain the culture

Sterile applicator(s) in a sterile culture tube(s), or a Culturette.* The type of culture tube will vary depending on the specific organism that is suspected. Check with your laboratory to ensure accuracy. Most laboratories request that an anerobic Culturette* be used for wound cultures. Always check the expiration date on the outside wrapper before using to assure stability of the culture medium at the time of use. See Chapter 22 for additional information on cultures and materials used.

To change the dressing

Sterile dressing tray or a prepackaged sterile dressing set containing the following:
- Tissue forceps
- Hemostat
- Scissors
- Gauze sponges 2 × 2 inch, or cotton balls, or antiseptic swabs
- Dry dressings, for example, 4 × 4 inch gauze, Topper sponges, Sof-wik sponges
- Small container for antiseptic solution
- Antiseptic solution

Additional equipment

Antiseptic solution, if not supplied in the prepackaged dressing set, such as povidone-iodine, hydrogen peroxide, alcohol 70%; 1:750 aqueous benzalkonium chloride

Tape, preferably hypoallergenic

Waxed paper or plastic bag for soiled dressing and disposable equipment

Sterile disposable gloves

Draping materials, as needed

Laboratory requisition

Optional equipment

Acetone or benzine or commercial tape remover to moisten tape on old dressing for easier removal

Sterile saline to moisten a dressing that has stuck to a wound, to allow for easier removal

Sterile towels

Additional dressing supplies appropriate to the condition of the wound site, for example, Telfa, adhesive bandages, Steripak, Surgipads, Adaptic dressing, roller gauze bandage, Kling elastic gauze bandage

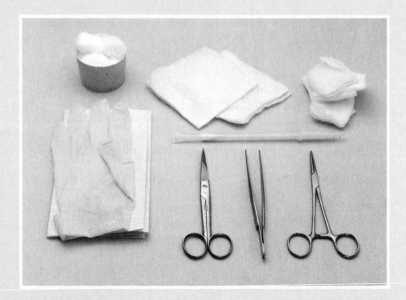

Figure 21.23
Supplies and instruments for dressing change with wound culture.

Procedure	*Rationale*

1. Wash your hands.
2. Assemble your equipment.

3. Identify the patient, and explain the procedure.

Place the supplies on a flat, clean surface, convenient for use.

Provide reassurance, and gain the patient's cooperation. Explain that you will remove the soiled dressing, obtain a culture of the discharge from the wound, and apply a clean sterile dressing. The culture will then be sent to the laboratory for study. When the physician receives the laboratory report, the appropriate medication to eliminate the causative organism(s) of the infection may then be prescribed.

4. Have the patient put on a patient gown if necessary. Position the patient, providing for comfort and relaxation. Drape if and as needed, exposing the area in which the wound is located. When the wound is on the arm or leg, place a towel under the area to be dressed. Remind the patient not to touch the open wound once the dressing has been removed and not to talk over it, because microorganisms can spread into the wound.

Gowning, positioning, and draping will vary with the location of the wound. The important thing to remember is that the part of the body from which the culture is to be obtained and the dressing changed must be well supported and exposed. In addition, the patient's modesty must be protected.

5. a. Open the dressing set. Using sterile transfer forceps, arrange supplies in their order to use.
   b. Open waxed paper or plastic bag.

   c. Pour the antiseptic solution into the sterile container located on the sterile field.

   d. Cut pieces of tape that will be used to secure the clean sterile dressing when applied.
6. Loosen tape on the present dressing (Figure 21.24).

Use aseptic technique at all times. The wrapper on the dressing set is used for the sterile field.

Place the bag in a convenient place to receive the soiled dressing and used disposable supplies.

NOTE: When the antiseptic solution is supplied in the dressing tray set, do not pour the solution until after you have donned sterile gloves.

These may be tagged onto the side of your dressing tray.

Loosen and pull tape gently, going toward the wound so you do not tear newly formed tissue. When the tape does not pull away easily moisten it with a sponge soaked with acetone, benzine, baby oil, or a commercial tape remover.

Figure 21.24
Technique for loosening tape on dressing.

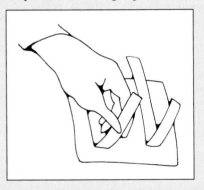

7. Loosen and remove the soiled dressing with a sterile forcep or a gloved hand. Do not pull on the dressing. A dressing can also be removed by placing your hand inside a plastic bag. Then grasp and lift the dressing off, inspect for drainage, and invert bag over the dressing.

Handle all dressings as if they are contaminated. The forceps or glove is to be used for this step on, then set aside or, if disposable, discarded in the bag with the soiled dressing. If a dressing is difficult to remove, sterile saline may be applied to help loosen it.

Continued.

Procedure for Dressing Change with a Wound Culture—cont'd

Procedure	*Rationale*
8. Inspect the dressing, and then discard it in the waxed paper or plastic bag.	Observe the amount and type of drainage on the dressing.
9. Observe the wound.	Note the location, type, and amount of drainage coming from the wound, and the presence of pus, necrosis, and/or a putrid odor. Note the degree of healing, and when sutures are present, if they are intact.
10. Remove the sterile applicator from the sterile culture tube or Culturettte. Swab the drainage area of the wound to obtain a specimen. If you need more of the drainage for culturing, you must use another application.	Swab only the draining area of the wound. Do not spread the infection to a clean area on the wound. Swab the wound only once in one direction. Never go back and forth over the area.
11. Place the applicator(s) in the culture tube(s), and set aside.	Secure the lid tightly to prevent air from getting into the tube. Air would cause the specimen to dry, thus destroying the microorganisms.
12. Don sterile gloves as described previously.	Gloves are donned to prevent any microorganisms that may be on your hands from entering the wound and also to keep your hands clean.
13. Pick up gauze sponge with forceps or hemostat (whichever is most comfortable for you to use).	
14. Dip the sponge into the antiseptic cleansing solution to wet through.	Do not oversaturate the sponge. Keep sponge and forceps facing downward.
15. Gently, but thoroughly, cleanse the wound using single strokes over and parallel to the incision, *one sponge per stroke.* Starting at the center of the wound, stroke toward the ends. Cleanse the side farthest from you, working outward from the incision, and then repeat on the side closest to you (Figure 21.25)	Do not go back and forth over a cleansed area. Do not touch forceps to skin. Bacterial count is usually lowest at the center of the incision and greatest at the edges. Always work from the least contaminated areas to most contaminated areas to avoid contaminating uncontaminated sites.
16. Discard each sponge in the bag for waste after use.	Do not touch the bag with the forceps.
17. Repeat the process directly over the wound until it is cleansed to your satisfaction.	Use a clean sponge for each single stroke.
18. When cleansing a drain site or a very small wound, move the antiseptic sponge in a circle around the site (Figure 21.26).	Cleanse around and away from the wound in an ever-widening circle. Do not go back over a clean area.
19. Discard the sponge, and repeat.	
20. Apply the sterile dressing. Center it over the wound area.	Forceps or gloved hands are used to apply the dressing. Additional layers of dressings are added as indicated by the type of wound and amount of drainage (when present).
21. Discard disposable forceps and gloves in waste bag. Put reusable forceps and gloves to the side of the sterile field or in a container for used supplies.	Remove gloves by pulling on the cuff and turning inside out.
22. Secure the dressing with tape applied so that it conforms to body contours and movement. Ensure that it is adequately spaced; do not cover all the dressing with tape (Figure 21.27). Place each strip of tape over the middle of the dressing and press down gently on both sides, working toward the ends.	Hypoallergenic tape is preferred. Have equal lengths of tape on both sides of the dressing—not too short or too long. Tape is not to cover the whole dressing, as it would interfere with air circulation. Distribute tension away from the incision. Do not tape too snugly, as this may constrict blood flow to the wound and interfere with the healing process.

Figure 21.25

Cleansing wound starting at center and moving toward end. Use one sponge per stroke.

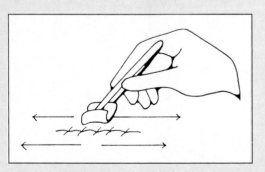

Figure 21.26
Cleanse small wound or drain site using circular strokes, working from center to outside portion of wound site.

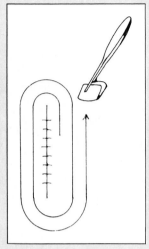

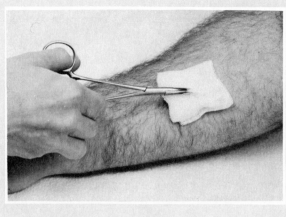

Figure 21.27
Correct method of securing dressing to conform to body contour and movement.

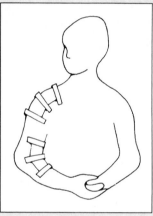

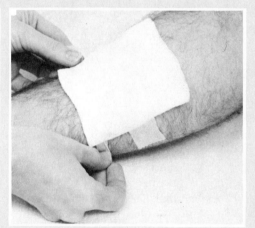

23. Attend to the patient's comfort; you may reposition the patient if necessary. Observe the patient for any undue reaction. Provide further instructions as indicated or as ordered by the physician.
24. Label culture tube(s) or Culturette(s) completely and accurately. COmplete and attach the appropriate laboratory requisition.

25. Take or send the culture to the laboratory.
26. Remove used items from the treatment room; dispose of correctly.

27. Wash your hands.
28. Replace supplies as needed. Leave the treatment room clean and neat.
29. Record the procedure and observations on the patient's chart, using correct medical abbreviations.

Check if the patient has any questions. Inform the patient if he/she is free to leave. Help the patient dress when necessary.

The label should include the following:
- Patients name
- Physician's name
- Date
- Source of specimen
- Test requested

Avoid delay to prevent drying of the specimen.

Discard soiled items and disposable equipment in a covered container. Rinse reusable instruments under running water and then soak in detergent and water until you are ready to prepare them for sterilization.

Prevent cross-contamination.

Charting example:
   March 4, 19_____, 1 PM
Rt. forearm dressing changed. Moderate amount of thick, yellow, purulent drainage on lower end of laceration. Culture taken and sent to lab for C & S [culture and sensitivity]. Wound cleansed and dry dressing applied.
   Ann Michaelson, CMA

*Marion Scientific Corp, Kansas City, Mo.

Figure 21.28
A, Triangular bandage. **B,** Triangular bandage used for arm sling.

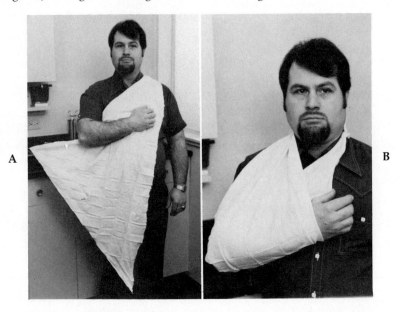

Bandages

Bandages are strips of soft, pliable materials used to wrap or cover a body part. When used correctly, bandages serve these four basic purposes:

- To hold dressings or splints in place;
- To immobilize or support body parts;
- To protect an injured body part; and
- To apply pressure over an area.

Bandaging materials should be clean, but necessarily sterile, because they should never come in direct contact with an open wound as do dressings.

Bandaging materials

There are several types of bandages prepared commercially.

Adhesive and elastic tape. Adhesive and elastic tape are supplied in rolls of various widths. When tape is used for a bandage, it is applied directly to the skin. Caution must be taken when wrapping a body part with tape so that circulation is not cut off by tape that has been wrapped too tightly. Elastoplast is an example of an elastic adhesive bandage.

Roller bandages. Roller bandages are available in various widths and materials. *Gauze,* a porous, lightweight, nonstretch material has little absorbency, does not self-adhere, and does not conform readily to body contours. However, it is relatively inexpensive.

A preferred type of gauze bandage is the *elastic gauze bandage,* such as Kling. Kling conforms to all body contours, stretches, adheres to itself, and is absorbent; it will not slip with movement, therefore eliminates frequent rebandaging. It is nonocclusive, allowing for wound aeration; thus it will not interfere with wound healing.

Elastic bandages. Elastic bandages, made of woven cotton with elastic fibers, are particularly useful for bandaging areas that require firm support, immobilization, or the application of pressure. Frequently used are the Ace bandage or the Peg bandage, which is self-adhering. Once wrapped around the body part, nonadhering elastic bandages are secured with bandage clips. Figure 21.30 illustrates the application of a Peg bandage.

Triangular bandages. Triangular bandages are large pieces of cloth, usually cotton, in the shape of a triangle. These bandages are usually used for slings on an injured arm, but can be adapted for use on almost any part of the body (Figure 21.28). A cravat bandage can be made by folding the point of a triangular bandage to the midpoint of the base and continued to fold it lengthwise until the desired width is obtained (Figure 21.29). A cravat bandage can be used to hold a dressing in place, to help support an injured joint, to hold a splint in place, and if necessary, as a tourniquet.

Tubegauz. Tubegauz, a seamless, tubular-knit-

Figure 21.29
Cravat bandage.

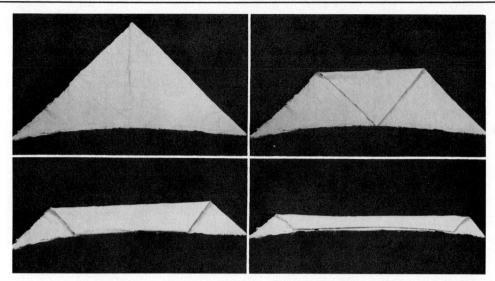

ted, cotton bandage, is adaptable and conformable to all body areas. Because Tubegauz is tubular, it stays in place with little or no adhesive tape. A finger or cage-type appliance is used in the application of Tubegauz to provide a neat and strong bandage. Figure 21.32 has instructions for applying Tubegauz bandages.

Application of bandages

Important criteria for acceptable bandaging techniques are that the bandage perform its function and that it not cause additional problems or pain. The following measures promote safety and comfort when applying bandages:

- Observe the principles and practices of medical asepsis when applying a bandage.
- Select a bandage of appropriate size for the area to be bandaged.
- Apply bandages to areas that are clean and dry. When an open wound is present, apply a bandage over a dressing.
- Do not have two skin surfaces touching each other under a bandage. Use absorbent material between touching skin surfaces under a bandage. For example, when bandaging two fingers together, place a padding between them to prevent the skin from rubbing together. Other areas that need similar techniques include the axillary areas, because an individual's perspiration provides a moist environment that is conductive to the growth of microorganisms, the areas under the breast, areas in the groin or folds of the abdomen, and areas between the toes.

- Pad bony prominences and joints over which a bandage must be placed to prevent skin irritation, to provide comfort, and to maintain equal pressure on body parts.
- Apply bandages on a body part while in its normal functioning position, and when placed in a resting position (1) so that deformities will not result and (2) to avoid muscle strain. Joints should be slightly flexed rather than extended or hyperextended.
- Apply bandages with sufficient pressure to attain the intended function, that is pressure, support, or immobilization. However, do not apply the bandage too tightly as this will interfere with circulation to the area. Ask the patient if the bandage feels comfortable.
- Wrap the bandage from the end of a limb toward the center of the body to avoid congestion and circulatory interferences in the distal part of the extremity.
- When possible, leave a small portion of an extremity, such as a finger or toe, exposed so that any change in circulation can be observed. Signs that indicate that the bandage is too tight include coldness and numbness to the part, pain, swelling, cyanosis, and pallor. If any of these signs occur, the bandage must be loosened immediately.
- Apply bandages so that they are secure and do not move about over the area causing irritation or the need for rebandaging frequently.
- Apply chest bandages so that they do not interfere with breathing.
- Avoid unnecessary layers of bandages, it will

Figure 21.30
Bandage wrapping techniques illustrating circular, spiral, and figure-eight turns.
The Peg self-adhering elastic bandage is used in these illustrations.
Courtesy Becton-Dickinson, Div of Becton, Dickinson and Co, Rutherford, NJ.

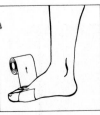

Foot and ankle Use 3-inch width. Hold foot at right angle to leg. Start bandage on ridge of foot just back of the toes.

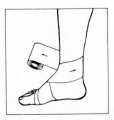

Pass bandage around foot from inside to outside. After two or three complete turns around foot, ascending toward the ankle on each turn, make a figure eight turn by bringing bandage up over

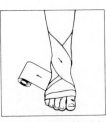

the arch—to the inside of the ankle—around the ankle—down over the arch—and under the foot.

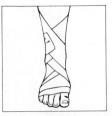

Repeat the figure eight wrapping two or three times. Fasten end by pressing the last 4 to 6 inches of <u>unstretched</u> bandage to the preceding layer.

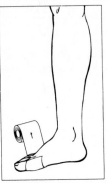

Lower leg Use 3- or 4-inch width depending on the size of the leg. A leg wrap requires two rolls of bandage. Hold foot at right angle to leg. Start bandage on ridge of foot just back of the toes.

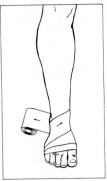

Pass bandage around foot from inside to outside. After two complete turns around foot, make a figure eight turn by bringing bandage up over the arch—to the inside of the ankle—around the ankle—

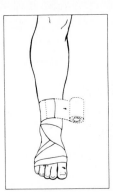

down over the arch—and under the foot. Start circular bandaging, making the first turn around the ankle. To begin the second roll of bandage, simply overlap the <u>unstretched</u> ends by 4 to 6 inches, press firmly, and continue wrapping.

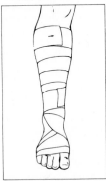

Wrap bandage in spiral turns to just below the kneecap. Fasten end by pressing the last 4 to 6 inches of <u>unstretched</u> bandage to the preceding layer.

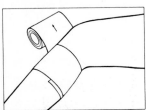

Knee Use 4-inch width. Bend knee slightly. Start with one complete circular turn around the leg just below the knee.

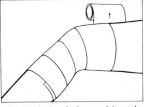

Start circular bandaging, applying only comfortable tension. Cover kneecap completely.

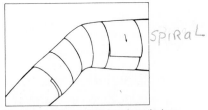

Continue wrapping to thigh just above the knee. Fasten end by pressing the last 4 to 6 inches of <u>unstretched</u> bandage to the preceding layer.

Continued.

not be comfortable for the patient. Use only the amount of bandage material to accomplish its purpose.
- Place securing materials, such as clips, pins, knots well away from the wound or inflamed area to avoid undue pressure and irritation to the area.

- Check (or inform the patient to check) the bandage at regular intervals to note the circulation to the part and to see if the bandage needs to be reapplied, as when it has slipped out of place or loosened to the point where it would no longer be accomplishing its purpose. Also with injuries or burns involving swelling,

Figure 21.30, cont'd

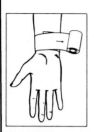

Wrist Use 2- or 3-inch width. Anchor bandage loosely at the wrist with one complete circular turn.

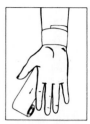

Carry the bandage across the back of the hand, through the web space between the thumb and index finger,

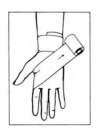

and across palm to the wrist. Make a circular turn around the

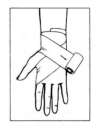

wrist and once more carry the bandage through the web space and back to the wrist.

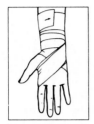

Start circular bandaging, ascending the wrist. Fasten end by pressing the last 4 to 6 inches of <u>unstretched</u> bandage to the preceding layer.

Elbow Use 3- or 4-inch width, depending on the size of the arm. Two rolls of bandage are required to complete the wrap. Start with a complete circular turn just below the elbow.

Wrap bandage in loose figure eights—

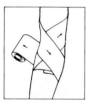

to form a protective bridge across the front of the elbow joint.

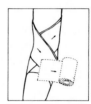

Fasten end by pressing 4 to 6 inches of <u>unstretched</u> bandage to preceding layer. Start second bandage with a circular turn below the elbow—

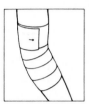

over the first wrap. Continue spiral bandaging over the elbow, ascending to the lower portion of the upper arm. Fasten end with a circular turn.

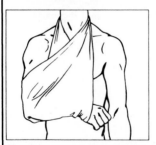

Shoulder A shoulder wrap is used to provide additional support for an arm in a sling. Use 4- or 6-inch width. One or two rolls of bandage may be used. Start under the free arm.

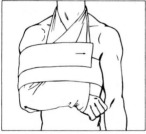

Carry the bandage across the back, <u>over the arm in the sling</u>, across the chest and back <u>under the free arm</u> in complete circular, overlapping turns. Fasten the end by pressing 4 to 6 inches of <u>unstretched</u> bandage to underlying bandage.

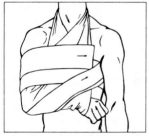

Additional support can be obtained with a second bandage. Start at the back just behind the flexed elbow in the sling. Carry the bandage under the elbow up over the forearm, around the chest and back, and repeat. Fasten end.

it is very important to check bandages frequently to ensure that they are not becoming too tight.
• Replace clean bandages as required. Many bandages can be washed or autoclaved and then reused. Gauze should be discarded and replaced with clean gauze.

Basic wrapping techniques

There are five basic turns used alone or in combination when applying a *roller bandage*. The type of turn used depends on the purpose and the area being bandaged.

When beginning a wrap with a roller bandage, you may anchor it by placing the outer portion on a bias next to the patient's skin; the bandage is circled around the body part, allowing the corner edge to protrude; the protruding edge is then folded down over the first turn and covered with the second encircling turn of the bandage.

The *circular turn* encircles the part with each layer of bandage overlapping the previous one. This turn is used most frequently for anchoring a bandage at the start and at the end, and on body parts that are even in size, such as the hand, fingers, toes and circumference of the head.

The *spiral turn* is applied by angling the turns of the bandage in a spiral fashion with each turn overlapping the previous one by one-third to one-half the width of the bandage. This turn is used on body parts that increase in size where circular turns are difficult to make, and on cylindrical shaped parts, such as the forearm, fingers, legs, chest, and abdomen.

The *figure-eight turn* consists of diagonal turns that ascend and descend alternately around a part, making a figure eight. This turn is used over joint areas such as the wrist, ankle, elbow, or knee to support the joint, support a dressing, or apply a pressure bandage.

Figure 21.30 illustrates the circular, spiral, and figure-eight turns along with wrapping techniques for the Peg self-adhering elastic bandage.

The *spiral-reverse turn* is a spiral turn in which reverses are made halfway through each turn; the bandage is directed downward and folded on itself, wrapped around that part so that when it circles around, it is parallel to the lower edge of the previous turn. Each turn overlaps the previous one by two-thirds the width of the bandage. Spiral-reverse turns allow for a neater fit because they take up the slack on the lower ends of the bandage applied to cone-shaped parts or parts that vary in width, such as the leg, thigh, or forearm.

The *recurrent turn* is a series of back-and-forth turns anchored by circular or spiral turns. After the bandage has been anchored, it is folded at right angles and passes across and back over the center of

Figure 21.31
Bandage wrapping technique: recurrent turn used for head bandage.

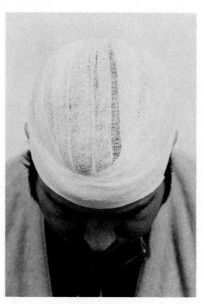

the part. Each subsequent fold is slightly angled and overlaps the previous fold by two-thirds the width of the bandage, first on one side and then on the other side of the center fold. To finish the bandage, a circular turn is made around the part and secured with tape, clips, pins, or a knot. The recurrent turn is used to bandage the head, fingers, toes, or the stump of an amputated limb (Figure 21.31).

Tubegauz bandages

Tubegauz is a seamless, tubular, knitted cotton bandage. It may be used for bandages on the arm, palm of the hand, finger, leg, toe, head, and shoulder. When a Tubegauz bandage is applied, there is one basic method used for application to any body part being bandaged. Figure 21.32 outlines basic instructions for all Tubegauz applications.

Figure 21.32
Tubegauz bandage applications.
Courtesy Scholl, Inc, Hospital Products Div, Chicago, Ill.

BASIC INSTRUCTIONS FOR ALL TUBEGAUZ APPLICATIONS.

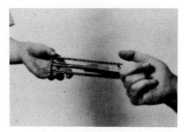

1 To apply any Tubegauz, first select a cage-type applicator that fits comfortably over the area to be bandaged.

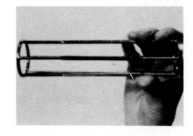

2 Next, select the size Tubegauz as printed on the cage-type applicator. For example, use Tubegauz size 01 for applicator No. 1.

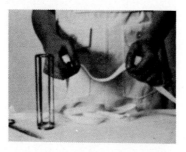

3 To load the Tubegauz onto the applicator, place the "channeled end" of the applicator on a flat surface and pull several feet of Tubegauz from the dispenser box.

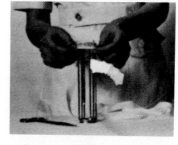

4 While spreading open the end of the tubular knit, slip the Tubegauz over the "smooth end" of the applicator.

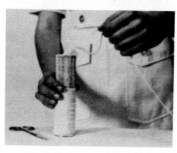

5 Complete loading by gathering sufficient Tubegauz to complete the bandage, onto the applicator and cut off near the dispenser box opening.

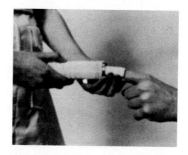

6 With the applicator loaded, pass the channeled end of the applicator over the limb to the middle of the dressing.

Continued.

Figure 21.32, cont'd

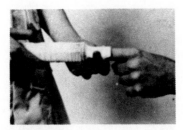

7 Pull the Tubegauz over the channeled end of the applicator, holding it lightly in place around the dressing.

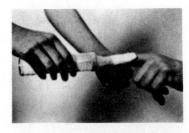

8 Continue to secure the dressing and Tubegauz end with one hand while slightly rotating clockwise to anchor as you withdraw the applicator over the limb.

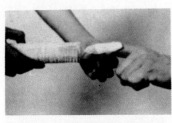

9 Withdraw the applicator several inches below the dressing or to the extremity, then rotate one full clockwise turn to anchor or close.

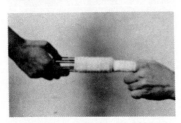

10 Move the applicator forward past the starting point and anchor with slight rotation several inches above the dressing.

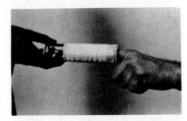

11 Continue this "back and forth" action until the desired layers of Tubegauz have been applied. Complete the last layer by stopping at the end of the bandage nearest the mesial plane.

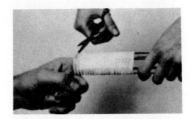

12 To finish, snip a small hole in the channeled rim, and continue cutting the Tubegauz from the applicator using the channeled rim as a cutting guide. If necessary, adhesive tape may be used to secure either end.

REMEMBER.....
   Tubegauz is often applied over a sterile dressing which covers broken skin. Tubegauz is not sterile, but can be autoclaved on or off a metal applicator if desired.

   Always load sufficient Tubegauz onto the applicator. It is difficult to complete a neat bandage when you have run out of Tubegauz in the middle of a procedure.

Figure 21.32, cont'd

SIMPLE ARM OR LEG BANDAGE

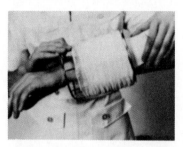

1 With applicator loaded as directed, bring the Tubegauz over the channeled end over sterile dressing.

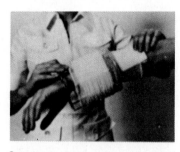

2 Hold the Tubegauz on the dressing with one hand and withdraw the applicator with the other hand letting the Tubegauz roll off the applicator to cover the desired area (usually just below the sterile dressing).

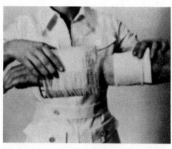

3 Rotate clockwise about ½ to ¾ turn to anchor slightly and proceed in opposite direction to above dressing.

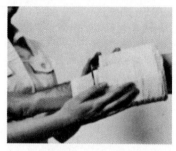

4 Rotate again in the same direction and return to base of bandage.

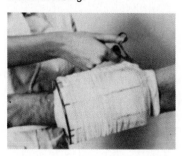

5 Cut Tubegauz off in channeled rim.

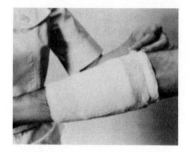

6 Secure with adhesive or slit and tie.

Adhesive tape may be applied at center of bandage by allowing a little more Tubegauz so that, after anchoring at base, the raw edge finishes in the center.

Conclusion

Strict aseptic technique is needed at all times when handling supplies and assisting with sterile or surgical procedures. Never be reluctant to admit a possible break in technique.

Be honest and admit contamination of sterile equipment, even if you are the only one who realizes that the equipment is not sterile. It is no disgrace to contaminate sterile equipment. The only disgrace is to use it after you know it is contaminated, because you would then subject the patient to the great danger of infection.

Learn the principles and practice the sterile techniques to be used when handling sterile supplies and equipment and when assisting with sterile procedures. Practice handling instruments so that the physician can grasp them in the way most convenient to use during a procedure. Be prepared to select and arrange the supplies and equipment required for the minor surgeries listed in this chapter.

When ready to accurately demonstrate your skills, arrange with your instructor to take a performance test.

Review Questions

1. Having opened a sterile suture removal kit for use, the physician then decides not to remove the patient's sutures. What would you now do with these instruments?
2. When pouring a solution into a sterile container on a sterile field, you accidentally spill some of the solution on the sterile field. What would you do to remedy this contamination?
3. While directly assisting with a minor surgical procedure, you accidentally puncture your sterile glove with a needle. What should be your next actions?
4. When assisting with a minor surgery, the physician asks for the thinnest back silk suture material. What size (number) of suture material would you provide?
5. List 15 of the principles and practices of aseptic (sterile) techinque.
6. Why do you open envelope-wrapped sterile packages with the top flap going away from your body?
7. List the supplies and equipment that you would assemble and prepare when the physician is to do the following:
   a. Incise and drain an abscess
   b. Remove sutures
   c. Repair a laceration by suturing
   d. Obtain an aspiration (needle) biopsy of breast tissue
   e. Remove a wart on the patient's left hand
   f. Insert an IUD
8. Describe how to prepare a patient for minor surgery.
9. List and explain four terms that describe the character of drainage from a wound.
10. List eight purposes of dressings and four purposes of bandages.

SUGGESTED READINGS

Hill G: Outpatient surgery, ed 2, Philadelphia, 1980, WB Saunders Co.

Meshelany CM: Post-op wound dressing, RN 42:22, May 1979.

Chapter 22

Collecting and Handling Specimens

- Specimens
- Urine specimen collection
- Stool specimen collection
- Hemoccult slide test on a stool specimen
- Respiratory tract specimens
- Wound culture

- Smears for cytology studies
- Smears for bacteriology studies
- Gram stain
- Bacterial culture and sensitivity (C and S) testing
- Vaginal smears and culture collection

Objectives

On completion of Chapter 22 the medical assistant student should be able to:

1 Define and pronounce the vocabulary terms listed.

2 Discuss the proper care, handling, and storage of all specimens.

3 List the purposes, the basic equipment and supplies required, and the medical assistant's usual assisting responsibilities for each procedure described in this chapter.

4 State and define seven types of urine specimens and discuss at least 10 general facts relating to the collection of urine for examination.

5 Discuss the hemoccult slide test for stool specimens, stating why and how it is done, the special diagnostic diet that the patient may be on before and during the test, and medications that would interfere with the test.

6 Differentiate between a smear, a culture, and a culture medium.

7 Briefly discuss the Gram stain and the culture and sensitivity tests performed for bacteriological studies.

8 List six types of smears that may be done to detect vaginal disorders and diseases.

9 Demonstrate correct technique and proper communication to the patient for collecting the following specimens, preparing them to be sent to the laboratory, and completing the appropriate requisition form:

- Urine specimen
- Stool specimen
- Sputum specimen
- Throat culture
- Nasopharyngeal culture
- Wound culture
- Vaginal smears and cultures

10 Demonstrate the correct procedure for performing a Gram stain.

11 Demonstrate the correct procedure for performing a hemoccult slide test on a stool specimen.

12 Demonstrate the correct technique for making a smear for cytology studies and a smear for bacteriology studies.

13 Demonstrate the correct technique for inoculating a culture medium with a specimen obtained on a cotton-tipped applicator.

14 Demonstrate the correct method for completing various types of laboratory requisition forms that accompany a specimen sent to the laboratory.

Vocabulary

bacteriology (bak-te′-re-ol′o-jē) The study of bacteria.

bacteriolysis (bak-te′-re-ol′i-sĭs) The destruction of bacteria.

biochemistry (bi-′o-kem′is-trē) The study of chemical changes occurring in living organisms.

culture (kul′tūr) The reproduction or growth of microorganisms or of living tissue cells in special laboratory media (the material on which the organisms grow) conducive to their growth. Various types of cultures include the following:

blood culture Used in the diagnosis of specific infectious diseases. Blood is withdrawn from a vein and placed in or on suitable culture media; then it is determined whether or not pathogens grow in the media. If organisms do grow, they are identified by bacteriological methods.

gelatin culture A culture of bacteria on gelatin.

hanging drop culture A culture in which the bacteria are inoculated into a drop of fluid on a coverglass and then mounted into the depression on a concave slide.

negative culture A culture made from suspected material that fails to reveal the suspected microorganisms.

positive culture A culture that reveals the suspected microorganisms.

pure culture A culture of a single microorganism.

smear culture A culture prepared by smearing the specimen across the surface of the culture medium.

stab culture A bacterial culture made by thrusting a needle inoculated with the microorganisms under examination deep into the culture medium.

streak culture A bacterial culture in which the infectious material is implanted in streaks across the culture media.

tissue culture The growing of tissue cells in artificial nutrient media.

type culture A culture that is generally agreed to represent microorganisms of a particular species.

Culturette A commercially prepared bacterial culture collection/transport system, consisting of a sterile plastic tube with applicator. Modified Stuart's transport medium is held in a glass ampule at the bottom end to assure stability of medium at the time of use. Transport medium is released only after the sample is taken, by crushing the ampule. A moist environment (not immersion) is maintained up to 72 hours to preserve the specimen (see Figure 22-7).

Culturette II culture collection system This is identical to the Culturette, with the exception that the plastic tube contains two applicators and the ampule contains twice the medium (1 ml) (see Figure 22-7).

anerobic Culturette culture collection system This system offers the same basic properties of the Culturette, plus a standardized and dependable anaerobic environment for transport of anaerobic bacteria. The transport medium, once released, maintains an anaerobic environment for up to 48 hours. Many laboratories request that the anaerobic culture system be used when taking a wound culture.

culture medium A commercial preparation used for the growth of microorganisms or other cells. (Types of culture media are described in this chapter.)

cytology (sī-tol′ō-jē) The study of the structure and function of cells.

dysplasia (dis-plā′ze-ah) An abnormal development of tissue.

histology (hīs-tol′o-jē) The study of the microscopic form and structure of tissue.

incubation (in-kū-bā′shun) When pertaining to bacteriology, this terms refers to the period of culture development.

inoculate (ĭ-nok′-ū-lāt) In microbiology, this refers to introducing infectious matter into a culture medium in an effort to produce growth of the causative organism.

macroscopic (mak-rō-skop′ĭk) examination An examination in which the specimen is large enough to be seen by the naked eye.

medical microbiology The study and identification of pathogens and the development of effective methods for their control or elimination.

microorganism (mī-krō-or′gan-ism) A minute living body not perceptible to the naked eye, especially a bacterium or protozoon; these are viewed using a microscope.

microscopic (mī-krō-skop′ik) examination An examination in which the specimen is visible only with the aid of a microscope.

pathogen (păth′ō-jĕn) A disease-producing substance or microorganism.

pathogenic (path′o-jĕn′ic) Pertaining to a disease-producing microorganism or substance.

serological (sē-rō-lŏj′ik-al) test A laboratory test involving the examination and study of blood serum.

smear (smēr) Material spread thinly across a slide or culture medium with a swab, loop, or another slide in preparation for microscopic study.

fixation of a smear Spraying with or immersing a slide into a special solution, drying the slide over a flame, or air drying to harden and preserve the bacteria for future microscopic examination.

specimen (spec′ĭ-men) A small part or sample taken to show kind and quality of the whole, as a specimen of urine, blood, or other body excretions, or a small piece of tissue for macroscopic and microscopic examination.

sputum (spū′tŭm) A mucous secretion from the trachea, bronchi, and lungs, ejected through the mouth, in contrast to saliva, which is the secretion of the salivary glands.

stool (stool) Body waste material discharged from the large intestine; synonyms: feces, bowel movement.

swab (swŏb) A small piece of cotton or gauze wrapped around the end of a slender stick used for applying medications, cleansing cavities, or obtaining a piece of tissue or body secretion for bacteriological examination; synonym: cotton tipped applicator.

urine (ū′rine) The fluid containing certain waste products and water that is secreted by the kidneys, stored in the bladder, and excreted through the urethra.

viable (vī′ah-bl) Able to maintain an independent existence.

The science of laboratory technology is becoming increasingly sophisticated in methods used to process specimens obtained from a patient. Thus it is rare if not obsolete that a medical assistant will be required to perform the actual tests on collected specimens in a physician's office or health agency, other than simple tests that may be performed several times a day, such as routine urinalysis. Most physicians use the services of professional laboratories, which perform tests under controlled conditions using expensive equipment that is impractical for the physician's office. Commonly, the patient will be referred to a clinical laboratory, at which the specimen is obtained and processed and the results prepared for report to the physician. At other times it will be necessary for the medical assistant to collect the specimen or to assist the physician in obtaining the specimen. Once the specimen has been properly obtained, the medical assistant's responsibility is to ensure that it is preserved and labeled correctly for submission to the laboratory for examination. It is therefore imperative that the medical assistant know how to collect various types of specimens and prepare a smear or culture from the specimen so that specimens arrive at the laboratory in good condition for processing. When collecting specimens, the medical assistant must also be aware of any special preparation that is required by the patient, ensure that the patient is thoroughly informed (for example, collect the first morning specimen, or fast 12 hours before collection of the specimen), ascertain that this preparation has been followed, and be certain that the correct equipment is used for the specimen obtained. Most professional laboratories furnish manuals on request that outline the specific requirements for each study to be performed. In this chapter you will learn techniques for obtaining and for helping the physician obtain different types of specimens, smears, and cultures, in addition to the care and handling of specimens.

SPECIMENS

Samples of body fluids, secretions, excretions, or tissues can be removed from a patient's body for laboratory study. These materials, once removed, are called specimens. Serological, biochemical, and microscopic tests can be performed on all body specimens. These tests provide a means for evaluating the patient's health status and identifying pathogenic microorganisms and other abnormalities present. Once the suspected cause of a disease process is determined, appropriate methods of treatment can be provided.

It is important that a specimen be collected at the onset of a disease or condition and, when possible, before the administration of any antibiotics when an infectious process is suspected. Commonly, active participation of a patient is required to obtain a specimen, therefore appropriate instructions must be given. Explain the procedure that is to be used in collecting the specimen (such as urine, sputum, or stool) completely and accurately.

Some tests require preparation by the patient, and again the appropriate instructions must be given along with an explanation of the necessity for following these instructions. Special preparation usually means a modification in diet or a period of fasting before the specimen collection. The time of day the specimen is to be collected may be specific; for example, the first morning urine may be collected. For women, the use of vaginal medications, douches, or the time of the menstrual flow should be avoided when obtaining vaginal specimens.

Caring for, Handling, Transporting, and Storing Specimens

Essential considerations to remember with regard to each specimen follow. See Vocabulary for types of collection and transport systems used. (See also Chapter 20, "Universal Blood and Body Substance Precautions," p. 344.)

The specimen must be properly labeled and placed in the correct container. Each specimen is to be placed in the proper container or solution that is designed for the type of material collected with the lid fastened securely. The container with the specimen must be labeled with the patient's name, the date, the source of the specimen, and the attending physician's name.

The specimen must be protected when it is sent to outside laboratories or through the mail. Most outside laboratories will provide specific instructions for the transportation of specimens to them. Specimen containers sent by mail must be closed securely and wrapped in a protective covering such as corrugated cardboard or cotton, which will absorb shock and prevent leakage. The wrapped specimen container should then be placed in a watertight metal container (Figure 22.1), which is

Figure 22.1
Wrap specimen container for mailing in corrugated cardboard or cotton and place in watertight metal container.

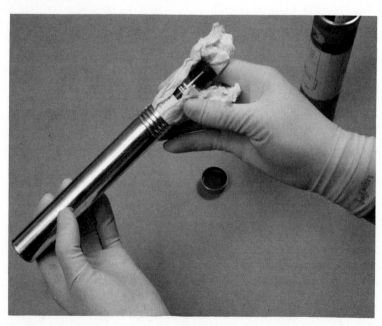

then placed with a laboratory requisition into a stiff cardboard mailing container that has shock-resistant insulating material (Figure 22.2). The outside of this container must have a label that identifies it as a medical specimen (see also Chapter 20, pp. 347-348).

The specimen must be uncontaminated. To prevent addition of microorganisms to the specimen obtained from the patient, sterile containers, sterile applicators, or other sterile devices and clean or sterile techniques are to be used to collect the specimen.

- Cracked or broken containers and applicators must not be used.
- Only regulation tops or plugs are to be used on stopper bottles and test tubes. Cotton balls or gauze, must not be used as a substitute. Many laboratories now use plastic-capped tubes, screw caps, and metal closure tubes; special vials or tubes with rubber stoppers are used for transporting suspected anerobic organisms.
- Plugs or the inner surface of tops that come in contact with an unsterile surface are to be discarded.
- Containers should be filled only half-way. The top or plug must not be permitted to become wet, either from the specimen or other sources, to prevent contamination to the specimen and to personnel handling it.
- Specimen material must not be spilled on the outside of the container or on any surface. This is for the protection of everyone handling the specimen or near the area. If a specimen is

accidentally spilled, call the laboratory to inquire how to destroy the pathogens that may be in the specimen and what to use. You must clean the work area immediately. A disinfectant such as 1:10 dilution of sodium hypochlorite (household bleach) or phenol or cresol is frequently used to clean the area.

The specimen must contain living organisms collected from the proper source and reach the laboratory in a condition suitable for culturing, incubating, or examining. Specimens collected for a smear or culture may be taken from any body opening, whether natural, surgical, or accidental, for example, material may be collected from the ear, eye, nose, throat, urethra, vagina, rectum, or a wound. Body fluids such as urine, blood, cerebrospinal fluid, and samples of tissue (biopsy) may also be obtained. To make sure that the pathogens remain viable (living), all specimens must be sent to the laboratory for processing without delay. If there is a delay, most specimens may be kept in a refrigerator for a few hours. Generally swabs from the throat, rectum, wounds, fecal (except when feces are to be examined for the presence of parasites) and sputum samples may be stored in a refrigerator for several hours. Spinal fluid may contain organisms that are sensitive to cold; therefore, this specimen should be placed in a bacteriological incubator.

Swabs of infectious matter must be prevented from drying before they are processed in the laboratory. Sometimes the sterile swab is moistened with a broth, or placed into tubes containing broth or a selected holding medium to prevent drying of

Figure 22.2
Place watertight metal container containing specimen and laboratory requisition into a stiff cardboard mailing container.

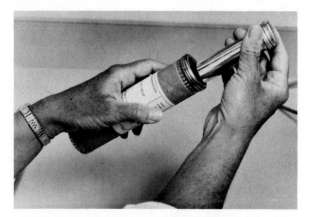

the specimen. The broth is used to keep the air around the swab moist and is *not* a culture medium.

Special procedures for preservation and growth are used when an anerobic organism (one able to live in the absence of oxygen) is believed to be the causative agent. Processing these specimens immediately is vital to maintaining the organism in a viable state. When there is a delay, inoculated culture plates may be placed in a candle jar (see Figure 22.15) and then sent to the laboratory.

Urine specimens should be examined or sent to the laboratory immediately. If this is not possible, they must be refrigerated. (See nos. 8 and 9 under "General Facts Relating To Urine Collection," which follows, and also Chapter 25, "Urinalysis.")

Most blood specimens must be examined within 8 hours or less from the time they were collected and preferably within 2 to 4 hours. Blood for bacteriologic studies must be collected in special containers and must not sit around. These specimens must be examined as soon as possible. Blood drawn for an electrolyte panel should be refrigerated if it is not tested immediately. Other blood samples may be left standing on the counter for 2 to 4 hours before testing, although some results may vary if the blood is left standing for 2 or more hours (see Chapter 26, "Hematology").

When a specimen is to be examined in the physician's office or clinic, it should be tested, cultured, or examined microscopically immediately.

The specimen should be handled and transported in an upright position and should not be shaken. Remember that failure to successfully identify pathogens may be caused by improper collection, care, and handling techniques.

Avoid and prevent contamination to yourself and other personnel who will be handling the specimen. All specimens obtained for microbiologic study are presumed to contain potentially dangerous pathogens. Always keep in mind the possibility of spreading the infectious pathogen, know the necessary protective measures that must be adhered to (as listed), and utilize excellent aseptic technique when obtaining the specimen. Gloves should be worn for handling specimens when contamination of the hands is anticipated. Care must be taken when collecting specimens to avoid contamination of the outside of the container and the laboratory slip. In addition:

- *Do not* eat, drink, or smoke while handling specimens because you could transmit pathogens to yourself by hand-to-mouth contact.
- *Do not* lick the label that will be placed on the specimen container.

- Cover any cut or scratch that you have with a Band-Aid.
- If you accidentally touch some of the specimen collected, immediately wash the contact area thoroughly with an antiseptic soap. If the contact area was on a cut or scratch, apply tincture of iodine or another antiseptic solution to the area. *Report the incident to your supervisor or employer.*
- At the end of each work day, clean the work area with a disinfectant solution.

All blood specimens from all patients, whether known to be infected or not, should be handled with caution.

All specimens from AIDS patients must be labeled with "H/A (hepatitis/AIDS) Precautions" labels, placed in ZipLoc bags, and sealed for transport to prevent spills from broken tubes. A laboratory requisition should also be labeled and attached to the outside of the bag.

A laboratory requisition to accompany the specimen must always be filled out completely and accurately. The following information must be included:

- Date (time of day if relevant, for example, an early-morning specimen);
- Name of the patient, address, age, and sex;
- Name and address of the attending physician;
- Source of the specimen;
- Name of laboratory test(s) to be performed; and
- If the patient is already taking antibiotics, a notation must be made.

Additional information will depend on the type of specimen obtained and may include the following:

- Clinical history;
- Previous normal or abnormal results;
- Previous surgery;
- X-ray treatment; and
- Clinical diagnosis.

For vaginal and cervical specimens the following, if applicable, is also added:

- Hormone treatment;
- Date of last menstrual period (LMP);
- Postpartum;
- Postmenopausal; or
- Pregnant.

URINE SPECIMEN COLLECTION

A specimen of urine is collected to perform a urinalysis (u'rĭ-nal'ĭ-sis), which is an analysis of the physical, chemical, and microscopic properties of urine. The results of these examinations help determine the renal functions of the body, which in turn helps the physician diagnose and provide the appropriate treatment required for a disease process.

Many types of tests are used in analyzing the urine to determine whether it contains abnormal substances indicative of disease. (See Chapter 25 for urinalysis procedures.) The most significant substances normally absent from urine and detected by a urinalysis are protein, glucose, acetone, blood, pus, casts, and bacteria.

Types of Urine Specimens
Random or spot specimen

To collect a random or spot specimen, the patient voids at any time of the day or night, collecting a portion of the urine in a clean container.

Fasting specimen

To collect a fasting specimen, the patient voids 4 or more hours after ingestion of food and discards this urine. The next voided specimen is collected and regarded as the fasting specimen.

First morning specimen

To collect a first morning specimen, the patient voids and discards the specimen before going to bed. On arising the next morning, the patient collects the first morning specimen.

Postprandial specimen

To collect a postprandial specimen, the patient voids after eating and collects this specimen.

Midstream specimen

To collect a midstream specimen, the patient starts to void into the toilet or bedpan; then, without stopping the process of voiding, a portion of the urine is collected in a clean container. The last part of the urine flow is passed into the toilet or bedpan.

Clean-catch specimen

To collect a clean-catch specimen, the patient is instructed to wash the external genitalia using soap and water or some mild antiseptic solution. Then a midstream urine specimen is collected in a clean, dry container or in a sterile container if the specimen is being collected for bacterial examination. This yields a specimen with limited contamination by skin bacteria.

Multiple-glass specimens

The multiple-glass test is performed on men to evaluate a lower urinary tract infection. The man must have a full bladder, as three samples of urine will be collected. To collect a multiple-glass specimen, the patient is instructed to wash the area around the urinary meatus with an antiseptic solution. Then he is to void about 100 ml (approximately 3½ ounces) into a clean, dry container. This specimen contains microorganisms and sediment "washed" from the urethra. Without interrupting the voiding process, another 100 ml of urine is then voided into a second clean, dry container. This specimen contains microorganisms and sediment representative of that in the bladder and kidney. Then the man is to stop voiding and the physician will gently massage the prostate gland. After this, the third urine specimen is collected in a clean, dry container. This last specimen contains secretions from the prostate gland.

Timed specimens (24-hour specimen)

To collect a timed specimen, the patient discards the first morning specimen and then collects all urine for exactly 24 hours (see no. 12, p. 418).

• • •

A specific type of urine collection can provide optimum information when performing certain tests; for example, postprandial urine can be used for testing sugar content, and first morning specimens can be used for testing protein content.

General Facts Relating to Urine Collection

1. To minimize bacterial and chemical contamination, use only clean, dry, or sterile collection containers. Disposable containers are ideal.
2. The early morning urine specimen is the most concentrated; therefore, if at all possible, this is the specimen that should be obtained for simple routine testing. The concentration of urine will vary during a 24-hour period, partly because of the patient's food and water intake and level of activity.
3. A freshly voided specimen is adequate for *most* urinalysis when the first morning specimen cannot be obtained, although collection of a clean-catch midstream specimen is the method of choice.
4. To collect a freshly voided specimen in the office, give the patient a clean, wide-mouthed bottle, and instruct him to void directly into it. Inform the patient how much urine you want in the bottle, that is, up to what point in the bottle you want collected (usually 2 to 4 ounces is sufficient).
5. When urine is required for bacterial cultures,

collect a clean-catch midstream specimen in a sterile container, and submit it to the bacteriology laboratory department as soon as possible for testing.

6. Ask patients if they are taking any medications, the type of medication, and if they are on a special diet. Certain medications and diets will affect the findings of a urinalysis. NOTE: A note of medications and/or special diet should be recorded on the laboratory requisition and the patient's chart.

7. Inquire if a female patient is menstruating when a urine specimen is collected. If blood is found in the urine it may be from the vaginal canal, rather than from the urinary tract. A note of this must also be recorded, and another specimen may be required when the patient has finished menstruating.

8. Voided specimens should not be left standing at room temperature, because they become alkaline as a result of contamination by urea-splitting bacteria from the environment. Explain to the patient that refrigeration of the specimen is necessary if collected at home, until time to submit it for analysis. If examination is delayed in your office or the laboratory, the specimen should also be refrigerated.

9. Microscopic examination of urine should be performed within 1 hour after collection. Waiting for longer than 1 hour will cause dissolution of cellular elements and casts and bacterial overgrowth, unless the specimen was obtained under sterile conditions.

10. When more than one specimen is required, number each specimen according to its sequence.

11. If the patient is to collect the specimen at home, the procedure should have been explained previously. The patient should be told to use a thoroughly clean 3- to 4-ounce container in which to collect the specimen. Instruct the patient to boil the container that will be used for the collection for 20 minutes before using it. It is advisable to instruct the patient not to use a container that has held drugs or other solutions that may make the specimen unsuitable for examination.

12. When a 24-hour specimen is required, it is vital that the patient understand the procedure. *All* urine must be collected within a 24-hour period.

    a. The first early-morning specimen is discarded.

    b. All subsequent specimens are collected, including the first early-morning specimen the next day.

    c. The last specimen is collected 24 hours after collection was started.

    d. Urine is collected in a clean bottle into which a preservative has been added (preservative is prescribed by the laboratory). This bottle must be refrigerated or kept cold by placing it in a bucket of ice.

Technique for Obtaining a Clean-Catch, Midstream Voided Specimen

Equipment

Antiseptic solution (such as benzalkonium chloride) *or* soap and water
Washcloth
Sterile gauze sponges 4 × 4 inch
Sterile specimen container (with cover if sending out to a lab)
Tissues
Laboratory requisition (Figure 22.3)

Figure 22.3
Sample urinalysis laboratory requisition that is sent with urine specimen to the laboratory.

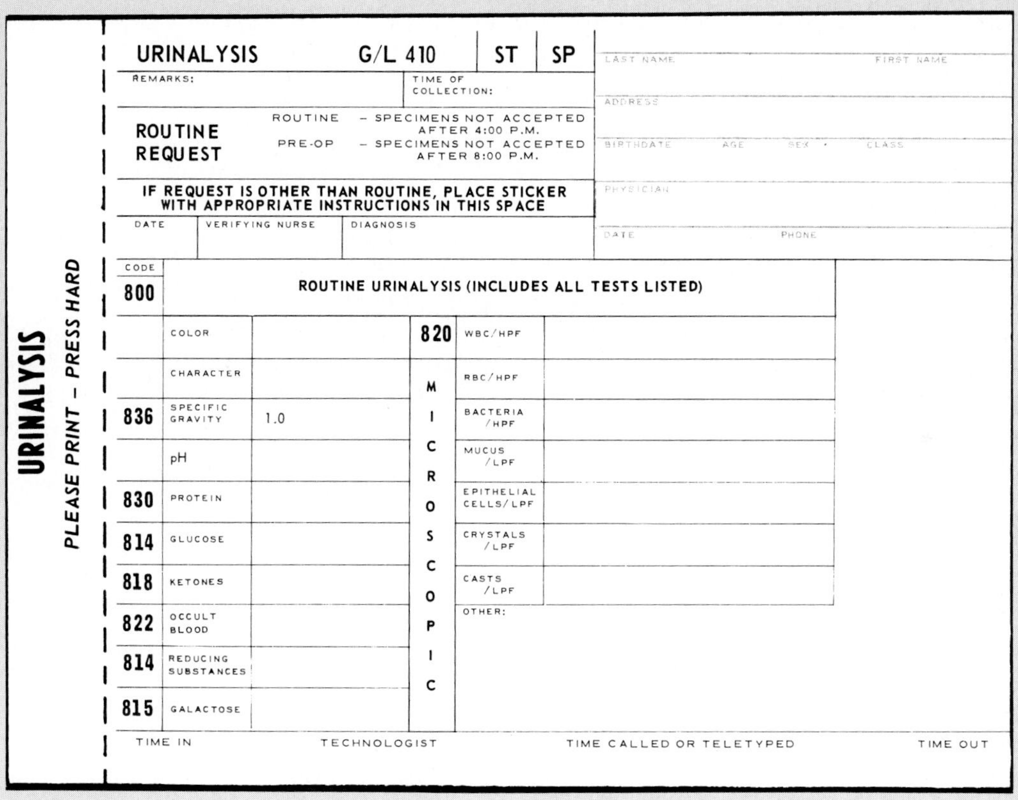

	URINALYSIS G/L 410 ST SP					
URINALYSIS PLEASE PRINT – PRESS HARD	REMARKS:		TIME OF COLLECTION:	LAST NAME	FIRST NAME	
	ROUTINE REQUEST	ROUTINE – SPECIMENS NOT ACCEPTED AFTER 4:00 P.M. PRE-OP – SPECIMENS NOT ACCEPTED AFTER 8:00 P.M.		ADDRESS		
				BIRTHDATE AGE SEX • CLASS		
	IF REQUEST IS OTHER THAN ROUTINE, PLACE STICKER WITH APPROPRIATE INSTRUCTIONS IN THIS SPACE			PHYSICIAN		
	DATE	VERIFYING NURSE	DIAGNOSIS	DATE PHONE		
	CODE **800**	ROUTINE URINALYSIS (INCLUDES ALL TESTS LISTED)				
		COLOR		**820**	WBC/HPF	
		CHARACTER		M	RBC/HPF	
	836	SPECIFIC GRAVITY	1.0	I	BACTERIA /HPF	
		pH		C R O S C O P I C	MUCUS /LPF	
	830	PROTEIN			EPITHELIAL CELLS/LPF	
	814	GLUCOSE			CRYSTALS /LPF	
	818	KETONES			CASTS /LPF	
	822	OCCULT BLOOD			OTHER:	
	814	REDUCING SUBSTANCES				
	815	GALACTOSE				
	TIME IN	TECHNOLOGIST		TIME CALLED OR TELETYPED	TIME OUT	

Procedure	**Rationale**
1. Wash your hands.	
2. Assemble supplies and equipment.	
3. Identify the patient, and explain the procedure.	Explanations help gain full cooperation from the patient, which is required to obtain a specimen successfully.

Continued.

Technique for Obtaining a Clean-Catch, Midstream Voided Specimen—cont'd

Procedure	*Rationale*
For a female patient	
a. Ask patient to wash her perineal area using soap, water, and washcloth; separate labia and cleanse the area around the urinary meatus.	Careful cleansing is necessary to obtain a satisfactory specimen. The urethral orifice is colonized by bacteria. Urine readily becomes contaminated during voiding.
b. Repeat step (a) using water and 4 × 4 inch sponges. NOTE: Rather than using soap and water, the patient may wash herself with 4 × 4 inch sponges soaked with a mild antiseptic solution such as benzalkonium chloride.	It is important to remove all the soap, as a soap residue changes the results of the specimen analysis.
c. Instruct patient to start voiding into the toilet; then after she has voided for a few seconds, to move the specimen container into the urinary stream to catch the midstream specimen in the sterile container.	This helps wash away uretheral contaminants. You will need approximately 2 to 4 ounces of urine for analysis. Instruct the patient to fill the container no more than three fourths full.
d. Instruct the patient to finish voiding into the toilet bowl.	Provide tissues for the patient to wipe herself and to wash the outside of the container if spillage should occur after collecting the specimen.
For a male patient	
a. Instruct the patient to take the penis, retract the foreskin (if uncircumcised) to expose the urinary meatus, and cleanse thoroughly with soap and water, and a washcloth.	Careful cleansing is necessary to obtain a satisfactory specimen. The urethral orifice is colonized by bacteria. Urine readily becomes contaminated during voiding.
b. Repeat step (a) using 4 × 4 inch sponges and water. NOTE: Rather than using soap and water, the patient may wash himself with 4 × 4 inch sponges soaked with a mild antiseptic solution such as benzalkonium chloride.	It is important to remove all soap, as a soap residue will change the result of the specimen analysis.
c. Instruct the patient to start voiding into the toilet and, after he has voided for a few seconds, to move the specimen container into the urinary stream in order to catch the midstream specimen.	This helps cleanse the urethral canal. Instruct the patient to fill the container no more than three fourths full, as you will need only 2 to 4 ounces for the analysis.
d. Instruct the patient to then finish voiding into the toilet.	The patient is to avoid collecting the last few drops of urine, as prostatic secretions may be introduced into the urine at the end of the urinary stream.
4. Have the patient signal you when the specimen has been obtained or instruct the patient where to place the specimen container.	
5. Send properly labeled specimen, with the correct laboratory requisition, to appropriate laboratory; or refrigerate it until it can either be tested or sent to the lab (Figure 22.3).	Do not allow a urine specimen to stand at room temperature for any length of time, because it becomes worthless. It is best to put a cover on the container.
6. Perform the urinalysis if this is required of you.	See Chapter 25 for this procedure.
7. Wash your hands.	Avoid contamination.
8. Record on chart the appropriate information. Always record on the chart if the urine appeared abnormal, that is, if blood appeared to be present, or if the urine was cloudy, and so on. Record the results if you have performed the analysis (as described in Chapter 25).	Charting example: February 25, 19_____, 4 PM Clean-catch urine specimen obtained and sent to the laboratory for routine UA [urinalysis]. Betty Bittinger, CMA

STOOL SPECIMEN COLLECTION

A stool specimen is collected for macroscopic, microscopic, and chemical examination to help diagnose the presence of parasites and ova, occult blood, fecal urobilinogen, pus or mucus, membranous shreds, worms, infectious diseases, foreign bodies, and to detect the amount of fat being eliminated and various disorders of metabolism.

The stool is examined macroscopically for its amount, consistency, color, and odor. Normal color varies from light to dark brown depending on urobilin content, a product formed from bilirubin. Various foods, medications, and conditions affect the color of the stool. For example, when a person has ingested the following, the color of the stool may be affected:

- Meat protein—the stool may be dark brown;
- Spinach—the stool may be green;
- Cocoa—the stool may be dark red or brown;
- Bismuth, iron, or charcoal—the stool may be black; or
- Barium—the stool may be milky white.

In conditions in which a patient is having upper gastrointestinal bleeding. the stool is tarry black; in lower gastrointestinal bleeding, bright red bloody; and in biliary obstruction, clay-colored. Other clinical conditions in which the stool has certain characteristics include the following:

- Steatorrhea (excess fat in the feces from a malabsorption state caused by disease of the intestinal mucosa or pancreatic enzyme deficiency)—the stool will appear bulky, greasy, foamy, foul in odor, and gray or clay-colored with a silvery sheen.

- Chronic ulcerative colitis—mucus or pus may be visible in the stool.
- Constipation, obstipation, and fecal obstruction—the stool will appear as small, dry, rock-hard masses.

As with most specimens, a fresh specimen is absolutely necessary and should be obtained before the administration of antibiotic therapy. Stool containing barium, mineral oils, or magnesia is usually unsuitable for diagnosis.

To best demonstrate parasitic infection, three fresh specimens collected on three different days are usually required. These must be sent to the laboratory immediately so that the parasites can be observed under the microscope while they are fresh, viable, and warm. Stool for occult blood testing should not be more than 1 hour old.

Some laboartories now prefer the new collection system that no longer requires that specimens be warm. The specimens are placed into two separate vials, each containing a special preservative, and then are to be sent to the laboratory as soon as possible.

When forwarding the specimen to a hospital or large laboratory, send specimens to be tested for occult blood to the hematology laboratory, specimens for culture and acid-fast bacilli to the bacteriology laboratory, and specimens for parasites and ova to the parasitology laboratory. All specimens are to be accompanied by the appropriate clinical laboratory slips with accurate and complete information (see box on pp. 422-423).

Technique for Obtaining a Stool Specimen

Equipment

Stool specimen container of waxed paper with a lid of glass
Wood tongue depressor or spatula
Clean bedpan with cover
Label for container
Small paper bag
Laboratory requisition
Rubber gloves

Procedure	*Rationale*
1. Wash your hands, and obtain a clean bedpan with a clean cover to give to the patient for use.	
2. Identify the patient. Explain to the patient that a stool specimen is needed and that a bedpan must be used.	Have the patient empty the bladder first if required, as urine should not be collected in the bedpan with the stool specimen. Explanations help gain the patient's full cooperation, which is essential for proper specimen collection.
3. Prepare the label for the specimen container. Fill out the laboratory requisition accurately and completely.	You can do this while the patient is collecting the specimen.
4. After the patient has used the bedpan, cover it and remove it to your work area.	Provide means for the patient to wash the hands.
5. Don gloves and transfer a portion (1 to 2 teaspoons) of the stool into the specimen container by using the clean tongue depressor or spatula as a spoon. Place the lid on the container securely.	Be sure that there is no toilet tissue in the stool specimen. Do not smear the specimen on the edge or outside of the container. You may scrape the tongue depressor or spatula only on the inside of the container to rid it of feces.
6. Place the tongue depressor or spatula in the paper bag, and wrap it securely for proper disposal.	*Do not* throw it in the wastebasket, as it may be contaminated with infectious disease organisms. You will have a special container for used equipment such as this.
7. Empty and clean the bedpan. Avoid contaminating yourself or your work area.	*Before* emptying the bedpan observe the feces for anything that appears abnormal to you, and report it at once.
8. Remove gloves and wash your hands thoroughly.	
9. Label the container and attach the correct completed laboratory requisition to the container (Figure 22.4).	The purpose of the examination must be stated on the requisition.
10. Send or take the labeled specimen to the laboratory immediately. If there is a delay, try to place the specimen for parasite examination in a warm place until it can be delivered to or picked up by the laboratory. Refrigerate specimens for other examinations until delivered to the laboratory. NOTE: If more than one specimen is to be sent, indicate No. 1, No. 2, and so on.	A stool specimen should be warm when it arrives in the laboratory for examination. This is especially important when looking for parasites so that they may be examined under the microscope while viable, fresh, and warm. Specimens for tests other than parasite detection can generally be refrigerated for a few hours when not sent immediately to the laboratory.
11. Wash your hands again.	Because of the chance of having disease organisms on your hands, wash them again to be safe.
12. Record on the patient's chart. If relevant, describe the appearance of the stool when charting.	Charting example: Feb. 27, 19_____, 10 AM Stool specimen No. 1 sent to laboratory for ova and parasites, and fat content examinations Connie Hanks, CMA

HEMOCCULT SLIDE TEST ON A STOOL SPECIMEN

The Hemoccult test is a rapid, convenient, and virtually odorless qualitative method for detecting fecal occult blood. It is not a test for colorectal cancer or any other specific diseases.

Hemoccult detects excess blood loss, which may have significance when related to certain diseases, such as colorectal cancer. A positive test usually indicates blood in excess of normal and should be followed up medically. A negative test usually indicates that no blood, in excess of normal, is apparent in the fecal specimen tested. The accuracy of the test depends upon the status of the patient at the time the specimen is taken and may be affected by interfering substances.

Hemoccult is recommended for use as a diagnostic aid during routine physical examinations, when hospital patients are first admitted, to monitor for bleeding in patients recuperating from sur-

Figure 22.4
Sample laboratory requisition for fecal specimen.

FECES - SEMEN

FECES – SEMEN LABORATORY

DATE Feb. 27, 19__.
Patient's name
Physician's name and address

Routine Feces Consists Of • Gross Description • Ova & Parasites • Occult Blood
☐ CULTURE REQUIRED (ALSO SUBMIT BACTERIOLOGY REQUEST)

☐ ROUTINE FECES	☐ UROBILINOGEN (QUAL.)	☐ SEMEN ANALYSIS
☑ OVA & PARASITES	☑ FAT (QUAL.)	☐
☐ OCCULT BLOOD	☐ STARCH	☐
☐ BILE PIGMENT (QUAL.)	☐ TRYPSIN	☐

COMMENTS: Stool spec #1

FECES – SEMEN

FINDINGS	STOOL EXAMINATION		FINDINGS			FINDINGS	SEMEN ANALYSIS
	COLOR			OVA & HELMINTHS	PARASITES		APPEARANCE
	CONSISTENCY			DIRECT	PARASITES		VOLUME (cc)
	MUCUS			CONC.	PARASITES		COUNT 100-150 M/cc
	PUS CELLS			TROPHOZOITES	AMEBAE		RBC
	RED BLOOD CELLS			CYSTS	AMEBAE		WBC
	BENZIDINE	OCCULT BLOOD		NEUTRAL FAT	Fats		CRYSTALS
	GUAIAC	OCCULT BLOOD		STARCH			% MOTILITY (INIT.)
	UROBILIN	BILE PIGMENT		TRYPSIN			MORPHOLOGY
	BILIRUBIN	BILE PIGMENT					
	UROBILINOGEN (QUAL.)	BILE PIGMENT					

ADDITIONAL RESULTS:

DATE | TECHNOLOGIST'S SIGNATURE

gery and other conditions, and in screening programs for colorectal cancer.

Because Hemoccult testing requires only a small fecal specimen, offensive odors are minimized and storage or transport of large fecal specimens is unnecessary.

See Figure 22.5 for more information, special instructions for the patient, and the equipment and procedure for performing this test. The American Cancer Society recommends that a stool blood test be performed every year on patients 50 years or older.

Figure 22.5

A, Hemoccult test and procedure.

Hemoccult Single Slides are convenient for use when single stool specimens are to be tested.

Hemoccult II Slides, in cards of three tests, are designed so your patient can collect serial specimens at home over the course of three bowel movements. After the patient collects the specimens, the Hemoccult II test may be returned to a laboratory, a hospital, or a medical office for developing and evaluation. Serial fecal specimen analysis is recommended when screening asymptomatic patients (**B** and **D**).

Hemoccult Tape is designed to complement Hemoccult slides and is best suited for "on-the-spot" testing for occult blood during rectal or sigmoidoscopic examinations.

The Hemoccult test and other unmodified guaiac tests are *not recommended* for use with gastric specimens.

SUMMARY, EXPLANATION AND LIMITATIONS OF THE TEST
The Hemoccult test is a simplified, standardized variation of the guaiac test for occult blood. It contains specially prepared guaiac-impregnated paper and is ready for use without additional preparation.

When a small stool specimen containing occult blood is applied to Hemoccult test paper, the hemoglobin comes in contact with the guaiac. Application of Hemoccult Developer (a stabilized hydrogen peroxide solution) creates a guaiac/peroxidase-like reaction which turns the test paper blue within 60 seconds if occult blood is present.

The test reacts with hemoglobin released from lysed cells. When blood is present, hemolysis is promoted by substances in the stool, primarily water and salts. Typical positive reactions for occult blood are shown under READING AND INTERPRETATION OF THE HEMOCCULT TEST. As with any occult blood test, results with the Hemoccult test *cannot* be considered conclusive evidence of the presence or absence of gastrointestinal bleeding or pathology. Hemoccult tests are designed for *preliminary screening as a diagnostic aid* and are not intended to replace other diagnostic procedures such as proctosigmoidoscopic examination, barium enema, or other x-ray studies.

A

BIOLOGICAL PRINCIPLE
The discovery that gum guaiac was a useful indicator for occult blood is generally credited to Van Deen. The test depends on the oxidation of a phenolic compound, alpha guaiaconic acid, which yields a blue-covered, highly conjugated quinone structure. Hemoglobin exerts a peroxidase-like activity and facilitates the oxidation of this phenolic compound by hydrogen peroxide.

REAGENTS
Natural guaiac resin impregnated into standardized, high-quality filter paper.

A developing solution containing a stabilized dilute mixture of 4.5% hydrogen peroxide and 75% denatured ethyl alcohol in aqueous solution.

PERFORMANCE MONITORS
The function and stability of the slides and Developer can be tested using the on-slide Performance Monitor. Both a positive and negative Performance Monitor are located under the flap and below the specimen windows on the back of the Hemoccult II and Hemoccult single slides.

The positive Performance Monitor contains a hemoglobin-derived catalyst which, upon application of Developer, will turn blue within 10 seconds.

The negative Performance Monitor contains no such catalyst and should not turn blue upon application of Developer.

The Performance Monitors provide additional assurance that the guaiac-impregnated paper and Developer are functional.
In the unlikely event that the Performance Monitors do not react as expected after application of Developer, the test results should be regarded as invalid. The manufacturer will provide further assistance should this occur.

PRECAUTIONS
For *in vitro* diagnostic use. Do not use after expiration date which appears on each slide or tape dispenser.

Prolonged exposure to some air pollutants and light may cause slides to turn blue. This does not affect the performance of the test and results can be read in the usual manner.

Hemoccult Developer should be protected from heat and the bottle kept tightly capped when not in use. It is flammable and subject to evaporation.
Hemoccult Developer is an irritant. Avoid contact with skin.

Do Not Use In Eyes. Should such contact occur, solution should be rinsed out promptly with water.

Do not use after expiration date on bottle.

STORAGE AND STABILITY
Do not refrigerate or freeze. Store at controlled room temperature 15°–30°C (59°–86°F) in original packaging. Protect from heat and light. Do not store with volatile chemicals (e.g., iodine, chlorine, bromine, or ammonia).

The Hemoccult test, stored as recommended, will maintain its sensitivity until the expiration date on the slide. The expiration date appears on each slide and tape dispenser.

Hemoccult Developer, stored as recommended, will remain stable until the expiration date on the bottle. The expiration date appears on each bottle.

SPECIMEN COLLECTION
Only a very small stool sample, about the size of a match-head, thinly applied, is necessary in preparing either slide or tape. When specimen is to be collected from toilet bowl, the patient should flush the toilet before defecating. The slides may be prepared and developed immediately or prepared and stored for up to 14 days at room temperature (20°–25°C).

Patients with bleeding from other conditions which may affect test results (e.g., hemorrhoids, menstrual bleeding, hematuria) are not appropriate test subjects while such bleeding is active.

Since bleeding from gastrointestinal lesions may be intermittent, it is recommended that stool smears for testing be collected from three consecutive bowel movements. To increase the probability of detecting occult blood, Greegor recommends that samples be taken from two different sections of each stool especially from darkened or discolored areas of the stool.

Patient Preparation
Whenever practicable, patients should be placed on the Special Diagnostic Diet (see below) starting two days before and continuing through the test period. Such a diet may increase the accuracy of the test and at the same time provide roughage to help uncover "silent" lesions which may bleed only intermittently.

An alternative procedure is to omit the special diet initially. Then if a patient has one or more positive tests in the initial three-slide series, he should be placed on the special diet and retested for three days.

```
Special Diagnostic Diet
(two days before and during the test period)
Foods to avoid
    Rare red meat (beef, lamb, etc.)
    Turnips
    Horseradish
    Melons
Drugs & Vitamins to avoid
    Vitamin C in excess of 250 mg per day
    Aspirin or aspirin-containing products
    Anti-inflammatory drugs
    Iron supplements
Foods to eat
    Well-cooked meats, poultry and fish
    Bran cereal daily
    Cooked fruits and vegetables
    Peanuts and popcorn
If any of the above are known from past
experience to cause discomfort, patient is
instructed to inform the physician.
```

Interfering Substances
Some oral medications (e.g., aspirin, indomethacin, phenylbutazone, corticosteroids, reserpine, etc.) can cause GI irritation and occult bleeding in some patients. These substances should be discontinued on the advice of the physician two days prior to and during testing.

Ascorbic acid (Vitamin C) in excess of 250 mg/day may cause false-negative results and should also be eliminated before testing.

Therapeutic dosages of iron can yield false-positive fecal occult blood test reactions. On the advice of the physician use of iron preparations should be suspended before and during testing for fecal occult blood.

PROCEDURE: HEMOCCULT SLIDES

Identification

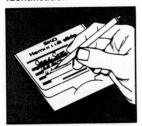

Write, or have patient write his or her name, age, address, phone number, and date specimen was collected in space provided on front of each slide.

Preparation

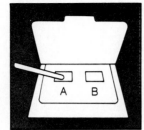

1. Collect small stool sample on one end of applicator.
2. Apply thin smear inside box A.
3. Reuse applicator to obtain second sample from different part of stool. Apply thin smear inside box B.
4. Close cover. Return slide to physician or laboratory as soon as possible.
CAUTION: Protect from heat, light, and volatile chemicals.

Development of Test

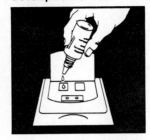

1. Open flap *in back* of slide and apply two drops of Hemoccult Developer to guaiac paper directly over each smear.
2. Read results within 60 seconds.
ANY TRACE OF BLUE ON OR AT THE EDGE OF THE SMEAR IS POSITIVE FOR OCCULT BLOOD.

Development of Performance Monitors

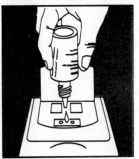

1. Apply ONE DROP ONLY of Hemoccult Developer between the positive and negative Performance Monitors.
2. Read results within 10 seconds.
A BLUE COLOR WILL APPEAR IN THE POSITIVE PERFORMANCE MONITOR, AND NO BLUE WILL APPEAR IN THE NEGATIVE PERFORMANCE MONITOR, IF THE SLIDES AND DEVELOPER ARE FUNCTIONAL.

IMPORTANT NOTE: Follow the procedure exactly as outlined above. Always develop the test, read the results, interpret them and make a decision as to whether the fecal specimen is positive or negative for occult blood BEFORE you develop the Performance Monitors. Do not apply Developer to Performance Monitors before interpreting test results. Any blue originating from the Performance Monitors should be ignored in the reading of the specimen test results.

READING AND INTERPRETATION OF THE HEMOCCULT TEST

Negative Smears*

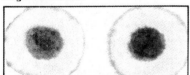

Negative and Positive Smears*

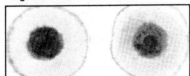

Positive Smears*

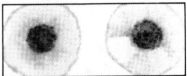

Specimen report: negative
No detectable blue on or at the edge of the smears indicates test is negative for occult blood.

Specimen report: Positive
Any trace of blue on or at the edge of one or more of the smears indicates test is positive for occult blood.

On-Slide Performance Monitors*

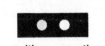

positive   negative

A blue color in the positive Performance Monitor will appear within 10 seconds if test system is functional.

No blue color will appear in the negative Performance Monitor if the test system is functional.

Neither the intensity nor the shade of the blue from the positive Performance Monitor should be regarded as an indication of what the blue from a positive fecal specimen should look like.

* The illustrations are an artist's rendition. Each specimen illustration is of two smears from a single stool specimen as displayed on a single Hemoccult test slide. A reaction on Hemoccult Tape may appear as any one of the illustrated smears.

PROCEDURE FOR HEMOCCULT TAPE

Preparation

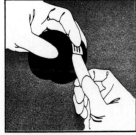

1. Tear strip of tape from dispenser.

2. Apply thin stool smear.

Development

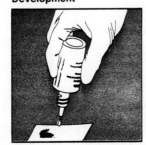

1. Apply two drops of Hemoccult Developer to side opposite smear.
2. Read results on side opposite smear within 60 seconds.
ANY TRACE OF BLUE ON OR AT THE EDGE OF THE SMEAR IS POSITIVE FOR OCCULT BLOOD.

Figure 22.5, cont'd
B, Hemoccult II slides. **C,** Hemoccult II Dispensapak with on-slide performance monitors. **D,** Instructions to the patient for collecting fecal specimens for Hemoccult II slide test and Hemoccult II procedure.
Courtesy SmithKline Diagnostics, Inc, Sunnyvale, Calif.

MATERIALS SUPPLIED (see panel **C**)
- Hemoccult guaiac paper slides (or tape in convenient dispenser)
- Specimen applicators (supplied with slides only)
- Patient envelopes with instructions for specimen collection and diet (supplied with Dispensapak™ units only)
- Hemoccult Developer (in plastic bottles)
- Hemoccult Identification Card

SATISFACTORY LIMITS OF PERFORMANCE; EXPECTED RESULTS
Results with the Hemoccult test are visually determined. The Hemoccult guaiac test paper should be observed for color change within 60 seconds after Developer has been applied.

This reading time is important because the color reaction may fade after two to four minutes.

If any trace of blue on or at the edge of the smear is seen, the test is positive for occult blood. For typical positive reaction, see READING AND INTERPRETATION OF THE HEMOCCULT TEST.

NOTE: Because this test is visually read and requires color differentiation, it should *not* be read by the visually impaired.

The function and stability of the Hemoccult slides and Developer can be tested using the on-slide Performance Monitors. The Hemoccult Tape may be tested by applying a drop of diluted whole blood (1 : 5,000 in distilled water) to an unused portion of the tape. Add Developer to opposite side. If any blue appears, the guaiac-impregnated paper and Developer are functional.

B

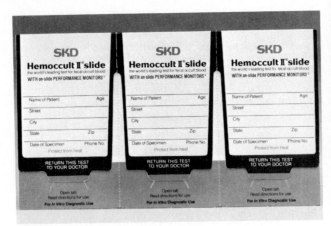

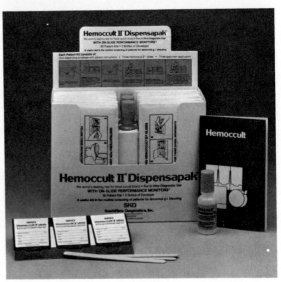

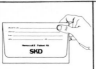

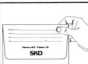

1. Fill in patient information on Hemoccult II* test. Give kit to patient.

2. Patient, at home, opens a cover flap and applies a thin stool smear to Box A, a second smear from a different site to Box B. Patient performs procedure for three consecutive bowel movements.

3. Patient returns prepared slides to doctor's office or lab.

4. Doctor or medical assistant applies two drops of Developer on the back of the slide directly over each smear.

5. Doctor or medical assistant reads results within 60 seconds. Any trace of blue on or at the edge of the smear is positive for blood.

6. Doctor or medical assistant applies ONE DROP ONLY of Developer between the positive and negative Performance Monitors*. A blue color will appear within 10 seconds in the positive Performance Monitor, no blue in the negative Performance Monitor, if the slides and Developer are functional.

INSTRUCTIONS TO THE PATIENT FOR COLLECTING FECAL SPECIMENS FOR THE HEMOCCULT II SLIDE TEST

Hemoccult slides are used routinely to check the intestinal tract. Please follow these instructions carefully. Before you begin, put your name, address, age, and telephone number on the front of each of the three slide sets. Date each pair of specimens on the day that the two specimens are collected.
1. With wooden applicator stick, collect a small stool specimen from the toilet bowl.
2. Spread a very thin smear on box A of first slide. Repeat from a different portion of the stool for box B.
3. Repeat these instructions for the other two slides after your next two bowel movements.
4. Mail the 3 slides as soon as possible in the addressed envelope provided. You will need to add a 22¢ stamp.

IMPORTANT
1. Fecal specimens should not be collected during a menstrual period or while suffering from bleeding hemorrhoids.
2. Protect slides from heat, sunlight, and fluorescent light. Also, do not refrigerate the slides.
3. Follow the special diagnostic diet if your physician has instructed you to do so at least 48 hours before you collect the first stool specimen. Stay on this diet until all slides have been prepared.
4. Mail the 3 completed slides (or as many as you have completed) back to the laboratory *no later than 6 days from the time you collected the first stool specimen.*

RESPIRATORY TRACT SPECIMENS
Sputum Specimen Collection

Sputum specimens are examined to help determine the presence of infectious organisms or to identify tumor cells in the respiratory tract. The laboratory findings provide relevant information to the physician when making a diagnosis and initiating treatment.

Other specimens that may be obtained if patient is unable to produce sputum include tracheal aspirates, collected by aspiration with a suction catheter, and bronchial washings and transtracheal aspirates, collected by the physician or a pulmonary technician. These specimens are of more value diagnostically than sputum, since they are not likely to become as contaminated with oropharyngeal flora. Nevertheless, because sputum is easy to collect and causes little discomfort to the patient, it is usually the first type of lower respiratory tract specimen to be obtained for examination and culture.

Procedures ordered on sputum specimens when sent to the laboratory include direct smears, routine culture and sensitivities, culture for acid-fast bacilli (tuberculosis), fungus cultures, and sputum cytology (exfoliative cytology), which is performed to identify tumor cells.

Periodic sputum examinations may also be done on patients receiving antibiotics, steroids, and immunosuppressive agents for prolonged periods, as these agents give rise to opportunistic pulmonary infections.

When you collect sputum specimens, it is essential that you understand the physician's order. For example, if the order states "sputum cultures × 3," this means that you should collect three different specimens at different times or on three successive days. This order *does not* mean that you should collect one specimen and divide it into three different containers. Even though these specimens would each be cultured, the findings will show that they were duplicates, and the whole procedure would have to be repeated (see box on pp. 428-429).

Technique for Obtaining a Sputum Specimen

Equipment

Sterile specimen container
Glass jar for acid-fast bacilli culture
Cardboard sputum container may be used for other studies
Label
Laboratory requisition
Paper bag and tape

Procedure	*Rationale*
1. Wash your hands, and assemble the supplies.	
2. Identify the patient, and explain the procedure. Give the sterile specimen container to the patient. Instruct the patient not to touch the inside of the container with the hands.	Obtain freshly expectorated sputum. If feasible, the specimen should be collected in the morning before eating or drinking. Usually a minimum of 5 ml of sputum is required by the laboratory for testing.
3. Instruct the patient to cough deeply and expectorate directly into the container, avoiding contamination to the outside of the container with the sputum.	Sputum (lung and bronchial specimen) is produced by a deep cough. You do not want a specimen of saliva from the mouth.
4. Label the container, and indicate test(s) required on the laboratory requisition (Figure 22.6).	Accurate, complete information is always required: date, time, patient's name, type of specimen, test(s) to be performed, name of attending physician and, when availble, probable diagnosis.
5. Send the specimen to the laboratory. a. Secure the sputum container lid with tape. b. Place the container in a paper bag and attach the laboratory requisition.	Specimens for culture and cytology should be sent to the laboratory within 30 minutes of collection, as any delay can cause organisms to multiply, which would result in misleading findings. Refrigerate the specimen to prevent bacteria overgrowth when it is not sent to the laboratory immediately.
NOTE: Specimens must be as fresh as possible except when accumulation over a specific length of time is ordered. Clearly mark on the label if the specimen is a 24 hour collection.	If a 24-hour specimen is to be obtained, instruct the patient to wrap a paper towel around the jar and secure it with a rubber band. Always keep the lid of the container closed except when in use.
6. Wash your hands.	Avoid contamination.
7. Record on chart. Note any abnormal quality that you may have observed, such as sputum that appeared to be blood tinged.	Charting example: February 25, 19_____, 8 AM Sputum specimen obtained: sent to laboratory for C & S [culture and sensitivity] Marjory Alving. CMA

Throat and Nasopharyngeal Cultures

Upper respiratory secretions most often obtained for examination are throat and nasopharyngeal cultures.

The throat is defined as the area of the body that includes the larynx and pharynx, passageways that link the nose and mouth with the respiratory and digestive systems. A sore throat is caused by inflammation, irritation, or infection of tissue in one or more of the areas in the pharynx or larynx. The common cause of throat infection is the invasion of the tissues by bacteria, such as streptococci, staphylococci, or pneumococci. Inflammation and discomfort in the throat are often caused by tonsillitis, as well as by just an overuse of the voice or excessive smoking.

Throat cultures are performed to determine the presence and the type of microscopic organism that is the cause of an infection. They are frequently ordered for patients suspected of having streptococcal pharyngitis and also for those with suspected cases of pertussis (whooping cough), diphtheria, and gonococcal pharyngitis. The nasopharynx (na′zo-far′ingks) is the part of the pharynx above the soft palate that is connected with the nasal cavities and provides a passage for air during breathing.

Usually nasopharyngeal cultures are ordered on infants and children (when a sputum specimen cannot be obtained) who are suspected of having whooping cough, pneumonia, or croup. They may also be ordered for patients suspected of being carriers of pathogenic organisms that cause meningitis, diphtheria, scarlet fever, pneumonia, rheumatic fever, and other diseases.

Figure 22.6
Sample laboratory requisition for sputum specimen for culture and sensitivity tests.

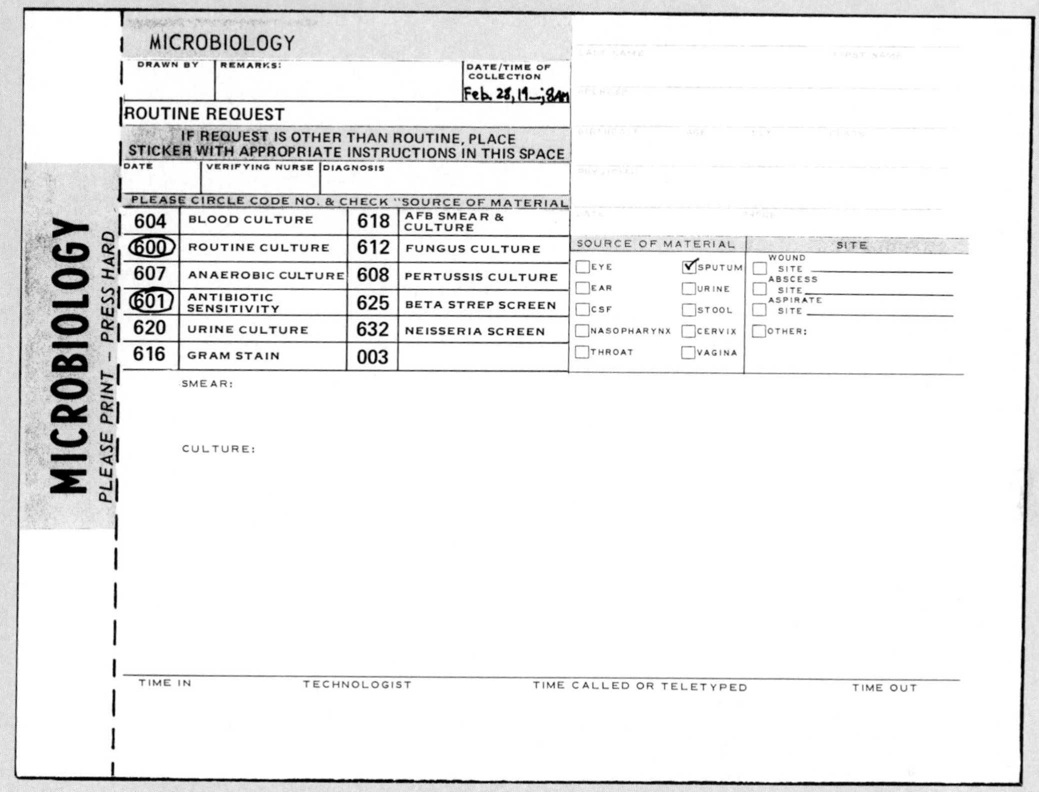

MICROBIOLOGY

DRAWN BY | REMARKS: | DATE/TIME OF COLLECTION Feb. 28, 19__; 8AM

ROUTINE REQUEST

IF REQUEST IS OTHER THAN ROUTINE, PLACE STICKER WITH APPROPRIATE INSTRUCTIONS IN THIS SPACE

DATE | VERIFYING NURSE | DIAGNOSIS

PLEASE CIRCLE CODE NO. & CHECK "SOURCE OF MATERIAL"

604	BLOOD CULTURE	618	AFB SMEAR & CULTURE
(600)	ROUTINE CULTURE	612	FUNGUS CULTURE
607	ANAEROBIC CULTURE	608	PERTUSSIS CULTURE
(601)	ANTIBIOTIC SENSITIVITY	625	BETA STREP SCREEN
620	URINE CULTURE	632	NEISSERIA SCREEN
616	GRAM STAIN	003	

SOURCE OF MATERIAL		SITE
☐ EYE	☑ SPUTUM	☐ WOUND SITE
☐ EAR	☐ URINE	☐ ABSCESS SITE
☐ CSF	☐ STOOL	☐ ASPIRATE SITE
☐ NASOPHARYNX	☐ CERVIX	☐ OTHER:
☐ THROAT	☐ VAGINA	

SMEAR:

CULTURE:

TIME IN | TECHNOLOGIST | TIME CALLED OR TELETYPED | TIME OUT

MICROBIOLOGY
PLEASE PRINT – PRESS HARD

Nasopharyngeal Culture

To obtain a better specimen with more organisms, you may induce the patient to cough by taking a throat culture first. Coughing can force organisms from the lower respiratory tract up to the nasopharyngeal area.

Procedure	*Rationale*
1. Obtain a throat culture first (if desired), then:	
2. Insert a sterile cotton-tipped applicator through the nose into the nasopharyngeal area.	
3. Gently rotate the applicator to obtain the specimen.	
4. Remove the applicator and place it into the sterile culture tube; secure the lid.	
5. Label and send the specimen to the laboratory with the correct laboratory requisition.	To prevent the drying of the specimen on the applicator, avoid delay.
6. Record the procedure on the patient's chart.	Charting example: February 27, 19_____, 1 PM Throat and nasopharyngeal specimens obtained and sent to the laboratory for C & S [culture and sensitivity] Abby Nelson, CMA

Throat Culture

Equipment

Sterile cotton-tipped applicator(s) in a sterile culture tube(s) or Culturette(s) (Figure 22.7)
Clean tongue depressor
Laboratory requisition(s)

Procedure	*Rationale*
1. Wash your hands.	Avoid contamination
2. Assemble the required equipment.	
3. Identify the patient, and explain the procedure.	Tell the patient that you are going to swab the back of the throat with the cotton-tipped applicator to obtain a specimen that will then be examined in the laboratory. This will help determine the cause of the patient's sore throat.
4. Have the patient assume an upright sitting position facing you.	The area where you are working should be well lighted. You may use an examination light that is positioned to give maximal illumination of the patient's throat.

Figure 22.7
A, Culturette II. **B,** Culturette bacterial collection/transport systems. See the vocabulary for an explanation of these systems.
Courtesy Marion Scientific Corp, Kansas City, Mo.

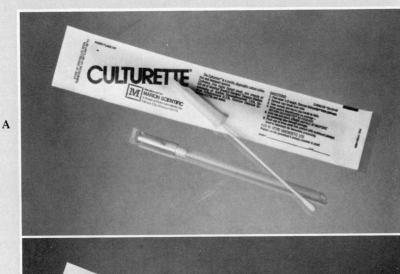

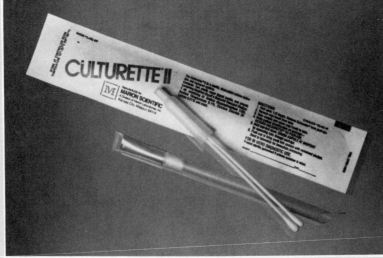

Throat Culture—cont'd

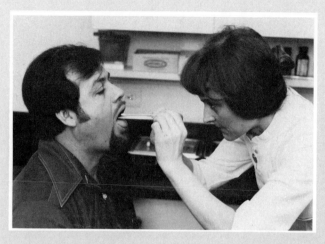

Figure 22.8
Obtaining a throat culture.

5. Ask the patient to open the mouth as wide as possible, to extend the tongue, and to say "ah."
6. Remove the sterile cotton-tipped applicator(s) from the culture tube.
7. Depress the patient's extended tongue with the tongue blade until the back of the throat is clearly visible (Figure 22.8).
8. Using the cotton-tipped applicator, swab the area at the very back of the throat on both sides. Particular attention should be taken to swab any red, raw, or raised bumps along the side and any areas coated with pus.

9. Remove the applicator quickly but gently, and place it into the culture tube, securing the lid. If a Culturette has been used, release the transport medium by crushing the ampule. NOTE: On occasion, two cultures will be required—one from both the right and left tonsillar areas. Two culture tubes with applicators will be used when doing this, and each must be labeled specifically. Use a quick downward stroke, first on one side and then with *another* applicator, on the opposite side. Keep the tongue depressed while obtaining both specimens.
10. Remove the tongue blade, and discard into covered waste container.
11. Attend to the patient's comfort; you may reposition the patient if necessary.
12. Wash your hands.
13. Label the culture tube(s) completely and accurately.

14. Complete and attach the appropriate laboratory requisition.
15. Send the culture tube to the laboratory. Avoid delay, so that your specimen will not dry out before the laboratory can transfer it to a culture medium.
16. Record on chart.

Saying "ah" will help relax the patient's throat muscle and minimize the gag reflex.

There are commercially prepared culture tubes in which the applicator stick is secured in the lid of the tube.

Place the tongue blade over two thirds of the tongue. This will help prevent the patient's tongue from touching the applicators as you are obtaining the throat specimen.

Care must be taken not to swab the tongue, but only the part of the throat from which the specimen should be obtained. Saliva must be avoided, as this will dilute the specimen, lead to overgrowth of nonpathogens, or inhibit the growth of the pharyngeal flora. Heavy mucus draining down the back of the throat from the nose is also undesirable culture material.

Patient's name, physician's name, date, and source of culture.

The above information is to be included, as well as the type of examination required.

In the laboratory the culture will be transferred by the technician to a culture medium, which enables growth of the infectious organisms for future examination.

Charting example:
  February 27, 19_____, 1 PM
  Throat culture obtained and sent to laboratory for C & S [culture and sensitivity]
    Marcia Edwards, CMA

WOUND CULTURE

When it is suspected that a wound is infected, a wound culture is done to determine the presence and the type of microorganism that is causing the infection. Cultures can be obtained from wounds on any part of the body.

The procedure for obtaining a wound culture is described in Chapter 21.

SMEARS FOR CYTOLOGY STUDIES

Obtaining a Cytology Smear

Equipment

Sterile cotton-tipped applicators or Ayer spatulas (number depending on the number of smears to be obtained)
Frosted-end glass slide(s)
Fixative spray, such as Cyto-Fix (a water soluble antiseptic), Spray-Cyte, or bottle of fixative solution (solution of 95% isopropyl alcohol preferred; however, formalin 10% may also be used)
Cardboard or plastic slide holder, rubber band, and envelope provided by the laboratory if the slide is to be mailed
Laboratory requisition
(Rubber gloves optional)

Procedure

1. Wash your hands.
2. Write the patient's name and the date on the frosted end of the slide.
   You may wish to wear rubber gloves for steps 3 through 10.
3. When the physician has obtained the specimen on the applicator or spatula, be prepared to hold the slide while the physician makes the smear, *or*
4. Take the applicator from the physician with your dominant hand, grasping the distal end of the stick.
5. Hold the glass slide between your thumb and index finger of your nondominant hand.
6. Starting near the unfrosted end of the slide, spread the specimen longitudinally along the slide by rotating the applicator in the opposite direction of spreading motion, that is, when spreading the specimen from right to left over the slide, rotate the cotton applicator clockwise (Figure 22.9).
7. Spread the specimen onto the slide evenly and moderately thin so that individual cells will be identifiable under a microscope.
8. *Do not touch* your thumb or fingers with the contaminated cotton-tipped applicator.
9. Discard the applicator in a covered waste container.
10. Fix the smear by immediately spraying it with the fixative spray or by immersing it in the bottle of fixative solution obtained from the laboratory. This should be done within 4 seconds to prevent drying and death of cells. Spray 5 or 6 inches away. With a continuous flow, make a stroke from left to right, then right to left. Allow to dry 4 to 6 minutes.
11. Remove gloves if you wore them for this procedure. Wash your hands.
12. Send the smear in the designated container to the laboratory for cytological tests with the correct and completed requisition. NOTE: If you are to mail the slide to a particular laboratory, place the slide inside the cardboard slide holder provided, once the fixative is dry. Close it with a rubber band. Fill out the requisition, giving the patient's name, age, last menstrual period, hormonal or other medication or treatment, pertinent clinical data, and history of any previous atypical Pap smears if this is a vaginal or cervical smear. Insert the slide and requisition into the envelope provided, seal, and mail (see Figure 19.15).

Rationale

Gloves should be worn for handling specimens when contamination of hands is anticipated.

Figure 22.9
Making a smear for cytology studies.

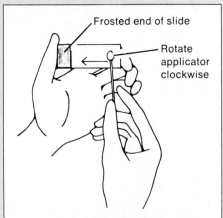

In the laboratory, the smear will be incubated for a prescribed time (24 to 72 hours) at 37° C or room temperature, because excessive heating of the smear destroys the microorganisms. To identify specific organisms, the laboratory personnel will use various staining procedures and then examine the smear microscopically.

SMEARS FOR BACTERIOLOGY STUDIES

Obtaining a Bacteriology Smear

The procedure for making a smear for bacteriology studies is the same as that for cytology smears (Steps 1 to 9), *except* to fix the smear.

Procedure	*Rationale*
10. Place the smear on a flat surface and allow to air dry for appoximately a half hour.	Air drying allows the specimen cells to dry slowly.
11. Grasp the slide with slide forceps, and pass it quickly through the flame of a Bunsen burner three or four times to *heat fix* the slide. *Do not* overheat the slide, as this will distort the cells present.	Microorganisms are destroyed with the heat and attached to the slide so that they will not wash off when the slide is stained in preparation for examination.
12. Forward the slide to the laboratory in the container provided with the completed laboratory requisition.	

GRAM STAIN

Once a smear is sent to the laboratory it will be treated in various ways so that visualization of microorganisms under a microscope is possible. A method commonly used to identify bacterial organisms is the Gram stain. This staining method permits the classification of bacteria into four basic groups: gram-positive or gram-negative rods and gram-positive or gram-negative cocci. The technique involves the treatment of the smear with Gram crystal violet, Gram iodine solution, 95% ethyl alcohol-acetone decolorizer, and safranin counterstain, after which the forms and structure of the microorganisms can be visualized. Differentiation of bacteria is done on the basis of their color reaction to the above stains. Gram-positive organisms stain purple, for example, staphylococci,

streptococci, and pneumococci. Gram-negative organisms are decolorized with the alcohol-acetone solution and will retain only the red color of the counterstain, safranin, for example, gonococci, meningococci, and *Escherichia coli (E. coli)*. Such a classification has important clinical implications, as it immediately narrows down the differential diagnosis, thus guiding treatment until additional tests, such as culture and sensitivity, are completed. The type of groups in which bacteria are arranged, such as chains, pairs, and clusters, can also be seen on the Gram stain. This is another important guide for treatment.

The Gram stain is usually followed by a culture and sensitivity test to help determine definitive diagnosis and appropriate treatment of an infectious process (see box on p. 434).

Procedure for a Gram Stain (Figure 22.10)

Equipment

Smear on a glass slide that has been *heat-fixed*
Slide forceps
Staining rack
Wash bottle containing distilled water
Gram crystal violet
Gram iodine solution
95% ethyl alcohol-acetone decolorizer
Safranin counterstain
Bibulous paper pad (absorbent paper pad)

Procedure

1. After making the smear and heat-fixing it as described above, place the slide on the staining rack, smear side facing up.
2. Cover the slide with Gram crystal violet. Allow it to react for 1 minute (Figure 22.10, A).
3. Grasp the slide with slide forceps and tilt it about 45 degrees to allow the Gram crystal violet to drain off (Figure 22.10, B).
4. Rinse the slide thoroughly with distilled water for about 5 seconds (Figure 22.10, C).
5. Replace the slide on the staining rack.
6. Cover the smear with Gram iodine solution, allowing it to react for 1 to 2 minutes.
7. Grasp the slide with the slide forceps and tilt it to a 45-degree angle to allow the Gram iodine solution to drain off.
8. Rinse the slide in this position with distilled water from the wash bottle for 5 seconds.
9. With the slide still tilted at a 45-degree angle, slowly pour the alcohol-acetone solution over it. This will decolorize the smear. Gram-posi-

tive bacteria are resistant to decolorization and will retain the Gram crystal violet stain. These bacteria will remain purple. Gram-negative bacteria will now be clear or colorless as they are unable to retain the stain.
10. Rinse the slide with distilled water for 5 seconds.
11. Replace the slide on the staining rack, cover it with the safranin counterstain, and allow it to react for 30 to 60 seconds. The gram-negative bacteria must be counterstained to be seen under the microscope. The safranin counterstain will stain them pink or red.
12. Grasp the slide with the slide forceps and tilt it to a 45-degree angle to allow the safranin counterstain to drain off.
13. Rinse the slide thoroughly with distilled water for 5 seconds.
14. Blot the smear dry between the pages of the bibulous paper pad with the smear side facing down. *Do not* rub the slide because you could rub the smear off of the slide (Figure 22.10, D).
15. The slide is now ready to be examined microscopically. Position the slide on the microscope using the oil-immersion objective. Adjust the microscope for the examination of the smear, ensuring that the slide was prepared properly (Figure 22.10, E). (Refer to Chapter 24 for instructions on using a microscope.)
16. Notify the physician that the smear is ready to be examined.

BACTERIAL CULTURE AND SENSITIVITY (C AND S) TESTING

Identification of bacteria may be done by means of a culture. A specimen is put on a culture medium that is conducive to the growth of microorganisms (Figure 22.11). The culture is then incubated for 24 to 48 hours to allow for the growth of the microorganisms. After this period the appropriate tests are performed to identify the microorganisms present. Most commonly the identification of a specific microorganism is accompanied by a sensitivity study. A sensitivity study determines the sensitivity of bacteria to antibiotics. The disc-plate method is most commonly used clinically (Figure 22.12). This method measures the inhibition of growth of a microorganism, on the surface of an

inoculated culture medium plate, by an antibiotic diffusing into the surrounding medium from an impregnated disc. The organism is reported as being either sensitive, intermediate, or resistant to the antibiotic. When the organism is sensitive to the antibiotic, there will be a clear zone around the impregnated disc. This indicates that the antibiotic was effective in destroying the organism. When there is growth around the impregnated disc, this indicates that the organism cannot be destroyed or inhibited by that antibiotic. The results obtained from a C and S provide the physician with information used to determine which antibiotic can be used to destroy pathogens causing a patient's infectious condition.

Figure 22.10
Gram stain procedure. **A,** With smear side facing up on the staining rack, cover it with gram crystal violet. **B,** Grasp slide with slide forceps, tilt it 45 degrees for gram crystal violet to drain off. **C,** Rinse slide with distilled water. **D,** Blot the smear dry between pages of bibulous paper. **E,** Position slide on microscope using the oil immersion objective for examination.

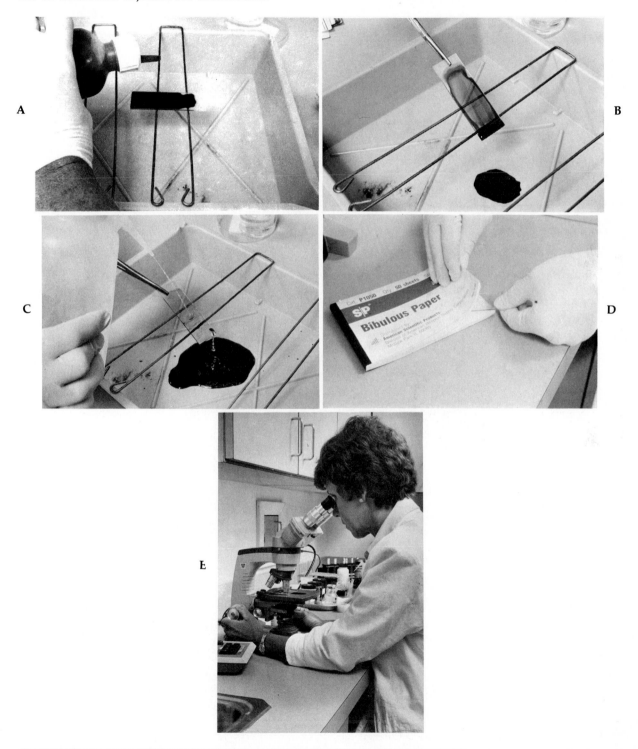

Figure 22.11
Blood agar culture media contained in a Petri dish showing growth of bacterial colonies.

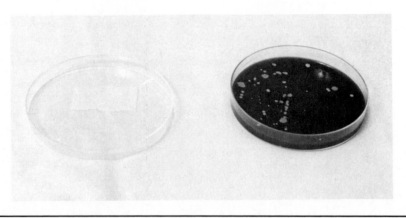

Figure 22.12
Disk-plate method for sensitivity test. Microorganism being tested is inoculated on the agar medium. Paper disks containing antibiotics are placed on the medium. Clear zones represent inhibition of growth of the microorganism by the specific antibiotic. Zone size is significant. If zone size is smaller than prescribed for clinical effectiveness, the microorganism will be reported as *resistant* to the drug. When the microorganism is *sensitive* to the antibiotic, there will be a clear zone around the impregnated disk. (Gloves are optional but strongly suggested.)

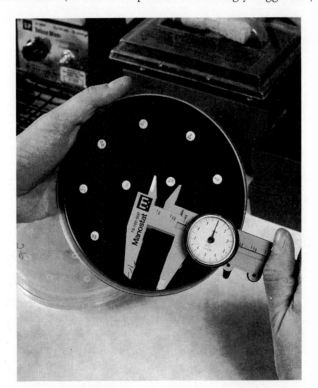

Culture Media

A culture medium is a sterile commercial preparation used for the growth of microorganisms or other cells. The most commonly used media are broths (liquids), gelatin (solid), and agar (solid). The liquid media are usually prepared in test tubes; solid media are prepared in test tubes or in Petri dishes or plates (round, flat, covered dishes) (see Figure 22.11).

Liquid media (broths) may be used for the growth of most organisms and for studying the production of gas, odor, and pH changes. Solid media (agar and gelatin base) are used for the growth of organisms, which then allows for the observation of colony size, shape, and color.

The classification of media according to their function and content follows.

Enrichment media

Enrichment media contain substances that inhibit the growth of various bacteria. They are used especially to isolate organisms that grow in the intestines and to prepare cultures from stool specimens. Examples include chocolate agar and blood agar.

Selective media

Selective media contain substances that suppress the growth of some organisms while enhancing the growth of others. They are used for the examination of stool and sputum specimens, for example, mannitol salt agar and the modified Thayer-Martin media, which are used mainly for suspected gonorrhea specimens and sometimes for detection of meningitis.

Differential media

Differential media contain substances that are used to distinguish between one microorganism and another. They are used to differentiate between forms of colony growth; for example, MacConkey agar is used for routine culturing of stool specimens, and eosin-methylene blue (EMB) agar is used for routine culturing of urine specimens.

Culture media are stored in a refrigerator and warmed to room temperature before being used. If the culture media are cold when used, the microorganisms placed on them will be destroyed. Petri plates are placed in the refrigerator with the media side facing up. Commercial plates come packaged in plastic bags that prevent the media from drying out. These plates will have an expiration date on them. If the expiration date has passed, these plates must not be used (see box on pp. 438-439).

Inoculating a Culture Medium

Equipment

Sterile cotton-tipped applicators in a sterile tube or Culturettes

Culture medium—this will vary with the type of specimen collected and the laboratory's preference; for example, Thayer-Martin (TM) culture medium is used most frequently for vaginal, cervical, and rectal cultures.

Bunsen burner and match

Sterile wire loop in container

Candle jar (see Figure 22.15)

Disposable rubber gloves

Procedure	*Rationale*
1. Wash your hands and put on disposable rubber gloves	Prevent contamination.
2. When you or the physician has obtained the specimen, remove the top cover lid of the culture plate and place it upside down on a flat surface.	Placing the lid in this manner avoids contamination to the inner surface of the lid, which will cover the culture.
3. Inoculate the culture plate by rolling the applicator in a large **Z** pattern on the culture medium (Figure 22.13).	This pattern provides adequate exposure of the organisms on the medium.
4. Discard the applicator in a covered container for waste materials.	
5. Replace the cover lid on the culture plate.	
6. Obtain the wire loop and the Bunsen burner.	
7. Light the burner, and place the wire loop over the flame until it is red hot.	Heating the loop destroys unwanted organisms. If these organisms are not destroyed, a contaminated growth of organisms would be found in the culture medium.
8. Allow the loop to cool.	If the loop is too hot, it will destroy the organisms that were inoculated on the medium.
9. Remove the lid of the plate, placing it upside down on a flat surface.	
10. Cross-streak the inoculated medium with the wire loop. With moderate pressure, criss-cross the **Z** with the wire loop (Figure 22.14).	Cross-streaking may be done in the laboratory. This spreads the organisms and isolates the colonies from the few contaminants that occasionally grow on selective media.

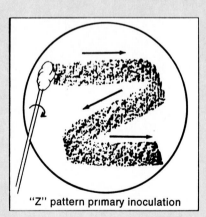

"Z" pattern primary inoculation

Figure 22.13
Method for inoculating culture medium.
From Criteria and techniques for the diagnosis of gonorrhea, U S Dept of HEW/Public Health Service, Center for Disease Control, Atlanta, Ga.

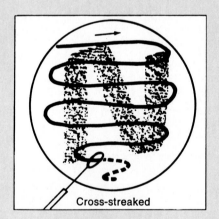

Cross-streaked

Figure 22.14
Cross-streaking inoculated medium with sterile wire loop.
From Criteria and techniques for the diagnosis of gonorrhea, U S Dept of HEW/Public Health Service, Center for Disease Control, Atlanta, Ga.

Inoculating a Culture Medium—cont'd

Procedure	Rationale

Figure 22.15
Inoculated culture medium plate placed in a candle jar for incubation. The jar provides an environment where bacterial colonies will grow.

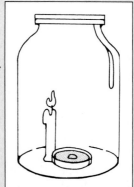

11. Replace the lid on the culture plate.
12. Reflame the loop to destroy any organisms that were picked up during the streaking process.
13. Return the loop to the storage place. Store the loop with the wire extending out of the container so that the delicate wire will not be destroyed.
14. Label the cover plate with the patient's name, date, and source of specimen.
15. Place the culture plate in a candle jar with the medium on the top side of the plate (Figure 22.15).

NOTE: A candle jar is a large gallon jar with a candle burning it it. The lid is tightly closed after the culture plate has been placed in it. When the oxygen in the jar is depleted, the candle will go out. An appropriate carbon dioxide environment is thus established. The gonococcus bacteria grows best in an environment enriched in carbon dioxide. Each time you place a culture plate in this jar or remove a plate, the candle must be relit.

16. Remove gloves and wash your hands.
17. Send the culture plate in the candle jar to the laboratory for incubation, along with the appropriate laboratory requisition completed correctly.

18. Record the procedure completely and accurately.

The jar will be kept at room temperature or 95° to 96.8° F (35° to 36° C). Incubation period is usually 20 to 24 hours. After this period the laboratory worker will examine the culture growth.
Charting example:
February 20, 19_____, 5 PM
Cervical and rectal specimens obtained by Dr. Edwards. Culture made and sent to the laboratory for C & S.
    Judy Dansie, CMA

19. NOTE: Following the determination of the type of organism that has grown on a culture plate, sensitivity tests are usually performed to determine the appropriate antibiotic to use for treatment. The organism grown is subjected to a special plate containing various samples of antibiotics. After a period of incubation, this plate is examined. When no growth is observed around a particular antibiotic sample, this indicates that the particular drug is effective in destroying or controlling the infectious organisms causing the disease process in the patient.

This same procedure is also used when inoculating a culture medium with specimens from the urethra and rectum and other sources.

VAGINAL SMEARS AND CULTURE COLLECTION

To assist the physician in diagnosing various gynecological conditions (for example, cancer of the uterus or cervic, dysplasia, infections, venereal diseases, and estrogen levels), smears and cultures for cytological and bacteriological tests are obtained from the vagina, cervix, and sometimes the rectum. Some of the more common gynecological laboratory tests include the Pap smear, vaginal smears for trichomoniasis and candidiasis (moniliasis) (common vaginal infections), vaginal smears to de-

termine estrogen levels, and smears and cultures for sexually transmitted diseases (STD), for example, gonorrhea, herpes simplex virus type II, and *Chlamydia trachomatis.*

General Instructions for Obtaining Vaginal Smears and Cultures for Cytologic and Bacteriologic Tests

1. Instruct the patient not to douche or use any vaginal medication for 24 hours before having a specimen taken (some physicians request absti-

nence from these for 3 days before the specimen is obtained).

2. Do not collect vaginal or cervical smears when a women is menstruating, because the microscopic readings can be invalid because of the blood cells that are produced during that period.

3. Avoid doing a Pap smear for at least 6 weeks if the cervix has been cauterized and for a longer period if the woman has undergone radiation therapy, as these procedures cause distortion to the cervical cells.

4. Call the laboratory for specific instructions when in doubt on how to collect a particular specimen. Many laboratories will provide all the necessary equipment and instructions.

5. Always wash your hands extremely well before and after assisting with any of these procedures. **Gloves should be worn for handling specimens when contamination of the hands is anticipated. Many now routinely recommend wearing gloves when obtaining and handling specimens.**

6. General preparatory and assisting techniques required are the same as those for assisting with a pelvic examination (Chapter 19).

7. Proper and accurate procedures must always be used to help the physician make a correct diagnosis and initiate the best treatment possible. It is the medical assistant's responsibility to see that specimens are handled and labeled correctly after the physician has collected them.

The Papanicolaou Smear (PAP Smear)

The Pap smear is probably the most common vaginal and cervical smear done, since the specimen is easily obtained at the same time that a woman is having a pelvic examination. The Pap smear is used to detect cervical or uterine cancer. The American Cancer Society recommends that:

all asymptomatic women age 20 and over, and those under 20 who are sexually active, have a Pap test annually for three or more consecutive satisfactory normal examinations and then at least every 3 years.

Women who are at high risk of developing cervical cancer because of early age at first intercourse, multiple sexual partners, or other risk factors may need to be tested more frequently.

A pelvic examination should be done as part of a general physical examination every 3 years beginning at age 20 and annually thereafter for sexually active women.*

Refer to Chapter 19 "Procedure for a Pelvic Examination with a Pap Smear," for more general information, the procedure, method, and assisting techniques used when obtaining this smear for examination.

Vaginal Secretions for Hormone Evaluation

Hormone evaluation is used to determine a woman's estrogen level. The specimen is obtained from the midlateral vaginal wall on a cotton-tipped applicator or spatula. A smear is then made and sent to the laboratory.

Smear for Trichomoniasis Vaginitis

Trichomonas is a genus of parasitic protozoa that occurs in vaginal secretions, causing a vaginal discharge, pruritus (itching), and sometimes a burning sensation on voiding. When trichomoniasis is diagnosed, specific medication such as metromidazole (Flagyl) will be prescribed for treatment. This organism is generally passed from one person to another through sexual contact; therefore the patient's partner, who may be a carrier of the infection but is presenting no symptoms, should also be treated.

When obtaining a smear to diagnose this condition, follow the procedure for assembling equipment and preparing and assisting the patient as outlined for obtaining a Pap smear during a pelvic examination (Chapter 19), *except* that a vaginal aspirator may be used rather than an applicator to collect the vaginal discharge, depending on the physician's preference. Follow steps 1 through 13-b as outlined for the pelvic examination in Chapter 19 then do the following. See also No. 5 in column at left.

---

*The American Cancer Society: Guidelines for the early detection of cancer in people without symptoms, 1989.

Obtaining a Smear for Trichomoniasis Vaginitis

Procedure	*Rationale*
1. Place a small amount of normal saline on a slide.	The physician will obtain a vaginal specimen by saturating the cotton-tipped applicator with the vaginal discharge (or collect the fluid with the vaginal aspirator).
2. You or the physician then dip the saturated cotton-tipped applicator into the saline solution on the slide (or place the fluid in the aspirator into the saline).	
3. Discard the applicator in a covered container for waste disposal.	
4. Place a coverglass over the depressed section in the middle of the slide.	A coverglass is a small, thin piece of glass that will cover the saline and the specimen obtained on the glass slide so that any movement of the live cells can be viewed when the slide is examined under a microscope.
5. Send the smear to the laboratory at once, because the organism, if present, will have to be identified immediately.	If the *Trichomonas* organism is present, the laboratory technician will observe a moving flagellated organism when the slide is viewed under the microscope.
6. Assist the patient as required.	
7. Assemble used equipment and dispose of it according to office or agency policy. Replace clean equipment as necessary.	Refer to Steps 14 through 25 as outlined in the pelvic examination procedure in Chapter 19.
8. Wash your hands.	
9. Record accurate and complete information on the patient's chart.	Charting example: February 9, 19_____, 1:15 PM Vaginal smear for *Trichomonas* obtained by Dr. Rouse. Specimen sent to the laboratory immediately. Patient sent home with a prescription to be filled pending positive test results from the lab. Mike King, CMA

Smear for Monilial Vaginitis

Monilia, now commonly referred to as *Candida,* is a yeastlike fungus. This is often referred to as simply a yeast infection by the general public. It is often in the female's vagina without causing any symptoms, and at other times it will produce an uncomfortable white, cheesy or curdlike vaginal discharge, itching, and irritation of the vulva.

Yeast infections are not commonly transmitted by sexual contact; the organisms are found everywhere. The infections tend to recur. The treatment generally includes the use of vaginal suppositories or creams that the physician will prescribe. The procedure for obtaining this smear is identical to the one just described for trichomoniasis, *except* the following three steps should be done first:

1. Place a small amount of saline on a slide.
2. Add (mix) 10% potassium hydroxide (KOH) to the saline.
3. Proceed as described in steps 2 through 9 above.

NOTE: If the *Monilia* organism is present on the smear, the laboratory technician will observe the branching arms of the fungus when it is viewed under a microscope.

Smears and Cultures to Detect Gonorrhea

Gonorrhea is a highly contagious, sexually transmitted disease caused by the bacterial organism *Neisseria gonorrhoeae,* or the gonococcus. Symptoms in a man usually occur within 1 week after exposure; a woman experiences no early symptoms. A man will have a burning sensation when voiding and a whitish fluid discharge or pus from the penis. Women may experience pain in the lower abdomen, with or without a whitish vaginal discharge or a burning sensation when voiding. Penicillin and other antibiotics or the sulfonamide drugs are all effective treatment. Cure for gonorrhea occurs relatively rapidly, although the patient is not considered cured until cultures taken of the discharge are negative for 3 to 4 weeks. Although gonorrhea is contracted through sexual contact, the gonococcus bacteria can infect the eyes (gonorrheal conjunctivitis) or a break in the skin or an open wound. Thus the importance of preventing contamination to yourself and others with specimens obtained from patients suspected of having gonorrhea cannot be overemphasized. Avoid touching your eyes and always wash your hands extremely well after assisting the physician when a specimen is obtained.

Procedure

For direct smears to be examined, urethral, endocervical, and vaginal specimens are collected and smeared evenly and moderately thin on two glass slides, then fixed and dried for 4 to 6 minutes (as described previously). Some physicians may obtain a specimen from the anal canal and also from the oropharynx, a common local source for disseminated gonococcal infection. The anal specimen is obtained by inserting a sterile cotton-tipped applicator approximately 1 inch into the anal canal. The applicator is moved from side to side; 10 to 30 seconds are allowed for absorption of the organisms on the applicator. A smear is then made and fixed. The oropharynx culture is obtained by swabbing the posterior pharynx and tonsillar crypts with a cotton-tipped applicator.

When a culture is desired, two sterile cotton-tipped applicators or Culturettes are used to collect the specimen. One is placed in a sterile culture tube or Culturette. The second applicator with the specimen is streaked across a special culture medium, such as the Thayer-Martin medium. Both specimens are sent to the laboratory together.

Chlamydia Trachomatis: The Direct Specimen Test*

The chlamydiae are a large group of obligate intracellular parasites closely related to gram-negative bacteria. There are two species: *Chlamydia trachomatis,* primarily a human pathogen, and *Chlamydia psittaci,* primarily an animal pathogen.

The chlamydial infections of trachoma, inclusion conjuctivitis, and lymphogranuloma venereum have been recognized and studied for many years. However, the chlamydiae have only recently been identified as important etiologic agents in sexually transmissible diseases. The prevalence of these *Chlamydia*-related diseases and the population at risk are thought to exceed those of gonorrhea. *Chlamydia trachomatis,* the nation's most common sexually transmitted disease, is now known to cause urethritis, epididymitis, proctitis, cervicitis, pelvic inflammatory disease, infant pneumonia, and conjunctivitis. It has also been implicated in Reiter's syndrome and premature birth. In both sexes the infection *may be asymptomatic.*

Females risk the most serious complication of chlamydial infection—acute salpingitis—and they can pass the infection to their newborn infants and sexual partners. Because of these risks, specific diagnosis of *C. trachomatis* in the large population of asymptomatic females is critical.

In addition to being undetected in large proportions of the female population, the organism is masked in another large population: men and women who have gonorrhea. Often *Chlamydia* cannot be differentiated from gonorrhea on the basis of symptoms alone. The result—gonorrhea is treated while the *C. trachomatis* goes undetected. Moreover, *Chlamydia* and gonorrhea may require different antibiotic treatment.

The common thread running through all of these aspects, and the most significant element in terms of control, has been the difficulty of diagnosis. Clinically visible signs (for example, macroscopic appearance of the cervix, amount of vaginal discharge) are not specific for chlamydial infection, nor are cellular changes seen on Pap smears. Tissue culture, though extremely sensitive and specific, requires a considerable technical and financial commitment and, hence, is unavailable to most physicians. Also, results from tissue cultures are not available until 4 to 6 days later.

Until recently efforts to control chlamydial infections have been limited by this lack of adequate diagnosis. Asymptomatic and recurrent infections have gone undetected and co-infections have been treated inappropriately.

Practical Screening: The Direct Specimen Test*

Screening for *Chlamydia* infections in asymptomatic women requires a diagnostic method that is less costly, less complex, and more available than tissue culture. The Syva MicroTrak *Chlamydia trachomatis* Direct Specimen test meets these criteria while retaining the sensitivity and specificity of tissue culture.

Using monoclonal antibodies labeled with fluorescein, the direct specimen test can detect and identify the smallest forms of the organisms, elementary and reticulate bodies, in direct urethral or cervical smears. Diagnosis can be made within 30 minutes after specimen receipt in the laboratory. No cell culture is required.

The procedure is as simple to perform as a Pap smear. The cervix (or, in the male, the urethra) is swabbed to remove a smear specimen. The specimen is rolled onto a glass slide, fixed with acetone, and sent to the laboratory at room temperature. In the laboratory the slide is stained with the MicroTrak antibody solution, causing *Chlamydia,* if present, to appear as individual bright apple-green

---

*Courtesy MicroTrak/Syva Company, Palo Alto, Calif.

*Courtesy MicroTrak/Syva Company, Palo Alto, Calif.

Figure 22.16
Procedure for *Chlamydia trachomatis* direct specimen test.
Courtesy MicroTrak, Syva Co, Palo Alto, Calif.

Collection

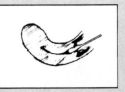

The specimen is swabbed from the urethra, endocervical canal, rectum or infant nasopharynx or neonatal conjunctiva and applied directly to the slide, where it is fixed and sent to the laboratory. (Recommended: MicroTrak® Specimen Collection Kit containing cytology brush, two swabs, slide with 8 mm well, methanol fixative, and transport pack.)

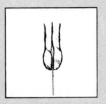

pinpoints on a background of reddish cells when viewed through a fluorescence microscope, a typical item available in most large laboratories. MicroTrak Mounting Fluid contains photobleaching retardant to inhibit fading of fluorescence during examination of the specimen (Figure 22.16).

This simple test design allows specific diagnosis of *Chlamydia trachomatis* in exactly the screening situations that must be tapped: prenatal clinics, family planning clinics, gynecologic offices, and abortion clinics. Further, any routine pelvic examination during which a Pap smear is taken can now be seen as an opportunity to screen for *C. trachomatis*. In populations of women under 25 years of age, where *C. trachomatis* is about 40 times more prevalent than abnormal cytology, the rationale for such Pap/MicroTrak testing is apparent. With the rapid results afforded by the new test, physicians can prevent further spread to sexual partners or neonates by beginning specific treatment immediately, even while patients are still in the clinic. Follow-up testing to document cure also becomes more convenient.

These advances will undoubtedly contribute to a more targeted therapy and an eventual reduction in the number of *Chlamydial* infections. Similar applications of monoclonal antibody technology have been developed for herpes simplex virus and are being developed for gonorrhea and other infectious diseases. The promise for improved diagnosis in these areas is equally great.

Staining

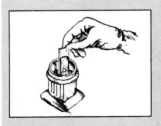

The fixed specimen is stained with MicroTrak® Reagent and incubated at room temperature for 15 minutes.

A rinse step removes unbound antibody. The slide is allowed to dry.

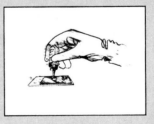

Mounting fluid (provided) is added and the coverslip is applied.

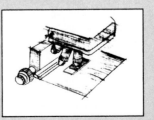

Viewed under the fluorescence microscope, positive specimens contain fluorescent apple-green chlamydial organisms.

See package insert for full instructions

Conclusion

You have now completed the chapter on collecting and handling specimens. When you have practiced the procedures sufficiently, arrange with your instructor to take a performance test. You will be expected to demonstrate accurately your ability to prepare for and to assist with all the procedures outlined in this chapter and to perform some of them. In addition, you will be expected to identify accurately the supplies and equipment by the proper name when questioned by your instructor.

Review Questions

1. List four types of material that can be obtained from a patient's body for laboratory examination.
2. What is meant by "special preparation" of the patient before collecting a specimen?
3. List three types of specimens for which active participation of the patient is required.
4. After obtaining a throat culture, you accidentally drop the lid of the culture tube on the floor. What action would you take before sending the specimen to the laboratory?
5. What specimens should be kept refrigerated if you cannot send them to the laboratory immediately, and why do you refrigerate them?
6. Itemize all the information that should be written on a laboratory requisition when submitting a specimen to the laboratory for examination.
7. You have obtained a specimen of material from a wound and have sent it to the laboratory for a C and S. Explain what types of testing will be performed on the specimen and the purpose of these tests.
8. Why is it important for you to wash your hands before and after obtaining any type of specimen from a patient?
9. List information that you should provide to patients who are to collect a urine specimen at home.
10. What is the purpose(s) of obtaining a sputum specimen from a patient? Describe the explanation that you would give to a patient who is to collect a sputum specimen.
11. Name two common vaginal infections that are diagnosed by means of vaginal smears.

SUGGESTED READINGS

McGucklin M: Tips for assisting with cultures of CSF and other body fluids, Nursing 76 7:17, April 1976.

McGucklin M: The problems with respiratory tract cultures—and what you can do about them, Nursing 76 7:19, February 1976.

Chapter 23

Principles of Pharmacology and Drug Administration

- Pharmacology and drugs
- Prescriptions
- Administer, dispense, prescribe
- Pharmaceutical preparations
- Professional responsibilities

- Routes and methods of drug administration
- Factors influencing dosage and drug action
- Injections

Objectives

On completion of Chapter 23 the medical assistant should be able to:

1 Define and pronounce the terms listed in the vocabulary.

2 List and briefly describe the uses, sources, names, classification, and types of drugs.

3 Differentiate between a controlled substance, a prescription drug, and a non-prescription drug.

4 Define *prescription* and list and explain the seven parts of a prescription.

5 Interpret abbreviations and symbols commonly used when administering medications.

6 State and discuss drug standards and the laws governing drug use.

7 Explain how drugs should be stored, handled, and labeled.

8 State and discuss the legal requirements for controlled substances inventory and the prescriber's record.

9 List 10 routes by which medication may be administered, briefly describing each.

10 List at least 15 general rules for administering medications and eight specific rules for administering injections.

11 List the five *rights* for preparing and administering medications.

12 List at least eight factors that will influence drug dosage and action.

13 State six reasons why medication is administered by an injection.

14 List six to eight dangers involved in giving injections and the sites that are to be avoided.

15 List three reasons for the administration of solutions by an intradermal injection.

16 Given medication orders, interpret them, and calculate the dosage of drug to be administered.

17   Given a medication order, prepare and administer safely and efficiently a subcutaneous, an intramuscular, an intramuscular Z-tract, and an intradermal injection using a sterile disposable syringe and needle of the correct sizes.

18   Demonstrate how to identify the correct sites for administering a subcutaneous and an intramuscular injection by palpating definite anatomical landmarks.

19   Given the *PDR* or other reference pharmacology book, obtain information on a variety of drugs.

Vocabulary

addiction (ah-dik'shun) An acquired dependence on a drug with tendencies to increase its use.

anaphylactic (an″ah-fi-lak′tik) shock An intense state of shock brought on by hypersensitivity to a drug, foreign toxin, or protein. Early symptoms resemble an allergic reaction, such as a rash, then increase in severity rapidly to dyspnea, cyanosis, and shock. This can be fatal if emergency measures are not taken immediately.

BNDD Bureau of Narcotics and Dangerous Drugs (a federal govenment agency of the DEA).

chemotherapy (kē″mo-ther′ah-pē) The use of drugs (chemicals) to treat disease; a type of therapy used for cancer patients in which powerful drugs are used to interfere with the reproduction of the fast-multiplying cancer cells.

contraindication (kon″tra-in″dĭ-kā′shun) A condition in which the use of certain drugs or treatments should be withheld or limited.

crude drug An unrefined drug.

cumulative action of a drug A drug accumulates in the body; it is eliminated more slowly than it is absorbed.

dilute To weaken the strength of a substance by adding something else.

drug idiosyncrasy (id″ē-ō-sing′krah-sē) An unusual or abnormal response or susceptibility to a drug that is peculiar to the individual.

drug tolerance The decreased susceptibility to the effects of a drug after continued use. In this case an increased dosage would be required to produce the desired effects, as the initial dose would be ineffective.

cross-tolerance Cross-tolerance can develop when tolerance to one drug increases the body's tolerance to drugs in the same category. For example, a tolerance to one depressant drug leads to a tolerance of other depressant drugs.

FDA Food and Drug Administration (A federal government agency).

habituation Emotional dependence on a drug caused by repeated use, but without tendencies to increase the amount of the drug.

placebo (plah-sē′bō) An inactive substance resembling and given in place of a medication for its psychological effects to satisfy the patient's need for the drug; it hopefully will produce the same effect as the real medication through psychological means. A placebo may also be used experimentally.

prophylaxis (prō″fi-lak′sis) The prevention of disease.

pure drug A refined drug; one that has been processed to remove all impurities.

side effect A response in addition to that for which the drug was used, especially an undesirable result.

untoward effect An undesirable side effect.

stock supply A large supply of medications kept in the physician's office or pharmacy.

toxicity (tok-sis′ĭ-tē) The nature of exerting harmful effects on a tissue or organism.

unit-dose A system that supplies prepackaged, premeasured, prelabeled, individual portions of a medication for patient use.

Among the many duties of a medical assistant, the administration of medications holds high responsibility. As a member of a professional team involved with the medical care of the public, it is important that the medical assistant seek all possible knowledge of drugs—their use or abuse, correct dosages, methods and routes of administration, symptoms of overdose, and abnormal reactions that may occur when they are administered. Although it is beyond the scope of this book to include a detailed presentation of pharmacology, general concepts, basic information on drugs, and procedures for the correct methods of administration will be discussed. Reference sources for more detailed information on drugs will be cited. It is the responsibility of the medical assistant to obtain adequate knowledge of a drug before administering it to a patient.

PHARMACOLOGY AND DRUGS

Pharmacon is Greek for drugs. Pharmacology is the science that deals with the study of drugs—their origins, properties, uses, and actions. Drugs are any medicinal substances or mixtures of substances that are used for therapeutic, prophylactic, or diagnostic purposes. Drugs are either medicinal, therefore therapeutic, or poisonous, depending on dosage and use. The therapeutic use of drugs includes the application of these substances to treat or cure a disease or condition, to relieve undesirable symptoms such as pain, and to provide substances that the body is not producing or not producing in sufficient amounts, for example, insulin, used for diabetes mellitus, and thyroid extract used for hypothyroidism. Prophylactically, drugs are used to prevent diseases, such as vaccinations given to prevent communicable diseases. Drugs can also help a physician diagnose an illness, as seen when dyes are given to a patient in a diagnostic x-ray procedure, or when antigens are used to detect skin allergies in a patient.

Pharmacology has undergone tremendous changes during the past few decades and continues to be dynamic. Through constant study and research, new drugs arrive on the market, and some old ones are withdrawn—either because newer ones are more effective or because complications arising from the use of the older drugs prove to be too hazardous to the patient's health.

Drugs are derived from four main sources, which are as follows:

- Plant sources—obtained from plant parts or products. Seeds, stem, roots, leaves, resin, and other parts yield these drugs; examples include digitalis and opium.
- Animal sources—glandular products from animals are used, such as insulin and thyroid.
- Mineral sources—some drugs are prepared from minerals, for example, potassium chloride and lithium carbonate (an antipsychotic).
- Synthetic sources—laboratories duplicate natural processes. Frequently this can eliminate side effects and increase the potency of the drug; examples include barbiturates, sulfonamides, and aspirin.

Drug Names: Brand (Trade), Generic, and Chemical

A typical drug may be known by as many as three names, as follows:

A brand or trade (proprietary) name;
The generic name; and
The chemical name.

When a drug is developed and marketed, it is assigned a specific name that is patented by the pharmaceutical company that has manufactured it. This is called the *trade or brand name* of the drug and is the exclusive property of the manufacturer. After a patent has expired (drug patents run 17 years), other companies may manufacture and sell the drug either under different brand names or under the drug's generic name. These exact copies of the original drug are often called generic drugs. Each drug has an official or nonproprietary name, which is also called the *generic name*. This name is often descriptive of the chemical composition or class of the drug and is assigned to the drug in the early stages of its development for general recognition purposes. Thus, every drug has a generic name. Generic names are established by the U.S. Adopted Name Council (USAN). Except in the case of older drugs, the generic (USAN) name is identical to the USP (United States Pharmacopeia) or NF (National Formulary) name. A generic drug may be manufactured by any number of companies and placed on the market under a different brand or trade name. Examples follow. Brand names are prominently used in advertising a drug to the medical profession, although the generic name must appear in advertising and labeling in letters at least half as big as that of the brand name.

Generic name	Brand or trade name	Pharmaceutical company
tetracycline	Tetracyn	Pfizer
meprobamate	Equanil	Wyeth
	Meprotabs	Wallace
	Miltown	Wallace
penicillin G	Bicilin	Wyeth
procaine penicillin	Crysticillin	Squibb

When prescribing a drug, the physician may use either the generic or the trade name. Currently the trend is to write more prescriptions using the generic name of the drug, if one is marketed (many trade names are still under patent protection and are not available from other manufacturers by the generic name), because it is generally less expensive for the patient to purchase. However, if the physician orders a specific trade name, most states now have laws that state that even though the prescription may be written under the trade name, the patient is entitled to ask the pharmacist for the medication under its generic name unless the physician has specifically directed otherwise, either orally or in handwriting. Also, the pharmacist filling the prescription order for a drug product prescribed by its trade or brand name may select another drug product of the same generic drug type (that is, the generic or chemical name of the drug that is considered to be therapeutically equivalent or "bioequivalent") unless the physician has specifically directed otherwise either orally or in handwriting, and only when the drug product selected costs the patient less than the prescribed drug product. Since both trade and generic named drugs represent the same chemical formula and must meet the same FDA standards, they can be used interchangeably according to most state laws. This provides one way to keep the cost of medical care down. When the substitution is made, the use of the cost-saving drug product dispensed must be communicated to the patient, and the name of the dispensed drug product must be indicated on the prescription label, except where the prescriber orders otherwise.

The third name a drug may be assigned is the *chemical name*. This represents the drug's exact formula, that is, the chemical make up or molecular structure. Generally, this name is used only by the manufacturer and on occasion by the pharmacy when compounding a drug, because, for most drugs, the chemical name is long and complex.

Official and Reference Books on Drugs

Established standards and up-to-date information on drugs are published in various books; some of the more common ones follow.

United States Pharmacopeia (USP)–National Formulary (NF)

Once two individual books, the USP and NF are now published as a single volume. The National Formulary was acquired by the U.S. Pharmacopeial Convention, Inc., in 1975 and now publishes the USP–NF approximately every five years. This is an authoritative book establishing the standards for drugs. Only "official" drugs are listed in this book. All drugs sold under the name listed in the USP–NF must legally conform to the standards set forth. Detailed information on the description of drugs, standards for purity, strength and composition, storage, use, and dosage are given. Drugs that meet the standards set by the *Pharmacopeia* will bear

the initials USP on their labels. Some drugs listed in the USP section of the book will be cross-referenced to the NF chapter. The NF chapter of the book deals primarily with the pharmaceutical ingredients of the drugs.

AMA Drug Evaluations

The book *AMA Drug Evaluations* is published annually by the American Medical Association (AMA). New drugs that are not yet listed in the USP but that have been evaluated by the Council on Drugs of the AMA are presented.

Physician's Desk Reference (PDR)

Although not official, the PDR is a very common reference book used by most medical personnel. It is published annually by Medical Economics Inc. and is automatically distributed free of charge to medical offices, agencies, and hospitals. The PDR has seven sections, which list the following:

1. Names, addresses, emergency telephone numbers, and a partial list of products available from the manufacturers who have provided information for the PDR.
2. Products by brand name in alphabetical order.
3. Products according to an appropriate drug category or classification.
4. Products under generic and chemical name headings.
5. Products shown in color and actual size under company headings and a directory of Poison Control Centers and emergency telephone numbers for the 50 states as well as Guam, Puerto Rico, and the Virgin Islands.
6. An alphabetical arrangement by manufacturer of over 2,500 products. Each is described as to composition, uses and action, administration and dosage, precautions, contraindications, side effects, form in which each is supplied, and the common names and generic compositions or chemical names.
7. An alphabetical arrangement by manufacturer of diagnostic products with descriptions for use.

Inside the back cover is a Guide to Management of Drug Overdose. Supplements that provide new or revised product information developed after the PDR was published for the current year are published and distributed as necessary.

American Hospital Formulary Service (AHFS)

The AHFS book is published by the American Hospital Formulary Service. Subscribed to by all hospital pharmacists, it contains extensive, unbiased drug information kept current by periodic supplements. The AHFS arranges drugs into therapeutic or pharmacological classes according to official (generic) names.

Medical assistants should be familiar with these publications and always keep one or more up-to-date copies in the physician's office as a reference source for both the physician and themselves.

Drug Standards and Laws Governing Use

When the physician or other qualified medical practitioners prescribe, administer, or dispense drugs, including narcotics, they must comply with federal and state laws that regulate such transactions. Comprehensive laws have been passed by the U.S. Congress and individual state legislatures to regulate the manufacture, sale, possession, administration, dispensation, and prescription of a range of drugs.

To assist physicians in complying with their legal obligations, medical assistants should know and understand the laws regulating drugs and narcotics in the state in which they are employed, because individual states may supplement federal legislation with their own laws.

All drugs available for legal use are controlled by the Federal Food, Drug and Cosmetic Act of 1938. This act contains detailed regulations to assure the purity, strength, and composition of food, drugs, and cosmetics. The general purpose of this act, based on interstate commerce, is to control movement of impure and adulterated food and drugs. Amended periodically, the Federal Food, Drug and Cosmetic Act is enforced by the Food and Drug Administration (FDA), a department with the Department of Health and Human Services (DHHS), formerly the Department of Health, Education, and Welfare (DHEW). There are also other federal and differing state laws that regulate the development, sale, and use of drugs.

Legal Classification of Drugs
Controlled substances

Drugs having the potential for addiction and abuse, including narcotics, stimulants, and depressants, are termed controlled substances. Control of these drugs at all levels of manufacturing, distribution, and use is mandatory. Federal legislation that outlines these controls is the Controlled Substances Act of 1970 (the Comprehensive Drug Abuse Prevention and Control Act), which supersedes the Harrison Narcotic Act of 1917 and became effective May 1, 1971. This act is enforced by the Drug Enforcement Administration (DEA) in the U.S. Department of Justice. The law is designed to improve the administration and regulation of manufacturing, distribution, and the dispensing of controlled substances by providing a "closed" system for legitimate handlers of these drugs. Such a closed system should help reduce the widespread diversion of these substances out of legitimate channels into the illicit market.

Under this act, drugs that are under federal control are classified into one of five schedules. Each schedule reflects decreasing levels of addiction and abuse potential, from Schedule I through Schedule V. Complete listings of the drugs in each schedule are available from district DEA offices. Only a few examples are included here. All controlled substances listed in the Physician's Desk Reference (PDR) are indicated with the symbol **C** with the Roman numeral II, III, IV, or V printed inside the **C** to designate the schedule in which the substance is classified.

Schedule I. Schedule I drugs, having the highest potential for addiction and abuse, have not been accepted for medical use in the United States. Their use is limited to research purposes only after the research facility has obtained government approval and agreement to research protocol to test drugs for medical indications. Examples are heroin, marijuana, LSD, and mescaline.

Schedule II. Schedule II drugs have a high potential for abuse and addiction, but have an acceptable medical use for treatment in the United States. Examples are amobarbital, amphetamine, cocaine, codeine, merperidine, methadone, methamphetamine, morphine, opium, and secobarbital.

Schedule III. Schedule III drugs have a potential for abuse less than the drugs in Schedules I or II and have a moderate or low addiction liability. They do have an acceptable medical use in treatment in the United States. Examples are APC with codeine, butabarbital, methyprylon, nalorphine, and paregoric.

Schedule IV. Schedule IV drugs have a lower potential for abuse than those in Schedule III and limited addiction liability relative to drugs in Schedule III. They do have an acceptable medical use in treatment in the United States. Examples are chloral hydrate, diazepam, meprobamate, paraldehyde, and phenobarbital.

Schedule V. Schedule V drugs have a low potential for abuse and a limited addiction liability relative to drugs in Schedule IV. They do have an acceptable medical use in treatment in the United States. Examples are drugs of primarily low-strength codeine (less than those compounds included in Schedule III) combined with other medicinal ingredients.

• • •

Under federal law, every practitioner who administers, dispenses, or prescribes a controlled substance (with the exception of interns, residents, law enforcement officials, and civil defense personnel who meet special conditions outlined in the Federal Code of Regulations) must be registered with the Drug Enforcement Administration. Medical practitioners must also have a valid license to practice medicine in their state. The practitioner's office location from which controlled substances are handled must be registered, and the certificate of registration is to be kept at this location. Applications for this registration can be obtained from any DEA regional office or from the DEA Section, PO Box 28083, Central Station, Washington, DC, 20005. Registration must be renewed every 3 years.

Only DEA-registered practitioners can order and purchase controlled substances. Schedule II substances must be ordered with the Federal Triplicate Order Form (DEA-222). Orders for Schedules III, IV, and V substances require only the practitioner's DEA registration number. In some states, when ordering Schedule II substances from out-of-state companies, a copy of the purchase agreement (not the Federal Triplicate Order Form) must be sent within 24 hours of placing the order to the office of the state attorney general.

Physicians who discontinue practice must return their Registration Certificate and any unused order forms to the nearest DEA office. It is suggested that the word "VOID" be written across the face of the order form before it is sent to the DEA. Physicians having controlled substances in their possession when they discontinue their practice should obtain information from the nearest field office of the DEA and from the responsible state agency on how to dispose of these drugs.

Some important duties of the medical assistant are to ensure that the physician is *currently* registered with the DEA, to obtain the correct federal forms for ordering and purchasing controlled substances, and to keep appropriate records of all transactions. Failure of the physician to comply with the laws regulating the use of controlled substances and other drugs could lead to considerable civil and criminal liability, in addition to the loss of the right to dispense or prescribe medications.

Prescription drugs

Prescription drugs may be obtained only when prescribed, administered, or dispensed by practitioners licensed by state law to prescribe drugs. The Federal Food, Drug and Cosmetic Act requires that these drugs bear on the label the legend *Caution: Federal Law prohibits dispensing without prescription*. Examples include digoxin and penicillin.

Nonprescription drugs

Drugs easily accessible to the general public fall into the category of nonprescription drugs. They are frequently referred to as "over-the-counter" (OTC) drugs, as they can be obtained without a prescription, for example, vitamin tablets and aspirin.

Classification of Drugs

Drugs are classified in various ways. These classifications include the following:
- Drugs that have a principal action on the body, for example, analgesics, antidiarrheals;
- Drugs used to treat or prevent specific diseases, for example, hormones, vaccines;
- Drugs that act on specific organs or body systems, for example, cardiovascular drugs, gastrointestinal drugs; and
- Forms of drug preparations, for example, solids or liquids.

You should be aware that frequently one drug may be used to treat varied conditions, because most drugs have multiple effects aside from the primary effects that they are assigned; or the same drug can affect different body systems by exerting its primary effect. For example, a broad-spectrum antibiotic can be used to treat various types of infectious processes, or a diuretic may be used to exert an effect on the cardiovascular system or urinary system.

Table 23.1 is a classification of drugs based on their primary actions or effects on the body.

PRESCRIPTIONS

A prescription is an order written by a licensed physician giving instructions to a pharmacist to supply a certain patient with a particular drug of specific quantity, prepared according to the physician's directions. It is a *legal document*. A prescription consists of the following seven parts (Figure 23.1):
1. Date, patient's name, and address (for children, the age should be given);
2. Superscription, consisting of the symbol ℞, from the Latin, recipe, meaning "take thou";
3. Inscription, specifying the ingredients and the quantities;

Text continued on p. 454.

Table 23.1
Classification of drugs based on actions or effects on body

Drug	Action	Examples
Amphetamine	Acts as stimulant on central nervous system; has temporary effect of increasing energy and mental alertness; sometimes used to depress the appetite	Amphetamine (Benzedrine), dextro-amphetamine (Dexedrine)
Analgesic	Relieves pain	Aspirin, Empirin Compound with codeine, codeine, acetaminophen (Tylenol), phenacetin
Anesthetic	Produces generalized or local loss of feeling	Thiopental sodium (Pentothal Sodium), tetracaine hydrochloride (Pontocaine Hydrochloride), lidocaine hydrochloride (Xylocaine Hydrochloride)
Angiotensin converting enzyme inhibitors	Used for hypertension	Capoten, Vasotec
Antacid	Counteracts acidity in stomach	Sodium bicarbonate, Maalox, Mylanta
Anthelminthics	Destructive to worms	Piperazine, mebendazole, Povan, Vermox
Antibiotic	Inhibits growth and reproduction of or eliminates pathogenic microorganisms	Penicillin, ampicillin, tetracycline
Antidiarrheal	Counteracts diarrhea	Lomotil, Kaopectate, codeine, paregoric
Anticoagulant	Inhibits blood clotting mechanism	Heparin sodium, dicumarol
Anticonvulsant	Inhibits convulsions, as in epilepsy. Prevents or reduces the frequency or severity of seizures related to idiopathic epilepsy, as well as seizures secondary to drug reactions, hypoglycemia, eclampsia, alcohol withdrawal, or traumatic brain injury	Phenytoin (Dilantin), bromides, ethotoin, phenobarbital, primidone, trimethadione
Antidepressant	Relieves depression; often called mood elevator or modifier	*Tricyclic antidepressants:* Imipramine (Tofranil), Amitriptyline (Elavil), Sinequan, Norpramin *Monoamine Oxidase Inhibitors (MAO):* Nardil, Parnate *Antimanic agents:* Lithium (Eskalith)
Antidote	Counteracts poison	Ipecac syrup
Antiemetic	Counteracts nausea and vomiting	Dimenhydrinate (Dramamine), prochlorperazine (Compazine), triethobenzamide (Tigan)
Antifungal	Destroys or checks the growth of fungi; controls Candida (Monilia) infections in vagina	Mycostatin, Nystatin

*From Zakus SM: Clinical skills and assisting techniques for the medical assistant, ed 2, St Louis, 1988, The CV Mosby Co.   *Continued.*

Table 23.1
Classification of drugs based on actions or effects on body—cont'd

Drug	Action	Examples
Antihistamine	Counteracts effect of histamine in the body; given to relieve symptoms of allergic reactions, such as hay fever, and also to relieve symptoms of common cold	Diphenhydramine (Benadryl), guaifenisen (Actifed), promethazine (Phenergan), chlorpheniramine (Chlor-Trimeton)
Antihypertensive (also referred to as hypotensive)	Reduces high blood pressure	Reserpine (Serpasil), guanethidine (Ismelin), hydrochlorothiazide (Esidrix)
Antiinflammatory agent	Reduces or relieves inflammation	Indomethacin (Indocin), triamcinolone (Kenacort), triamcinolone acetonide (Kenalog), piroxicam (Feldene)
Antiarthritic preparation	Acts against arthritic symptoms	Indomethacin (Indocin), phenylbutazone (Butazolidin), prednisone, Feldene, Naprosyn
Antiseptic Skin antiseptic Urinary antiseptic to be taken internally	Inhibits growth of microorganisms	 70% alcohol Nitrofurantoin (Furadantin), nalidixic acid (NegGram)
Antineoplastic	Inhibits growth and spread of malignant cells	Chlorambucil (Leukeran), busulfan (Myleran), melphalan (Alkeran)
Astringent	Constricts tissue and arrests discharges or bleeding	Silver nitrate, alum, zinc oxide
Beta-adrenergic blockers	Used to treat angina, hypertension, cardiac arrhythmias, myocardial infarctions. Act as a shield against excessive stimulation to the sympathetic nerve endings in the heart tissue. Slow down the heartbeat besides making the heart less responsive to stimulations. Thus the heart performs more work with less oxygen demand and pain can be prevented	Inderal, Corgard, Lopressor, Tenormin, Visken
Bronchodilator	Causes dilation of bronchi, eases breathing	Aminophylline, Bronkotabs, isoproterenol (Isuprel), epinephrine (Adrenalin)
Calcium channel blockers	Used for hypertension and angina	Cardizem, Ipoptin
Cardiogenic (heart stimulator)	Strengthens heart muscle action	Digitoxin, digitalis, digoxin (Lanoxin)
Cathartic	Relieves constipation and promotes defecation; often classified according to the increased intensity of their action as laxatives, purgatives, and drastic purgatives	Cascara, mineral oil, castor oil, bisacodyl (Dulcolax)
Contraceptive	Prevents or diminishes likelihood of conception	Enovid, Ortho-Novum

Table 23.1
Classification of drugs based on actions or effects on body—cont'd

Drug	Action	Examples
Cytotoxins	Toxic to certain cells. Used for treatment of cancer	Cytoxan, 6-mercaptopurine
Decongestant	Relieves swelling and congestion in upper respiratory tract	Ornade Spansule, Actifed, pseudoephedrine (Sudafed), phenylephrine (Neo-Synephrine)
Diuretic	Increases urinary output	Chlorothiazide (Diuril), furosemide (Lasix)
Emetic	Stimulates vomiting	Ipecac syrup
Expectorant	Liquifies mucus in bronchi and aids in the expectoration of sputum, mucus, or phlegm	Benylin expectorant, terpin hydrate, potassium iodide
Hemostatic	Arrests flow of blood by helping coagulation	Vitamin K
Hormone	Endocrine system produces hormones and secretes them directly into bloodstream. Commercial preparations are available for patients whose own glands are malfunctioning.	Cortisone, insulin, thyroxin
Hypnotic	Produces sleep	Glutethimide (Doriden), chloral hydrate
Laxative	Promotes movement of bowels	Mineral oil, docusate (Colace), senna (Senokot)
Miotic	Contracts pupils of eye	Pilocar ophthalmic solutions
Muscle relaxant	Relaxes muscles	Diazepam (Valium), carisoprodol (Soma) compound
Mydriatic	Dilates pupils of eye	Phenylephrine (Neo-Synephrine) solution, atropine sulfate ointment
Narcotic	Produces sound sleep, stupor, and relief of pain	Drugs derived from opium; morphine, codeine, meperidine (Demerol)
Psychedelic	Produces feelings of relaxation, freedom from anxiety, highly creative thought patterns, and perceptual changes; causes hallucinations, alters mental functions. Highly controversial, potentially very dangerous, and used only under controlled supervision for experimental purposes	LSD, mescaline
Sedative	Quiets and relaxes patient without producing sleep	Phenobarbital
Stimulant	Increases activity of an organ or body system	Caffeine, amphetamine (Benzedrine)
Styptic	Checks bleeding by means of astringent quality	Styptic pencil

Continued.

Table 23.1
Classification of drugs based on actions or effects on body—cont'd

Drug	Action	Examples
Sulfa preparations	Antibacterial	Sulfisoxazole (Gantrisin)
Tranquilizers (also called ataractics)	Calms or quiets patients who are anxious or disturbed without causing drowsiness that a sedative would produce or the stimulation that antidepressants produce	*Antianxiety (anxiolytic)—minor tranquilizers* *Benzodiazepines* Librium, diazepam (Valium), Ativan, Serax, Halcion, Xanax, Dalmane *Nonbenzodiazepines* meprobamate (Equinil and Miltown) *Antipsychotic (neuroleptic)—major tranquilizers:* *Phenothiazines* chlorpromazine (Thorazine), Mellaril, prochlorperazine (Compazine), Haldol, Navane, Stelazine, Trilafon
Vaccine	Prevents infectious diseases	Salk polio vaccine, tetanus and typhoid vaccines, measles, mumps, and hepatitis B vaccines
Vasoconstrictor	Constricts blood vessels to increase force of heartbeat, relieve nasal congestion, raise blood pressure, or stop superficial hemorrhage	Epinephrine (Adrenalin), norepinephrine (Levophed), ephedrine sulfate
Vasodilator	Dilates blood vessels and reduces blood pressure	Nitroglycerin reserpine (Serpasil), amyl nitrite
Vitamins	Organic substances found in foods that are necessary for body to grow and maintain health; commercial preparations of all these vitamins are available	Fat-soluble vitamins; A, D, E, K Water-soluble vitamins: B, C

4. Subscription, giving directions to the pharmacist on how to compound the drug(s);
5. Signa (Sig), from Latin, meaning "mark," which gives instructions to the patient indicating when and how to take the drug and in what quantities;
6. Physician's signature and address, registry number (this is the physician's license number), and, when prescribing controlled substances, the BNDD number (this is the same as the DEA number); and
7. Number of times, if any, that the prescription may be refilled; instructions to the pharmacist that the physician wants the drug identified on the label of the container.

Present-day prescription writing has been greatly simplified, as pharmaceutical companies now prepare most drugs ready for administration. These preparations have largely eliminated the need for the pharmacist to compound or mix drugs and solutions.

When the physician writes a prescription, it is given to the patient to take to a pharmacist, who will dispense the required medication. Once the prescription has been filled, the pharmacist must keep a record of that sale for 2 years (3 years in four states). These records are subject to inspection and copying at any time by authorized employees of state and federal law enforcement and regulatory agencies. When a prescription is written for a Schedule II controlled substance (narcotic), a few states require the physician to use an official triplicate prescription blank. Where this is the case, one copy is kept for the physician's office files, and the

Figure 23.1
Sample of a prescription.

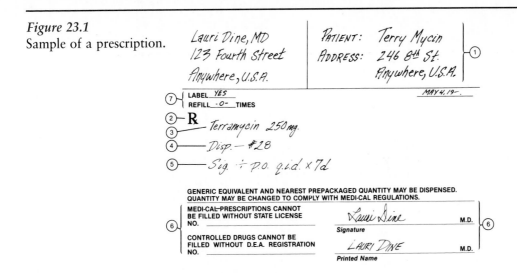

original and other copy are given to the patient to take to the pharmacist. After filling the prescription, the pharmacist retains the original and endorses the copy, which is forwarded to the Department of Justice at the end of the month in which the prescription was filled.

All prescriptions written for controlled substances in Schedule II must be wholly written and signed in ink or indelible pencil by the physician. A separate prescription blank is to be used for each controlled substance ordered. These prescriptions must contain the following information:

- Name and address of patient;
- Date of prescription;
- Name and quantity of controlled substance prescribed;
- Directions for use;
- Physician's DEA registration number (referred to as BNDD number); and
- Signature and address of physician.

Prescriptions for controlled substances in Schedule II cannot be refilled, and some states require that they be filled within 7 days of the date written.

In the case of a bonafide emergency, the physician may telephone a prescription order to a pharmacist for a Schedule II controlled substance. In these cases, the prescribed drug must be limited to the amount required to treat the patient during the emergency period. Within 72 hours the physician must furnish a written, signed prescription order to the pharmacy for the controlled substance prescribed. Pharmacies are required by law to notify the DEA if they have not received the written prescription order within the 72 hours. ("Emergency" means that the drug must be administered immedi-

ately for treatment, that there is no alternative treatment available, and that it is not possible for the physician to provide a written prescription form for the drug at that time.)

Prescriptions for controlled substances in Schedules III, IV, and V are written on the physician's standard prescription blank, and need only to be signed by the prescriber. These prescriptions are limited to five refills within a 6-month period with proper authorization. A prescription for any controlled substance must be issued for a legitimate medical purpose by physicians acting in good faith in the course of their professional practice. Keep in mind that regulations for prescribing and dispensing controlled substances differ for each of the five schedules and may also be subject to stricter controls passed by many states. It is therefore vital for medical assistants to learn what laws apply for their state.

Prescription pads should be kept in a safe place where they cannot be picked up easily by patients. Minimize the numbers of pads in use at any one time. They are to be used only for writing prescriptions; do not use them for notes or memos. A drug abuser could easily erase the note, and use the blank to forge a prescription. The Drug Enforcement Administration is to be contacted if your office experiences any theft or loss of controlled substances or official order forms. Contact a local police department if you are aware of forged prescriptions.

Although medical assistants do not write prescriptions, a knowledge of prescription abbreviations and terms used is valuable and may be required to carry out the physician's orders, tran-

Table 23.2

Common prescription abbreviations and symbols*

Abbreviation or symbol	Meaning	Abbreviation or symbol	Meaning	Abbreviation or symbol	Meaning
ā	before	kg	kilogram	qd	every day
āā	of each	L	liter	qh	every hour
ac	before meals	liq	liquid	q2h or q2°	every 2 hours
ad lib	as desired	m or min	minim	(q3h or q3°	every 3 hours
amt	amount	mcg	microgram	and so on)	
aq	aqueous	mEq	milliequiva-	qhs	every night
bid	twice a day		lent	qid	four times a
c̄	with	mEq/L	milliequiva-		day
cap(s)	capsule(s)		lents per	qod	every other
cc	cubic centi-		liter		day
	meter	mg	milligram	qs	quantity suf-
dil	dilute	ml	milliliter		ficient
Dx or Diag	diagnosis	mm	millimeter	℞	take thou
D/C or d/c	discontinue	npo (NPO)	nothing by	s̄	without
D/W	dextrose in		mouth	sc or subq or	subcutaneous
	water	NS	normal saline	SubQ	
dr	dram	noc(t)	night	Sig	directions
ʒ	dram	od	daily or once	sol	solution
ʒᵢ	one dram		a day	ss or s̄s̄	one half
d	day	OD	right eye	subling	sublingual
Dr	doctor	oint	ointment		(under the
fl or fld	fluid	OS	left eye		tongue)
gal	gallon	OU	both eyes	stat	immediately
g (or gm)	gram	oz	ounce	S/W	saline in wa-
gr	grain	ʒ	ounce		ter
gt or gtt	drop(s)	p̄	after, past	tid	three times a
H or hr	hour	per	by or with		day
hs	hour of sleep	pc	after meals	tinc or tr or	tincture
	or bedtime	po (or per	by mouth	tinct	
IM	intramuscular	os)		tab	tablet
IU	international	prn	whenever	tsp	teaspoon
	units		necessary	Tbsp	tablespoon
IV	intravenous	pt	pint (or pa-	ung or ungt	ointment
			tient)	U	units
		pulv	powder	wt	weight
		q	every		
		qam	every morn-		
			ing		

From Zakus SM: *Clinical skills and assisting techniques for the medical assistant*, ed 2, St Louis, 1988, The CV Mosby Co.

*According to the style established by the American Medical Association, medical and pharmaceutical abbreviations are to be written *without* the use of periods. That is, rather than writing b.i.d., as was done in the past, you will now write bid, and so on.

scribe medical notes, take telephone messages, answer questions for a patient regarding a prescription, verify information for a pharmacist, and understand instructions for the administration of medications. Table 23.2 is a list of the more common abbreviations and symbols used.

ADMINISTER, DISPENSE, PRESCRIBE

In the physician's office medications may be handled in one of three ways; that is, they may be administered, dispensed, or prescribed. A medication is administered when it is actually given to the patient to take by mouth or when it is injected, in-

Figure 23.2
Solid forms of drugs.

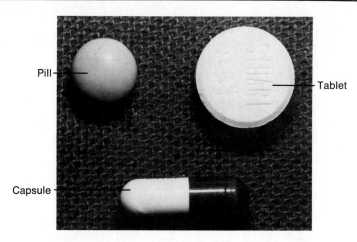

serted, or given by any other method used for administering medications. It is dispensed when it is given to a patient by the physician (or pharmacist at the pharmacy) to be taken at a later time; and it is prescribed when the physician gives the patient a written order, the prescription, to have filled by the pharmacist. Only the physician is licensed to prescribe medications. Depending on state law, varied medical personnel may administer medications, and the physician and pharmacist will dispense them. On occasion under the physician's order and supervision, the medical assistant may also dispense stock medications to a patient in the physician's office or health agency.

PHARMACEUTICAL PREPARATIONS

Because of the various properties and uses of different drugs, there are different ways in which they are prepared for patient use. Drugs are supplied in either a solid or liquid state.

Solid state (Figure 23.2)

pills	spansules
tablets	powders
caplets	suppositories
capsules	

Liquid state

solutions Liquid preparations consisting of one or more substances (solutes) that are dissolved or suspended in a substance (the solvent). The most frequently used solvents are distilled water, sterile water, normal saline, and alcohol. Solutes may be (1) a 100% full-strength or pure drug in a solid, liquid, or powder form, (2) tablets of a known specific amount of drug, or (3) stock solutions that are strong solutions of known strength used to prepare a weaker solution. To obtain a *true solution*, the solute must be completely dissolved in the solvent. If the solute is evenly dispersed throughout the solution but not dissolved, it is called a *suspension* or a *colloidal solution*. The difference between these two is determined by the molecular size of the particles of the solute, the colloidal solution containing very small particles. Drugs that are supplied in a suspension *must* be shaken before administering and will have on the label the instruction *Shake well*.

diluent A solution that is added to another to reduce the strength of the initial solution or mixture. Percentages or ratios are used to describe solutions. For example, a 15% solution means that 15 parts of the solute are mixed with 85 parts of the solvent. Some solutions come prepared for immediate use; others will have to be mixed before they are suitable for use. When a solution must be prepared for use, it may be necessary to convert the apothecary system of weights and measures to the metric equivalents. Table 23.3 presents the conversion equivalents for these systems. Table 23.4 presents the components to prepare a solution. Some solutions may be administered by injection, by mouth, inhalation, instillation, irrigation, or lavage; others may be used topically on the skin, on dressings, or for cleansing purposes.

emulsion	liniment
tincture	ointment
lotions	aerosol
elixirs	

Table 23.3

Metric doses with approximate apothecary equivalents*

Weights				Liquid measures†	
Metric	Approximate apothecary equivalents	Metric	Approximate apothecary equivalents	Metric	Approximate apothecary equivalents
2 grams (g or gm) = 30 grains (gr)		15 mg = ¼ gr		1,000 ml = 1 quart	
1.5 g = 22 gr		12 mg = ⅕ gr		750 ml = 1½ pints	
1 g = 15 gr		10 mg = ⅙ gr		500 ml = 1 pint	
0.75 g or 750 mg = 12 gr		8 mg = ⅛ gr		250 ml = 8 fl ounces	
0.6 g or 600 mg = 10 gr		6 mg = 1/10 gr		200 ml = 7 fl ounces	
0.5 g or 500 mg = 7½ gr		5 mg = 1/12 gr		100 ml = 3½ fl ounces	
450 mg = 7 gr		4 mg = 1/16 gr		50 ml = 1¾ fl ounces	
300 mg = 5 gr		3 mg = 1/20 gr		30 ml = 1 fl ounce	
0.25 g or 250 mg = 4 gr		1.5 mg = 1/40 gr		15 ml = ½ fl ounce (4 fl drams)	
200 mg = 3 gr		1.2 mg = 1/50 gr		10 ml = 2½ fl drams	
0.15 g or 150 mg = 2½ gr		1 mg = 1/60 gr		8 ml = 2 fl drams	
120 mg = 2 gr		0.8 mg = 1/80 gr		5 ml = 75 minims (1¼ fl drams)	
0.1 g or 100 mg = 1½ gr		0.6 mg = 1/100 gr		4 ml = 1 fl dram	
75 mg = 1¼ gr		0.5 mg = 1/120 gr		3 ml = 45 minims	
60 mg = 1 gr		0.4 mg = 1/150 gr		2 ml = 30 minims	
50 mg = ¾ gr		0.3 mg = 1/200 gr		1 ml = 15 minims	
40 mg = ⅔ gr		0.25 mg = 1/250 gr		0.75 ml = 12 minims	
30 mg = ½ gr		0.2 mg = 1/300 gr		0.6 ml = 10 minims	
25 mg = ⅜ gr		0.15 mg = 1/400 gr		0.5 ml = 8 minims	
20 mg = ⅓ gr		0.1 mg = 1/600 gr		0.3 ml = 5 minims	
				0.25 ml = 4 minims	
				0.2 ml = 3 minims	
				0.1 ml = 1½ minims	
				0.06 ml = 1 minim	

From Zakus SM: Clinical skills and assisting techniques for the medical assistant, ed 2, St Louis, 1988, The CV Mosby Co.

*The approximate dose equivalents in this table represent the quantities that would be prescribed, under identical conditions, by physicians trained, respectively, in the metric or in the apothecary system of weights and measures.

†A milliliter (ml) is the approximate equivalent of a cubic centimeter (cc).

PROFESSIONAL RESPONSIBILITIES
Storage and Handling of Drugs

If a physician keeps medications in the office, certain rules and precautions should be followed. Ideally, all medications should be stored in a separate room in a locked cabinet and all *must* be kept in their original container. Many medications must be stored in dark containers or dark areas or refrigerated. Some must also be in glass containers, because the chemical composition of the drug may react with plastic. Drugs that must be refrigerated will be labeled as such. Since drugs will deteriorate, it is necessary to have a review schedule so that outdated drugs can be discarded and then replaced with a new supply. When discarding outdated drugs, you should pour liquids down a sink; drugs

in the solid form should be crushed and then flushed down the sink. This method should also be used if you have taken a drug out of its original container and then are unable to use it, as it is *never* to be replaced in the container once removed. Using this method of disposal of medications eliminates the possible chance of drug abuse, as some people will take medications out of garbage containers and administer the drug to themselves or dispense it to others.

To avoid medication errors, drugs for external use must be kept well separated from those to be used internally. Disinfectants, cleansing preparations, and all drugs that would be poisonous if taken internally, must be stored in a location well separated from the other drugs. To facilitate easy

Table 23.4
Equivalents of common household weights and measurements and preparation of solutions

Household	Metric	Apothecary
Liquid		
1 drop (gtt)		= 1 minim (m)
15 drops	= 1 milliliter (ml or cc)	= 15 minims
1 teaspoon (tsp)	= 4 ml	= 1 fluid dram (fl dr)
1 dessert spoon	= 8 ml	= 2 fl dr
6 teaspoons or 2 tablespoons (tbsp)	= 30 ml	= 1 fluid ounce
1 measuring cup	= 240 ml	= 8 fluid ounces
2 measuring cups	= 500 ml	= 1 pint (pt) (16 fl oz)
4 measuring cups	= 1,000 ml	= 1 quart (qt) or 2 pts
1 tbsp	= 15 ml	= 4 drams (½ oz)
Dry		
⅛ teaspoon	= 0.5 gram (g)	= 7½ grains (gr)
¼ teaspoon	= 1.0 g	= 15 grs
1 teaspoon	= 4 g	= 60 grs or 1 dram
1 tablespoon	= 15 g	= 4 drams
2 tablespoons	= 30 g	= 1 ounce

Preparation of solutions

Prescribed strength	Amount of full-strength drug	Fluid to be added to make up
1:1,000	1 teaspoonful	1 gallon
1:1,000	15 drops	1 quart
⅒ of 1%	15 drops	1 quart
1:500	2 teaspoonsful	1 gallon
1:500	30 drops	1 quart
⅕ of 1%	30 drops	1 quart
1:200	5 teaspoonsful	1 gallon
1:200	1¼ teaspoonsful	1 quart
½ of 1%	1¼ teaspoonsful	1 quart
1:100 (1%)	2¼ teaspoonsful	1 quart
1:50 (2%)	5 teaspoonsful	1 quart
1:25 (4%)	2½ tablespoonsful	1 quart
1:20 (5%)	3 tablespoonsful	1 quart

From Zakus SM: Clinical skills and assisting techniques for the medical assistant, ed 2, St Louis, 1988, The CV Mosby Co.

access to the drugs, you should organize the central storage area. You may organize the drugs in an alphabetical arrangement or according to drug substance or classification, for example, antibiotics, contraceptives, diuretics, hormones, vaccines. It is also recommended to label storage areas as *external use only* and *internal use*. A further organizational system is to label areas for drugs to be used for oral administration, those for parenteral administration, and so on.

In addition, federal law requires that all controlled substances be kept in a substantially con-structed, separate, securely locked cabinet or safe. Some states require that these drugs be kept in a locked cupboard in a locked room. Extra security precautions must also be taken for the needles and syringes that will be used for administering parenteral medications. Any loss or theft of controlled substances must be reported by the physician upon discovery to the DEA field office in the area. The field office will provide information on what reports are required of the physician. Also, the physician is required to notify the local police department of such theft.

Emergency Tray

A special container or tray in a readily accessible location should be kept with drugs needed for emergencies. Sterile syringes, needles, alcohol sponges, diluents, and a tourniquet should also be kept in this container. In most offices and clinics, the physician will make a checklist of the drugs and supplies to be kept in the emergency tray, varying with the need of the office and the physician's preference. The medical assistant should be familiar with these specific drugs, knowing the use, usual dosage, and method of administration of each. This container or tray must be checked frequently to replace items that have been used and to discard outdated drugs or sterile supplies.

Listed below are examples of drugs that *may* be kept on the emergency tray. These will vary according to the type of patient and possible emergency that you may encounter at your facility.

Adrenalin (epinephrine) A vasoconstrictor and antispasmodic; used to counteract anaphylactic shock, to relieve symptoms of allergic reactions, and as an emergency heart stimulant.

aminophylline A bronchodilator; used to ease breathing as for asthmatic patients.

Benadryl An antihistamine; used to relieve symptoms of allergic reactions, itching, and anaphylactic shock.

Compazine An antiemetic; used to counteract nausea and vomiting.

dextrose 50% Used for severe hypoglycemia.

Digoxin A cardiac glycoside; used for congestive heart failure and certain cardiac arrhythmias.

Ipecac An emetic; used to stimulate vomiting in some poisoning cases.

Lasix A diuretic; used to promote the formation and excretion of urine.

Narcan A narcotic antagonist; used in emergency situations for narcotic overdose.

nitroglycerin A vasodilator, used commonly for angina patients.

pitocin A hypothalmic hormone; stimulates uterine contractions to control postpartum bleeding in obstetric patients.

steroids (such as hydrocortisone, Solu-Cortef, or Solu-Medrol) Used for their anti-inflammatory action.

Valium A muscular relaxant and an antianxiety, minor tranquilizer; used to relax muscles or calm and quiet extremely anxious patients.

Additional supplies that may be kept near this tray for emergency situations include the following:

- Airway equipment (Ambu bag, laryngoscopes and airways of different sizes, and resuscitation masks of various sizes to fit adults, children, and infants);
- Defibrillator;
- Intubation equipment and other related materials;
- Oxygen tank, mask and/or nasal cannula; and
- Suction equipment.

You should check the above equipment daily to make sure that it is in good working order and to ascertain that there is sufficient oxygen in the tank.

The following points must be kept in mind when oxygen is being adminstered:

- Do not use electrical appliances when oxygen is being adminsitered. Do not connect or disconnect plugs when oxygen is in use.
- Do not use acetone and alcohol in the presence of oxygen.
- Do not use oil or grease on oxygen equipment. Your hands must also be free of grease when you are turning oxygen equipment on or off.
- Do not use oxygen tanks as a clothes rack.
- Keep all flammable substances away from the area where oxygen is in use.
- Post "No Smoking" signs in areas where oxygen is being used.
- Patients *should not be allowed* to have cigarettes, lighters, or matches with them while oxygen is being used. This is because they may forget that these items should not be used while oxygen is being administered and use them.
- When transporting an oxygen tank, fasten it to the platform of a carrier designed for that purpose.

Labeling

All drugs and solutions must be clearly labeled. Poisons should be clearly labeled as such and kept separate from other medications. Leave all drugs and solutions in the original labeled containers until they are administered or dispensed. Never use, but discard, medications or substances that are not clearly labeled or are in unlabeled containers. When pouring liquids from bottles, hold the bottle so that the label is facing the palm of your hand. Using this technique will prevent soiling or obliterating the label if any of the liquid runs down the side of the bottle (see also p. 375, Pouring Sterile Solutions). If a label becomes loose, soiled, or torn, type a new label with the exact information that was provided on the original. It is advisable to have someone else in the office check the new label for accuracy before you affix it to the container.

Controlled Substances Inventory and Prescriber's Record

A running inventory of all narcotics and controlled substances must be kept. A special record—either a card for each type of drug or a daily log book—must be maintained for 2 years (3 years in some states), during which time this record is subject to inspection and copying by authorized employees of state and federal law enforcement and regulatory agencies.

Records kept on all Schedule II controlled substances dispensed, adminstered, or prescribed must show the date, name and address of the patient, character and quantity of the drug provided, and pathological condition and purpose for which the drug was provided. *All records for Schedule II substances must be stored separate from other files.*

Records kept on all Schedule III, IV, and V controlled substances administered or dispensed from the office or medical bag must show the date, name and address of the patient, and the quantity of the drug dispensed or administered. Schedule III, IV, and V records may be stored separate from other files or in such form that the information is readily retrievable from the practitioner's other business and professional records.

All these records are to be kept for 2 years (3 years in some states), subject to inspection and copying by authorized employees of state and federal law enforcement and regulatory agencies.

A physician who dispenses or regularly engages in administering controlled substances and is required to keep records as stated above must take an inventory every 2 years of all stocks of the substances on hand.

All inventories and records of controlled substances in Schedule II must be maintained separately from all other records of the physician. All inventories and records of controlled substances in Schedules III, IV, and V must be maintained separately or must be in such form that they are readily retrievable from the ordinary professional and business records of the physician.

Medical assistants should play a major role in helping the physician keep all the appropriate records, guarding prescription pads, securing medication storage areas to prevent theft, ensuring the proper type of storage and correct labeling for all medications, and discarding and destroying outdated drugs.

ROUTES AND METHODS OF DRUG ADMINISTRATION

Drugs are supplied in various forms for different purposes (Table 23.5). Certain drugs can be administered in a variety of ways, and others must be administered in a specific way to be effective. Methods of administration are divided into two general categories: (1) drugs used for local effect, which are applied directly to the skin, tissue or mucous membrane involved, and (2) drugs used for a systemic or general effect. A drug applies in this manner must be absorbed and circulate through the bloodstream to produce an effect on the body cells or tissues.

Rules for Administering Medication

There are certain rules to follow when preparing and administering medications. Additional guides and rules that apply specifically to medications given parentally (by injection) are described later in this chapter.

You must know and always adhere to the five *rights* of proper medication administration, which are as follows:

- *Right* drug;
- *Right* dose;
- *Right* route for administration;
- *Right* time; and
- *Right* patient.

It is the patient's *right* to expect the five *rights*.

General instructions

1. Wash your hands before preparing medications.
2. Give only medications for which you have the physician's order. A safe practice is to follow only written orders.
3. Prepare the medication in a well-lighted area away from distractions and interruptions. Give full attention to what you are doing.
4. Read the label of the medication three times:
   - When removing from the storage area;
   - Before pouring the desired amount; and
   - When replacing the container in the storage area.

   Do not use unlabeled or illegibly labeled medications.
5. Know the drug that you are giving. Check the *PDR* or other reference books if you are unsure of the usual actions, uses, dosage,

Table 23.5
Routes and methods used for administering medications

Routes of administration	How drug is administered	Form drug supplied in
Oral	The patient is given the drug by mouth to swallow. This is the simplest method and the method most desirable to patients.	Pills, tablets, capsules, spansules, or solutions. These are supplied in bulk form or as a unit dose.
Sublingual	The drug is placed under the patient's tongue and left to dissolve and be absorbed. It is *not* to be chewed or swallowed.	Tablets
Buccal	The drug is placed between the cheek and gum to dissolve and be absorbed.	Tablets
Inhalation	The drug is given via the respiratory tract. The patient inhales the drug using a nebulizer or a special mechanical apparatus.	Aerosols, sprays, mists, or steams medicated with drugs
Rectal	The drug is inserted into the rectum. This method is used when a patient cannot tolerate the drug orally; or if unconscious; or if the drug would be destroyed by digestive enzymes. Also may be administered by proctoclysis, a drip method.	Suppositories, enemas, or other solutions
Inunction	The drug is applied or rubbed into the skin. Rubber gloves should be used when applying drugs such as nitroglycerin, or those containing mercury, to prevent absorption of the drug into your system.	Ointments, lotions, sprays, solutions, powders, tinctures, liniments
Vaginal	The drug is inserted into or applied to the vagina.	Suppository; solution, as in a douche; or liquids or ointments to be applied for local effect on the cervix or vaginal canal; also contraceptive foams and creams
Instillation	The drug is applied in drops to a membrane, as into the eye or ear.	Solutions
Irrigation	The drug is flushed through a membrane or body cavity.	Solutions
Parenteral	The drug is given by injection through a needle. Types of injections include the following: a. *Subcutaneous:* under the skin. b. *Intramuscular:* into a muscle. c. *Intradermal* or *intracutaneous:* into the upper layers of the skin. Used chiefly for skin reactions, as in allergy or tuberculosis testing. d. *Intraarticular:* into a joint for local effects. e. *Intraarterial:* into an artery; used in certain diagnostic procedures. f. *Lumbar puncture* or *intraspinal:* into the spinal canal between two vertebrae; used to administer drugs for diagnostic techniques or for spinal anesthetics. g. *Intravenous:* into a vein; used for immediate effect of a drug, for blood transfusions, or parenteral feeding.	A drug solution supplied in ampules for single use; in vials for single or multiple use; and in syringes or cartridges prefilled by the manufacturer. Drugs that deteriorate in solutions may be supplied in vials in powdered form to which a specified amount of diluent is to be added when prepared for use. Sterile hypodermic tablets that are to be dissolved before the drug is administered are also available. Larger amounts of solutions for intravenous use are supplied in bottles of 250 ml, 500 ml or 1,000 ml, such as dextrose in water and normal saline, to which other drugs may be added. Plasma and blood are also used for intravenous transfusions.

From Zakus SM: Clinical skills and assisting techniques for the medical assistant, ed 2, St Louis, 1988, The CV Mosby Co.

Figure 23.3
A, Hold the medicine or graduate at eye level so you can measure accurately as you pour the medication. **B,** Shake or drop tablet into cap of container.

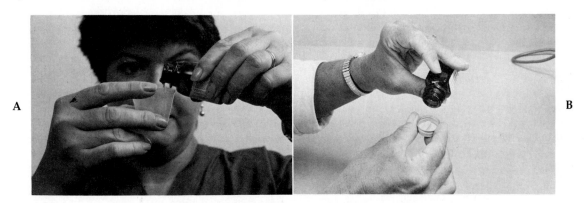

route of administration, and undesirable side effects.

6. Calculate a dosage accurately, when this is necessary. Consult another competent person for verification when you doubt your answer.

7. Liquid medications: (Review p. 375, Pouring Sterile Solutions)
   - Shake well any medication that is in the form of an emulsion or suspension.
   - Do not use medications that have changed color, turned cloudy, or have sediment at the bottom (except suspensions).
   - Hold the bottle with the label in the palm of your hand to avoid damaging the label if the liquid runs or spills.
   - Hold the medicine or graduate at eye level so that you can measure accurately as you pour the medication (Figure 23.3, *A*)
   - Wipe the neck of the container before replacing the cap.
   - Do not mix liquid medications unless specifically ordered to do so.

8. Tablets, pills, capsules, or spansules: Shake or drop the tablet or other preparation into the cap of the container; then drop it into a medicine cup. You must *not* handle the medication with your fingers (Figure 23.3, *B*).

9. Do not leave poured medications unattended.

10. Do not administer medications prepared by others. If an error is made, the person administering the medication is responsible.

11. Take both the drug and container to the physician for additional identification when you have prepared a medication to be administered by the physician.

12. Know your patient. You may ask the patient to state his name to ensure correct identification.

13. Make sure that the patient is not allergic to the medication before administering it.

14. Stay with the patient until you are certain that an oral medication has been swallowed.

15. Observe the patient for any unusual reactions to the drug administered.

16. Discard a medication that the patient refuses. Never replace a medication into the original container once it has been removed.

17. Report immediately to the physician if the patient refuses the medication or if an error was made so that appropriate action can be taken promptly or adjustments made for the patient's care.

18. Record as soon as possible on the correct patient's chart the date, time, drug, and amount given, route of administration, and your signature. *(Errors in administering drugs must be recorded, describing the incident in full.)* Body locations must be recorded for drugs administered parenterally. In addition, if the medication administered was a narcotic or other controlled substance, you must record this information in the physician's controlled substances records.

Dosage: Weights, Measurements, Calculations

A complete understanding of basic arithmetic is essential when preparing solutions or administering medications. A review of mathematical calculations is recommended at this time before you prepare to calculate dosages and administer medications.

The two primary systems of weights and measures used for describing dosages for medications are the apothecary system and the metric system. The *apothecary* system is our oldest system of measurement, the term being an ancient word meaning pharmacist or druggist. Today the trend is to use the metric system, the standard system of weights and measurements set up by the International Bureau of Weights and Measures, although it has not been completely adopted for use by everyone at this time. Therefore it is necessary to have an understanding of both systems.

The apothecary system units of fluid measurements are minim, fluid dram, fluid ounce, pint, quart, and gallon. The units of solid measurement are the grain, dram, ounce, and pound. Roman numerals and fractions are used for this system, for example, HC1 gtt X (Hydrochloric acid drops ten); or nitroglycerin gr 1/150 (nitroglycerin grains one/one hundred fifty).

In the metric system, the units of fluid or volume measurements are the milliliter, cubic centimeter, and liter. Units of weight or solid measurements are the milligram and gram. Arabic numbers and the decimal system are used with this system. Example: 1/1,000 = 0.001, 1/100 = 0.01, 1/10 = 0.1, for example, tetracycline 250 mg/ml or cc.

See Tables 23.3 and 23.4 for the equivalent values of apothcary and metric measurements for liquids and solids, and the equivalents of common household weights and measurements for these systems.

At times you may be required to calculate the dose of a medication that you are to administer. A simple formula to use is as follows:

$$\frac{\text{Dose you } want}{\text{Dose you } have} = \text{Dose you } give$$

EXAMPLE: The physician has ordered 500 mg tetracycline, by mouth (po). The dose of tetracycline that you have on hand is labeled 250 mg/tablet. Therefore:

$$\frac{\text{Dose you want (500 mg)}}{\text{Dose you have (250 mg)}} = \text{Tablets to give (2)}$$

You would therefore give the patient two tablets of tetracycline 250 mg/tablet, so that the patient would receive 500 mg of tetracycline as was ordered.

The same formula can be used when preparing drugs supplied in a solution form.

EXAMPLE: The physician has ordered 500 mg of tetracycline to ge given intramuscularly (IM). The bottle you have on hand is labeled tetracycline 250 mg/ml. Therefore:

$$\frac{\text{Dose you want (500 mg)}}{\text{Dose you have (250 mg/ml)}}$$
$$= \text{Dose in ml that you give (2ml)}$$

When this formula is used, both the dose you want to give and the dose you have on hand must be expressed in the same measurements. That is, to give so many milligrams, the dose on hand must be in milligrams per milliliter for a solution, or in milligrams per tablet or capsule for drugs supplied in the solid form. If this is not the case, you will have to convert one measurement into the equivalent value of the other. You should be familiar with the methods used for converting one system of measurements into the other.

It is recommended that you refer to some of the many books available with practice problems in the mathematics of drugs, solutions, and dosages to gain competence in this. Use the tables of weights and measurements for a reference. When you doubt your calculations, always seek help from another competent person or the physician.

FACTORS INFLUENCING DOSAGE AND DRUG ACTION

Not all individuals will respond to a given medication in the same manner. When prescribing a drug for a patient, the physician will take into account the following, as each will influence the prescribed dosage and anticipated action.

Age

Infants, young children, and the elderly will usually require a smaller dosage of a medication.

Sex

The average woman will be given a smaller dosage than the average man because of the difference in body structure and overall weight. Also when a woman is pregnant, drugs and the dosage will be monitored very closely to prevent harmful effects on the fetus.

Weight

The usual rule is the smaller or lighter the patient, the smaller the dosage of drug. Certain medication dosages will be determined according to the weight of the patient.

Past Medical History and Drug Tolerance

If a patient has been taking a medication regularly for an extended period of time, a tolerance to the drug may have developed, and a larger dosage may be required to obtain the desired results. This is frequently seen with the use of narcotics, barbiturates, sedatives, and analgesics.

Physical or Emotional Condition of the Patient

A patient who has excruciating pain will require a larger dose of an analgesic than a patient who experiences intermittent pain. A severely depressed patient will require a larger dosage of an antidepressant than a patient suffering from mild depression.

Drug Idiosyncrasies or Allergies

At times the patient may experience an abnormal susceptibility or reaction to a drug. Alternate drugs with similar actions could then be prescribed.

Type of Action Desired or Produced

Drugs can produce local, systemic, selective, or cumulative actions. A *local action* occurs when the drug is absorbed and produces an effect at the site to which it was administered, as a local anesthetic administered to deaden sensation in the body area to be worked on. A *systemic action* occurs when the drug is absorbed and circulates in the blood stream to produce a general effect, such as central nervous system stimulants and depressants. A *selective action* is a more specific effect of a drug on one special body area than on other areas, as bronchodilators. A *cumulative* action happens when a drug accumulates in the body and exerts a greater effect than the initial dose; the drug accumulates in the body faster than it can be metabolized and excreted, such as alcohol does when a person drinks two or three drinks in 1 hour.

Route of Administration

Although there are exceptions, generally medications administered parenterally are given in smaller dosages than those given by mouth. Larger amounts of medications are used for topical application than for internal administration. Drugs administered parenterally will produce their effects much more rapidly than drugs administered orally. When a systemic effect is desired from an irritating drug, it should be given intramuscularly rather than by other parenteral routes.

Time of Administration

For optimal effects, some drugs must be taken before meals; two, three, or four times a day; or after meals to avoid irritating the lining of the stomach. Drugs will be absorbed more quickly and have a more rapid effect if taken on an empty stomach.

Interactions of Drugs

Some drugs, when taken together, may enhance or counteract the effect of the other. If the interaction is *synergistic,* one drug augments the activity of the other drug; the action of the drugs is such that their combined effect is greater than the sum of their individual effects. For example, barbiturates taken with alcohol have up to four times the depressant effect that either drug would have if taken alone. A *potentiating* interaction is a synergistic action in which one drug increases the effect of another drug when taken simultaneously, producing a combined effect that is greater than the sum of the effects of each drug taken separately. Drugs can also create an *antagonistic* interaction. This is when one drug neutralizes or counteracts the action of the other drug when they are taken together. Another type of drug interaction is termed *additive.* This is when the combined effect produced by the action of two or more drugs is equal to the sum of their separate effects.

Thus, it is vital to know if the patient is taking any other medication and, in some cases, any alcoholic beverage, before a new medication is prescribed. It is also important to know if the patient takes nonprescription drugs, for often patients do not consider drugs that they purchase over the counter as medications. Nonetheless, these drugs are medications that may possibly interact adversely with a prescription drug.

Summary

It must be remembered that drugs are potent substances that can provide individuals with extremely beneficial results when used properly and with care, but are also capable of producing hazardous or fatal results when used indiscreetly. Toxic effects, such as allergic reactions, adverse effects on the blood or blood producing tissues, drug dependence, accidental poisoning, or drug overdose, can be the result of careless or uninformed use of any drug on the market for legal use or from illegal drugs obtained in the streets. Always handle and administer drugs with extreme care, as a life may depend on their proper use.

INJECTIONS

Injections are a very important means of administering chemotherapy treatment. Because two foreign objects, the medication and the needle, are being introduced into the patient's body, these procedures must be performed with extreme care and excellent technique. The effectiveness of the medication is influenced by the correct choice of injection site and the use of precise technique. Any injection administered into an inappropriate body site or with incorrect technique may interfere with the body's use of the medication, and more important, may cause irreparable damage. The practices of aseptic (sterile) technique (see Chapter 21) must be observed when administering injections to minimize the danger of causing an infectious process.

Reasons Physicians Order Injections

1. To achieve a rapid response to the medication. When injected, a medication will enter the bloodstream quickly and therefore be more effective.
2. To guarantee the accuracy of the amount of medication given.
3. To concentrate the medication in a specific area of the body, such as into a joint cavity, fracture, or lumbar puncture.
4. To produce local anesthesia to a specific part of the body.
5. To administer the medication when it cannot be given by mouth or by other methods, either because of the physical or mental condition of the patient or the nature of the drug.
6. To administer the medication when its effect would be destroyed by the digestive tract or lost through vomiting or when it would irritate the digestive system.

Dangers and Complications Associated with Injections

1. Injury to superficial nerves or to a vessel.
2. Introduction of infection because of the im-proper sterilization of the injection site, needle, or syringe, or caused by an operator with unclean hands.
3. Breakage of a needle in a tissue.
4. Injecting a vein rather than a muscle.
5. Hitting a bone in a very thin patient.
6. Allergic reactions that may be mild, severe, or even fatal.
7. Toxic effects produced by the medication.
8. Too much air entering the bloodstream in a venipuncture.

Body Areas to Avoid when Administering Injections

- Burned areas.
- Scar tissue.
- Edematous areas.
- Cyanotic areas.
- Traumatized areas.
- Areas near large blood vessels, nerves, and bones.
- Areas in which there has been a change in skin texture or pigmentation.
- Areas in which there are other tissue growths, such as a mole or wart.

Supplies and Equipment for Administering Injections
Syringes

Disposable plastic or glass and nondisposable glass syringes are available in several standard sizes and shapes. The most common sizes used in the physician's office are 2 cc, 3 cc, 5 cc and 10 cc. The parts of a syringe are the barrel, the outside portion; the plunger, the portion that fits inside the barrel; and the tip, the point at which the needle will be attached, which will be either a plain tip or a Luer-Lok tip (Figure 23.4). Other variations of syringes include the insulin syringe (Figure 23.5), tuberculin syringe (Figure 23.6), Tubex metal syringe for use with a disposable needle-cartridge unit, and a disposable syringe unit-dose system. Sterile disposable syringes come supplied in a paper wrapper or a rigid plastic container. Calibrations, usually in cubic centimeters (cc) and minims, are marked on the barrel of the syringe.

Needles

Needles come in various lengths ranging from ¼ inch to 6 inches, and with various gauges ranging from 13 to 27. The gauge of the needle and the length are indicated on the outside of the sterile protective cover or wrapper. Some manufacturers

Figure 23.4
Parts of a syringe.
Courtesy Becton-Dickinson, Div of Becton, Dickinson, and Co,
Rutherford, NJ.

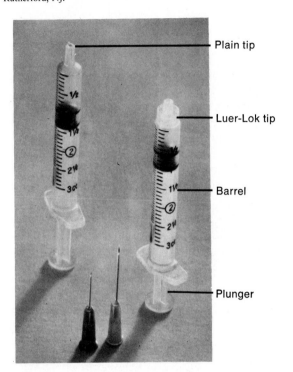

— Plain tip

— Luer-Lok tip

— Barrel

— Plunger

Figure 23.6
Tuberculin syringe with fine calibrations up to 1 cc.
Courtesy Becton-Dickinson, Div of Becton, Dickinson, and Co,
Rutherford, NJ.

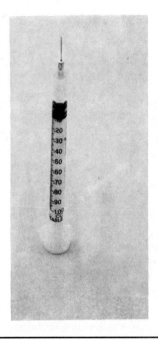

Figure 23.5
Insulin syringe. Calibrations are marked in units
per cubic centimeter.

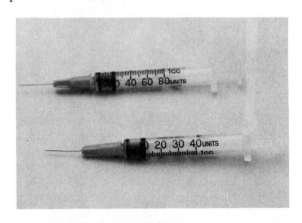

The size and length of a needle govern its use.

Today most practitioners use disposable needles
and syringes to prevent all danger of cross-infec-
tion, although the reusable type is still available.

Skin antiseptic

Before an injection is administered, the skin must
be cleansed with an antiseptic. The most commonly used is isopropyl alcohol placed on a sterile
cotton ball, or a prepackaged sterile alcohol
sponge.

Medications and diluents

Most medications for parenteral use are in an
aqueous solution or in a suspension, although
some are in an oil solution or suspension, and a
few are in tablet or powdered form. When a sterile
hypodermic tablet or powdered drug is to be dissolved before parenteral use, sterile water or bacteriostatic normal saline will be used as the diluent.
The type and amount to be used will be indicated
on the container in which the drug is supplied.

Medication solutions are supplied in single or
multiple dose form. Those for *single use* will be
supplied (1) in syringes or cartridges that are prefilled by the manufacturer, (2) in an ampule, a
small glass container with a constricted neck that is

also color code the wrappers for quick and easy
identification. The parts of a needle are the point,
the cannula or shaft, and the hub, which fits onto
the tip of a syringe (Figure 23.7). The smaller the
gauge of the needle, the larger the lumen or inside
diameter. For example, an 18-gauge needle has a
large lumen; a 26-gauge needle has a small lumen.

Figure 23.7

Various sized needles with parts labeled.
Courtesy Becton-Dickinson, Div of Becton, Dickinson, and Co, Rutherford, NJ.

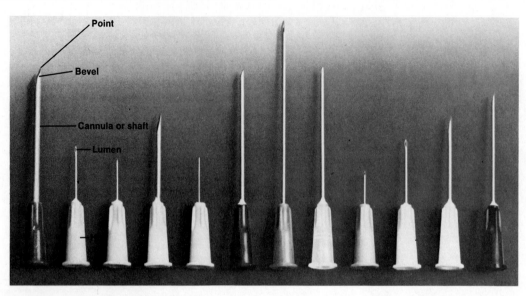

to be broken off when the drug is to be used, or (3) in a single-dose vial.

Containers with *multiple doses* of a medication are called vials. These are small bottles containing from 10 to 50 ml of a drug solution. Vials are usually covered with a soft metal cover and have a rubber, self-sealing stopper. At the time of use, this rubber stopper is cleansed with an alcohol sponge and then punctured with the needle to inject air and withdraw an equal amount of drug (Figure 23.8). Procedures to withdraw solutions from an ampule and vial are discussed under the procedure "Administration of an Intramuscular Injection."

Selection of Syringe and Needle Size

The smaller the amount of medication to be given, the smaller the size of syringe to use. In special circumstances, such as the administration of insulin, it is essential that an insulin syringe be used. For measuring a very small amount of drug, use a tuberculin syringe.

Needles with large lumens are required when the medication to be injected is oily or very thick. Needles with small lumens are used for aqueous solutions. Shorter needles with a larger gauge number may be used on children and very thin patients; longer needles may be required for obese patients to ensure that the needle reaches muscular or subcutaneous tissue.

Figure 23.8

Drugs supplied in liquid form. *Left to right:* Cartridge, vial, ampule.

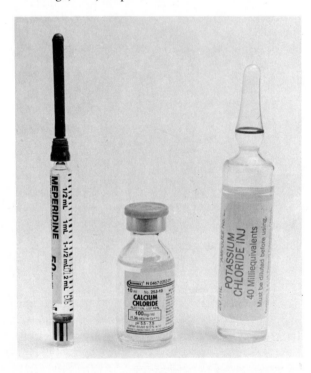

Figure 23.9
Gluteus medius IM injection site.

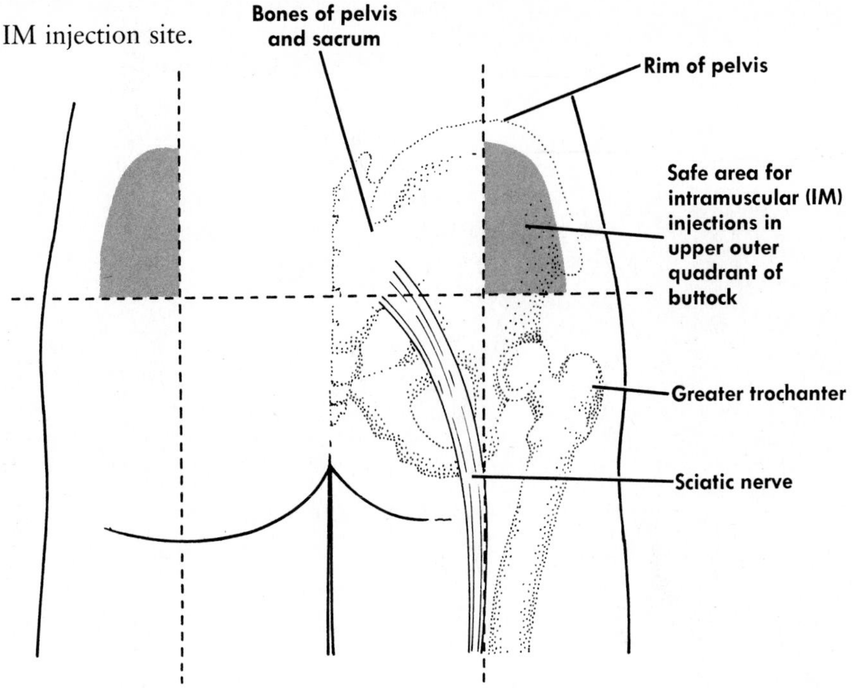

Bones of pelvis and sacrum

Rim of pelvis

Safe area for intramuscular (IM) injections in upper outer quadrant of buttock

Greater trochanter

Sciatic nerve

Common sizes of syringes and needles used for various injections are given in each following procedure.

Anatomical Selection of Injection Sites
Intramuscular injections

The main objective when administering an intramuscular medication is to inject it deep into the muscle for gradual and optimal absorption into the bloodstream. The usual amount of solution to be given by this method is 2 to 5 ml. It is recommended to divide a 4 or 5-ml dose in half, using two different sites for injecting the medication. Identification of suitable sites for an injection is based on the use of definite anatomic landmarks, located by palpation. Four anatomic sites commonly used follow.

Gluteus medius. The most common site for intramuscular injections, the gluteus medius is located in the upper outer quadrant (UOQ) of the buttock. Have the patient assume a prone position, toes pointed inward, and the buttock clearly exposed. This position allows for best relaxation of the muscles and best exposure of the area. Injecting a needle in a tense muscle causes pain. Undergarments must be completely removed. Under no circumstances must you deviate from using the cor-

rect technique. Palpate for and then draw a diagonal line from the greater trochanter of the femur to the posterior superior iliac spine. The injection is to be given well above and outside of this diagonal line. Extreme care must be taken to locate the correct site to avoid hitting the sciatic nerve or the superior gluteal artery (Figure 23.9).

Middeltoid area. The middeltoid site is located on the upper, outer aspect of the arm, below the lower edge of the acromion and above the axilla. Although there is easy access to this site when the patient is standing, sitting, in a prone or supine position, the actual area that can be used for the injection is limited, as there are major vessels, nerves, and bones to be avoided in the upper arm. It is therefore recommended to limit the use of this site for injections, because of the small area available, which can tolerate only small amounts of medication and infrequent injections. In addition, patients often experience more pain and tenderness in this area (Figure 23.10).

Ventrogluteal area (von Hochstetter's site). Growing in recognition for use, the ventrogluteal site is removed from major blood vessels and nerves. To locate this site, have the patient in a supine or side position. Palpate for the greater trochanter of the femur, the iliac crest, and the anterior superior iliac spine. Then place the palm of

Figure 23.10
A, Mid-deltoid IM injection site. **B,** Giving intramuscular injection. Hold syringe and needle in pencil or dartlike grip; insert at 90-degree angle with quick thrust. *Do not* hit skin with hub of needle.

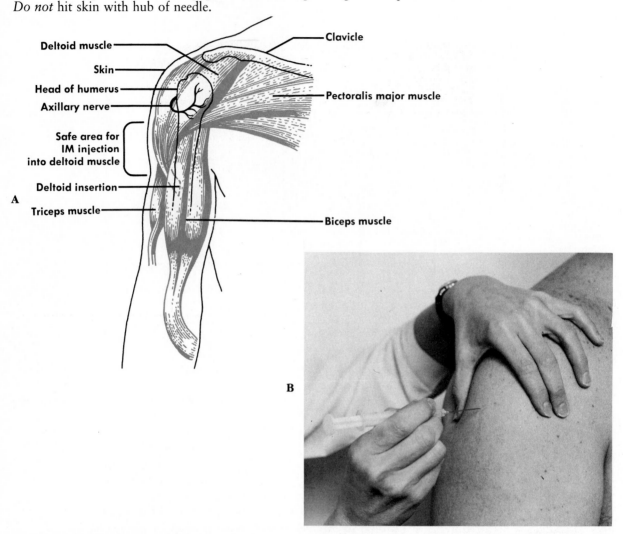

your right hand on the patient's left greater trochanter, your index finger on the anterior superior iliac spine, and move your middle finger posteriorly along the iliac crest as far as possible. (Do this with your left hand when injecting into the patient's right side.) A V space is now formed between your index and middle finger. The injection is to be given in the middle of this V space

Vastus lateralis.* The vastus lateralis, a thick muscle on the upper side of the leg, is also being used more frequently, as it is free of major blood vessels

and nerves. With the patient in a supine position, locate this site by palpating the greater trochanter of the femur and the lateral aspect of the patella. Divide the distance between these two landmarks into thirds. The needle is to be inserted into the middle third of this area (Figure 23.11).

Subcutaneous injections

The objective of a subcutaneous (sc) injection is to deposit a relatively small amount of an aqueous solution under the skin for rapid absorption into the bloodstream. The amount of the solution given by this method should not exceed 2 ml. To avoid overdistention of the tissues, the medication should

---

*When intramuscular injections are administered to children, both the ventrogluteal and vastus lateralis sites are recommended.

Figure 23.11
Vastus lateralis IM injection site.

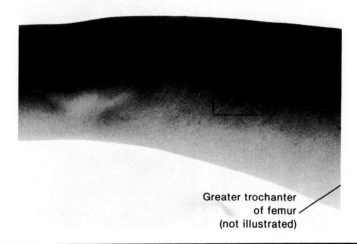

Greater trochanter
of femur
(not illustrated)

be administered slowly. The most common and preferred sites for a subcutaneous injection are the following:

- Outer surface of the upper arm, usually half-way between the shoulder and elbow;
- Lateral aspect of the thigh; and
- Upper two thirds of the back.

Additional sites that may be used, especially when the medication is self-administered, as a diabetic may do, include the following:

- Areas on the abdomen;
- Front aspect of the thigh.

When frequent subcutaneous injections are given, sites of administration should be rotated to prevent damaging a tissue, excessive pain, and possibly disfigurement (Figure 23.12).

Intradermal injections

The objective of the intradermal injection is to inject a minute amount of solution between the layers of the skin. The amount of drug given by this method is usually 0.1 ml to 0.3 ml. A tuberculin syringe (Figure 23.6) is to be used because of its fine calibrations, which provide the best means for measuring minute amounts of a drug. Drugs must be administered slowly in this method; they produce a small pale bump on the skin when given correctly.

The most common and preferred site for intradermal injections is the dorsal surface of the forearm, about 4 inches below the elbow. The lateral and posterior sides of the arm can also be used if

Figure 23.12
Subcutaneous injection sites.

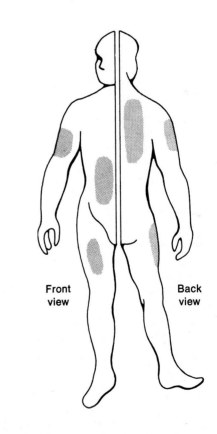

Front
view

Back
view

Figure 23.13
Angles of insertion for parenteral injections.

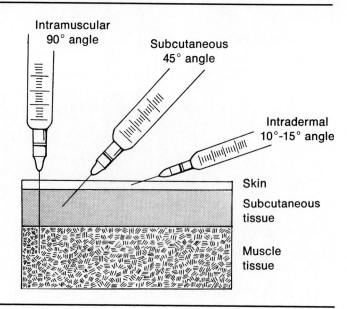

and when required. These sites are used because they can be easily observed for reactions resulting from the drug injected and also can be kept free of irritation from clothing. Intradermal injections are used for various skin tests to determine allergies (sensitivities) to drugs and various other foreign substances, such as food substances, dust, and grass; to determine the patient's susceptibility to an infectious disease, such as tuberculosis (the Mantoux test) and diphtheria (the Schick test); or to aid in the diagnosis of infectious diseases. In addition to their frequent use for these tests, intradermal tests are used in the diagnosis of parasitic infections such as schistosomiasis and fungal diseases.

Instructions for Administering Injections

In addition to the rules listed previously, the following apply to injections:

1. Select the injection site carefully. You must avoid major blood vessels, nerves, and bones.
2. Use only sterile, preferably disposable, syringes and needles.
3. Select the correct size of syringe according to the amount of medication to be given and the appropriate size and length of needle according to the type of solution to be given and the size and condition of the patient.
4. Insert the needle using the correct angle (Figure 23.13).
5. After inserting the needle, but before injecting the medication, always pull the plunger back to determine if you have entered a blood vessel.
6. If you entered a blood vessel, withdraw the needle a bit, redirect and again insert the needle. Pull the plunger back to determine if you have entered a second blood vessel.
7. If a large amount of blood returns in the syringe when you pull back on the plunger, remove the needle and begin the procedure again using new medication, syringe, and needle.
8. Rotate injection sites on patients receiving frequent injections.
9. Aseptic technique *must* be used when administering all injections.
10. For care of used equipment see Chapter 20, "Universal Blood and Body Substance Precautions—Barrier Precautions: Sharps," on p. 346.

Administration of an Intramuscular Injection

Equipment

Appropriate size sterile needle and syringe, depending on amount and type of drug to be given (usually a 2 cc or 3 cc syringe, and a 21- or 22-gauge, 1½-inch needle *or* a 1-inch needle for thin or small patients, a 2-inch needle for obese patients *or* a hypodermic metal syringe when the medication is supplied in a prefilled sterile cartridge-needle unit, such as a Tubex hypodermic metal syringe

A 23-gauge, 1-inch needle may be used when administering the drug into the deltoid muscle

Sterile alcohol sponges

Medication ordered

Small tray

Procedure	*Rationale*
1. Wash your hands.	
2. Assemble the equipment.	
3. Prepare the syringe and needle for use. When using a separate syringe and needle, remove them from the wrappers, and leave the cover (sheath) on the needle intact. Grasping the hub of the needle and the barrel of the syringe, attach the hub of the needle to the tip of the syringe. Secure by turning the hub ¼ inch clockwise.	Avoid touching the tip of the syringe and the open end of the hub of the needle with your fingers. These parts are to remain sterile.
4. Compare the physician's order with the label on the medication.	These must be the same. At times you may have to calculate the dosage to be given.
5. Check the label of the medication three times during the preparation of the medication to ensure that you have the correct medication and strength.	Check the label three times: • When removing the medication from storage area, • When filling the syringe, and • When replacing the medication in the storage area. The same medication is often supplied in different strengths.
6. Take an alcohol sponge to cleanse the rubber stopper of the vial or the neck of the ampule; then discard this sponge. Withdraw medication into the syringe. *If an ampule is used:*	Cleansing helps prevent the introduction of microorganisms into the vial and prevents contamination of the needle.
a. Tap the tip of the ampule to dislodge any medication there.	
b. Cleanse the neck at the marked line	
c. File across this line.	Files are supplied with ampules.
d. Hold the ampule; with your other hand, cover the top end with a sponge, and break the top off going away from you (Figure 23.14). The medication is now ready for use.	The sponge is used to protect your fingers when the top is broke off.
e. Remove the needle cover (sheath)	Do not touch the opening of the ampule with the needle. The needle is contaminated if it touches the outside or entrance of the ampule. In this instance, you must obtain another sterile needle for use.

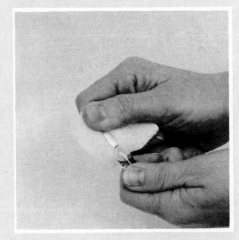

Figure 23.14
Technique for breaking top off ampule.

Continued.

Administration of an Intramuscular Injection—cont'd

Procedure

f. Insert the needle into the ampule (Fig. 23.15).

g. Pull back on the plunger of the syringe to withdraw the required amount of medication.

h. Remove the needle from the ampule.

i. Replace the needle cover (sheath) over needle.

j. Place this unit on a small tray.

k. Check the label, and then discard the ampule.

l. Proceed to the patient, carrying this medication and a sterile alcohol sponge on the small tray.

If a vial is used:

a. Take the syringe and pull the plunger back to obtain a measured amount of air equal to the amount of medication to be withdrawn from the vial.

b. Remove the needle cover.

c. Insert the needle through the cleansed rubber stopper, keeping it above the solution.

Rationale

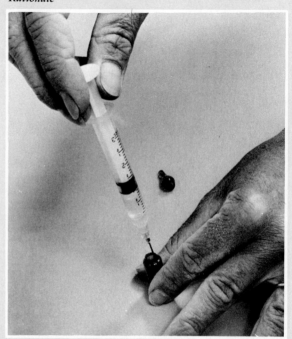

Figure 23.15
Insert needle into ampule and pull back on syringe plunger to withdraw the medication.

d. Push the plunger of the syringe down to the bottom of the barrel.

This gives air replacement, which prevents the creation of a vacuum in the vial when the medication is withdrawn. If a vacuum is created, it makes it difficult to withdraw the medication. Do not inject more air than is required, as the pressure in the vial will then force the solution into the syringe, making it difficult to obtain an accurate dosage.

e. Invert the vial; have the vial and syringe at eye level.

f. With the needle opening in the solution, pull the plunger of the syringe back gently until the required amount of medication has been obtained (Figure 23.16).

Keep the vial and syringe at eye level to ensure correct measurement of the drug withdrawn.

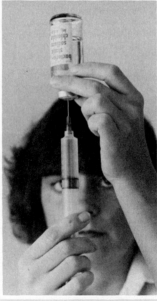

Figure 23.16
Withdrawing medication from vial. Hold syringe at eye level to ensure correct measurement of medication.

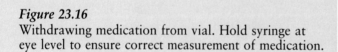

Procedure	*Rationale*
g. Remove the needle from the vial.	
h. Replace the needle cover over the needle.	
i. Place the filled syringe with the covered needle on a small tray.	
j. Check the label on the vial and replace the vial in the correct storage area.	Ensure that the correct medication will be administered.
k. Proceed to the patient, carrying the medication and a sterile alcohol sponge on the small tray.	
7. Identify the patient and explain the procedure.	Correct patient identification is crucial. Explanations help gain the patient's cooperation and relaxation.
8. Select the injection site and position the patient accordingly, exposing the site clearly.	Refer to pp. 469-472, Anatomical Selection of Injection Sites. Your view and accessibility to the injection site must not be obstructed by the patient's clothing or any drape sheet. Be sure that you have ample lighting when administering the injection.
9. With the alcohol sponge, cleanse the injection site, starting at a central point and moving out to an area approximately 2 inches square, allow it to dry.	
10. Remove the needle cover.	
11. Hold the syringe with the needle facing upward; slowly push on the plunger until a tiny drop of medication comes to the needle tip.	This helps get rid of air bubbles, which must be expelled from the syringe before injecting the medication. Also, the tiny drop of medication obtained at the top of the syringe ensures that the needle is clear and not plugged.
12. Using the index finger and thumb of your nondominant hand, spread or tense the skin around the injection site.	
13. Using your dominant hand, hold the syringe and needle as if you were holding a pencil, with the bevel of the needle facing up.	Your index finger and second finger may surround the top part of the needle hub with your thumb placed on the end of the syringe; or all three fingers may surround the bottom end of the syringe near the needle, but not touching the needle.
14. With a quick thrust, insert the needle at a 90-degree angle to about ¾ of the needle length. Do not hit the skin with the hub of the needle (Figure 23.10, *B*).	Hold the needle perpendicular to the skin and insert quickly in a dartlike thrust.
15. Steady the syringe with your dominant hand. Using your other hand, pull back on the plunger to see if any blood can be aspirated into the syringe.	Aspiration must be done to check if you have entered a blood vessel. If a blood vessel is entered, withdraw the needle slightly, redirect and reinsert; then pull back on the plunger again to check for blood. Some recommend complete withdrawal of the needle if a blood vessel is entered, then beginning the procedure again with a new needle.
16. Continue to steady the syringe with your dominant hand. With your other hand push on the plunger slowly to inject the medication.	Injection of the medication slowly allows the solution to disperse into the tissues. Discomfort, caused by pressure, will result if the medication is injected too quickly.
17. Using your nondominant hand, apply pressure at the injection site with the alcohol sponge, and quickly remove the needle with your dominant hand (the hand that has constantly been on the syringe and needle unit).	Applied pressure and the quick withdrawl of the needle reduces discomfort and the risk of medication leaking into the subcutaneous tissues and possibly forming abscesses.
NOTE: By keeping your dominant hand in constant contact with the syringe and needle unit, rather than switching hands after inserting the needle (some suggest inserting the needle with your dominant hand, then changing hands and steadying the syringe with your nondominant hand, then using your dominant hand to aspirate and push on the plunger), you help prevent further discomfort to the patient and tissue irritation that may occur if the syringe is jiggled or moved during a hand change.	
18. Massage the injection site. Move the tissue as you massage, not merely the sponge.	Massaging the area helps spread the medication in the tissue. If rapid absorption is desired, continue to massage the area for about 2 minutes.
19. Help the patient assume a comfortable and safe position.	

Continued.

Procedure

20. Observe the patient for any unusual reactions, such as a rash or shock.
21. Inform the patient if he is free to leave or if the physician requires additional consultation time.
22. Place a disposable needle and syringe in a puncture-resistant container without breaking or recapping the needle. The needle box should be in the room or as close as possible to the area of use (Figure 23.17).

Rationale

To protect the physician, medical assistant, and janitorial staff. Needle recapping and disposal are frequent causes of needlesticks.

Figure 23.17
Placing a used disposable syringe and needle in the rigid puncture-resistant disposable container. This puncture-resistant container must be located as close as practical to the area where needles and other sharps will be used. (Gloves are not needed when giving injections, but are to be worn when doing venipunctures and disposing of that needle and syringe.)

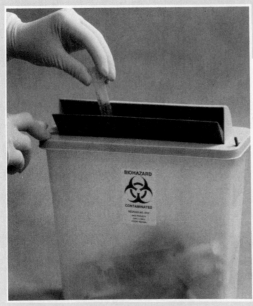
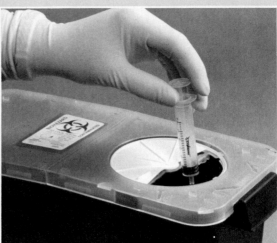

Guidelines for preventing needlesticks

a. Slow down and *think* when using or disposing of needles.
b. DO NOT *recap* needles unless absolutely necessary. If necessary, place cap on table top before inserting needle (insert needle into cap without holding cap).
c. Never put a needle down—dispose of it promptly in approved container.
d. Never put needles or other sharp instruments in trash cans.
e. Never leave needles or other sharp instruments on counter tops, examination tables, or disposable procedure trays.
f. Never push a needle into the red plastic needle disposal box with your hand. If the needle does not go into the opening easily, use a large syringe to push it in.
g. Never try to remove a needle or syringe from the red plastic needle box.
   If using a reusable syringe and needle:
   • After using a reusable syringe and needle, flush tap water through both until clean.
   • Separate the needle, barrel, and plunger, and place each in a designated cleansing solution until ready to prepare all for sterilization. See also "Sharps" in Chapter 20, pp. 346 and 348.
23. Wash your hands.
24. Record the procedure on the patient's chart.

Charting example:
June 3, 19_____, 4 PM
Penbritin-S 500 mg IM in ROQ [right outer quadrant] of buttock, for respiratory tract infection.
Brooke Thomas, CMA

Intramuscular Z-Tract Technique

The alternate intramuscular injection technique is called the Z-tract technique. It may be used for medications such as Imferon, which may cause irritation of subcutaneous tissue and discoloration from leaking medications, or when complete absorption of the medication by the muscle is crucial. The preferred site for this technique is the upper outer quadrant of the buttock.

In this technique the tissue is pulled down and toward the median before, during, and after the injection. When the tissue is released the needle track that is created is a Z pattern rather than the straight needle track that is created in other intramuscular injections. The Z pattern tract keeps the medication deep in the muscle and prevents seepage up through the tissues.

Use a 2-inch needle if the patient weighs approximately 200 pounds. If you do not use a needle this long on a patient of this weight, you will need to insert the needle its full length and then indent the tissue with the hub of the needle to ensure deep muscle penetration.

Use a 1¼- to 1½-inch needle if the patient weighs around 100 lb. Use a ¾- to 1-inch needle on children weighing around 50 lb.

Follow Steps 1 through 11 as outlined on pp. 473-475, under "Administration of an Intramuscular Injection," with the **exception** that you should change needles after you have drawn the medication into the syringe. This eliminates the chance of medication left in the needle leaking into the tissue during the injection or of an extra "needle's worth" of medication being given. This minute extra amount of drug is of less concern with adult patients than it is with children for whom even minute quantities of drug may be significant. Now proceed as follows:

Procedure	*Rationale*
12. Move the skin downward and toward the median.	The skin and subcutaneous tissue of an average adult will move about 1 to 1.6 inches. The underlying muscle within the selected injection site remains stationary.
13. Insert the needle at a 90-degree angle while maintaining traction on the tissue.	
14. Extend the thumb and index finger of the hand that is displacing the tissue to support the base of the syringe and aspirate by pulling back on the plunger using your other hand. Maintain traction on the tissue. If blood appears, select a new site and use a new needle.	You may damage subcutaneous tissue and cause pain if traction is released while the needle is in place.
15. Inject slowly and smoothly while maintaining traction on the tissue.	
16. Wait 10 seconds, then withdraw the needle and immediately release the skin, creating a Z pattern, which blocks any infiltration of the medication into the subcutaneous tissue.	Waiting provides time for the medication to disperse into the muscle and gives the muscle time to relax.
17. DO NOT MASSAGE THE INJECTION SITE. If bleeding occurs, gently wipe the area with a dry sterile cotton ball or gauze.	
18. Advise the patient not to exercise or wear tight clothing immediately after the injection.	This will minimize the chance of the medication spreading into other layers of tissue.
19. Continue with Steps 19 through 24 under the procedure "Administration of an Intramuscular Injection."	

If a metal syringe and medication in a prefilled sterile cartridge-needle unit are used, the method for giving the medication is basically the same as when using a disposable or reusable syringe. After use, you should clean the metal syringe with an antiseptic solution. Sterilization is not required, as the syringe does not come in direct contact with the patient.

Administration of a Subcutaneous Injection

Equipment

Sterile needle and syringe; usually a 2, 2½, or 3 cc syringe, ½- or ⅝-inch, 25-gauge needle
Sterile alcohol sponges
Medication ordered
Small tray to transport prepared medication to the patient

Preparation of the needle, syringe, and medication follows the same procedure that was outlined under Administration of an Intramuscular Injection. Remember to wash your hands before beginning the procedure, check the medication label three times, measure dosage accurately, identify your patient and explain the procedure, position the patient, and select injection site correctly before administering the medication. Follow Steps 1 through 11 as outlined under the intramuscular injection technique, then do the following.

Procedure

12. Grasp the skin surrounding the injection area between your thumb and index finger *or* spread the skin and hold it taut.

13. Hold the barrel of the syringe between your thumb and other fingers of your dominant hand, letting the hub of the needle rest on your index finger. The bevel of the needle should be facing upward.
14. Insert the needle at a 45-degree angle into the skin using a quick, forward thrust (Figure 23.18).

Rationale

The decision of which method to use will depend on the size of the patient and the size of the needle. Grasping the skin may be done on small, very thin, or dehydrated patients; spreading the skin may be used on large, well-nourished patients. Whichever method you use, be sure that you enter subcutaneous tissue when inserting the needle.

The needle should be inserted almost to its full length. Do not touch the skin with the hub of the needle.

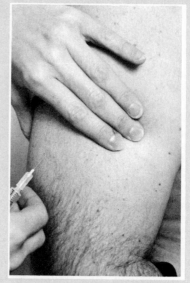

Figure 23.18
Technique for administering a subcutaneous injection. Insert needle at a 45-degree angle.

15. Release the skin.
16. Keep your dominant hand on the syringe for support. With your other hand, pull back on the plunger to see if you aspirate any blood.
17. Inject the medication slowly.
18. With an alcohol sponge, apply pressure to the injection site, and quickly remove the needle.
19. Massage the injection site with the alcohol sponge, and observe the patient for any unusual reaction.
20. Leave the patient safe and comfortable, providing any further instructions.
21. Remove and dispose of used equipment properly.
22. Wash your hands. See no. 22, p. 476.
23. Record the procedure on the patient's chart.

Refer to Steps 15 through 22 as outlined in the procedure for administering an intramuscular injection for full explanations of the remaining steps.

See no. 22, p. 476.

Charting example:
   June 2, 19_____, 2 PM
     Thiomerin [a diuretic] 1 ml, sc in left upper arm.
      Kathy Kron, CMA

Administration of an Intradermal Injection

Equipment

Alcohol sponge or skin antiseptic and cotton ball
Tuberculin syringe, as fine calibrations are needed (0.5 or 1.0 ml)
Needle ⅜- or ½-inch, 26- or 27-gauge (See Figure 23.6)
Solution to be injected
Commercial trays of prepackaged sterile syringes are available for intradermal allergy tests (Figure 23.19)

Procedure

1. Wash your hands.

2. Assemble the equipment.
3. Prepare the syringe and needle for use.
4. Compare the physician's order with the medication label.
5. Check the medication label three times during preparation.
6. Cleanse the vial rubber stopper, insert the needle, and withdraw the needed amount of solution into the syringe.
7. Identify the patient, and explain the procedure.
8. Select the injection site, and position the patient comfortably.

9. Cleanse the injection site with the alcohol sponge and allow to dry.
10. Remove the needle cover.
11. Expel air bubbles from syringe.
12. Stand in front of the patient. With your nondominant hand, grasp the middle of the patient's forearm on the posterior side, and pull the anterior skin taut.

Rationale

Steps 1 through 11 listed here correspond to Steps 1 to 11 under intramuscular injection technique, pp. 473-475.

For intradermal injections, the dorsal surface of the forearm, about 4 inches below the elbow, is used. For patients over 60 years of age, loss of skin turgor in this area can contribute to bruising or to extravasation of the testing solution. To prevent these problems, inject the solution into the area over the trapezius muscle (on the back), just below the acromial process.

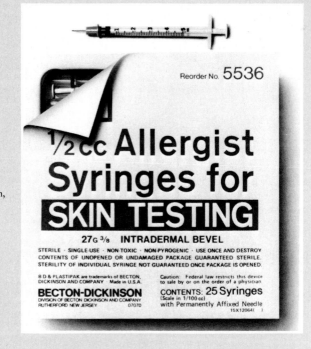

Figure 23.19
Prepackaged tray of sterile intradermal syringes for allergy testing.
Courtesy Becton-Dickinson, Div of Becton, Dickinson and Co, Rutherford, NJ.

Continued.

Administration of an Intradermal Injection—cont'd

Procedure

13. Hold the barrel of the syringe between your thumb and other fingers of your dominant hand; have the bevel of the needle facing upward.
14. Insert the needle into the skin at a 10- to 15-degree angle (Figure 23.20; see also Figure 23.13).

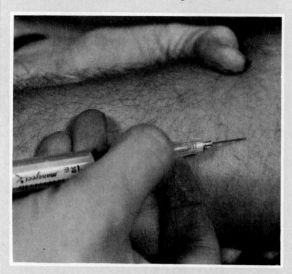

Rationale

The angle used to insert the needle is almost parallel to the skin. The point of the needle is inserted into the most superficial layers of the skin.

Figure 23.20
Administering intradermal injection at 10- to 15-degree angle.

15. Inject the solution slowly. NOTE: This type of injection does not require aspiration before the solution is injected.

As the drug is injected, a small pale bump will rise over the point of the needle in the skin. If the injection is given subcutaneously (that is, no bump forms), or if a significant part of the solution leaks from the injection site, the test should be repeated immediately at another site that is at least 2 inches (5 cm) away.

16. Withdraw the needle, and wipe the injection site very gently with the alcohol sponge.
17. Observe the patient for any unusual reaction, such as general febrile reaction, faint feeling, and shock.
18. Position the patient for safety and comfort, and provide further instructions.
19. Tell the patient when the test results will be read. Schedule a future appointment when necessary. The patient may be dismissed if the results are not to be read until a day or two later. If the test result is to be determined within the next half hour or so, let the patient rest comfortably and safely.
20. Remove and dispose of the used syringe and needle correctly.

Do *not* apply pressure or massage the skin. The medication is *not* to be dispersed into the underlying tissues.

Have the patient lie down if feeling faint, or sit for a few minutes to ensure that no unusual reaction will occur.
The skin reaction is read at various times, depending on the test done. Check with the physician or the literature that accompanies the drug used. Most allergy skin tests will be read within 20 to 30 minutes; the Mantoux test for tuberculosis will be read within 48 to 72 hours, and other tests at varying times within 48 hours.
Place a disposable syringe and needle in the puncture-resistant, disposable container without breaking or recapping the needle (see no. 22, p. 476). Reusable syringes and needles should be flushed with water, then separated and placed in a designated cleaning solution until prepared for sterilization (see Chapter 20).

21. Wash your hands.
22. Record the procedure on the patient's chart.

23. Read the skin reaction.

24. Record the reaction on the patient's chart.

When several skin tests are given, record the site of each injection with the name of the substance injected. This avoids confusion when the results are read.
Many tests are read as either positive or negative depending on the amount of redness (erythema) or hardening (induration). For some tests the areas of redness or induration must be measured in millimeters. Follow the directions provided with the test solution.
Charting example:
August 5, 19_____, 4 PM
Reaction of Mantoux test given August 3, 19_____,
4 PM is negative.
       M.E. Burgdorf, CMA

Conclusion

Having completed this chapter, you should be able to discuss the laws regulating the distribution and administration of medication, in addition to the responsibilities and rules governing the administration of all types of medication. Certain legal stipulations are set forth that a physician must meet before using narcotics. You should be familiar with the specific laws of your state of practice and know how you can best help your physician comply with the state and federal laws applying to the dispensing, administering, and prescribing of medications, including narcotics and controlled substances. Knowledge of and familiarity with resource reference books on drugs are required to ensure adequate knowledge of any medication you are required to administer. There are numerous references providing information on improved medication techniques and current pharmacological products. Check with your instructor for additional assignments and reference sources in areas of your own particular interest and need.

A variety of ways in which medications may be administered have been discussed in this chapter. You must be able to describe all nine routes of administration and demonstrate your ability to administer an intramuscular, a subcutaneous, and an intradermal injection. When you feel competent in this knowledge and these three techniques, arrange with your instructor to take a performance test. You will be expected to accurately demonstrate your ability to prepare for and administer subcutaneous, intramuscular, and intradermal injections to a patient, in addition to identifying the equipment used and the care of such equipment after use.

Review Questions

1. Explain what a drug is; list three uses for drugs and four sources from which drugs are derived.
2. Describe the difference between the trade name and the generic name of a drug and give two examples of each.
3. Describe the difference between the following three classifications of drugs:
   a. Controlled substances
   b. Prescription drugs
   c. Nonprescription drugs
4. List one use for each of the following:
   a. Analgesics
   b. Anticoagulants
   c. Antidotes
   d. Antiseptics
   e. Bronchodilators
   f. Diuretics
   g. Emetics
   h. Hemostatics
   i. Miotics
   j. Narcotics
   k. Tranquilizers
   l. Vasodilators.
5. Describe how and where medications should be stored.
6. When the label of a medication is torn and soiled so that the name of the drug cannot be clearly identified, what should you do with it?
7. List the information that must be kept on the office record for Schedule II controlled substances after they have been administered to a patient in the office.
8. Discuss at least 10 rules and responsibilities that you must be concerned with when administering medications.
9. The following orders have been written by the physician for patients. Using the abbreviation lists, transcribe these orders into English:
   a. Compazine 15 mg × 12 caps
      Sig i̅ cap po, tid, ac & hs, prn
   b. Digitoxin 0.1 mg × 30 tabs
      Sig i̅ tab po, od
   c. Digoxin 0.25 mg × 30 days
      Sig i̅ tab po, bid for 10 days, then ½ tab bid po for 10 days
   d. Benadryl 50 mg × 8 caps
      Sig i̅ cap po, qid for 2 d
   e. Dramamine 25 mg × 30 tabs
      Sig 25 mg, po, tid, ac, prn
   f. Vitamin B$_{12}$, 2 mcg, IM, qd
   g. Ampicillin 500 mg × 28 caps
      Sig 500 mg, po, q6h for 7 days
   h. Streptomycin 3 g, qd, IM for 7 days
10. Solve the following problems to determine the amount of drug that is to be administered:
    a. Give ASA gr 10 po; bottle reads 5 gr/tablet

b. Give Compazine 10 mg IM; ampule reads 5 mg/ml

c. Give digitoxin 0.4 mg po; bottle reads 0.2 mg/tablet

d. Give ascorbic acid 0.5 g po; bottle reads 500 mg/tablet

e. Give Kantrex 15 gr IM; bottle reads 1 g = 3 ml

f. Give Maalox 1 ounce. How many ml do you give?

g. Give tetracycline 500 mg, po; bottle reads 250 mg/capsule

h. Give Valium 5 mg po; bottle reads 10 mg/tablet

SUGGESTED READINGS

Asperheim M: Pharmacology for practical nurses, ed 4, Philadelphia, 1975, WB Saunders Co.

Lambert M: Drug and diet interactions, Am J Nurs 75:402, March 1975.

Lang S, Zawacki A, and Johnson J: Reducing discomfort from IM injections, Am J Nurs 76:800, May 1976.

Chapter 24

Laboratory Orientation

- The typical laboratory
- Liaison of the medical assistant with laboratories
- Diagnostic and therapeutic procedures
- The microscope
- Centrifuges

Objectives

On completion of Chapter 24 the medical assistant student should be able to:

1 State the importance of the information gathered from clinical laboratory tests.

2 State the reason why most laboratory tests are performed in a commercial clinical laboratory rather than in a physician's office or health care agency.

3 List six types of workers in a clinical laboratory, indicating the basic functions or responsibilities of each.

4 List six specialized departments common to all clinical laboratories and describe the function of each department.

5 List five additional special departments that may be part of some clinical laboratories and describe the function of each department.

6 Discuss the medical assistant's responsibilities when dealing with a clinical laboratory.

7 List seven items that are to be included on a laboratory requisition that accompanies a specimen to the laboratory.

8 Discuss the organization of diagnostic reports that are to be placed in the patient's chart.

9 Demonstrate proficiency in using a microscope.

10 Identify the parts of a microscope.

11 Demonstrate proficiency in using a clinical centrifuge.

Vocabulary

Vocabulary terms are presented in the specific sections to which they apply throughout this chapter.

Medical practice is based on information obtained from various sources. Chapter 18 discussed information obtained from a patient history and from a general or specific physical examination. Another important source of information to help diagnose and treat disease processes is gathered from clinical laboratory tests. It is important to remember that the physician evaluates all data gathered before a diagnosis is made or treatment initiated. Commonly, information from a combination of sources is required, as one source may not be sufficient. Repeat tests may be needed to confirm initial findings and establish the progress of a disease process or the elimination of it.

Scientific and technological discoveries have aided medicine tremendously by making accessible abundant data on numerous types of body specimens with a speed and accuracy that previously were not available. Laboratory medicine can determine changes in the chemical or physical characteristics of body fluids, excretions, and tissues, and in turn reflect changes in the anatomy and physiology of various organs. Changes noted may indicate a disease process at the site from which the specimen was obtained: for example, a wound culture may identify the presence of bacteria and an infectious process. At other times, the changes in the characteristics of the specimen may indicate a disease process in another part of the body: for example, the presence of excessive sugar in the urine may indicate diabetes mellitus, a disorder in carbohydrate metabolism, and not a disorder of the urinary system; elevated levels of certain blood enzymes may indicate a heart attack or a liver disease.

Thus with laboratory techniques specific data concerning the status of certain body functions and conditions may be determined. Normal values for the physical and chemical characteristics of body substances have been predetermined; each technique used has its own normal value ratio. Deviations from these set norms aid in the diagnosis and treatment of abnormal disturbances in body function and structure.

THE TYPICAL LABORATORY

Initially, many clinical laboratory procedures were performed in the physician's office. Over the years, as numerous tests were developed that were more time-consuming and required more specialized equipment, specially trained personnel became necessary. As a result, most laboratory procedures were transferred from the physician's office to a hospital or a private or public health department laboratory. Many physicians' offices still perform very basic routine tests but find it more economical, efficient, and accurate to have most tests performed by the trained personnel of a larger clinical laboratory.

There are various types of workers in a clinical laboratory. These may include a physician who is certified as a pathologist acting as the director of the laboratory; medical technologists, who are trained at a college for 4 years and are able to perform specialized tests; medical technicians, trained for 2 years at a junior or community college, who assist and perform tests under the supervision of the medical techonologist. A cytotechnologist, trained for 2 years at a college, is a highly specialized worker who examines cells and tissues microscopically for the presence of cancer. A histological technician, trained for 1 or 2 years in a technical training program, is also a specialized worker who is involved with the preparation of various types of tissues for microscopic examinations performed by the pathologist. The clinical laboratory assistant, usually trained at a technical level or below that of a 2-year college program, performs basic and routine tests under the direct supervision of the medical technologist or the director of the laboratory. Frequently, medical technologists become specialized in one or two fields in the clinical laboratory and devote all their working time to the area of their expertise.

All clinical laboratories have certain specialized departments in common. They are divided into areas based on function and types of tests performed. These areas usually include hematology, urinalysis, serology, blood banking, medical microbiology, and clinical chemistry. Parasitology and examination of feces may be special departments or they may be included in one of the other departments. Some laboratories may also have special areas for histology, mycology, immunochemistry, and cytology.

Hematology deals with the study of blood. Examination for the total cell number, the types and number of different cells, cell morphology (shape and size), and the important aspects of the functions of blood in addition to coagulation studies are all part of hematology.

Urinalysis deals with the examination of the physical, chemical, and microscopic properties of urine.

Serology involves laboratory tests that examine blood serum. Reactions involving antibodies and antigens are observed and used to determine various types of infections, such as tests for infectious mononucleosis. The tests for pregnancy and syphilis are also serology tests, as they involve immunological reactions.

Blood banking deals with the processing of blood and blood products that will be used for transfusions. It is also known as immunohematology because antigen-antibody reactions are involved in the typing of blood.

Medical microbiology deals with isolation and culture, microscopic identification, and biochemical tests to detect microorganisms that cause disease. Depending on the classification of the microorganism under investigation, the field of medical microbiology is generally divided into areas of specialization that include the following:

bacteriology (bak-te″-re-ol′o-je) The study of bacteria.
virology (vi-rol′o-je) The study of viruses.
mycology (mĭ-kol′o-je) The study of fungi.
rickettsiology (rĭ-ket″sĭ-ol′o-je) The study of rickettsiae.
protozoology (pro″to-zo-ol′o-je) The study of protozoa, the simplest forms of animals.
phycology (fi-kol′o-je) The study of algae.
parasitology (par″-ah-si-tol′o-jē) The study of parasites. These may be protozoans or even larger organisms that have microscopic stages in their development.

Parasitology may be an area apart from microbiology. Stool and blood specimens are examined for the presence of eggs or parts of a variety of roundworms, tapeworms, and flukes.

Clinical chemistry examines body fluids, such as blood, urine, and cerebrospinal fluid, for any change in their chemical content. Glucose and electrolyte levels are determined, as well as the presence of uric acid or urea in the urine or blood.

Histology involves the study of specimens of tissue from any source in the body. Form and structural changes are observed microscopically.

Immunochemistry is the study of the chemistry involved with immunity.

Cytology involves the microscopic study of cells shed from a body surface to detect any malignant change.

Cost Containment

Cost containment is a factor that must be considered when ordering or performing laboratory tests. Generally speaking, it is less expensive for the patient if simple routine laboratory tests are performed in the physician's office or health care agency. There are two reasons for this. First, you can collect and perform simple laboratory tests with relative ease on samples collected at the time the patient is at your facility. Second, the physician or health care agency can avoid the costs of extensive laboratory equipment and the high salary of laboratory technicians or technologists. The next less expensive situation for patients is when you obtain the sample in your facility and forward it to a commercial laboratory or when you refer patients directly to a commercial laboratory to have

the test performed. The larger the laboratory or organization, the less expensive the procedure is for the patient, because large laboratories perform tests on a large volume of samples using more sophisticated equipment. The specialized instruments available in large laboratories can perform multiple tests at the same time, thereby reducing the cost to each patient. The most expensive situation for patients is when you refer them to a hospital laboratory to have the required test performed. This cost results from the general high cost of operating a hospital, which must be shared by all departments. An example to illustrate this follows. When a laboratory test is performed in the physician's office or in a health care agency, it may cost the patient $10. When the same test is performed at a commercial clinical laboratory it may cost the patient $12, and when the test is performed at a hospital laboratory it may cost $17. Thus when laboratory tests other than the very simple procedures that you can easily perform in your facility are ordered, it is suggested that you refer patients to a commercial laboratory that is qualified and with which you have established a business relationship. This is the most cost-efficient procedure to follow.

LIAISON OF THE MEDICAL ASSISTANT WITH LABORATORIES

Because the information obtained from laboratory tests is a very important source of data for the physician when treating a patient, the medical assistant must have an understanding of and establish a good communication with this branch of clinical medicine.

The medical assistant has certain responsibilities when dealing with a laboratory. These include a basic knowledge of the various tests available, proper collection and handling of specimens that are to be forwarded to a laboratory, instructions to the patient when preparing for certain tests (see Chapters 22 and 26), and the handling of completed reports as they return to the office. To help prevent errors, good communication between all parties involved is vital. When you are not sure of the procedure for collecting or handling a specimen or what instructions are to be given to the patient, never hesitate to contact the laboratory for this information. By doing this, you avoid errors and inconveniencing the patient, who would have to return to give another specimen if the initial procedure was performed incorrectly.

Correct labeling of the specimen and completion

of the laboratory requisition are other important responsibilities of the medical assistant. The container in which the specimen has been collected should always be labeled with the date, the patient's name, and the source of the specimen. The items to be included on the laboratory requisition that accompanies the specimen include the following:

- The patient's full name, age, sex, and address;
- The physician's full name (also address when sending specimens to outside laboratories);
- Date the specimen was collected; date the specimen was sent to the laboratory if this differs from the date of collection; time the specimen was collected;
- Source of the specimen;
- Test(s) requested;
- Possible diagnosis when feasible, as this will alert the laboratory for specifics to watch for; and
- Medications or treatments the patient is receiving that may interfere with test results.

Most laboratories will provide specific requisitions for the various types of tests that will be performed in different areas of the laboratory (see sample requisitions in Chapters 22 and 26). Be certain that you use the correct requisition for the test(s) requested on the specimen. EXAMPLES: A blood specimen will be sent to the hematology department when a complete blood count is ordered; therefore you must complete the hematology laboratory requisition. A cytology requisition is sent with a cervical smear for a Pap test.

Medical assistants should know the normal ranges of test results so that when abnormal results are reported, they can be brought to the physician's attention immediately. Depending on the office or health agency's policies, you may circle or underline abnormal results in red. This helps to bring it to the physician's attention quickly. Commonly, physicians will sign or put a check on a laboratory report after reviewing it. This gives you an indication that it may be filed in the patient's chart. Never file a report before it has been reviewed by the physician. To hasten the physician's awareness of abnormal test results, many laboratories will report these by telephone immediately, then forward the written report later, signed by the laboratory worker who performed the test. Accuracy in reporting test results cannot be stressed enough, because commonly the diagnosis and treatment for a patient are contingent on these reports.

DIAGNOSTIC AND THERAPEUTIC PROCEDURES

Earlier in this book it was stated that the physician arrives at a diagnosis by employing and reviewing multiple factors and information obtained on the patient's condition; that is, the physician uses various studies to arrive at a diagnosis. Three reasons for diagnostic studies follow:

- To determine (diagnose) the condition from which the patient is suffering so that treatment, if feasible, may be initiated.
- To discover disease in its early stage before the patient experiences any signs or symptoms. This is called screening. Screening for disease often permits the cure of the disease, because treatment can be started in the early stages of the disease process (for example, cancer), or early treatment can delay the progression of the disease (for example, hypertension).
- To evaluate past or ongoing treatment received by the patient.

As the field of medical science continues to expand, newer and more accurate and sophisticated techniques are continually made available to help physicians diagnose disease processes. Diagnostic procedures and studies include but are not limited to physical examinations, surgical intervention, and laboratory technology. Other procedures used in diagnosing and treating disease processes require some elaboration. These involve the areas of radiology (roentgenology), the specialized field of nuclear medicine, physical medicine and physiotherapy, special skin tests, and electrocardiography.

To completely understand all these diagnostic and therapeutic procedures, special courses of study are necessary. Nevertheless, the following chapters give the medical assistant an exposure to various additional tests that the physician may order for a patient. (Physical examinations and minor surgery are discussed in preceding chapters of this book.) It is hoped that the descriptions of the following diagnostic and therapeutic studies and procedures will help the medical assistant understand the nature and purpose(s) of the numerous clinical entities available to health care practitioners for the treatment and care of patients.

Various studies, related vocabulary, and procedures are presented along with special patient preparation when it is required. It is important to remember that the medical assistant is not expected to also be a laboratory, x-ray, nuclear medicine, or electrocardiography technician or physical therapist but is expected to be familiar with the vocabulary and the nature and purpose(s) of diagnostic or therapeutic procedures and studies performed by these specialists. At times the medical assistant may be called on to assist with procedures performed by these medical specialties or to perform the more routine and simplified procedures, such as routine urinalysis, the application of heat or cold, and electrocardiograms. Additional medical assistant responsibilities may be to explain the nature and purpose of the procedure to the patient, to record the procedure on the patient's record, and to file or store the reports and films received after the test or treatment has been completed.

The next two chapters are devoted to information on urinalysis and hematology, because urine and blood, being the two most abundant body fluids, provide a wealth of information on the health status of an individual. Reference tables for various urine and blood tests with related information and the normal evaluation ranges for their results are also presented.

No attempt will be made in this book to give detailed instructions for the procedures involved in performing all of these laboratory tests, *as most must only be performed by certified laboratory personnel or physicians.* The purpose of the following information and Chapters 25 and 26 is to prepare the medical assistant for performing basic routine procedures that may be done in the physician's office or health care agency, and to make the medical assistant aware of some of the many laboratory tests, special equipment, and supplies that are available, along with the normal ranges for test results. The medical assistant is expected to know how to collect and handle specimens, the special instructions, when applicable, to give to the patient before the collection of a specimen, and the normal test results. By attaining this knowledge and these skills, patient care can be enhanced, and the medical assistant's value to the physician, patient, and laboratory is vastly increased.

The remainder of this chapter is devoted to a discussion on two major pieces of laboratory equipment, the microscope and centrifuge. The medical assistant should be familiar with this equipment if simple laboratory procedures are performed in the physician's office or health care agency and also when blood samples are to be prepared for transport to a commercial laboratory. It is suggested that the medical assistant also review

"Universal Blood and Body Substance Precautions" in Chapter 20, p. 344.

THE MICROSCOPE

The microscope (Figure 24.1) is a precise scientific instrument used in the laboratory when an enlarged image of a small (microscopic) object is required. When using the microscope, details of structure not otherwise distinguishable are revealed. Microscopes vary greatly in quality. For maximum efficiency the operation of a microscope must be studied carefully. Complete instructions for assembling and using the microscope are provided by each manufacturer. Read these instructions completely before you use the microscope for laboratory procedures.

Parts of the Microscope
Eyepieces

Eyepieces fit into the eyepiece tubes. The eyepieces in common use today are marked $5\times$, $6\times$, or $10\times$. The latter has the greatest magnifying power. Since the exterior surface of the eyepiece is exposed, it is likely to become dusty; therefore it should be carefully cleaned before use. This cleaning can be done with a special lens paper or with a very soft cloth.

Nosepiece and objectives

The microscope is provided with a revolving nosepiece into which the various objectives are screwed. Care must be used in properly attaching the objectives to the nosepiece. Follow the procedure provided by the manufacturer of the microscope. The objectives make up the lens system on the nosepiece. *Never* at any time force the objective or allow its lower end (the lens) to touch the metal stage. Lenses are very expensive and are easily damaged by contact with any other objects— slides, cover glasses, specimens.

Objectives have different magnifying powers. The following are in common use:
- The lowest power objective, marked 16 mm or $10\times$;
- The intermediate power, frequently called the high dry power, marked 4 mm, $43\times$, or $45\times$; and
- The highest power, the oil-immersion objective, marked 1.8 mm., $97\times$, or $100\times$.

In becoming familiar with the different objectives, remember that the low power is the shortest

Figure 24.1

A, Nikon Optiphot microscope. **B,** Nikon Labophot microscope.
Courtesy Nikon, Inc, Instrument Div Garden City, NY.

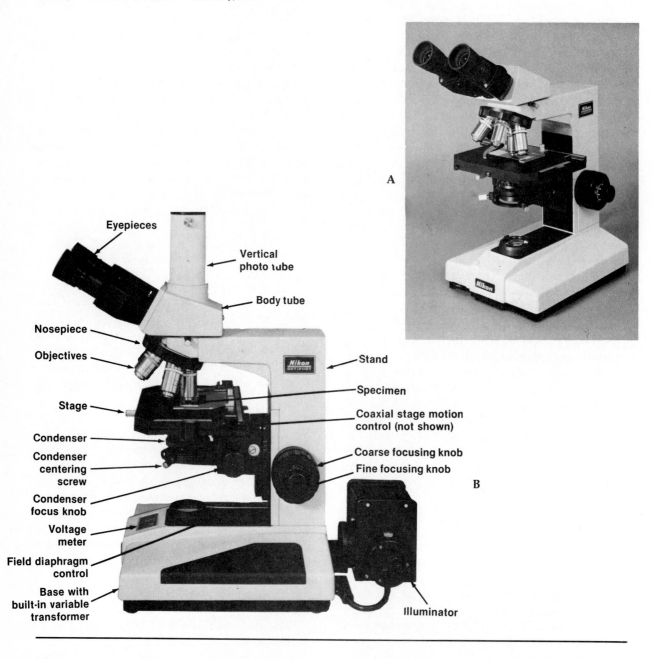

of the three objectives, whereas the oil immersion is the longest of the three. Another point of differentiation is the size of the opening in the smaller end of the objectives. The objective with the widest lens is the lowest power, and conversely the one with the smallest lens is the highest power, the oil-immersion lens. Some examples of magnification power are as follows.

Eyepiece	Objective	Magnification
5×	10×	50
10×	10×	100
5×	45×	225
10×	45×	450
5×	100×	500
10×	100×	1,000

Arm or stand

The arm or stand (Figure 24.1) is used for carrying the microscope. When carrying the microscope, place one hand on the arm and support the base of the microscope with your other hand.

Body tube

The body tube directs the path of light from the light source to the eyepieces.

Stage

The stage is the flat heavy part on which slides are placed for examination. On the stage are found two slide clips. In place of these clips, it is more convenient to apply an attachable mechanical stage, which is used to move the slides more precisely. This mechanical stage is almost indispensable in laboratory work, especially when the work requires high-power magnification.

Substage

Fitting into the opening on the stage, and immediately below it, is the substage. This part holds the substage condenser, a necessity in microscopic work. Its purpose is to condense the light upon the object under examination. For best results you should focus the proper amount of light onto the object by lowering and raising the substage by means of the pinion adjustment (or condenser focus knob). On the lower part of the substage will be found the shutter or diaphragm. This shutter is to close off light or to admit more light. Since the amount of light required varies, adjustment of the substage in connection with specific uses of the microscope will be described.

Other parts of the microscope

The *pinion head* or *coarse-focusing knob*, the larger one, is used for coarse adjustment of the microscope. The *fine-focusing knob*, the smaller one, is used in fine adjustment and focusing. These two knobs are very important because they must be used every time the instrument is used. When you are looking for the field, it is always necessary to lower the head of the microscope by means of the course adjustment. After this is accomplished, the fine adjustment is then used. This is absolutely essential when using high-power magnification. Another part is the *light source* or *illuminator*.

Care, Cautions, and Maintenance

1. When carrying the microscope, hold it by the arm with one hand, supporting the bottom of the microscope base with the other.

2. Handle the microscope gently, taking care to avoid sharp knocks.

3. Do not try to adjust the microscope yourself if you do not fully understand its mechanism. You may throw the instrument out of balance and adjustment or damage the lens by hitting it on the stage.

4. Never force the adjustment knobs if they do not turn easily. They may need oiling or simple adjustment.

5. Never force a high-powered objective on a microscope slide. Doing so may break the slide, scratch the objective, or damage the lens.

6. Be sure that the lens of the objective is clean before attempting to do microscopic work. Do not leave dust, dirt, or finger marks on the lens surfaces. To clean the lens surfaces, remove dust using a soft-hair brush or gauze. Only for removing finger marks or grease should a soft cotton cloth, lens tissue, or gauze lightly moistened with absolute alcohol (methanol or ethanol) be used. For cleaning the objectives and immersion oil, use only xylene. For cleaning the surface of the entrance lens of the eyepiece tube, use absolute alcohol. Observe sufficient caution in handling alcohol and xylene.

7. Avoid the use of any organic solvent (for example, thinner, ether, alcohol, or xylene) for cleaning the painted surfaces and plastic parts of the instrument.

8. Avoid the use of the microscope in a dusty place or where it is subject to vibrations or exposed to high temperatures, moisture, or direct sunlight.

9. Never attempt to dismantle the instrument, so as to avoid the possibility of impairing its operational efficiency and accuracy.

10. Attention must be given to protect the objective lenses. Never leave immersion oil on the objective when the instrument is not being used. Before you put the microscope away, rotate the nosepiece so that the low-power objective is in position.

11. Remove the eye lens at regular intervals to clean out the dust and dirt particles that may have collected there.

12. When the microscope is not in use, cover it with the accessory vinyl cover and store it in a place free from moisture and fungus. It is especially recommended that the objectives and eyepieces be kept in an airtight container containing desiccant.

13. Contact the salesperson for any serious problems you may have with the instrument.

Figure 24.2
Technologist using a microscope.

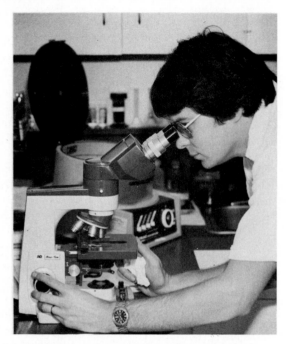

Space for Using the Microscope

The microscope should be kept set up and ready for use. However limited the office laboratory area is, sufficient space must be allotted exclusively for the use of the microscope. It need be no more than a shelf wide enough to accommodate the equipment. Added to this should be a convenient seat *of proper height.* A kitchen stool will suffice. Attempting work with the microscope handicapped by improper relationship between the height of the worktable and stool is fatiguing and may lead to unreliable work.

Use of the Microscope (Figure 24.2)

The material to be examined under the microscope will be placed on a glass slide. The slide is then placed on the microscope stage and fastened with the clips or held in place by the mechanical stage. Using the lowest power objective and a $10\times$ eyepiece, slowly lower the microscope head by using the coarse-focusing knob. When you find the field, adjust the light by raising or lowering the pinion attached to the substage. Next, open or close the diaphragm to admit just the proper amount of

light to give a clear, distinct field. To make the field of vision clear, use the fine-adjustment knob. From this point on, you can obtain a higher power of magnification by changing the objective.

Proper Adjustment of Illumination

The problem of obtaining maximum efficiency of illumination remains. Two factors enter into this problem: the light itself and the manipulation of the diaphragm, which controls the amount of light admitted to the condenser.

To know when the illumination has been properly adjusted, place a slide on the microscope and focus the low-power lens upon it. Remove the ocular and look down the tube of the microscope at the lenses of the objective. If shadows appear in this field, try to eliminate them by raising and lowering the condenser.

The most difficult part of illumination seems to be the proper manipulation of the iris diaphragm. Two cardinal principles should be remembered. *First,* the lower the power of the objective used, the more the light should be cut. In using the 16 mm lens to examine urine sediment or to count leukocytes, close the diaphragm almost completely; when the 4 mm objective is brought into play, the opening should be slightly increased; and when using the oil-immersion objective, the diaphragm may be opened wide. *Second,* the more brilliantly stained the object being viewed, the more light you can admit. As an example, if a differential blood count is being made with the 4 mm lens (the high dry power), the diaphragm may be at least half open, whereas during the examination of urinary sediment, especially if seeking hyaline casts, the light should be cut almost completely off. If this is not done, these hyaline structures will not be seen. *The diaphragm should be constantly adjusted while an examination is being made to get the most revealing picture. It is controlled by a little lever below the condenser. You should learn to seek this out and manipulate it subconsciously, as the fine adjustment is kept in constant use while focusing. If you are having trouble with an examination and things are not seen as clearly as they should be, examine the amount of light being admitted. The trouble is not infrequently caused by improper adjustment of the diaphragm.*

Focusing

In the microscopes illustrated in Figure 24.1, a coarse- and fine-adjustment control will be seen, the coarse adjustment being the larger knob and placed behind the smaller, which is for fine adjustment. The coarse adjustment is for finding the relative focus; the fine adjustment is for bringing out the details clearly. *Do not use these interchangeably.* Using the coarse adjustment for fine focusing will result in broken cover glasses and slides; *trying to find a field with the fine adjustment will place too much strain on it and quickly wear it out.*

Place a slide on the stage and bring the low or high, dry power objective down until it almost touches. Then, while looking into the microscope, slowly raise it with the coarse adjustment until the image is seen. Then, using the fine adjustment, bring out the details as described. It is a good plan never to turn the fine adjustment more than two thirds of one revolution. It is frequently desirable to keep the slide moving on the stage while attempting to focus. If this is not done, you may find that you are trying to focus on a spot where there is no material.

If it is found impossible to obtain a clear image although the illumination has been found satisfactory, the eyepiece should be rotated. If the blur is seen to rotate, the eyepiece is the source of the trouble. Remove it and wipe it thoroughly. The upper portion should be frequently cleaned, as it becomes soiled from contact with the eyelashes. In the event that the difficulty is not in the ocular, it is possible that the back of the objective has become fogged. This is not an infrequent occurrence if the instrument has been brought into a warm room from a cold one. Again, it is possible that the objective has been dipped into some fluid—immersion oil or water—and this has dried and caused fogging. Water can be removed with moistened lens tissue, and the lens can then be polished dry. If oil has dried on the lens, it must be cautiously removed with the smallest possible amount of xylene and the excess of this reagent wiped away with lens tissue.

Never focus down while looking through the microscope. This is inviting disaster to slides and cover glasses as well as possible damage to the lens. Observe from one side when you do focus down.

Use of Objectives

Of the three objectives, designated 16 mm, 4 mm, and 1.8 mm respectively, the 16 mm is the shortest in length and has the widest lens. The objective is used for low-power work, principally examining urine sediment, counting leukocytes, and inspecting the counting chamber of red cells for irregularity of distribution *(but only an expert should use it for counting these cells)*. The 4 mm lens, the high dry, is mostly used for close inspection of the urinary sediment, counting red blood cells, and making routine differential blood cell counts.

Always use a cover glass when using the high, dry power objective for examining urinary sediment. Do not dip the lens into the fluid without this protection. When using a 4 mm objective for differential blood counts, spread a thin film of immersion oil on the slide, over the stained blood, before making the examination.

The oil-immersion lens (1.8 mm) is used for obtaining the highest magnification in a conventional light microscope. Used with the eyepiece that gives a magnification of 10 diameters (marked 10×) the object as seen is about 1,000 times its actual size. To use this lens, place a drop of oil (such as Nujol) on the slide and focus down with coarse adjustment until the tip of the lens just touches the oil. Now, look through the microscope and focus upward very slowly with the coarse adjustment. When the object is seen, bring it into proper detail by use of the fine adjustment. This lens is used for all types of bacteriological work, for seeking malarial parasites, and for all other purposes demanding high magnification.

Practical Pointers for Microscope Use

If a single-tube microscope is used, learn to work with both eyes open. Squinting or closing one eye causes unnecessary strain. If much work is done, frequently shift from one eye to the other.

If you wear glasses, learn to do microscopy without them if possible. The instrument will focus to compensate for your visual defects if you are nearsighted or farsighted. On the other hand, if astigmatism is your difficulty, glasses will have to be worn, as this difficulty cannot be corrected by the microscopic lens.

CENTRIFUGES

Centrifuges are motorized devices that rotate at a high speed (Figures 24.3 and 24.4). The speed is stated as *revolutions per minute (rpm)*. Centrifuges are used to separate components of varying densities contained in liquids by spinning them at high speeds. Through centrifugal (moving away from a center) force, heavier or solid components move to the lower part of the container, and the lighter substances move to the upper part of the container. By

Figure 24.3
Centrifuge used for blood and urine separations.

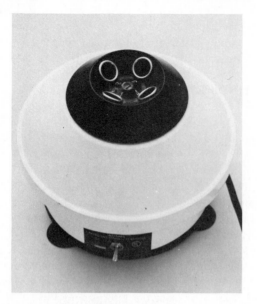

this process the two substances, solid material and fluid supernatant, are separated.

Centrifuges are used in every department of a clinical laboratory. In a physician's office or health care agency, centrifuges will be used if a microscopic analysis of urine is performed and also when serum is required for hematology or blood chemistry laboratory tests.

There are numerous types of centrifuges available. Each must be selected according to the intended use. Centrifuges commonly used in a physician's office or clinic are table models. One type is used for routine blood and urine separations (Figure 24.3), and another type is used for microhematocrit applications (Figure 24.4). The speed at which these centrifuges operate varies from 3,200 rpm for the routine blood and urine separations to 11,500 to 15,000 rpm for the microhematocrit centrifuges. Special centrifuge tubes should be used in the centrifuges for serum or urine separations. These tubes are either conical or round-bottomed in shape and made of a special quality glass. Some Vacutainer tubes used for blood collection may also be put into the centrifuge. Capillary tubes are

to be used in the microhematocrit centrifuges. It is important that you always use tubes that are the correct size and strength for the required application.

In the centrifuge there are special centrifuge cups with rubber cushions that are used to hold the tubes containing the blood or urine samples. Be certain that the cushions are at the bottom of the holders before you place the tubes into them.

Placement of Tubes in the Centrifuge

When you place a tube containing a specimen into the centrifuge you must counterbalance it with a tube of similar design and weight. This other tube must be placed directly opposite the tube containing the specimen and should contain a liquid of equal weight. Water can usually be used for this purpose. If you do not balance the load in a centrifuge, severe vibration of the centrifuge may occur and you may possibly lose the specimens. *Do not* use tubes that are cracked or badly scratched, because they may break under the stress of the centrifugal force. If breakage does occur, immediately turn the centrifuge off. Don rubber gloves and clean the centrifuge cushion and cup. You must clean these areas before using the centrifuge again to avoid additional breakage of tubes.

Operating the Centrifuge

When you operate the centrifuge you must close the cover. (Many newer models will not work if you do not close the cover.) If you are using an older model centrifuge, *do not* open the cover until the rotor has completely stopped. *Do not* brake sharply when using centrifuges that operate with hand brakes. Always use tubes that are the correct size and strength for the required application. Electrical appliances such as the centrifuge should have three-pronged grounding plugs, and there should be sufficient grounded outlets available. Frequent lubrication, calibration, and cleaning are required for the proper operation of all centrifuges. Specific instructions for operating each centrifuge are provided by the manufacturer. Read these instructions completely and carefully before you operate any centrifuge.

Figure 24.4
A and **B,** Centrifuges used for microhematocrit applications. **C,** View inside the
TRIAC centrifuge. Capillary tubes will be placed inside the numbered columns.
D, Enlargement of columns shown in **C.**

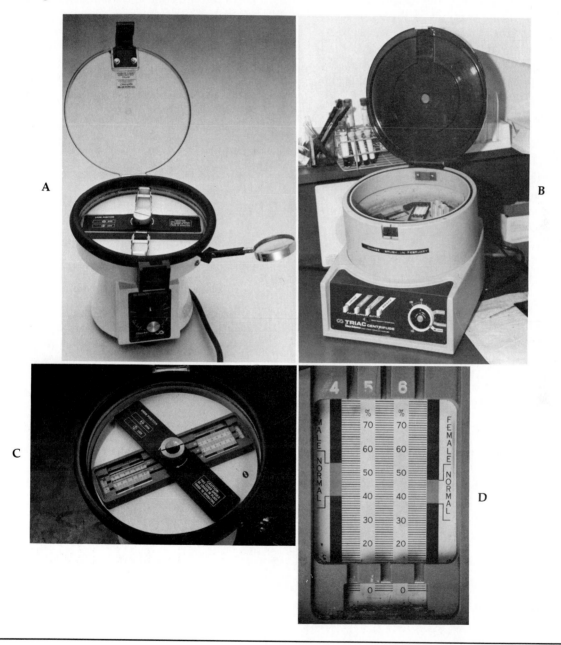

Conclusion

With the advances in the knowledge of physiology and improved technology, scientific diagnostic and therapeutic procedures have increasingly become valuable aids to the physician and the patient. From all the diagnostic and therapeutic procedures presented in the preceding chapters and Chapters 25 through 29, it can be readily seen that modern medicine offers many methods to physicians for arriving at a diagnosis and treating disease processes. The functional and structural alterations of body tissues, organs, and systems in disease can be studied and treated. Great strides have been made, and even greater achievements are expected as the mysteries of scientific research continue to unfold. At the opposite end of the spectrum from the concept of disease is health. For the body to remain healthy, the functions of the body systems must be normal. A primary requirement for survival of the human organism is the maintenance and safeguarding of the anatomical and physiological equilibrium of the individual cells that make up the sum of the body and its parts.

There are numerous sources you may refer to for expanding your knowledge on the topics discussed in the following chapters. Check with your instructor for additional enrichment assignments and references in areas of your own particular need and interest.

Review Questions

1. State the importance of the information gathered from clinical laboratory tests.
2. List six specialized departments common to all clinical laboratories. Describe the function of each department.
3. Describe the medical assistant's responsibilities in dealing with a commercial clinical laboratory.
4. List seven items that are to be included on a laboratory requisition that accompanies a specimen to the laboratory.
5. Define the following:
   a. Microscope
   b. Centrifuge
6. State how you should carry a microscope.
7. State what type of tubes should be used in a centrifuge.

SUGGESTED READINGS

Garb S: Laboratory tests in common use, ed 6, New York, 1976, Springer Publishing Co, Inc.

Lee LW: Elementary principles of laboratory instruments, ed 4, St Louis, 1978, The CV Mosby Co.

Wittman KS and Thomas JC: Medical laboratory skills, New York, 1977, McGraw-Hill Book Co.

Chapter 25

Urinalysis

- Urinary system—formation and components of normal urine
- Routine urinalysis

Objectives

On completion of Chapter 25 the medical assistant student should be able to:

1 Define and pronounce the vocabulary terms listed.

2 Briefly describe the formation of urine, list the main normal components of urine, and give a description of normal urine.

3 Define *routine urinalysis*, listing the three basic categories into which it is divided, along with the major observations and examinations made in each category; and list the fourth category of tests that may now be included in a routine urinalysis.

4 Identify normal and abnormal findings obtained on a complete urinalysis. Relate the abnormal findings to the most probable or possible causes.

5 Describe a reagent strip that is used for doing chemical tests on a urine specimen; explain how reagent tablets and strips are to be stored.

6 List the organized and unorganized sediment that may be present in a urine specimen, indicating if they are normal or abnormal findings.

7 Identify urine tests, other than those performed on a routine urinalysis.

8 Demonstrate the correct procedure for performing a physical and chemical analysis of a urine specimen and for preparing a urine specimen for a microscopic examination.

9 Demonstrate the correct procedure for testing a urine specimen for the presence of glucose, acetone, and bilirubin using the Clinitest, Acetest, and Ictotest reagent tablets.

10 Demonstrate the correct procedure for testing a urine specimen for the presence of glucose using the Tes-Tape.

11 Discuss the advantage and use of the Tek-Chek system.

Vocabulary

acetonuria (as″ĕ-tō-nu′rē-ah) or **ketonuria (kē″tō-nu′rē-ah)** The presence of acetone or ketone in the urine

albuminuria (al-bū″mi-nu′rē-ah) The presence of serum albumin in urine.

anuria (ah-nu′rē-ah) The absence of urine.

bacteriuria (bak-te″rē-u′rē-ah) The presence of bacteria in urine.

dysuria (dis-u′rē-ah) Painful or difficult urination.

glucosuria (gloo″kō-su′rē-ah) or **glycosuria (glī″kō-su′rē-ah)** Abnormally high sugar content in urine.

hematuria (hēm″ah-tu′rē-ah) The presence of blood in urine.

oliguria (ol″i-gu′re-ah) Scanty amounts of urine.

polyuria (pol″e-u′re′ah) Excessive excretion of urine.

proteinuria (pro″te-in u′re-ah) An abnormal increase of protein in urine.

pyuria (pi-u′re-ah) The presence of pus in urine.

qualitative tests Used for screening purposes. These tests provide an indication as to whether or not a substance is present in a specimen in abnormal quantities. A qualitative test does not determine the exact amount of a substance present in a specimen. Color charts are usually used to interpret qualitative tests. *Sometimes they are called semiquantitative tests.* Results are reported in terms such as trace, small amount, moderate, large amount, or 1+, 2+, 3+, and so on, or simply as positive or negative.

quantitative tests More precise tests. They determine accurately the amount of a specific substance that is present in a specimen. A high level of skill and sophisticated equipment are required to perform these tests. Results are reported in units such as grams (gm) per 100 milliliters (ml), or milligrams (mg) present, or milligrams per deciliter (dl).

URINARY SYSTEM—FORMATION AND COMPONENTS OF NORMAL URINE

The organs of the urinary system include the two kidneys, two ureters, one bladder, and one urethra. Urine is formed in the kidneys and passes through the ureters into the bladder, where it remains until the individual voids, and then it is excreted through the urethra. The kidneys, located in the retroperitoneal cavity (which means they lie behind the peritoneum), lie anterior and lateral to the twelfth thoracic and first three lumbar vertebrae; they are relatively small, approximately 4½ inches long, 2 inches wide, and 1¼ inches thick. Being highly complex and discriminatory organs, they help maintain the state of homeostasis in the internal environment by selectively excreting or reabsorbing various substances according to the needs of the body. You should recall from your studies in anatomy and physiology the nephron unit, which is the functional unit of the kidney. Each kidney has approximately 1,000,000 nephron units working together to selectively retain or excrete the substances passing through them. Blood, entering the kidneys by the way of the renal arteries, eventually reaches the nephron unit for this process to occur. Approximately 1,200 ml (30 ml = 1 ounce) of blood flows through the kidneys each minute. This represents about one fourth of the total blood volume in an adult. As blood enters the glomerulus of the nephron, water and the low molecular weight components of the plasma filter through to Bowman's capsule, then to Bowman's space, and on through the various parts of the tubules. It is in the tubules that reabsorption of some substances, secretion of others, and the concentration of the urine occur as a mechanism for conserving body water. Many components of the plasma filtrate, such as water, glucose, and amino acids, are partially or completely reabsorbed, and potassium, hydrogen ions, and other substances are secreted. On the average, nearly all the water that passes through this network is reabsorbed; approximately 1 liter (1,000 ml) or so is secreted as the largest component of urine (Figure 25.1). The main normal components of urine follow:

- Water—about 95% of urine is water;
- Nitrogenous waste substances of the organic compounds, that is, urea, uric acid, and creatinine;
- Mineral salts or the inorganic compounds, such as sodium chloride, sulfates, and phosphates of different kinds; and
- Pigment—derived from certain bile compounds, it gives color to the urine.

Many physiologic changes in the body can lead to an upset in the normal functions carried out by the kidneys. Urine, which is continuously formed in and excreted from the body, provides important information with regard to many diseases and disorders. Accordingly, it is widely studied as an aid

Figure 25.1

A, Coronal section through right kidney. **B,** Nephron unit with its blood vessels. Blood flows through nephron vessels as follows: intralobular artery → afferent arteriole → glomerulus → efferent arteriole → peritubular capillaries (around tubules) → venules → intralobular vein.
From Anthony CP and Thibodeau GA: Textbook of anatomy and physiology, ed 11, St Louis, 1983, The CV Mosby Co.

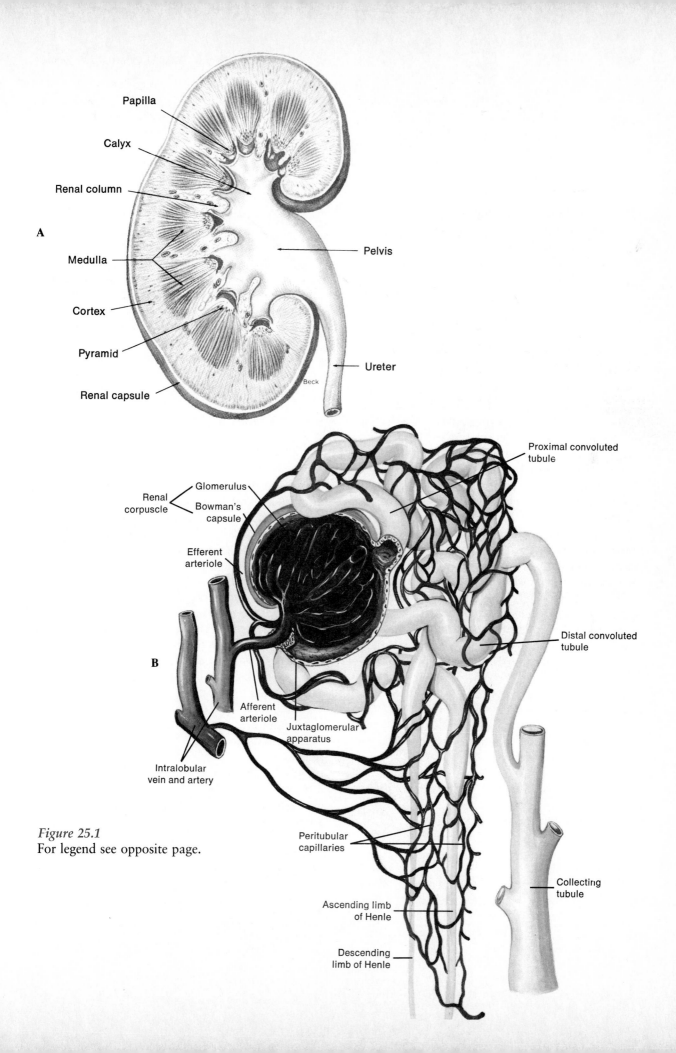

Papilla

Calyx

Renal column

A

Medulla

Cortex

Pyramid

Renal capsule

Beck

Pelvis

Ureter

Proximal convoluted
tubule

Renal
corpuscle

Glomerulus

Bowman's
capsule

Efferent
arteriole

Distal convoluted
tubule

B

Afferent
arteriole

Juxtaglomerular
apparatus

Intralobular
vein and artery

Peritubular
capillaries

Collecting
tubule

Ascending limb
of Henle

Descending
limb of Henle

Figure 25.1
For legend see opposite page.

in diagnosis, in monitoring the course of treatment of disease, and in providing a profile of the patient's health status. Urine has been referrred to as a mirror that reflects activities within the body and as such provides much varied information as a result of many chemical, physical, and microscopic measurements. The analysis of urine can provide information on the whole body as well as its many parts. Kidney disorders modify the composition of urine and may also affect many other body functions. The study of urine may also reflect the situation in which kidney function is normal but other parts of the body are functioning incorrectly.

ROUTINE URINALYSIS

A routine urinalysis, or basic urinalysis as it is often called, can be easily and quickly performed. It is a basic test, but it provides the physician with a tremendous amount of information when a disease process is present. This test can help confirm or rule out a suspected diagnosis. All patients having a physical examination or entering the hospital for treatment will have a urinalysis performed. It is a routine test for many patients seen in the physician's office or clinic and will be repeated annually or as frequently as is necessary to evaluate the patient's health status.

A routine urinalysis is divided into three basic categories, and a fourth category—detection and semiquantitation of bacteriuria—can now also be done easily in the microbiology and urinalysis laboratories. These categories and the major observations and examinations for each follow:

1. General physical characteristics and measurements
   a. Appearance
   b. Color
   c. Odor
   d. Quantity
   e. Specific gravity
2. Chemical examinations
   a. Reaction (pH)
   b. Protein
   c. Glucose
   d. Ketone
   e. Bilirubin
   f. Blood
   g. Nitrite
   h. Urobilinogen
   i. Special tests when indicated, such as for pregnancy, phenylketonuria, and porphyrinuria
3. Microscopic examination of centrifuged sediment
   a. Cells (epithelial, red blood cells, and white blood cells)
   b. Casts
   c. Bacteria
   d. Parasites and yeasts
   e. Spermatozoa
   f. Crystals
   g. Artifacts and contaminants
4. Detection and semiquantitation of bacteriuria
   a. Culture plate methods—require the special facilities and personnel of a microbiology laboratory; tests should be done immediately, or the specimen should be refrigerated and tested within 8 hours
   b. Nitrite test and culture strip methods—can now be done in the urinalysis laboratory
   c. Collect a clean-catch midstream specimen in a sterile container for these tests (See Chapter 22 for this procedure.)

Standard Procedures

A freshly voided random urine specimen is collected in a dry, clean container. (Review types of urine specimens outlined in Chapter 22, "Collection and Handling of Specimens," and also review Chapter 24, "Laboratory Orientation.") This specimen should be examined within 1 hour to avoid changes or deterioration to the contents. If the examination cannot be performed within this time, the specimen should be refrigerated at 41°F (5°C) to preserve the specimen.

When you are doing the examination, the first procedure is to note the physical characteristics of the urine; the second is to measure the specific gravity; the third is to perform the series of chemical tests; and the fourth is to prepare the specimen for the microscopic examination. This fourth step is accomplished by centrifuging 10 to 12 ml of a thoroughly mixed urine specimen. The residual sediment is then resuspended in 0.25 to 1 ml of urine on a slide for the microscopic examination. The remainder of the urine specimen should be kept until all the procedures are completed, in case any of the tests have to be repeated, or if other special tests have to be performed, when indicated.

Tests performed on a random specimen of urine are qualitative. Only the concentration of a substance in this particular specimen can be measured. The total amount of a substance excreted can be measured only when urine is collected over an accurately measured period of time, such as a 24-hour specimen.

General Physical Characteristics and Measurements
Appearance

The appearance is generally the first observation made on a urine specimen by virtue of just handling it.

Normal, fresh urine is usually transparent or clear. If the specimen is alkaline, it may appear white and cloudy because of the presence of carbonates and phosphates, but will clear when a small amount of acid is added to the urine. Urate crystals may be present in an acid urine, giving the specimen a pinkish, cloudy appearance, which usually clears on heating to 140°F (60°C). Both these appearances are normal.

Abnormal cloudiness in urine may be seen in patients who have a urinary tract infection. This may be caused by the presence of pus cells, leukocytes, and bacteria, or by the alkalinity of the urine. Also important to note when observing the appearance of urine is the presence of any sediment (solid particles) in the urine. When red blood cells, white blood cells, or casts are present in large amounts, this could indicate renal disease or bladder or urinary tract infection.

Color

Normal fresh urine color ranges are described as straw-colored, yellow, or amber, the result of the presence of the yellow pigment, urochrome. The concentration of normal urine determines the degree of the color: very concentrate urine is dark; dilute urine is pale. Various other factors affect the color of urine, for example, medications, dyes, blood, and food pigments. In many disease states, color changes are caused by the presence of pigments that normally do not appear.

Medications such as multivitamins may make the urine a very pronounced dark yellow; nitrofurantoin (Furadantin) (used in the treatment of urinary tract infections) may make the urine brown; and phenazopyridine (Pyridium) (an analgesic used for relief of pain, frequency, urgency, and other discomforts arising from irritation of the lower urinary tract mucosa) produces a reddish orange discoloration of the urine. The presence of hemoglobulin in the urine may make it reddish brown; bile pigments may turn urine yellow to yellow-brown or greenish. Melanins (dark pigments that occur abnormally in certain tumors), when excreted in urine, cause it to turn brown-black if left standing. If the patient is eating large amounts of carrots, the urine may turn a bright yellow. In hepatitis the urine may be a very pronounced orange (when the urine is shaken, even the bubbles will be orange if the patient has hepatitis). Also, when an individual eats a fair amount of rhubarb, the urine may be red to red-brown.

Odor

Normal urine has a characteristic aroma that is thought to be caused by the presence of certain acids. An ammoniacal odor will develop when urine is left standing for any length of time. This is caused by the decompression of urea in the specimen.

Urine containing acetone, as seen in patients with diabetes mellitus, may have a fruity odor. Urinary tract infections may cause the urine to be foul-smelling or putrid.

Although you will usually record the odor of urine when performing a routine analysis, it is generally thought to be of little significance in diagnosing a patient's condition.

Quantity

The normal quantity of urine voided by an adult in a 24-hour period varies somewhat, depending on the individual's fluid intake, the temperature and climate, the amount of fluid output through the intestines (as in diarrhea), and the amount of perspiration. The average quantity is about 1,500 ml and ranges from 750 to 2,000 ml. The quantity voided by children is somewhat smaller than the amounts excreted by adults, but the total volume is greater in proportion to body size.

To measure the quantity of urine, pour the specimen into a large graduated cylinder and record the quantity in cubic centimeters or milliliters. The amount recorded is reported as urine quantity per unit of time (usually 24 hours). Measuring the quantity of urine output is an important aid in diagnosing conditions or diseases related to polyuria, oliguria, or anuria.

Anuria is the absence of urine. At times it may be described as the dimunition of urine secretion to 100 ml or less in 24 hours. This may be seen in shock, severe dehydration, and urinary system disease.

Oliguria is the dimunition of urinary secretions to between 100 and 400 ml in 24 hours; more commonly defined as scanty amounts of urine. This is seen in drug poisoning, deep coma, and cardiac insufficiency and after profuse bleeding, vomiting, diarrhea, and perspiration. Oliguria is also present with decreased fluid intake and with an increased ingestion of salt.

Polyuria is an excessive excretion of urine. This

occurs in diabetes mellitus, diabetes insipidus, and chronic nephritis and following the ingestion of diuretic medications or an excessive amount of fluids. It also may be present during periods of anxiety or nervousness.

Dysuria is painful or difficult urination, symptomatic of many conditions such as cystitis, prolapse of the uterus, enlargement of the prostate, and urethritis.

Specific gravity

The specific gravity of urine is its weight compared with the universal standard weight of an equal mount of distilled water (expressed as 1.000). This measurement indicates the relative degree of concentration of dilution of the specimen, which in turn helps determine the kidney's ability to concentrate and dilute urine.

Normal specific gravity of urine is generally between 1.010 and 1.025, although it may range from 1.005 to 1.030, depending on the concentration of the urine. The first morning specimen has the highest specific gravity, generally being greater than 1.020. It will then vary throughout the day, depending largely on the individual's fluid intake.

Abnormally low specific gravity values may be seen in patients who have diabetes insipidus, pyelonephritis, glomerulonephritis, and various kidney anomalies. In these conditions, the kidneys have lost effective concentrating abilities.

Abnormally high values will be seen in patients with diabetes mellitus, congestive heart failure, hepatic disease, and adrenal insufficiency. The specific gravity will also be elevated when the patient has lost an excessive amount of water through the gastrointestinal tract, as with diarrhea and vomiting, or through the skin during excessive perspiration. High amounts of glucose and protein in the urine, as seen in patients with diabetes mellitus, will also increase this value.

There are several methods by which the specific gravity of urine can be measured. The newest and easiest method is by using one of three of the Ames Company's Multistix reagent strips. The strip is dipped into a urine specimen and then is compared with the color chart. The test strip will reflect specific gravity as it changes color from blue (low specific gravity) through shades of green to yellow (high specific gravity) (see also "Chemical Examinations of Urine Using Reagent Strips").

Specific gravity can also be measured by using a refractometer [Total Solids (TS) Meter], a delicate, hand-held instrument that requires calibration daily. Only one to two drops of urine are required when using this meter. *Wear disposable rubber gloves when performing this procedure.* The procedure for use is as follows (Figure 25.2):

1. Clean and dry the surface of the prism and cover, and close the cover.
2. Using an eye dropper, place a drop of urine at the notched end of the cover. The urine should be drawn over the prism by capillary action (Figure 25.2, *A*).
3. Pointing the meter toward a light source, rotate the eyepiece to focus on the calibrated scale. You will observe a light and a dark area (Figure 25.2, *B*).
4. Read the results on the specific gravity scale at the line that divides the light and dark areas (Figure 25.2, *C*).
5. Record the results.
6. Clean the prism with a damp cloth and then dry it.

The specific gravity of urine can also be determined by using a urinometer, a weighted, bulb-shaped instrument that has a stem with a scale calibrated from 1.000 to 1.040. The procedure for using the urinometer follows on p. 502.

The urinometer should be placed in distilled water and checked daily to test its reliability. If it does not read 1.000 when in the distilled water, the urinometer must be replaced. Also, if an unusually high reading is found when testing a urine specimen, remove the urinometer and rinse it under cool water to remove all urine residual; test in distilled water, and then retest the urine specimen. These extra steps are important in case someone had previously left an unclean urinometer, which would lead to abnormal testing results when used again.

Figure 25.2
Using a refractometer to determine the specific gravity of urine. **A,** Using eye
dropper, place drop of urine at the notched end of the cover. **B,** Point meter
toward light source, rotate eyepiece to focus on calibrated scale, and read results.
C, Read results on the specific gravity scale at the line that divides the light and
dark areas.

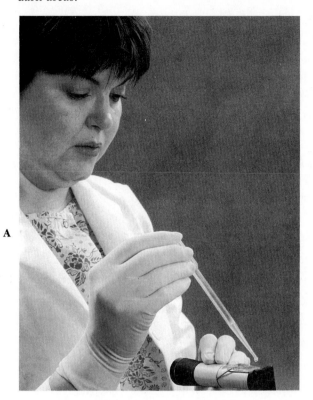

A

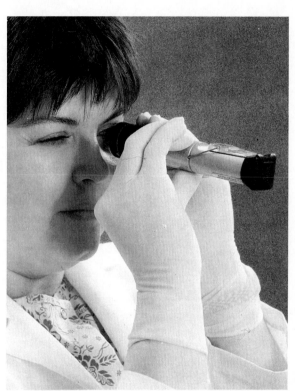

B

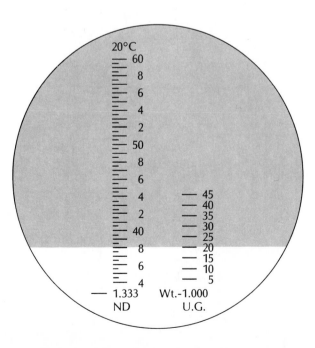

Procedure for Determining Specific Gravity (Figure 25.3)

Equipment

One 5-in—high glass cylinder

One urinometer (a weighted bulb-shaped instrument that has a stem with a scale calibrated from 1.000 to 1.040)

Figure 25.3

A, Items for determining the specific gravity of urine. **B,** Urinometer scale for determining specific gravity of urine. Specific gravity as shown would be 1.017. To read specific gravity, place the cylinder so that the lower line of the meniscus is at eye level.

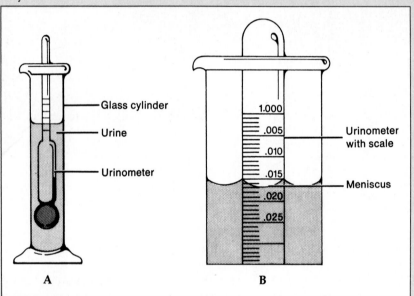

Procedure	Rationale
1 Wash your hands and assemble the equipment, then don disposable rubber gloves.	
2. Pour well-mixed urine into the cylinder to the three-quarter mark.	
3. Place the urinometer in the urine, and spin it gently.	The urinometer will float in the urine. When there is insufficient urine to float the urinometer, the specific gravity cannot be read. You would then simply record *quantity insufficient.*
4. Place the cylinder so that the lower line of the meniscus is at eye level.	The meniscus is a crescent-shaped structure appearing at the surface of a liquid column.
5. Read the specific gravity by noting the point at which the lower middle part of the meniscus crossed the urinometer scale.	
6. Record the reading.	
7. Discard the urine. Rinse the urinometer and cylinder with water. Wipe the urinometer dry before using it again.	
8. Remove gloves and wash your hands.	

Figure 25.4
Using a reagent strip. **A,** Dip test areas into urine. **B,** Remove immediately and
tap to remove excess urine. **C,** Comparing results of chemical analysis of urine
when using reagent strip.

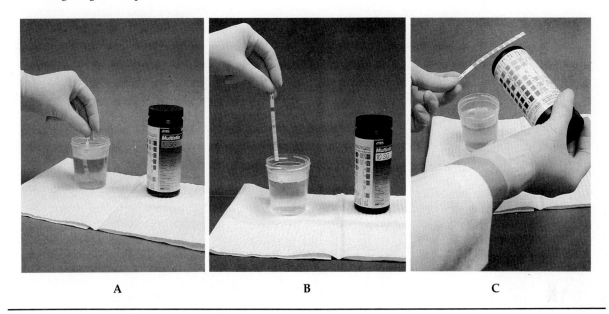

A   B   C

Chemical Examinations of Urine Using Reagent Strips

Chemically impregnated reagent strips have viru-
ally replaced older, more cumbersome methods for
performing a urinalysis. They provide an easy and
rapid method for obtaining the results of tests done
in a routine or basic urinalysis, thus are especially
practical and convenient for use in a physician's
office or clinic. In addition to these strips, other
special paper tapes, chemical tablets, selectively
treated slides, and simplified culture tests are available for special examination.

The pH of urine and several other components
can be easily and rapidly determined with the use
of a variety of specially prepared reagent strips and
a color chart. The reagent strip is a clear plastic
strip with up to ten pieces of colored filter paper
attached, each used to identify different components in the urine. Every piece of filter paper is impregnated with various chemicals and will change
color when dipped in the urine. Color changes on
the filter papers will depend on the presence and
amount of the substance that is being measured.
The most complete reagent strip is the Multistix 10
SG,* which is used for determining the pH, the
specific gravity, the presence and amount of urobil-

inogen, nitrite, blood, bilirubin, ketone, glucose,
protein, and the presence of intact and lysed leukocytes (white blood cells) in urine. There are various
other Multistix reagent strips available. The Multistix product name includes a number suffix that indicates the number of urine tests on the strip. In
addition, strips that test specific gravity have an SG
suffix.

Reagent strips are supplied in plastic bottles
containing 100 strips with directions for use. The
color chart and specified times used to read the results of the tests are presented on the sides of the
bottle. Both open and unopened product expiration dates are established for these strips to ensure
maximum product quality.

Since the pH of urine is usually determined as
part of a complete urinalysis, it is desirable to use a
multiple reagent strip such as the Multistix 10 SG,
which measures ten components of the urine; the
N-Multistix,* which measures eight components;
the Multistix,* which measures seven components;
the Labstix,* which measures five components; the
Hema-Combistix,* which measures four components; or the Combistix,* which measures three
components in the urine. All of these strips measure the pH as well as other components.

*Ames Co., Elkhart, Ind.

Figure 25.5

Multistix 10 SG chart used for determining amounts of ten factors when performing urinalysis.

Courtesy Ames Div, Miles Labs, Elkhart, Ind.

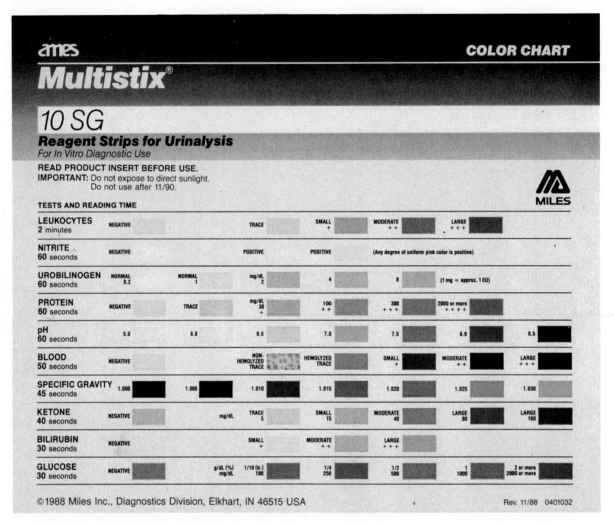

Procedure for using a reagent strip

1. Don disposable rubber gloves. Dip the test areas of the strip into a freshly voided urine specimen; remove immediately and tap to remove excess urine (Figure 25.4, *A* and *B*).
2. Compare the test areas to the appropriate color chart on the bottle at the specified times (Figure 25.4, *C*).
3. Record the results.

For best results, reading urine tests at the proper time is critical. Multistix reagent areas are designed to be read from the bottom up. After removing the Multistix 10 SG reagent strip from the urine, read the results at the following specified times (Figure 25.5):

- Glucose—read at 30 seconds;
- Bilirubin—read at 30 seconds;
- Ketone—read at 40 seconds;
- Specific gravity—read at 45 seconds;
- Blood—read at 50 seconds;
- pH—read at 60 seconds;
- Protein—read at 60 seconds;
- Urobilinogen—read at 60 seconds;
- Nitrite—read at 60 seconds; and
- Leukocytes—read at 2 minutes.

For screening positive from negative specimens only, all reagent areas except leukocytes may be read between 1 and 2 minutes.

The addition of a leukocyte test to dry reagent strips may reduce the need for microscopic analy-

Figure 25.6
Clinitek 10 urine chemistry analyzer. A semi-automated instrument designed to
read the reagent strip. Results show up on the display panel.

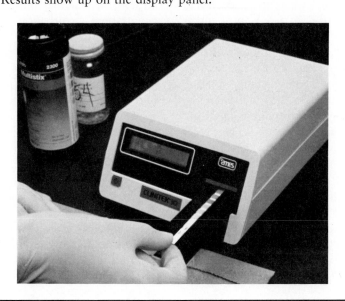

sis. Chemical testing for leukocyte esterase detects
lysed white blood cells that cannot be detected
microscopically. Since leukocyte esterase will be
present hours after sample colleciton, false nega-
tives are reduced.

Microscopic analysis of urine is not indicated
when negative findings are obtained by leukocytes,
nitrite, protein, and occult blood. Time-consuming
microscopics can be reduced to those specimens
where positive chemical results suggest that more
specific information is needed.

Urine Chemistry Analyzers for Use with Reagent Strips

The Ames Multistix reagent strips are also designed for use with instrumentation, such as with
the Ames Clinitek 200 urine chemistry analyzer for
moderate to large volume urine testing, or the
Clinitek 10 urine chemistry analyzer for small to
medium volume urine testing (Figure 25.6). These
instruments are demi-automated and are designed
to *read* the reagent strips. Readings are standardized for improved precision through the elimination of visual color discrepancies and operator and
environmental variables. Both of these analyzers
are very easy to use. Directions for use are supplied
with the instruments, and they must be followed
explicitly.

Clinitek 10

When the Clinitek 10 analyzer is turned on, the
feed table automatically moves out to the *load* position; then the instrument goes through a self-test
cycle. After this cycle is completed, the name of the
Ames strip programmed to read is displayed (see
Figure 25.6).

After properly immersing the reagent strip in
urine and removing the excess urine by blotting,
slide the strip onto the feed table, pad side up,
within 10 seconds after pressing the "Start" button. Be sure that the tip of the strip lies flat on the
table and is touching the end stop of the feed table
insert.

Record the test results shown on the display
panel; then remove and discard the used reagent
strip.

Significance of Test Results

Multistix 10 SG reagent strips may provide diagnostically useful information about the status of
carbohydrate metabolism, kidney and liver function, acid-base balance, bacteriuria-pyuria, and
many other conditions as follows:

Reaction (pH).   pH is the symbol for the hydro-
gen-ion concentration that expresses the degree of
acidity or alkalinity of a solution. The pH is measured on a scale ranging from 0 to 14, with 7 being

neutral; 0 to 7 is acidic, and 7 to 14 is alkaline. Usually freshly voided normal urine from patients on normal diets is acidic, having a pH of 6.0, although normal kidneys are capable of secreting urine that may vary in pH from 4.5 to slightly higher than 8.0.

Excessively acidic urine may be obtained from patients on a high-protein diet or who are taking certain medications such as vitamin C or ammonium chloride and from patients who are retaining a large amount of sodium. In the conditions of uncontrolled diabetes mellitus and acidosis, you will also find the patient's urine to be very acidic.

Alkaline urine is seen in patients who have ingested a large meal and in those who consume a diet high in milk and other dairy products, citrus fruits, and vegetables. Certain medications, such as sodium bicarbonate, will help produce alkaline urine. Urinary tract infections, specimens contaminated by bacteria, and specimens left standing for any length of time will also produce highly alkaline urine.

Protein. Normal urine may contain protein, mostly albumin, after exposure to cold, excessive muscular activity, or ingestion of large amounts of protein. *Albuminuria* (al-bu-mŭ-nu-re-ah) is the presence of serum ablumin or serum globulin in the urine. It is usually a sign of renal impairment; however, it can also occur in healthy individuals following vigorous exercise. *Proteinuria* (prō'te-in-u'rē-ah) is an abnormal increase of protein in the urine. This is an important indicator of renal disease. Also it is seen in congestive heart disease, constrictive pericarditis, multiple myeloma, and toxemia of pregnancy. Functional proteinuria is seen in fever, excessive exercise, emotional stress, exposure to heat or cold, and fad diets.

Glucose. Normal urine does not contain any detectable glucose unless the concentration of blood glucose exceeds 160 to 180 mg/100 ml; at that point, glucose begins to spill into the urine. *Glucosuria* (gloo'kō-su'rē-ah) or *glycosuria* (glī"kō-su'rē-ah) is abnormally high sugar content in the urine. The major cause of this is diabetes mellitus. Other common causes of glucosuria include an excessive carbohydrate intake, pain, excitement, liver damage, shock, and sometimes general anesthesia. Ingestion of large amounts of vitamin C may interfere with glucose testing and produce a false positive result.

Ketone. Normally, ketone bodies do not appear in urine unless the patient is on a carbohydrate-deficient diet or a diet that is very rich in fat content. *Acetonuria* (as"ĕ-tō-nu'rē-ah) or *ketonuria* (kē"tō-nu'rē-ah) is the presence of acetone or ketone bodies in the urine. This is an important symptom in diabetes mellitus. Ketonuria is also seen in patients whose carbohydrate intake is decreased, such as with fasting or anorexia, in gastrointestinal disturbances, and after general anesthesia.

Bilirubin. Normally, no bilirubin appears in the urine. *Bilirubinuria* (bĭl"ĭ-roo"bĭ-nu'rē-ah) is the presence of bilirubin in the urine. This occurs in liver disease, bile duct obstruction, and cancer of the head of the pancreas.

Blood. A few red blood cells noted in urine when examined under the microscope are normal. The Multistix 10 SG does not determine the number of red blood cells present, but provides an indication of the presence of occult blood conditions. *Hematuria* (hēm"ah'tu-rē-ah) is the presence of blood in the urine. The urine may be slightly blood-tinged, grossly bloody, or a smoky brown color. This is symptomatic of injury, disease, or calculi in the urinary system. Certain drugs, such as anticoagulants or sulfonamides, may also cause hematuria.

Nitrite. Normal urine should yield negative results for nitrite testing; a positive result is a reliable indication of significant bacteriuria. *Bacteriuria* (bak-te"rē-u'rē-ah) is the presence of bacteria in the urine. A positive nitrite test is indicative of a urinary tract infection.

Urobilinogen. Normal urine contains a small amount of urobilinogen. Biliary obstruction leads to the absence of urobilinogen in the urine; reduced amounts are seen during antibiotic therapy; and increased amounts of urobilinogen in the urine are present in liver tissue damage and in congestive heart failure.

Leukocytes. Positive results are clinically significant. Positive and repeat trace results indicate that further testing of the patient and/or sample is needed, according to the medically accepted procedures for pyuria (see also p. 514, "Significance of Microscopic Test Results").

Specific gravity. See p. 500.

Tests for Glucose, Acetone, and Bilirubin Using Chemical Reagent Tablets
Clinitest

When the presence of glucose is determined by using a reagent strip, a more quantitative determination may be required. This can be accomplished by using the Clinitest* reagent table 5-drop method

---

*Ames Co., Elkhart, Ind.

Figure 25.7
Clinitest procedure. **A,** Place 10 drops of water into test tube containing 5 drops
of urine. **B,** Add one Clinitest tablet to test tube. **C,** Compare contents in test
tube with color chart.

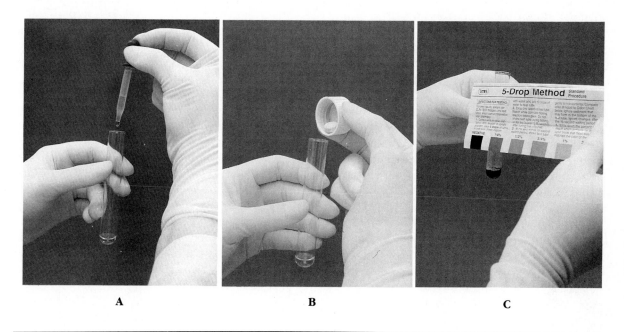

             A   **B**   **C**

(Figure 25.7). *Wear disposable rubber gloves when
doing this procedure.*

1. Place 5 drops of urine into a test tube.
2. Rinse dropper; add 10 drops of water to the
   test tube.
3. Add one Clinitest tablet to the test tube.
4. Wait 15 seconds while the spontaneous boiling occurs; this is the normal action seen
   when the tablet is added to the urine and water mixture. Do not touch the bottom of the
   test tube, as intense heat is generated during
   this reaction.
5. Once the boiling stops, shake the tube gently
   and compare the color of the contents with
   the color chart that accompanies the bottle
   of tablets. Do not wait longer than 15 seconds to compare the colors, as results seen
   after this period are invalid. There are six
   color blocks ranging from dark blue (indicating a negative reading) through green and
   tan up to orange, which is read as 2% or 4+,
   indicating the presence of large amounts of
   sugar. The results are interpreted and recorded as negative, trace, 1+, 2+, 3+, or
   4+, *or* 0%, ¼%, ½%, ¾%, 1%, or 2%.

Test result	Color change	Interpretation
Negative (0%)	Dark blue	No glucose present
Trace (¼%)	Green	250 mg/dl*
1+ (½%)	Olive green	500 mg/dl
2+ (¾%)	Greenish-brown	750 mg/dl
3+ (1%)	Tan	1000 mg/dl
4+ (2%)	Orange	2000 mg/dl

*1 deciliter (dl) = 100 milliliters (ml)

Observe the solution in the test tube carefully
during the reaction and the 15-second waiting period to detect rapid, pass-through color
changes caused by large amounts of sugar
(over 2%). Should the color *rapidly* pass
through green, tan, and orange to a dark
greenish brown, record as over 2% (4+)
sugar without comparing the final color development with the color chart.

6. Record the results.
   NOTE: The use of this method is not advisable
   for patients receiving the drugs nalidixic acid
   (NegGram), cephalothin (Keflin), cephalexin
   monohydrate (Keflex), cephaloridine (Lori-
   dine), probenecid (Benemid), or large

amounts of ascorbic acid, as they may cause a false positive. The preferred method in these situations is testing the urine by the Tes-Tape* method. This will be discussed later in this chapter.

A modification of the above standard (5-drop) procedure is the Clinitest reagent table 2-drop method, also used for quantitative determination of reducing sugars, generally glucose, in urine. Directions for use are identical to the standard procedure *except,* use 2 drops of urine and 10 drops of water. For this specific tablet, the results are identified by comparing the contents in the test tube with a color chart having seven color blocks ranging from dark blue through green and tan up to orange. The results are interpreted and recorded as 0, trace, ½%, 1%, 2%, 3%, or 5% or more.

Acetest

To detect the presence of acetone and acetoacetic acid in urine, you may use the Acetest* reagent tablet. *Wear disposable rubber gloves when performing this procedure.*

1. Place one tablet on a clean piece of paper, preferably white.
2. Place 1 drop of urine on the table.
3. At 30 seconds, compare the test results with the color chart. Colors will range from buff to lavender to purple. The four color blocks indicate negative, small, moderate, or large concentrations being present.
4. Record the results.

NOTE: This tablet may also be used to test serum, plasma, or whole blood. Serum or plasma ketone readings are made 2 minutes after application of the specimen to the tablet. When testing whole blood for ketones, apply the specimen to the tablet, wait 10 minutes, then remove clotted blood and read the results immediately.

Ictotest

To detect liver function, a simple test on urine to determine the presence of bilirubin may be done with the use of the Ictotest* reagent tablet. *Wear disposable rubber gloves when performing this procedure.*

*Ames Co., Elkhart, Ind.

1. Place 5 drops of urine on the piece of special mat that is provided with the tablets.
2. Place a tablet in the center of the wet area.
3. Put 2 drops of water onto the tablet.
4. Determine any color change on the mat around the tablet within 30 seconds, and compare with the color chart. The presence of a blue or purple color indicates a positive reaction.
5. Record the results.

Summary

These three reagent tablets and the reagent strips must be kept in the bottles in which they are supplied with the cap secured tightly. Exposure to the air or moisture for any length of time will cause them to deteriorate, and they would then be unfit to use for testing urine. Do not remove the desiccants from the bottles. Store at temperatures under 86°F (30°C). Do not store in a refrigerator. Do not use after the expiration date indicated on the bottle.

Controls for Routine Urinalysis

The various qualitative (or semiquantitative) tests for urinary pH, protein, blood, glucose, ketones, bilirubin, nitrite, urobilinogen, and specific gravity should be checked from time to time using solutions containing known quantities of these substances. A convenient quality control system to help determine if Ames urinalysis tests are properly performed and interpreted is available. This control system is called Tek-Chek. It is particularly valuable in instituting a quality control system or making an existing system more convenient by the use of ready-made controls. There are four different Tek-Chek packages, each consisting of four vials which provide different controls (results). When purchased, each package comes supplied with a summary of the Tek-Chek system, instructions for use, and the expected values that should be obtained when using the control vials. The boxed material on pp. 509-510 shows the table of expected values that should be obtained when using Tek-Chek #1—No. 1301, a summary of the system, and the instructions for use.

TEK-CHEK® Controls for Routine Urinalysis

Summary and explanation:

TEK-CHEK® Controls for Routine Urinalysis are lyophilized human urine specimens, designed for use with Ames Reagent Strip and Tablet Tests in routine urinalysis.

TEK-CHEK is reconstituted by the addition of 15 ml of water. Specific chemical additions are made to the pooled urines prior to lyophilization so that, when reconstituted, each of the two TEK-CHEK Control Urines will react to one or more of AMES Reagent Strips or Tablets to yield the results listed in the Table of Values in this insert. The bottles are designated as No. 1 and No. 4. TEK-CHEK No. 4 contains a combination of natural and artificial ingredients to give positive results with Ames products.

Major areas of use of TEK-CHEK Control Urines in a quality control program to upgrade urinalysis are,

Knowns:

1. For demonstration and teaching purposes.

2. To determine if the test reagents are reacting properly.

3. To confirm the user's ability to properly perform and reliably interpret the Ames tests.

Unknowns:

1. To develop proficiency in routine urinalysis performed in the laboratory, from sample handling through test procedures to reporting of results.

2. To provide confidence in obtaining good results in routine urinalysis.

Each laboratory should define its own standards of acceptable performance after a period of routine use of an established quality control program. Quality control has become an integral part of several sections of the clinical laboratory and should be more widely used in routine urinalysis.[1,2] Establishment of quality control programs as a means of helping to assure good results has been recommended by the accreditation groups involved with the Clinical Laboratories Improvement Act of 1967 and by scientific associations involved with clinical laboratory personnel such as the CAP, ASCP, AACC and ASMT.

Reagents:

TEK-CHEK Control Urines are of two kinds, each with specific characteristics. After reconstitution of the lyophilized material with 15 ml of water, results may be expected as follows:

TEK-CHEK 1: Normal urine with negative reactions for glucose, protein, ketone, bilirubin, occult blood, and nitrite, with normal urobilinogen, and defined pH and specific gravity.

TEK-CHEK 4: Composite positive with positive reactions for glucose, protein and occult blood; normal urobilinogen; negative ketone, bilirubin, and nitrite; and a defined pH and specific gravity.

Warnings and precautions:

TEK-CHEK Control Urines are for *in vitro* diagnostic use. Improper storage may cause TEK-CHEK to become darkened or discolored. Such material may give misleading results and should not be used.

Instructions for reconstitution:

Remove cap from vial, add 15 ml of water and swirl gently to reconstitute lyophilized urine. Do not shake solution as shaking will denature protein.

Storage:

TEK-CHEK 1 should be stored at temperatures under 30°C. TEK-CHEK 4 must be stored under refrigeration (2°-8°C). TEK-CHEK 1 and 4 must be used within the expiration date and are stable for 5 days after reconstitution if stored under refrigeration (2°-8°C). Allow to warm to room temperature before use. Do not mix controls or make any chemical additions. Chemical additions to reconstituted controls may seriously affect results due to chemical interference, dilution or both.

Procedure:

Each laboratory should define its own quality control program utilizing control urines in the routine urinalysis schedule. Controls should be used as knowns to check procedure and technique, to check product reactivity and for teaching and demonstration purposes. Unknowns should be hidden in each series of specimens and tested with the regular urine specimens, using the same reagents, personnel and handling procedure. A typical routine urinalysis quality control program has been described[1] as follows:

Quality Control Supervisor: 1.) Reconstitute one bottle of TEK-CHEK Urine Control #1 (negative) and one bottle of TEK-CHEK Urine Control #4 (composite positive). 2.) Place the negative and the composite positive control into the same type of urine specimen container used in the laboratory and place one or both of these controls as "hidden" specimens in each batch of specimens tested on all shifts. Retrieve controls before specimens are centrifuged for microscopic examination and reuse at random in each series making sure to check them each time to make sure no change in reactivity has occurred. 3.) At intervals during the day, or at the end of the day, tabulate the "hidden control" results obtained on a quality control chart which can be maintained a month at a time as charts are for blood chemistries.

Analyst: 1.) Test, as knowns, the negative specimen and the composite positive and record the results in the laboratory urinalysis record book as "tests on reference specimens." 2.) Record results on unknown or "hidden" specimens in the laboratory notebook and/or on the request slip as for any routine urine.

Results:

Results using TEK-CHEK Control Urines either as knowns or as hidden unknowns should be recorded in the same terms used for routine testing.

Expected Values: Table of Values

For use only with Control No. 2 <u>0001022</u>

Test	Expected Results with TEK-CHEK No. 3 <u>1301</u>	Ames Reagent Strips and/or Tablets
pH	5	COMBISTIX® HEMA-COMBISTIX®, LABSTIX®, BILI-LAB-STIX®, MULTISTIX®, N-MULTISTIX®, N-MULTISTIX®-C, MULTISTIX® SG, N-MULTISTIX® SG
Protein	NEGATIVE	ALBUSTIX®, URISTIX®, N-URISTIX,® COMBISTIX, HEMA-COMBISTIX, LABSTIX, BILI-LABSTIX, MULTISTIX, N-MULTI-STIX, N-MULTISTIX-C, MULTISTIX SG, N-MULTISTIX SG
	NEGATIVE	BUMINTEST®
Blood	NEGATIVE	HEMASTIX®, HEMA-COMBISTIX, LABSTIX, BILI-LABSTIX, MULTISTIX, N-MULTISTIX, N-MULTISTIX-C, MULTISTIX SG, N-MULTISTIX SG
Glucose	NEGATIVE	DIASTIX®, KETO-DIASTIX®, URISTIX, N-URISTIX, COMBIS-TIX, HEMA-COMBISTIX, LABSTIX, BILI-LABSTIX, MULTI-STIX, N-MULTISTIX, N-MULTISTIX-C, MULTISTIX SG, N-MULTISTIX SG
	NEGATIVE	CLINISTIX®
	NEGATIVE	CLINITEST®
Ketone	NEGATIVE	KETOSTIX®, KETO-DIASTIX, LABSTIX, BILI-LABSTIX, MUL-TISTIX, N-MULTISTIX, N-MULTISTIX-C, MULTISTIX SG, N-MULTISTIX SG
	NEGATIVE	ACETEST®
Bilirubin	NEGATIVE	BILI-LABSTIX, MULTISTIX, N-MULTISTIX, N-MULTISTIX-C, MULTISTIX SG, N-MULTISTIX SG
	NEGATIVE	ICOTEST®
Nitrite	NEGATIVE	N-URISTIX, MICROSTIX®-NITRITE, N-MULTISTIX, N-MUL-TISTIX-C, N-MULTISTIX SG
Phenylketones (PKU)	NEGATIVE	PHENISTIX®
Urobilinogen	0.1 to 1.0 EU/dl	UROBILISTIX®, MULTISTIX, N-MULTISTIX, N-MULTISTIX-C, MULTISTIX SG, N-MULTISTIX SG
Specific gravity*	1.015 to 1.020	MULTISTIX SG, N-MULTISTIX SG
	1.015	(T.S. Meter)

*Because of the manner in which TEK-CHEK 4 Control is processed and the constituents added to the Control, specific gravity values determined using Ames Reagents Strips are approximately 0.007 higher than values determined using the T. S. Meter. Equivalent results are obtained using both methods with TEK-CHEK 1.

Bibliography:

1. Free HM and Free AH: Quality control of urinalysis in large hospitals and small laboratories. In Aneido G, Van-Kampen EJ, and Rosalki SB, editors: Progress in quality control in clinical chemistry, Transactions of 5th International Symposium, Bern 1973, Hans Huber, p 332.
2. Becker ST, Ramirez G, Pribor H, and Gillen AL: A quality control product for urinalysis. Am J. Clin. Pathol. 59:185, 1973.

Courtesy Ames Division, Miles Laboratories, Inc.

Figure 25.8

A-C, Test for glucose in urine using the Tes-Tape.

Courtesy Eli Lilly and Co, Indianapolis, Ind.

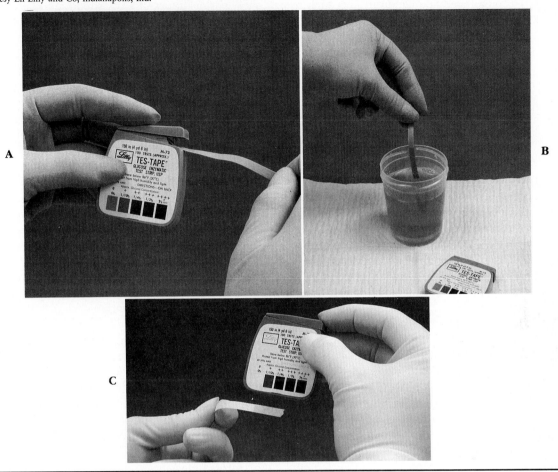

Test for Glucose Using the Tes-Tape
Instructions for use

The Tes-Tape* is a roll of paper that is treated specifically for the analysis of glucose in urine. It comes packaged in a small plastic dispenser, with directions for use and a color chart for comparing the test results on the sides. *Wear disposable rubber gloves when performing this procedure.*

1. Tear off 1½ inches of Tes-Tape paper (Figure 25.8, *A*).
2. Dip one end of tape into the urine specimen, and remove (Figure 25.8, *B*).
3. Wait 1 minute, then compare any color change on the tape with the color chart on the dispenser (Figure 25.8, *C*). If the tape indicates 3+ or higher, make a final comparison 1 minute later.
4. Record the results.

Microscopic Examination of Centrifuged Urine Sediment

The third part of the routine urinalysis is the microscopic examination of the sediment present in the urine. The purpose of this examination is to identify the type and the approximate number of formed elements present, which in turn helps the physician determine the presence of a disease process. The sediment in urine is usually classified as organized or unorganized sediment. Organized sediment includes red blood cells, white blood cells, epithelial cells, casts, bacteria, parasites,

*Eli Lilly & Co., Indianapolis, Ind.

yeast, fungi, and spermatozoa. Unorganized sediment is usually chemical and includes crystals of various components and other amorphous (having no definite shape) material. The urine specimen to be used in the microscopic examination must be freshly voided, preferably a clean-catch voided specimen, and examined without excessive delay so that cellular deterioration is prevented. Microscopic examination of urine is performed after the urine is centrifuged. Centrifugation produces a solid portion called sediment.

Preparation and microscopic examination of specimen

Equipment
Fresh urine specimen
Conical centrifuge tubes
Clinical centrifuge
Droppers
Glass slides
Cover glass
Microscope
Disposable rubber gloves
See Chapter 24 for information on microscopes and centrifuges.

Procedure. *(Always wear disposable rubber gloves when working with specimens.)*

1. To obtain the sediment, place 10 to 15 ml of thoroughly mixed urine in a centrifuge tube and centrifuge for 5 minutes at the standard speed of 1,500 rpm (revolutions per minute).
2. Pour off the supernatant fluid.
3. Allow the several drops of urine that remain along the side of the tube to flow back down into the sediment, then tap the tube with your finger to mix the contents.
4. Place a drop of this sediment on a slide, and cover with a cover glass. The slide is now ready to be examined.
5. Position the slide on the microscope stage.
6. Adjust the low-power objective of the microscope and examine the slide for casts in at least 10 different fields; then examine for other elements that are present in just a few fields. Reduce the light to a minimum by almost completely closing the diaphragm beneath the stage of the microscope, and scan the entire slide to obtain an overall picture of the sediment. It is necessary to vary the intensity of the light source on the microscope so that correct identification of the various components may be obtained.
7. Next adjust the microscope to the high-power objective to identify the specific types

of cells, such as red blood cells, white blood cells, crystals, and other elements present in the sediment. Further identification of the various types of casts should also be done at this time.

8. Estimate the approximate number of the various structures identified. Casts are counted per low-power field; epithelial cells, white blood cells, and red blood cells are reported in terms of cells per high-power field (hpf), for example, 10 to 15 WBC/hpf. To determine the number of elements present, count the number of each type seen in at least 10 fields. The average of this number is then used for the reported value. The other elements (crystals, bacteria, parasites, and spermatozoa) are reported as none, rare, occasional, frequent, many, or numerous.

There is no easy way to learn how to identify these structures (Figure 25.9). A great deal of practice and training is required to master this skill. Reference charts and books should always be used without hesitation. Usually this examination is performed by laboratory personnel; on occasion the physician may do it in the office or clinic laboratory. It is not commonly a responsibility of the medical assistant to do the actual examination, although you may be required to prepare the slide for the examination.

Significance of microscopic test results

Normal urine sediment contains a limited number of formed elements. The presence of one or two white blood cells and red blood cells and a few epithelial cells per high-power field is usually not considered abnormal. At times an occasional hyaline cast may also be considered as a normal finding. Mucous threads in moderate amounts are normal.

Organized sediment
1. Cells
   a. Red blood cells (RBC): The presence of more than one or two RBC per hpf is an abnormal finding. This may be caused by a variety of kidney and systemic diseases, as well as from trauma to the urinary system, violent exercise, or possible contamination from menstrual blood. Hemorrhagic diseases such as hemophilia may also produce hematuria. The presence of red blood cells in the urine must always be reported, as this is a very significant finding.

Figure 25.9
Atlas of urine sediment.
Courtesy Ames Div, Miles Labs, Elkhart, Ind.

Crystals found in acid urine (× 400)

| Uric acid | Amorphous urates and uric acid crystals | Hippuric acid | Calcium oxalate | Tyrosine needles Leucine spheroids Cholesterin plates | Cystine |

Crystals found in alkaline urine (× 400)

  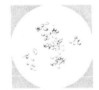 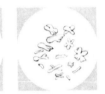

Triple phosphate Ammonium and magnesium   Triple phosphate going in solution   Amorphous phosphate   Calcium phosphate   Calcium carbonate   Ammonium urate

Sulfa crystals

Sulfanilamide   Sulfathiazole   Sulfadiazine   Sulfapyridine

Cells found in urine

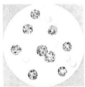

RBC and WBC   Renal epithelium   Caudate cells of renal pelvis   Urethral and bladder epithelium   Vaginal epithelium   Yeast and bacteria

Casts and artifacts found in urine (× 400)

Granular casts fine and coarse   Hyaline cast   Leukocyte cast   Epithelial cast   Waxy cast   Blood cast

Cylindroids   Mucous thread   Spermatozoa   *Trichomonas vaginalis*   Cloth fibers and bubbles

b. White blood cells (WBC): The presence of large numbers of WBC in the urine usually indicates the presence of a bacterial infection in the urinary tract, and/or pyuria. Pyuria (pī-u′rē-ah) is the excretion of urine containing pus. This indicates renal disease that may be either infection or lesions in the bladder, urethra, ureters, and kidneys.

c. Epithelial cells: The presence of large numbers of renal epithelial cells and bladder-type epithelial cells is abnormal and should always be reported. The presence of a large number of renal epithelial cells may indicate degeneration of the renal tubules. Proteinuria and casts are frequently seen in this condition.

2. Casts: It is essential that casts be correctly identified, as the presence of these structures is a very significant laboratory finding. Inflammatory disorders or damage to the glomerulus, tubules, or general renal tissue are usually associated with the presence of casts and are usually accompanied by albuminuria. The various types of casts include red blood cell casts, white blood cell casts, epithelial cell casts, hyaline casts, granular casts, and waxy and fatty casts.

3. Bacteria: Normal urine does not contain bacteria unless the specimen was contaminated by improper collection techniques and handling or by vaginal secretions in the female. The presence of numerous bacteria in the urine may indicate a urinary tract infection. A true infection can be differentiated from contamination if the specimen also contains white blood cells.

4. Yeasts and parasites: Yeast may be seen as a contaminant in the urine of females who have vaginal moniliasis, or it may indicate a urinary moniliasis, especially in patients who have diabetes mellitus. Parasites seen in the urine are usually contaminants from vaginal or fecal excretions.

5. Spermatozoa: Spermatozoa may appear as contaminants in the urine. They commonly are present in urine after sexual intercourse or nocturnal emissions.

Unorganized sediment

1. Crystals: The type and quantity of crystals in the urine vary with the pH of the specimen. Normally, most crystals are of little importance and will form in urine as it cools.

   Crystals seen in normal acid urine are uric acid, amorphous urates, hippuric acid, and calcium oxalate. Crystals seen in normal alkaline urine include triple phosphate, ammonium, magnesium, calcium phosphate, calcium carbonate, and ammonium urate. Abnormal crystals found in acid urine include cholesterin, cystine, leucine, and tyrosine.

2. Artifacts and contaminants: These include hair, cloth fibers, mucous threads, and other contaminants. It is important to differentiate these structures from other elements in the sediment that may indicate the presence of a disease process.

Other Urine Tests
Protein determinations

Bence Jones protein is the name of an abnormal protein in the urine that is commonly seen in patients who have multiple myeloma and a few other abnormalities. This protein is characterized by the fact that during special testing methods (the Bence Jones Protein Test) it precipitates when urine is heated, but disappears once the urine is cooled. Many feel that this is not a very sensitive test, because it can miss detecting small amounts of the Bence Jones protein or other similar types of abnormal protein. Thus many laboratories have discontinued using this test and are now doing the urine-protein electrophoresis. This test determines the relative concentration and also the type of abnormal protein present in the urine. It can be performed on a random urine specimen, although it is preferable to collect a 24-hour specimen in most cases.

Hormone determinations

These urine tests help detect metabolic and endocrine conditions or disorders. One very common test performed is the pregnancy test in which urine is tested for the presence of the human chorionic gonadotropin (HCG) hormone. There is a wide range of tests on the market that are used for this purpose. Many are slide tests that provide results within a few minutes. Complete instructions for use are provided with the test equipment when purchased. Although these are highly reliable tests, incorrect results may be obtained at times because of the presence of protein or blood in the urine or when the urine is too dilute. For most reliable results, the urine should have a specific gravity of at least 1.015. The first morning specimen is preferred for testing.

Multiple-glass test

The multiple-glass test is performed on men to evaluate a lower urinary tract infection. See p. 417 in Chapter 22 for the procedure used to collect three specimens for this test.

Conclusion

Numerous other tests can be performed on urine to aid the physician in diagnosing and treating a patient's condition. It is not within the scope of this book to discuss all of them in detail. *Most must be performed in a laboratory by qualified personnel.* Having completed the chapter on urinalysis, prac-

tice the procedures. When you feel that you know the equipment and steps of the procedures, arrange with your instructor to take a performance test. You will be expected to demonstrate accurately your ability to prepare for and perform all of the procedures that have been presented.

Review Questions

1. List the four major components of normal urine.
2. Why and when is a routine urinalysis performed?
3. List five physical characteristics of urine and eight chemical examinations that are part of a routine urinalysis.
4. List and classify urine microscopic sediment as either organized or unorganized sediment.
5. Indicate if the following urinalysis results are normal or abnormal findings:
   a. Specific gravity of 1.035
   b. Red
   c. Glucose 4+
   d. Acetone, negative
   e. Numerous bacteria
   f. Foul odor
   g. Cloudy
   h. Quantity, 3500 ml in 24 hours
   i. pH 6.5
   j. Protein, trace amounts
   k. Ketones, large amount
   l. Blood, negative
   m. Urobilinogen 0.1 to 1, small amount
   n. Nitrite, positive
6. For each of the following, list two conditions or diseases in which each may be detected:

   a. Albuminuria   f. Bacteriuria
   b. Glucosuria   g. Polyuria
   c. Acetonuria   h. Oliguria
   d. Bilirubinuria   i. Anuria
   e. Hematuria   j. Dysuria

   k. Excessively acid urine
   l. Excessively alkaline urine
   m. Very low specific gravity
7. Name three items used for measuring the specific gravity of urine.
8. Differentiate between normal and abnormal sediment and contaminants that may be observed during a microscopic examination of urine.
9. You are asked to perform the chemical analysis on a urine specimen and find the bottle of reagent strips in the refrigerator with the cap removed. Is this the proper storage method for these reagent strips? Would you use one of these strips to perform the tests? Explain the reason for your answer.
10. A urine specimen that was collected at 10 AM for a microscopic examination was placed in your laboratory on the shelf. It is now 3 PM. What would you do with this specimen? Explain the reason for your answer.

SUGGESTED READINGS

Ames Co: Urodynamics: concepts relating to routine urine chemistry, Elkhart, Ind, 1978, Ames Co.

Btesh S, editor: Disease of the urinary tract and male genital organs, Geneva, 1974, Council for International Organization for Medical Sciences.

Shuman D: Doing it better: tips for improving urine testing techniques, Nursing 76 6:23, Feb 1976.

Chapter 26

Hematology

- Blood components, functions, and formation
- Obtaining blood samples
- Blood tests
- Automation in the clinical laboratory

Objectives

On completion of Chapter 26 the medical assistant student should be able to*:

1. Define and pronounce the listed vocabulary terms and define the listed laboratory abbreviations.

2. List the components of blood; state where each is formed in the body and the functions of each.

3. List and locate body sites used for obtaining capillary and venous blood for testing. List body sites to avoid when obtaining blood samples.

4. Explain the difference between a collection tube with an additive and one without an additive, indicating the preferred use for each.

5. List seven factors that should be considered before performing a venipuncture.

6. List the general order of draw when more than one tube of blood is to be obtained during a venipuncture for various different tests.

7. Discuss how a blood specimen should be handled after collection.

8. List at least five blood tests that require the patient to be in a fasting state before having a blood sample drawn.

9. Given the laboratory results on blood tests that are presented in this chapter, determine if they represent normal values, and relate the abnormal findings to the most probable or possible causes.

10. List six blood tests that are performed for a complete blood count (CBC) and the normal values for each.

11. Explain the terms *multiphasic tests*, *test panels*, and *profiles*.

12. Discuss automation in the clinical laboratory and the advantages this provides.

13. Demonstrate the correct procedure for obtaining a blood sample from a patient by performing a skin puncture and a venipuncture.

14. Demonstrate the correct procedure for obtaining multiple blood samples using the Vacutainer holder and needle, and evacuated blood collection tubes.

15. Demonstrate the correct procedure for determining the presence of glucose in

---

It is suggested that you review Chapter 24 before proceeding with this chapter.

blood by using a Dextrostix; by using the One Touch™ blood glucose meter and test strip.

16 Demonstrate the correct method for recording information relevant to hematology procedures and findings.

Vocabulary

agglutination (ah-gloo″tĭn-nā′shun) A clumping together of cells, as of blood cells or bacteria. An example is when red blood cells (RBC) clump together as a result of an incompatible blood transfusion.

agranulocyte (a-gran′ū-lō-sīt″) A white blood cell (WBC) with a clear or nongranular cytoplasm. There are two types, monocytes and lymphocytes.

anemia (ah-nē′mē-ah) There are a variety of forms of anemia, but broadly speaking it is a lack of red blood cells in the circulating blood or a reduction of hemoglobin or both. Anemia is thought of as a symptom of a disease or disorder; it is not a disease.

anisocytosis (an-i″-sō-sī-tō′sis) A state of abnormal variations in the size of red blood cells in the blood.

blood dyscrasia (dis-krā′zē-ah) An abnormal or diseased condition of the blood.

electrophoresis (e-lek″tro-fo-re′sis) A laboratory method used to diagnose certain diseases by analyzing the plasma protein content.

erythrocytosis (ĕ-rith′-rō-sī-tō′sis) Increased numbers of red blood cells (erythrocytes).

granulocyte (gran′-ū-lō-sīt″) A white blood cell having granules in its cytoplasm. These types of WBCs are neutrophils, basophils, and eosinophils.

band-form granulocyte A granular WBC in a stage of development.

hemoglobin (hē″mō-glō′bin) A protein in an RBC that carries oxygen and carbon dioxide. The pigment in hemoglobin is what gives the blood its red color. The protein in hemoglobin is globin; the red pigment is heme. For the body to make hemoglobin, it must have iron, which is derived from the food we eat.

hemolysis (hē-mol′ĭ-sis) The destruction of red blood cells with the release of hemoglobin into the plasma.

hyperchromia (hi′per-kro′me-ah) An abnormal increase of the hemoglobin levels in red blood cells.

isocytosis (ī″sō-sī-tō′sis) A state in which cells are equal in size, especially equality of size of red blood cells.

leukocytosis (lū″kō-sī-tō′sis) An increased number of circulating white blood cells.

leukopenia (lū″kō-pē′nē-ah) A deficient number of circulating white blood cells.

macrocyte (mak′rō-sīt) The largest type of red blood cell; seen in cases of pernicious anemia (vitamin B_{12} deficiency) and folic acid deficiency.

microcyte (mī′krō-sīt) An abnormally small red blood cell, found in cases of iron deficient anemia and thalassemia.

poikilocytosis (poi″kĭ-lō-sī-tō′sis) The presence of red blood cells in the blood that show abnormal variations in shape.

polycythemia (pol″ē-sī-thē′mē-ah) An abnormal increased amount of red blood cells or hemoglobin.

reticulocyte (rĕ-tik′ŭ-lō-sīt) A nonnucleated immature red blood cell. Generally, of all the red blood cells in the circulating blood, less than 2% are reticulocytes.

serum (se′rum) The clear, straw-colored liquid portion obtained after blood clots; it consists of plasma minus fibrinogen, which is removed in the process of clotting.

thrombocyte (throm′bō-sīt) A blood platelet.

thrombocythemia (throm″bŏ-sī-thē′mē-ah) An increased number of platelets in the circulating blood.

thrombocytopenia (throm′bo-si″-to-pe′ne-ah) A decreased number of platelets in the circulating blood.

Hematology, the study of blood, covers vast areas and numerous tests. Today, in the physician's office, most of the tests will be performed by a trained laboratory worker, or blood samples will be obtained and then sent to a larger clinical laboratory for testing. At other times, the patient will be sent directly to the laboratory to have the blood sample drawn. Most laboratories use automated equipment in performing many of the tests. These modern advances in laboratory technology have made it possible to obtain quick and accurate results on a relatively small sample of blood.

For the most part, it will not be a duty of the medical assistant to perform blood tests, other than a few simple ones. Depending upon the laws of the state in which you practice, you may be called upon to perform a skin puncture or a venipuncture to obtain blood samples for testing at a clinical laboratory. Even though you may not do these procedures, it is important that you be familiar with the equipment and supplies that are needed so that you are capable of assisting the physician as required or explaining the procedure to a patient. These procedures, supplies, and some of the routine and basic blood tests will be discussed in this chapter.

BLOOD COMPONENTS, FUNCTIONS, AND FORMATION

Blood, a type of connective tissue, is composed of a clear yellow liquid portion, the plasma, in which the cellular or formed elements are suspended. Plasma makes up about 55% of the blood by volume. The remaining 45% consists of the formed elements, which are red blood cells (RBC), white blood cells (WBC), and platelets. The average adult has approximately 5 to 6 quarts of blood.

Blood has at times been referred to as the "river of life," because it is by way of this special tissue that numerous substances are transported to all the cells in our body for nourishment and function, and waste products are in turn carried to certain body systems for disposal. It is a transportation system in our body, helping also in the maintenance of acid-base, electrolyte, and fluid balance of the internal environment.

Plasma, which is 90% water, acts as the carrier for the formed elements and other substances, which include blood proteins, carbohydrates, fats, amino acids (proteins), mineral salts (the electrolytes), hormones, enzymes, gases, antibodies, and waste products such as urea and uric acid.

The formed elements all have special functions. The prime function of the red blood cell, or erythrocyte, is to transport oxygen from the lungs to the body cells and carbon dioxide from the cells back to the lungs to be exhaled. Each RBC contains a protein substance, hemoglobin (Hgb, Hg, or Hb), which gives red color to blood and transports the oxygen and carbon dioxide to and from the body cells. Anemia is the result of too few RBCs in the circulating blood, or RBCs with reduced amounts of hemoglobin, or both.

The five types of white blood cells, or leukocytes, are classified into two general groups, the granular and agranular. Granular WBCs, sometimes called polymorphonuclear leukocytes, include the eosinophils, basophils, and neutrophils. They are characterized by their heavily granulated cytoplasm and segmented nuclei. The agranular leukocytes are the monocytes and lymphocytes, both having a solid nucleus and a clear cytoplasm. The prime function of WBCs is to protect the body against infection and disease; some fight invading bacteria by their phagocytic activity (destroying and ingesting harmful microorganisms), and others play an important role in producing immunity to disease. Infection in the body is indicated when there is a marked rise in the WBC count. Also, in leukemia, the WBC count is greatly increased.

Platelets (thrombocytes), the smallest of the formed elements in blood, play a vital role in initiating the clotting process of blood. Thrombocytopenia may be accompanied by bleeding.

All blood cells are produced in hemopoietic (blood-forming) tissue. The agranular WBCs are produced mainly in lymph nodes and other lymphoid tissues. Granular WBCs, RBCs, and platelets are produced in the red bone marrow or myeloid tissue of bones such as the femur, humerus, sternum, vertebrae, and cranial bones.

OBTAINING BLOOD SAMPLES
Types and Sources

For most routine hematologic studies, there are two sources of blood for testing. Capillary or peripheral blood is obtained by performing a *skin puncture* on the palmar surface of the fingertip or on the ear lobe. For infants, the skin puncture is done on the plantar surface of the great toe or heel. You *must* avoid areas that are cyanotic, scarred, traumatized, edematous, and heavily calloused. A minimal amount of blood, just a few drops, is obtained by this method, but it is sufficient to perform some of the routine tests, such as the complete blood count (CBC), some coagulation studies, and some of the chemistry tests.

The *second* source for obtaining blood is a vein. This is called venous blood, and the procedure by which it is obtained is called a *venipuncture*. The most common sites for obtaining blood by this method are from the basilic and cephalic veins located in the antecubital area of the arm, which is at the inner aspect of the arm opposite the elbow. This is the more common method for obtaining a blood sample and is the method that must be used when larger amounts of blood are needed to perform several different tests. When you cannot obtain blood from a vein in the antecubital space because of stenosed or collapsed veins or if the patient has plaster casts on both arms, alternative sites to use are the veins on the top of the hand, in the wrist, or even in the foot. In extreme situations, blood may be obtained from the femoral vein. This site must be used *only* by physicians.

At times special blood studies, such as blood gases, will be ordered. In these circumstances, arterial blood (blood from an artery, usually the brachial or femoral) rather than venous blood is required. A physician or qualified laboratory personnel *must* obtain this blood sample. A situation in which this may be necessary in the physician's office is when an emphysemic patient has an acute episode of shortness of breath. The physician may draw arterial blood for blood gases while the patient is still breathing room air; then if oxygen is administered to the patient, the physician would draw another arterial blood sample for examination. In the latter case, it is important to indicate on the laboratory requisition how many liters of oxygen were administered to the patient so that this can be considered when the test results are interpreted.

Collection Tubes and Proper Handling of a Venous Blood Sample

Because of the multitude of tests that can be performed on a blood sample, there are certain requirements that must be met when collecting and handling the sample. Using excellent technique, you will collect the samples in either a plain tube without additives or in a tube that contains anticoagulant additives. *The type of test to be performed as well as the laboratory's preference will govern this choice.*

Tubes without additives

Generally speaking, a tube without an additive is used when you want a clot to form to obtain serum for testing. Once collected, the blood is left standing in an upright position at room temperature, usually for 30 to 60 minutes, to allow a clot to form. To separate the serum from the clot, the sample is then centrifuged for 10 minutes. After this, serum is removed from the tube and is ready for testing.

A more convenient method used when serum is required for testing is the use of a serum separator tube to collect the blood sample. Once collected, the sample is left standing at room temperature for 30 to 60 minutes and then centrifuged for 10 minutes. After centrifuging, a jellylike substance will be between the clot and the serum in the tube. The

sample can then be sent to the laboratory in this tube. This sample is used most commonly for most blood chemistries (varying with the laboratory's preference), serology tests, and Rh-factor testing.

Tubes with additives

Tubes containing EDTA anticoagulant additive are recommended for use when doing hematology studies. The WBCs and platelets are best preserved in this type of tube, and better red cell morphology results will be obtained. The additive has no adverse effects on the blood sample when a sufficient quantity of blood is obtained. Problems will arise if too little blood is drawn into tubes containing anticoagulant additives. Misleading results and therefore incorrect diagnoses will occur; for example, the hematocrit is lowered and poor red blood cell morphology results, because the red blood cell shrinks and produces a false appearance. All tubes with anticoagulant additives must be filled with blood.

A tube containing an anticoagulant additive, such as heparin, prevents the blood from clotting. Depending on methods used by the laboratory when performing certain tests, this is generally the preferred tube to use when collecting a sample for blood chemistries, and especially for potassium levels. *Do not* use this tube for hematology studies, as the heparin additive will distort the cells and lead to false results.

There are several other additives used in tubes for collecting venous blood. It is very important that the correct tube, plain or with an additive, be used. Most laboratories will supply these tubes with directions indicating which to use for various tests. *They are not interchangeable and must not be confused.*

Vacutainer system

Rather than using the conventional syringe, needle, and test tube when obtaining blood samples, newer, more convenient systems consisting of a disposable needle, a holder, and vacuum tubes are available. One such unit is the Vacutainer system, which consists of a holder-needle combination or separate needle and holder and evacuated glass tubes containing a premeasured vacuum to provide a controlled amount of blood draw. The tubes have color-coded rubber stoppers that indicate the type of test that they are best suited for, and are supplied plain or with additives, sterile or nonsterile. (The trend today is to use sterile tubes for all collections.) All are available in a variety of sizes, the most common being 3, 5, 7, 10, and 15 ml ca-

Figure 26.1
A, Vacutainer evacuated blood collection system. **B,** Sterile Vacutainer serum
tubes of various sizes without additive, used for chemistry tests.
Courtesy Consumer Products Div of Becton-Dickinson, and Co, Rutherford, NJ.

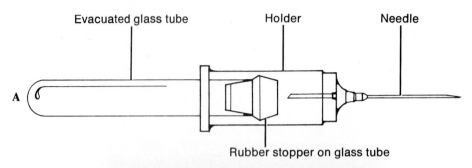

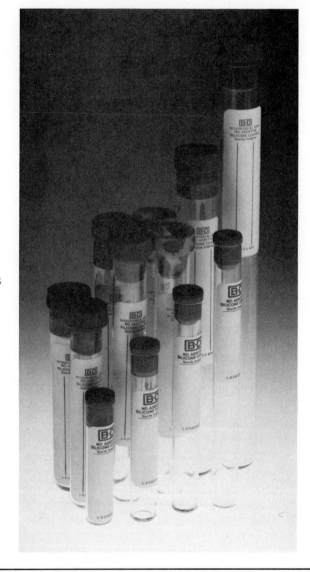

pacities. Vacutainers are supplied in packages with labels that indicate the additives present in the tubes, the expiration date, and the approximate draw amount (Figure 26.1).

The most frequently used vacuum tubes classified according to the tube top color, additive content, average amount of blood drawn, and recommended use are as follows:

Tube top color	Additive	Average amount of blood drawn	Common blood determinations
Red (most common)	No additive	10 ml	Used for tests done on serum: blood bank tests, e.g., blood typing (ABO and Rh factor) and cross-matching; serology tests; serum pregnancy test; most common chemistries; immunology tests; viral studies; AIDS antibody (HTLVIII antibody)
Lavender	EDTA (Ethylenediamine tetraacetic acid, an anticoagulant)	5 ml	Used for tests done on whole blood or plasma: hematologic tests, including a CBC, WBC, RBC, hematocrit, hemoglobin, platelet count, reticulocyte count, and sedimentation rate
Blue	Sodium citrate (an anticoagulant)	5 ml	Used for tests done on whole blood: coagulation studies, including prothrombin time (PT), partial thromboplastin time (PTT), and thrombin time (TT)
Green	Sodium heparin	5 ml	Used for tests done on whole blood or plasma: blood chemistry tests, especially potassium levels; electrolytes; blood gases
Gray	Potassium oxalate and sodium fluoride	5 ml	Used for tests done on whole blood or plasma: blood glucose; blood alcohol; the coagulation study activated clotting time (ACT)
Gray and red (mottled top) (serum separation tube)	Silicone serum separation material	5 ml	Used for tests done on serum: can be used for every test where you want the blood to clot *Do not use for blood bank tests*

When you are to draw more than one tube of blood the general order of draw is as follows:

- First draw—blood culture tubes (for example, sterile tubes with no additive, then blood should be transferred to a culture medium within 5 minutes);
- Second draw—tubes with no additives (for example, red tops);
- Third draw—coagulation tubes (for example, blue tops); and
- Last draw—tubes with additives (for example, lavender, green, and gray tops).

After the blood has been drawn, the tubes without an additive are *not* to be inverted or shaken, but are to be centrifuged as was discussed previously. Tubes that contain an additive should be gently inverted 8 to 10 times to mix the blood with the additive. *Do not shake these tubes,* as vigorous mixing may cause hemolysis. The amount of blood drawn will vary according to the size of the tube used.

Amount and handling of specimen

The amount of venous blood to be drawn is 3 to 30 ml, varying with the test(s) to be performed. Consult your laboratory for exact amounts that are needed for each specific test that is to be performed. Frequently 1 to 2 ml more blood than is required is drawn to avoid having a patient return for a second collection if the first battery of tests does not turn out.

A blood specimen must be tested on the same day of collection. Depending on the test(s) to be performed, blood should be examined within 8 hours or less from the time it was collected, and preferably within 2 to 4 hours from the time that it was drawn. Blood for bacteriologic studies must be collected in special containers and must not sit around. These specimens must be examined as soon as possible. Blood drawn for an electrolyte panel should be refrigerated if it is not tested immediately. Other blood samples may be left standing on the counter for 2 to 4 hours before testing, although some results may vary if the blood is left standing for 2 or more hours. On request, your laboratory will provide schedules that list specific sample requirements for each test they perform. The quality of a test is diminished if a blood sample stands for a long time before being tested; for example, glucose levels will decrease within a couple of hours, and potassium levels will rise if serum is left standing on the cells; the sedimentation rate will be lowered if left standing for over 2 hours, and the bacteria count will increase.

As with all specimens, blood samples must be accurately identified and labeled, and adequate amounts are to be forwarded to the laboratory as soon as possible. The time the sample was drawn should also be indicated on the laboratory requisition. To prevent errors, patient identification on the collection tube must be identical to that on the requisition. Correct patient preparation must be adhered to when required. Some tests (or the physician's preference) require the patient to fast 8 to 14 hours before having blood collected, such as for a fasting blood sugar. Other tests require timed samples; that is, samples may be collected every hour for 3 consecutive hours, as in a glucose tolerance test. Proper recording on the patient's chart is essential. This includes the date, time, sample(s) obtained, test(s) to be performed, and when the sample was sent to the laboratory. (See also "Care, Handling, Transporting, and Storing Specimens" in Chapter 22.)

Venipuncture Technique

Venipuncture is the preferred method for obtaining blood samples and must be used when a larger amount of blood is required for testing. From 3 to more than 30 ml may be drawn by this method. To spare the patient the pain of unsuccessful punctures, consider the following before doing a venipuncture:

1. Ask the patient if he/she has any preference as to which vein you should puncture. Patients often know where their better veins are and which sites should be avoided.
2. Palpate the vein before inserting the needle to determine if the vein is patent. *(stable)*
3. Use a sturdy-walled vein for the puncture. The walls of sturdy veins will feel firm when you touch them, and they will exhibit elasticity and resilience when pressure is carefully applied.
4. Fragile veins are usually narrow veins. If you must puncture these veins, use a 23-gauge needle rather than a 21-gauge needle.
5. Do not use a weak-walled vein. These veins are soft to the touch and lack the elasticity of a sturdy vein.
6. Do not use sclerosed veins. These veins will be resistant to pressure, even if they do look like good veins.
7. Do not use a vacuum apparatus to draw blood from a small or constricted vein because this will cause the vein to collapse.

Text continued on p. 530.

Venipuncture Using a Syringe and Needle

Equipment

· 70% alcohol and sterile cotton sponges; or disposable alcohol sponges
· Sterile cotton sponges
Tourniquet
Sterile disposable needle, usually 1-, 1½-, or 1¼-inch, 21 gauge
Sterile disposable syringe, either 5-, 10-, 20-, or 30-cc size, depending on the amount of blood to be obtained.

Test tube(s) with proper patient identification, with or without an additive, depending on the test that is to be performed; *or a vacuum tube (rather than the syringe and test tube, or vacuum tube, you may use the Vacutainer system with appropriate tube[s], needle, and holder; see Figure 26.1)*
A Band-Aid
Disposable rubber gloves

Procedure

1. Wash your hands.
2. Assemble required equipment.
3. Identify the patient and explain the procedure.
4. Have the patient sit with the arm well supported in a downward position (Figure 26.2).
5. Don disposable rubber gloves. Prepare equipment for use: attach the needle to the syringe (or to the Vacutainer holder [Figure 26.1, *A*]), leaving the needle shield in place. Label the collection tube with the patient's name, the date, and time (Figure 26.3).
6. Select the site for venipuncture by palpating the antecubital space.

Rationale

Explanations help gain the patient's cooperation.
This avoids movement by the patient.

If you are drawing blood from more than one patient, it is best to label the tubes after you have drawn the blood. Often when tubes are prelabeled, people have a tendency to use the wrong tube if they are in a rush or under pressure.
This site is located on the inner aspect of the arm, opposite the elbow. You must *avoid* the artery. At the antecubital site, the basilic and cephalic veins are used for drawing blood samples.

Figure 26.2

For a venipuncture, have the patient sit with the arm well supported in a downward position.

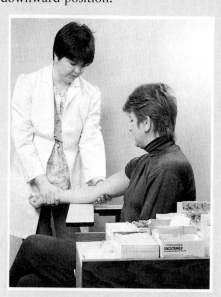

Figure 26.3

Label the collection tube with the patient's name, the date, and the time.

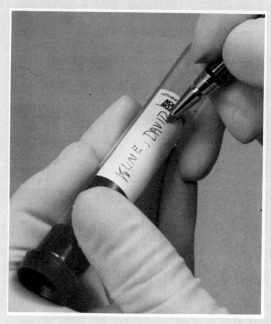

Continued.

Venipuncture Using a Syringe and Needle—cont'd

Procedure

7. Apply the tourniquet around the patient's arm 3 to 4 inches above the elbow. Palpate the vein again. (Figure 26.4).
8. Swab the venipuncture site with an alcohol sponge.
9. Remove the needle shield.
10. Using your nondominant hand, draw the skin over the puncture site until tense. Gently and slowly insert the needle at a 15-degree angle through the skin into the vein (Figure 26.5).

Rationale

You may ask the patient to open and close the hand several times to help produce engorgement of the vein in the arm.

Do not palpate the venipuncture area after cleansing with alcohol.

Countertension immobilizes the vein and exerts tension in the opposite direction to that of the needle. Thus the needle goes in more easily and less painfully. You will retain better control over the needle when the vein is immobilized by the countertension. The bevel of the needle should be facing upward because by doing this the sharpest point of the needle is inserted first.

Figure 26.4

A, Apply the tourniquet around the patient's arm 3 to 4 inches above the elbow. Cross the ends of the tourniquet and pull the ends away from each other to create tension. **B,** Secure the tourniquet by tucking the upper end into the band to form a half-bow. The tourniquet must be tight enough to obstruct venous blood flow.

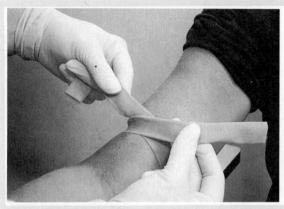

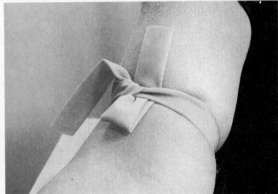

A

B

Figure 26.5

Gently and slowly, insert the needle at a 15-degree angle through the skin into the vein.

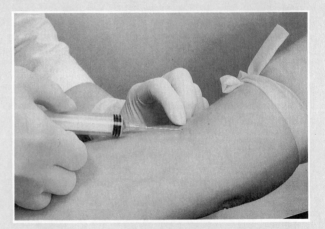

Venipuncture Using a Syringe and Needle—cont'd

Procedure	*Rationale*
11. Having entered the vein using your dominant hand, now use your nondominant hand to slowly pull on the plunger of the syringe to withdraw blood. As soon as blood starts to flow into the syringe, release the tourniquet.	Make sure that you do not move the needle and syringe after entering the vein. If you withdraw the blood too rapidly, you may cause the vein to collapse, and thus will be unable to obtain the required sample. Keep in mind that a nontraumatic venipuncture produces the most reliable results, because any tissue injury can falsely elevate some results, such as enzyme levels.
12. When you have obtained the required amount of blood, place a dry sterile sponge over the puncture site, and withdraw the needle, using a straight downward motion.	The tourniquet *must be off before the needle is withdrawn.*
13. Apply pressure with a sterile sponge over the puncture site for a few minutes; you may have the patient elevate the arm at this time.	You may ask the patient to hold the sponge over the puncture site and apply the pressure. Elevation prevents oozing of blood at the puncture site.
14. Remove the needle from the syringe and inject blood into the test tube(s). NOTE: When injecting blood into a vacuum tube from a syringe and needle system, leave the needle on the syringe, and gently insert the needle through the rubber stopper on the tube. The vacuum inside will draw the required amount of blood into the tube.	When using different tubes for multiple samples, first inject blood into the tubes that do not contain any additives, then inject blood into the coagulation tubes, then into tubes containing an additive.
15. Cap the tubes. Those that contain an additive should be *gently* inverted 8 to 10 times to mix the blood with the additive. *Do not shake these tubes.* Do not mix blood in the plain tubes (that is, tubes without an additive).	Vigorous mixing may cause hemolysis.
16. Apply an adhesive bandage to the puncture site if desired.	
17. Discard disposable syringe and needle in containers designated for disposal. (If you have used a nondisposable glass syringe rather than a disposable one, rinse it with cold water, separate the barrel and plunger, and soak in soap and water.)	
18. Remove gloves and wash your hands.	
19. Complete the laboratory requisition, and send it to the laboratory with the blood sample(s) obtained.	
20. Record on patient's chart.	Charting example: May 18, 19_____, 1 PM Venipuncture done on left arm. Two samples sent to lab for a CBC and blood chemistries. 　　Charles Rubin, CMA

Procedure

1. Complete steps 1 through 5 as described in "Venipuncture Techniques Using A Syringe And Needle."
2. Select the correct tube for the type of sample required and label it. Gently tap tubes that contain additives to dislodge any additive that may be trapped around the stopper.
3. Insert the tube into the holder up to the guideline; push the tube stopper onto the needle inside the holder.
4. Perform the venipuncture in the usual manner (steps 6 through 10 in venipuncture technique using a syringe and needle).
5. Place two fingers at the end of the holder; with your thumb, push the tube onto the needle to the end of the holder.
6. Release the tourniquet as soon as blood begins to fill the tube. Do not allow contents of tube to contact the stopper or the end of the needle during the procedure. NOTE: If blood does not flow into the tube or if the blood flow ceases before an adequate amount is collected, take the following steps:
   a. Check to see that the needle cannula is in the correct position in the vein.
   b. If a multiple sample needle is being used, remove the tube and place a new tube into the holder.
   c. Remove the needle and tube and discard. Start the procedure over again.

Single sample collection

7. Remove the needle from the vein when the vacuum is exhausted and blood stops flowing into the tube (Figure 26.6).
8. Apply pressure with a sterile sponge to the puncture site, and have the patient elevate his or her arm for a few minutes to prevent oozing of blood (Figure 26.6).
9. Remove the tube of blood from the holder.
10. For tubes that contain additives, *gently* invert eight to ten times to mix blood thoroughly with the additive. *Do not shake.*

11. Apply a bandage to the puncture site if required.
12. Discard the needle in a designated container; complete the laboratory requisition and forward with the blood sample to the laboratory. Discard Vacutainer holder in sharps container at the end of each day, or when soiled with blood.
13. Remove gloves and wash your hands.
14. Record on the patient's chart.

Multiple sample collection

7. Remove the tube from the holder when the vacuum is exhausted and the blood stops flowing. Keep the needle holder steady.
8. Place the second and succeeding tubes into the holder, puncturing the diaphragm of the stopper to initiate the blood flow. Keep the needle holder steady. Tubes without additives are drawn first, then coagulation tubes, and then tubes with additives.
9. While blood is flowing into succeeding tubes, gently invert previously filled tubes that contain additives 8 to 10 times to mix the additive with the blood. *Do not shake.* Vigorous mixing may cause hemolysis.
10. Remove the needle from the vein when blood stops flowing into the last tube (Figure 26.6).
11. Apply pressure with a sterile sponge to the puncture site (Figure 26.6), and have the patient elevate the arm for a few minutes to prevent oozing of blood.
12. Remove the tube of blood from the holder. *Gently* invert the tube 8 to 10 times if it contained an additive. *Do not shake.*
13. Apply a bandage to the puncture site if required.
14. Discard the needle in a designated container; complete the laboratory requisition and forward it with the blood sample to the laboratory.
15. Remove gloves and wash your hands.
16. Record on the patient's chart.

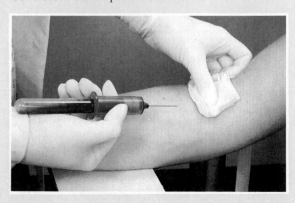

Figure 26.6
Remove needle from vein when vacuum is exhausted and blood stops flowing into tube. Apply pressure with a sterile sponge to the puncture site.

Equipment

A sterile disposable lancet
70% alcohol and cotton sponges; or disposable alcohol sponges
Clean blood pipette *or* capillary tube *or* Unopette *or* Microtainer (this piece of equipment will vary with your agency's preference, with the test(s) to be performed on the blood sample, and with the methods used by the laboratory)

or

A reagent strip if you are doing a simple test for blood glucose (see p. 533).
Disposable rubber gloves.

Procedure	*Rationale*
1. Wash your hands.	
2. Assemble equipment and supplies.	
3. Identify the patient and explain the procedure.	Explanations help gain the patient's cooperation.
4. Have the patient seated with the arm well supported.	This avoids movement by the patient.
5. Don disposable rubber gloves. Select the lateral part of the tip of a finger or the earlobe for the puncture site; use the heel or great toe for an infant.	Avoid the thumb and index finger as they are usually more calloused than the other fingers. Using the lateral part of a fingertip rather than the palm side will lessen discomfort for the patient.
6. "Milk" or gently rub the finger along the sides.	This promotes circulation. If the patient's fingers are cold, you may rub them or apply a warm pack to promote circulation. You may also instruct the patient to dangle his or her hand toward the floor to help force blood into the finger.
7. Clean the puncture site with an alcohol sponge; allow the area to dry.	Do not blot or blow on the puncture site. Allow it to air-dry.
8. Grasp the patient's finger on the sides near the puncture site with your nondominant thumb and forefinger.	
9. Hold the lancet with your dominant fingers and make a quick in-and-out puncture on the patient's fingertip. Hold the lancet at a right angle to the lines on the patient's finger (Figure 26.7).	Lancets are usually designed so that you can make a puncture to a depth of 3 to 4 mm., which is sufficient to obtain drops of blood.
10. Wipe away the first drop of blood with a clean cotton sponge.	The first drop of blood is not a desirable sample, as it will contain tissue fluid.
11. Apply gentle pressure above the puncture site to cause the blood to flow freely.	Do not squeeze the finger, as this liberates tissue fluid, which in turn dilutes the blood and causes inaccurate results.
12. Obtain the blood sample as required by the test to be performed. You may: • Use the pipette to take up the blood sample. Take up the blood sample to the desired level in the pipette. **or** • Lightly touch the blood drop to the test pad on the reagent strip, and continue the test according to the individual test directions.	

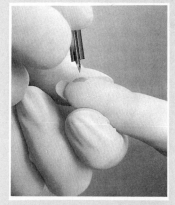

Figure 26.7
Fingertip skin puncture technique using a lancet.

13. When more than one sample is needed, wipe the finger with a clean cotton sponge and obtain fresh drops of blood in each pipette.	You may have to apply gentle pressure to the finger to obtain more blood.
14. When using bulb pipettes and Unopettes, make dilutions according to instructions for the specific test to be performed.	Blood collected in Microtainers and capillary tubes is not to be diluted, but is sent directly to the laboratory for testing.
15. Apply pressure to the puncture site with a dry cotton sponge.	

16. Label the blood samples and laboratory requisition correctly, and forward to the laboratory for testing.	Charting example:
	 April 21, 19_____, 11 AM
	     Finger puncture done on second finger, left hand. Blood sample sent to laboratory for a CBC (complete blood count).
	     Ann Patterson, CMA

17. Remove gloves and wash your hands.	
18. Record on the patient's chart.	

Fingertip Skin Puncture Using the Penlet Blood Sampling Pen* (Figure 26.8)

Equipment

Penlet with disposable caps (Figure 26.8, *A*)
Sterile lancet
70% alcohol and cotton sponges *or* disposable alcohol sponges
Disposable rubber gloves

Procedure

1. Wash your hands.
2. Assemble equipment and supplies.
3. Identify the patient and explain the procedure.
4. Have the patient seated with the arm well supported.
5. Don disposable rubber gloves. Load the Penlet with a sterile lancet. Remove the clear plastic cap and press the lancet straight into the lancet holder until it comes to a firm stop. This will leave the device cocked. *Do not twist* the lancet into position (Figures 26.8, *B*, and 26.8, *C*).
6. Select the lateral part of the tip of a finger for the puncture site.
7. "Milk" or very gently rub the finger along the sides.
8. Clean the puncture site with an alcohol sponge; allow the area to dry.

*Lifescan Inc., Mountain View, Calif.

9. Hold the end of the Penlet firmly with one hand and with the other hand twist off the lancet protective disk (Figure 26.8, *D*).
10. Replace the Penlet cap.
11. Grasp the patient's finger on the sides near the puncture site with your nondominant thumb and forefinger.
12. Position the opening of the Penlet's transparent cap over the skin area that will be punctured (Figure 26.8, *E*).
13. Press the trigger button. The depth of penetration of the lancet will depend on the amount of pressure with which the Penlet is held against the skin. The greater the pressure, the deeper the puncture will be (Figure 26.8, *E*).
14. Complete this procedure by following steps 10 through 18 of the fingertip skin puncture technique using a lancet.
15. To remove the lancet from the Penlet, take the cap off and insert the inside rim of the cap into the notched side of the lancet and pull the lancet out. Dispose of it in a container for used sharp instruments.
16. Put a clean cap on the Penlet and replace in the proper storage area.

Figure 26.8
A, Penlet automatic blood sampling pen to use for obtaining a skin puncture blood sample. **B, C, D,** and **E,** Technique for using the Penlet puncture device.

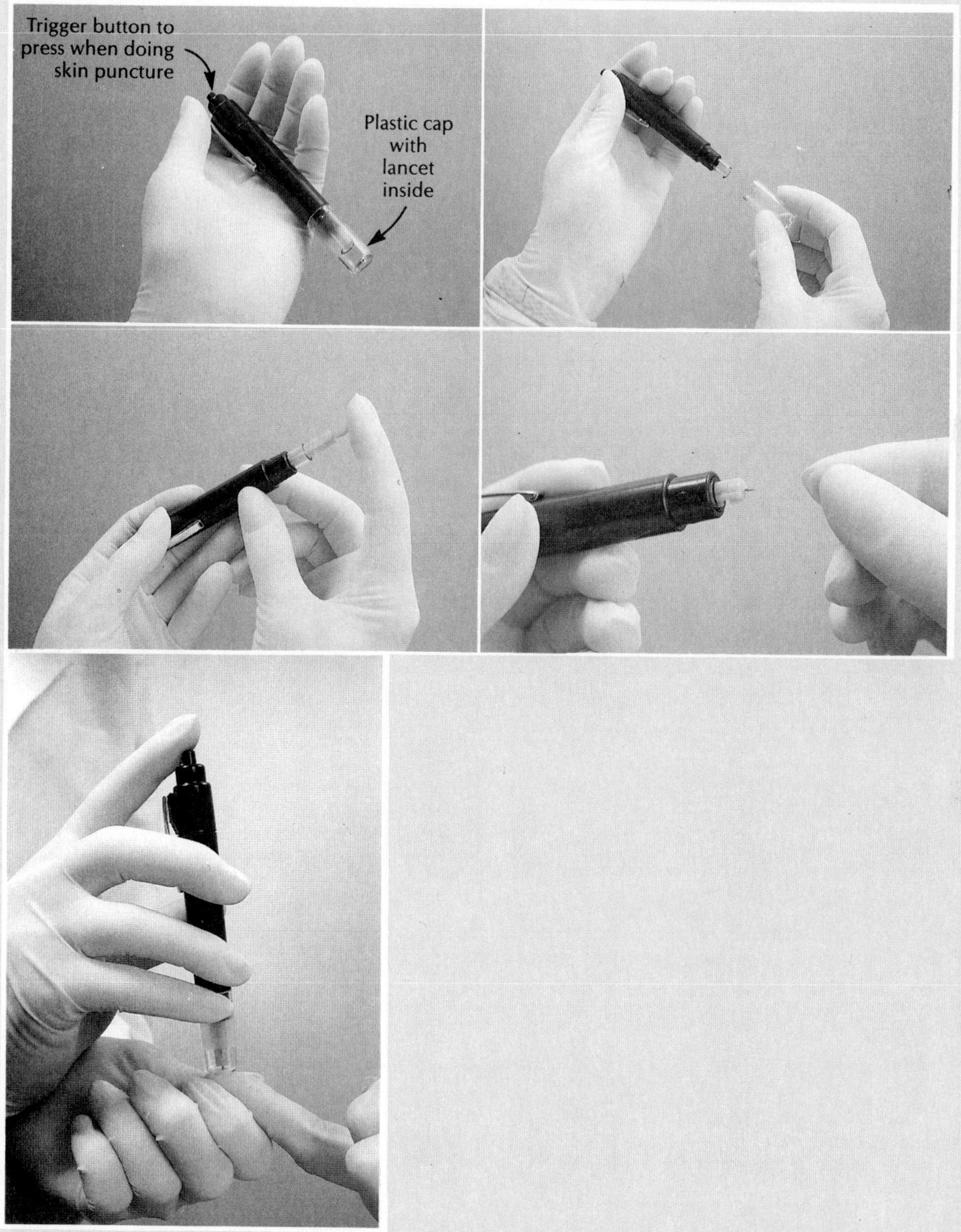

Unopette system

The Unopette system consists of a disposable self-filling diluting pipette and a plastic reservoir prefilled with a precise amount of diluent. These systems serve as a collection and dilution unit for microblood samples. There are various types of Unopette systems available that contain the appropriate diluting substances required for hematology and chemistry tests (Figure 26.9).

Figure 26.9

Techniques for using Unopette system for laboratory procedures.

Courtesy Becton-Dickinson, Div of Becton, Dickinson and Co, Rutherford, NJ.

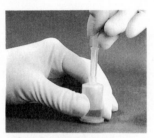

1. Puncture diaphragm

Using the protective shield on the capillary pipette, puncture the diaphragm of the reservoir as follows:
a. Place reservoir on a flat surface. Grasping reservoir in one hand, take pipette assembly in other hand. Push tip of pipette shield firmly through diaphragm in neck of reservoir, then remove.

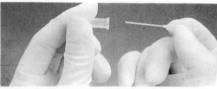

b. Remove shield from pipette assembly with a twist.

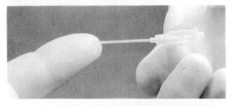

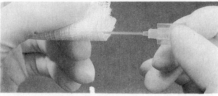

2. Add sample

Fill capillary with sample and transfer to reservoir as follows:
a. Holding pipette *almost* horizontally, touch tip of pipette to sample. (See alternate methods in illustrations above.) Pipette will fill by capillary action. Filling is complete and will stop automatically when sample reaches end of capillary bore in neck of pipette.

b. Wipe excess sample from outside of capillary pipette, making certain that no sample is removed from capillary bore.

c. Squeeze reservoir slightly to force out some air. Do not expel any liquid. Maintain pressure on reservoir.

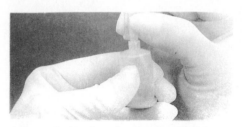

d. Cover opening of overflow chamber with index finger and seat pipette *securely* in reservoir neck.

e. Release pressure on reservoir. Then remove finger from pipette opening. Negative pressure will draw blood into diluent.

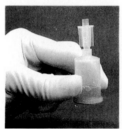

f. Squeeze reservoir *gently* two or three times to rinse capillary bore, forcing diluent into, *but not out of,* overflow chamber, releasing pressure each time to return mixture to reservoir.

CAUTION: If reservoir is squeezed too hard, some of the specimen may be expelled through the top of the overflow chamber.

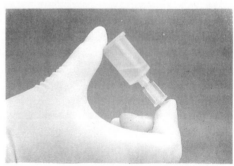

g. Place index finger over upper opening and gently invert several times to thoroughly mix sample with diluent.

Figure 26.9, cont'd

3. Count cells (option 1)

Mix diluted blood thoroughly by inverting reservoir (see 2g) to resuspend cells immediately prior to actual count.

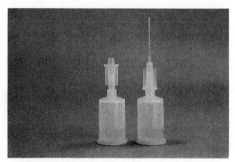

a. Convert to dropper assembly by withdrawing pipette from reservoir and reseating securely in reverse position.

b. Invert reservoir, gently squeeze sides and discard first three or four drops.

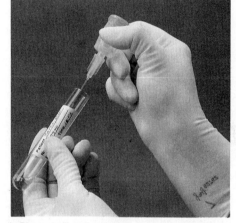

b. Place capillary tip into appropriately labeled test tube or cuvette which will accommodate 5.0 ml of reagent and squeeze reservoir to expel entire contents.

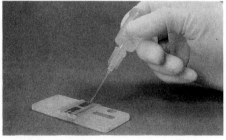

c. Carefully charge hemacytometer with diluted blood by gently squeezing sides of reservoir to expel contents until chamber is properly filled.

OR

3. Store diluted specimen (option 3)

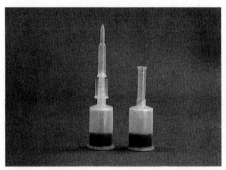

Cover overflow chamber with capillary shield or remove capillary and insert tip of shield firmly into reservoir opening. (Note time for which diluted specimen remains stable for each test.)

OR

3. Transfer contents (option 2)

Transfer thoroughly mixed contents of each reservoir to appropriately labeled test tubes or corresponding cuvettes as follows:

a. Convert reservoir to dropper assembly by withdrawing pipette and reseating securely in reverse position as shown above.

BLOOD TESTS

The results obtained from laboratory examinations performed on blood samples, combined with other clinical information, help the physician in various aspects of patient care, such as screening for or diagnosing a condition, evaluating body functions, making therapeutic decisions, and monitoring therapy provided.

There are numerous blood tests that can be performed to aid the physician in diagnosing, treating, or evaluating a patient's condition. Some of these tests are performed on whole blood, whereas others are performed on blood serum. A few simple procedures that may be performed in the physician's office or health agency, and a table of some common tests done routinely in laboratories by certified personnel with the aid of automated equipment follow on pp. 553 and 554. The actual performance of these tests is usually not a responsibility of the medical assistant, because in general *most state laws require that individuals performing laboratory procedures be certified laboratory technicians or technologists, or physicians, certified or licensed in the state of their practice.* Nonetheless, it is important for the medical assistant to be familiar with the type of tests available and the normal values for each and to have an understanding of the significance of normal and abnormal results. When aware of this information, the medical assistant will have a greater understanding and appreciation for the diagnosis, treatment, and evaluation of patients under the physician's care, in addition to being of greater value to the patient, physician, and laboratory.

At times, basic screening tests will be performed in the physician's office, and then the more detailed tests and precise results will be obtained from larger laboratories using automated equipment.

All tests have predetermined normal values or ranges that establish the limits within which the results indicate the absence of any pathological condition. Normal ranges are established on the basis of the procedures and equipment used by the laboratory. It is important to keep this in mind when reviewing laboratory reports received on specimens obtained from the patients under your physician's care. Often you may obtain a list of normal blood values from the laboratory that performs the procedures.

Generally speaking, hematology tests are done on whole blood and serological tests and blood chemistries are done on serum or sometimes on plasma. Blood banking and transfusion services use cells as well as serum for testing.

A conscientious medical assistant should be alert for new techniques available that may be valuable to the physician in the office. Manufacturers will provide brochures and catalogues with information on the latest developments. Medically oriented magazines are another good source for obtaining this type of information.

Patient Preparation for Blood Tests

There are very few blood tests that require any special preparation of the patient. Generally special preparation means that the patient should fast, that is, abstain from all solid foods and liquids, for up to 14 hours before the blood sample is drawn. This is required because food substances may alter the reliability of the test results. Water may be taken before some tests. The laboratory will provide you with specific directions. Usually you are to instruct the patient to take nothing by mouth (NPO) after midnight the night before the test is to be done.

The principal tests that require the patient to fast beforehand include fasting blood sugar; glucose tolerance test; any type of lipid analysis, such as cholesterol and triglycerides; and the sequential multiple analysis (SMA-12, SMA-18, SMAC-20, and SMAC-24), a series of 12, 18, 20, and 24 blood chemistries. Some laboratories also request that the patient be fasting before all enzyme and electrolyte tests. At other times fasting tests will be done according to the individual orders of the physician. Care must be taken to provide the patient with correct and adequate instructions in these situations.

Blood chemistries

Some basic blood chemistries can be performed easily in the physician's office with the use of chemically impregnated reagent strips to determine the presence of blood glucose and blood urea nitrogen (BUN). (Blood glucose testing is more accurate than urine tests for glucose, and is especially valuable in the management of diabetes.) In addition, there are compact and economical instruments on the market such as the Ames Seralyzer Blood Chemistry Analyzer. This instrument is a reflectance photometer that gives accurate quantitative results from blood serum or plasma for 15 routine diagnostic tests. Blood chemistries, certain therapeutic drug assays (TDA), and electrolytes are determined using special reagent test strips. The blood chemistry analyzer is particularly useful in the physician's office when on-site testing is desir-

Figure 26.10
Ames Seralyzer blood chemistry analyzer—a compact instrument that performs 15 routine diagnostic tests.
Courtesy Ames Co, Inc, Elkhart, Ind.

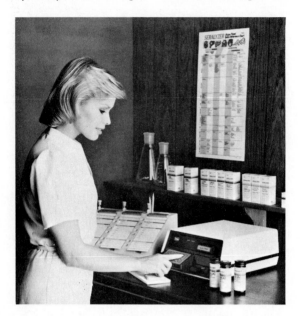

able so that test results can be viewed as an aid to prompt decision making, frequently while the patient is still in the office. Most tests require less than 15 minutes elapsed time, averaging 2 minutes of operator time. Once the test strip is placed on the specimen table you can read the test results on the digital display in less than 2 minutes. Complete instructions for specimen collection, preparation, and use are supplied with the instrument (Figure 26.10).

Test for blood glucose using Dextrostix

The Dextrostix* is a reagent strip that measures blood glucose levels over a range of 45 to 250 mg/100 ml of blood (or 45 to 250 mg/dl). It is supplied in glass bottles that have a color chart on the side that is used for determining test results. Only fresh whole blood is to be used on these strips, as plasma and serum will give false results.

Instructions
1. Don disposable rubber gloves. Do a skin puncture on a fingertip. Allow a large drop of blood to form.
2. Place a large drop of blood on the test area of the strip. (This may be done by putting the strip on the blood over the puncture site.)

3. Wait 60 seconds exactly, holding the strip horizontally to avoid blood runoff from the test area.
4. Holding the strip vertically, wash the blood off, using a sharp stream of water from a wash bottle. No more than 1 to 2 seconds is required.
5. Compare the color on the test area with the color chart on the bottle. There are five color blocks representing 45, 90, 130, 175, and 250 mg/100 ml of blood.
6. Record the results.
7. Remove gloves and wash your hands.

NOTE: If not enough blood is used, you will obtain lower values. If you overwash the strip, you can wash color off and obtain lower values.

To obtain more precise blood glucose results, the same manufacturer has marketed an instrument, the Eyetone Reflectance Colorimeter*, to be used with the Dextrostix. From a precisely calibrated meter that covers the range of 10 to 400 mg/100 ml blood glucose, rapid and accurate determination can be read. Complete instructions for use are provided with the instrument.

---

*Ames Co., Elkhart, Ind.

*LifeScan, Inc., Mountain View, Calif.

Test for Blood Glucose Using the One Touch™ Blood Glucose Meter Monitoring System
(Figure 26.11)*

One Touch blood glucose meters are portable, battery-operated meters that are used with One Touch

*Ames Co., Elkhart, Ind.

test strips to measure glucose concentrations in whole blood in a simple 45-second procedure. The One Touch meter will provide blood glucose readings between 0 and 600 mg/dl (0 and 33.3 mmol/L). Higher values are displayed as HIGH. This equipment can be used in the physician's office or by the patient at home. The purpose of testing with

---

Figure 26.11
One Touch™ blood glucose meter.
Courtesy LifeScan, Inc, Mountain View, Calif.

GETTING STARTED

Before you read about the test procedure, you should study the diagram on the front cover flap to become familiar with the various parts of your ONE TOUCH™ Meter.

POWER BUTTON–This is the main operating button. You will use it every time you perform a test. (We'll explain how in the detailed test instructions later on.)

CODE BUTTON–Each vial of test strips has a code number on the label. You will use the CODE button to set the meter to match the code number on the vial of test strips you are using.

MEMORY BUTTON–The ONE TOUCH Meter automatically stores your test results. You push this button when you want to recall past test results.

DATA PORT–Lets optional DATA MANAGER™ unit access test results in ONE TOUCH memory. (See *Recalling Tests From Memory.*)

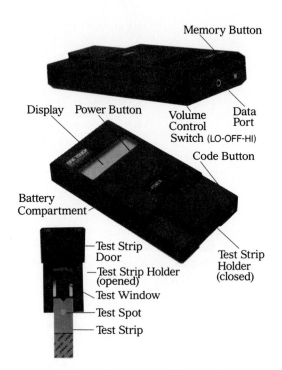

BATTERY COMPARTMENT–Holds the four size "N" batteries included with the meter. You will need to install these batteries before you can operate the meter.

TEST STRIP HOLDER AND TEST WINDOW–This is the area of the meter you will need to be most familiar with. When you open the door of the TEST STRIP HOLDER, you'll see a two-pronged metal clip that holds the test strip in place. Between the two prongs is a small hole which is directly above the TEST WINDOW. The meter reads the test strip through the test window (and the hole) to determine your blood glucose level.

DISPLAY–This is where your test results are shown, in addition to simple messages that help guide you through the test procedure. (See *Summary of Display Messages.*)

VOLUME CONTROL SWITCH adjusts the volume of the "beeps" that help you through the test procedure. In the middle position, the sound cues are OFF. For louder beeps, move the switch up to HI. For softer beeps, move it down to LO.

TEST STRIPS–(Use only ONE TOUCH™ Test Strips.) ONE TOUCH Test Strips come in a moisture-proof, light-protected vial. Because the test strips are sensitive to moisture and light, it's important to keep them in the vial–firmly closed–until you're ready to use them. Always replace the vial cap immediately after you remove a test strip.

As you can see, there is a small dot–called the TEST SPOT–in the center of each test strip. This is where you apply the blood sample.

the One Touch at home is to measure the amount of blood glucose in the blood. The results of this test help the patient determine how much insulin, food, and exercise are needed to control diabetes.

The new One Touch system makes reliable blood glucose monitoring easier than ever. With One Touch, results can be achieved by touching the reagent pad just once—to apply blood—because no wiping or blotting is required. One Touch eliminates three major stumbling blocks to reliable monitoring: starting the test, timing the test, and removing the blood. The opportunity for proce-

---

Figure 26.11, cont'd

Your ONE TOUCH™ Meter is shipped with four "N" (1.5 v) alkaline batteries. You need to install these batteries before operating the meter.

TO INSTALL BATTERIES

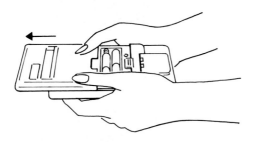

1. Hold the meter level or place on flat surface.

2. Slide top cover away from POWER button as far as it will go. (Do not force cover past battery compartment.)

3. Install new batteries as shown.

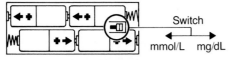

Note placement of batteries:

On the top row, the battery ends marked "+" point to the left.

On the bottom row, "+" ends point to the right.

4. Slide cover back to its original position.

"N" batteries are available from your Authorized LifeScan Distributor, directly from LifeScan, and at most photo supply stores.

When batteries are getting low, the display will flash continuously as long as the meter is ON. The meter will still provide accurate test results with low batteries, but you should replace them as soon as you can.

> **BATTERY**

When BATTERY appears in the display, the batteries are no longer usable, and you must replace them before you can perform another test.

Dead batteries or battery removal will *not* affect the information stored in the meter's memory as long as they are replaced with fresh batteries within fifteen minutes. (You will need to replace the batteries before you can recall test results.)

MEASUREMENT CONVERSION

A small switch located at the bottom of the battery compartment selects the unit of measure for all test results. In the U.S. the switch is set for mg/dL (right position) in the factory. Meters intended for use in Canada are preset for mmol/L (left position). To set your meter for the other unit of measure, simply move the switch to the opposite position.

SUMMARY OF DISPLAY MESSAGES

> **CODE** (number)

Appears for a few seconds after you press POWER button to turn meter ON; (number) is between 1 and 16, and should be reset to match the code number on the test vial. See *Coding the Meter.*

> **INSERT**
> **STRIP**
> **AND**
> **RESTART**

Appears if POWER is pushed before a test strip has been inserted. It remains on the display until a test strip is inserted, the test door closed, and POWER pressed again. See *Testing Your Blood,* Step III.

> **APPLY**
> **SAMPLE**

Appears when meter is ready for blood. See *Testing Your Blood,* Step III.

Continued.

Figure 26.11, cont'd

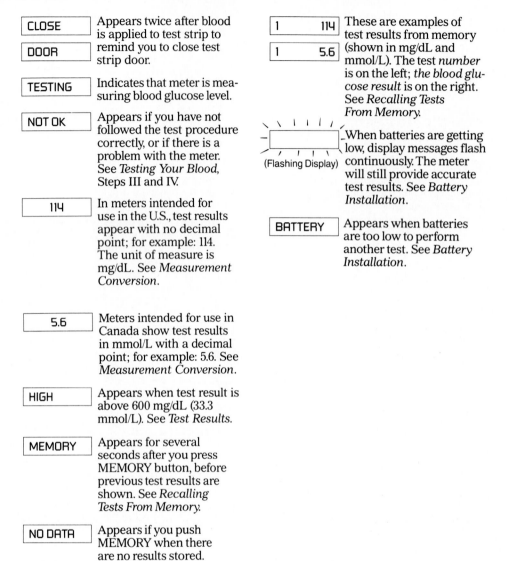

CLOSE / DOOR — Appears twice after blood is applied to test strip to remind you to close test strip door.

TESTING — Indicates that meter is measuring blood glucose level.

NOT OK — Appears if you have not followed the test procedure correctly, or if there is a problem with the meter. See *Testing Your Blood,* Steps III and IV.

114 — In meters intended for use in the U.S., test results appear with no decimal point; for example: 114. The unit of measure is mg/dL. See *Measurement Conversion.*

5.6 — Meters intended for use in Canada show test results in mmol/L with a decimal point; for example: 5.6. See *Measurement Conversion.*

HIGH — Appears when test result is above 600 mg/dL (33.3 mmol/L). See *Test Results.*

MEMORY — Appears for several seconds after you press MEMORY button, before previous test results are shown. See *Recalling Tests From Memory.*

NO DATA — Appears if you push MEMORY when there are no results stored.

1   114 / 1   5.6 — These are examples of test results from memory (shown in mg/dL and mmol/L). The test *number* is on the left; *the blood glucose result* is on the right. See *Recalling Tests From Memory.*

(Flashing Display) — When batteries are getting low, display messages flash continuously. The meter will still provide accurate test results. See *Battery Installation.*

BATTERY — Appears when batteries are too low to perform another test. See *Battery Installation.*

dural error is virtually eliminated. To perform the test, insert the test strip into the meter, press the Power button, then apply a blood sample to the test spot on the reagent pad at any time. At this point the meter takes over, starting the test automatically when it detects blood on the reagent pad. No blood removal, timing, wiping, blotting, or washing is required. Test results appear in just 45 seconds. The One Touch meter provides a stable platform for the test strip while you are applying the blood sample. The test spot is smaller, so less blood is required, and the wider test strip is easier to handle.

An added feature for convenience is that the One Touch system is the first to provide "conversational" messages in plain English to guide you through the test. Messages and results are shown on a large, easy-to-read display. With each test, numerous system self-checks are automatically performed to ensure that the meter is working properly. In addition, 250 previous results can be easily recalled from its memory.

Text continued on p. 544.

Procedure for using the One Touch Blood Glucose Meter

Coding the meter

Before you use your One Touch Meter for the first time—and every time you begin using a new vial of test strips—you must use the Code button to reset the meter to match the code number on the new vial of test strips.

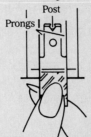

1. First, insert a test strip into the test strip holder as shown. It should slide under prongs, notched end first, "Lifescan" side up. Be sure that the notch rests firmly against the small post.

(Always check the expiration date on the label of the test strip vial. Do not use test strips if expiration date has passed.)

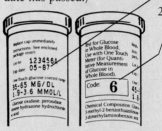

2. Note the code number on the test strip vial label.

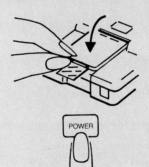

3. Close the test strip door. Push the Power button to turn the meter on. The word Code and a number between 1 and 16 will appear on the display for a few seconds:

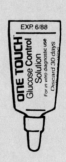

CODE 5   The number shown is the code number from your previous vial of test strips. If this is the first time you've used the meter, the number shown is the one programmed into the meter at the factory.

If it happens to be the same as the code number on your new test strip vial, there is no need to code a new number before you proceed with the test. If it is *not* the same, go on to Step 4.

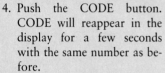

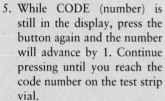

The display should now read APPLY SAMPLE. If the display reads NOT OK, there may be a problem with your meter. For technical assistance, call toll-free

In the U.S.   1 800 227-8862
In Canada   1 800 663-5521

4. Push the CODE button. CODE will reappear in the display for a few seconds with the same number as before.

5. While CODE (number) is still in the display, press the button again and the number will advance by 1. Continue pressing until you reach the code number on the test strip vial.

The meter is now properly coded, and you may proceed with the test. From now on, the meter will keep that code until you re-code for the next vial of test strips.

Checking the system

Your ONE TOUCH® System includes a clear GLUCOSE CONTROL SOLUTION you can use instead of blood to practice the test procedure, or to make sure your meter and test strips are functioning properly. Use only ONE TOUCH Glucose Control Solution. Refer to the glucose control solution insert for detailed instructions and other important information.

To test the system, follow the same procedure you would if you were testing your blood (as described in the next section), substituting control solution for the blood sample. The control solution should yield test results that are within the range printed on the label of the test strip vial.*

*The control range is shown in two different units of measure: mg/dL (used widely in the U.S.) and mmol/L (used in Canada and other countries). This range is for the glucose control solution only; it is not intended as a recommended range for your blood glucose test results.

Continued.

Procedure for using the One Touch Blood Glucose Meter—cont'd

When you begin using the meter for the first time, you should use the control solution until you can do three tests in a row that are within the expected glucose control range. When you can, you will know that you have mastered the test procedure.

Thereafter, you should test the meter with the control solution:
- At least once a week,
- When you begin using a new vial of test strips; and
- Whenever you suspect the meter or test strips may not be functioning properly.

Testing your blood

You can test your blood glucose by following just four simple steps:

Test Summary
Step I: Insert test strip and close door.
Step II: Obtain blood sample.
Step III: Press POWER.
Step IV: Open door; apply sample, and close door.

Be sure to read the following sections for details and additional information.

Step-by-step instructions

Choose a clean, dry work surface. Gather together all the materials you will need for a test:
ONE TOUCH™ Meter
ONE TOUCH™ Test Strips
PENLET™ Sampling Pen
     (or substitute)
Lancets

You should be prepared to move through the test procedure without interruption once you have inserted a test strip and turned the meter ON. To help conserve battery power, the meter turns itself off if blood is not applied to the test strip within two minutes.

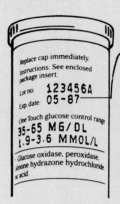

Check the expiration date on the test strip vial. If the date has passed, discard the vial and use a new vial of test strips. The test spot on each test strip should be white or ivory-colored, and free of tears or wrinkles. If it is any other color or appears damaged, discard the test strip and use another.

Step I. Insert test strip

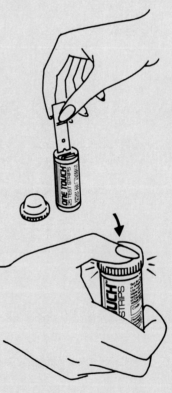

1. Remove test strip from vial. Replace vial cap immediately. **Do not push POWER button first. Do not apply blood to test strip yet.**

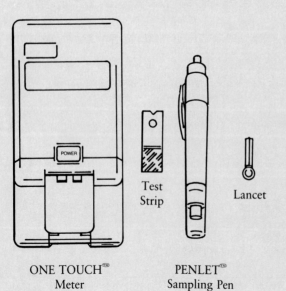

ONE TOUCH™
Meter

PENLET™
Sampling Pen

Test
Strip

Lancet

Procedure for using the One Touch Blood Glucose Meter—cont'd

2. Slide test strip into position under prongs as shown: notched end first. "LIFES-CAN" side up. Make sure notch rests firmly against small post.

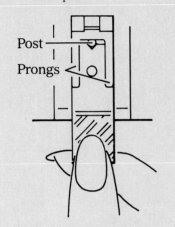

Post

Prongs

3. Close test strip door.

Most users find it quicker and easier to insert test strips with the door closed, but you may want to have the door open at first to make sure you're doing it right.

BE SURE THE DOOR IS CLOSED BEFORE YOU TURN THE METER ON.

Step II. Obtain blood sample

1. Insert a new lancet into the PENLET as shown at right. To reduce the chance of infection, always use a new lancet.

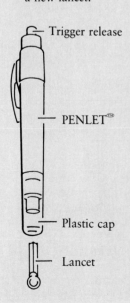

Trigger release

PENLET™

Plastic cap

Lancet

NEVER USE A LANCET THAT HAS BEEN USED BY SOMEONE ELSE.

To protect against possible infection, wash your hands with warm, soapy water; rinse and dry thoroughly. Hand-washing also stimulates the flow of blood to the fingers, making it easier to obtain a sample for the test. Letting your arm hand down at your side for 10-15 seconds before the finger-stick will make it easier, too.

To insert a new lancet in PENLET™

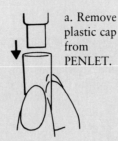

a. Remove plastic cap from PENLET.

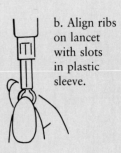

b. Align ribs on lancet with slots in plastic sleeve.

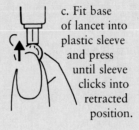

c. Fit base of lancet into plastic sleeve and press until sleeve clicks into retracted position.

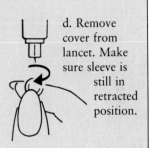

d. Remove cover from lancet. Make sure sleeve is still in retracted position.

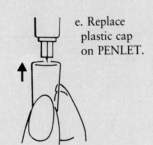

e. Replace plastic cap on PENLET.

Continued.

Procedure for using the One Touch Blood Glucose Meter—cont'd

2. Place PENLET™ against side of finger and press button at top.

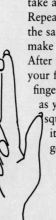

Choose a spot on the side of a different finger each time you take a blood sample. Repeated sampling in the same spot can make your finger sore. After you have pricked your finger, keep the finger pointed down as you gently squeeze or "milk" it to get a good-sized droplet.

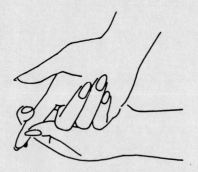

STEP III. Press POWER

1. Be sure test strip door is closed.

2. Press POWER button.

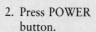

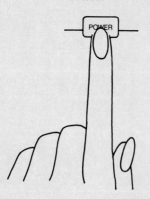

CODE 6

The word CODE and a number between 1 and 16 appear on display for a few seconds. The number should be the same as the code number of the vial of test strips you are using. If it's not, you must re-set the code number. (See *Coding the Meter*.)

APPLY

SAMPLE

APPLY SAMPLE appears on display, and remains until you apply blood to test spot on test strip. But if you take longer than two minutes to apply the blood, the meter will turn itself OFF (to conserve battery power). If it does, push POWER to turn meter back ON. Wait for *APPLY SAMPLE* to reappear, then continue with the test.

INSERT

STRIP

AND

RESTART

If you turn meter ON before you insert test strip, INSERT STRIP AND RESTART will appear after CODE (number). If it does:
insert test strip, close test strip door, then press POWER. In this instance,

POWER does not turn meter OFF, but returns you to CODE (number), followed by APPLY SAMPLE Continue to Step IV.

NOT OK

If NOT OK appears on the display, your meter may have a problem. For technical assistance, call the toll-free number.

Be careful not to change the position of the test strip after APPLY SAMPLE appears. If you do, CLOSE DOOR may appear before you have applied the blood sample. If this happens, do not apply blood. Instead:
  a. Push POWER to turn meter OFF.
  b. Reposition test strip properly.
  c. Push POWER to turn meter back ON.
  d. Wait for APPLY SAMPLE to reappear on display, then continue with Step IV.

Procedure for using the One Touch Blood Glucose Meter—cont'd

Step IV. Apply blood sample

1. Open door.

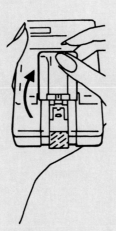

4. Note test results.

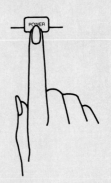

114

5. Press POWER to turn meter OFF.

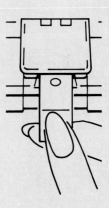

2. Apply blood to test spot.*

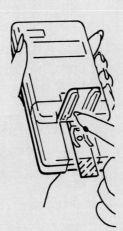

6. Remove test strip and discard it.*

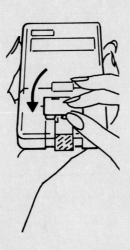

3. Close door:

correct incorrect

*After you do a test, take a look at the back of the test spot when you've finished and removed the test strip from the meter. There should not be any uncovered patches in the test spot. If there are, you should do the test over again with a new test strip. Remember to turn the meter OFF, then back ON again after the new test strip is in place.

If test strip becomes dislodged *before* you apply blood, return to Step I. If it is dislodged *after* you have applied blood, start over again with a new test strip.

CLOSE

DOOR

*You may be most comfortable holding the meter in one hand as you apply blood from the other (as illustrated). Or you may find it easier to keep the meter on a flat work surface when you apply blood.

Continued.

Procedure for using the One Touch Blood Glucose Meter—cont'd

As soon as you touch test spot with blood, the meter will beep. CLOSE DOOR will appear on display twice, followed by TESTING. (You have about 10 seconds to close the door before TESTING appears.)

> TESTING

The meter beeps twice when your test result appears.

> 114

> NOT OK

If NOT OK appears, something needs to be corrected. It could be one of the following:

- The door was not closed in time,
- The test strip moved and blocked the small window beneath it while you were applying blood, or
- The test strip was not inserted correctly.

Go back to Step I and start over with another test strip. Make sure you are following the instructions carefully. If NOT OK appears again, call the toll-free number for technical assistance.

Test results

Your test result will appear in 45 seconds. Results above 600 mg/dL (33.3 mmol/L) are displayed as HIGH.

If you think your test result may be wrong:

a. Before discarding test strip, turn it over and make sure there are no white or ivory-colored (uncovered) patches on the back of the test spot. If there is even one small uncovered patch, go back to Step I and repeat the test with a new test strip.

b. Make sure the CODE (number) diplay is the same as the code number on the test strip vial. If it isn't the same, reset CODE (number) on meter and repeat the test with a new test strip.

c. Check expiration date on test strip vial. If expiration date has passed, discard vial and repeat the test with a strip from a new vial, being sure to reset CODE (number).

d. Make sure test strip holder and test window are clean and lint-free.

e. Was the test performed in direct sunlight or very bright incandescent light? If so, shade the meter and repeat the test with a new test strip.

f. Did the temperature or humidity exceed the meter's operating specifications.

g. Was the test strip door closed (with test strip in place) when you turned meter on? If not, repeat the test with a new test strip.

h. If test result is a number below 34 and has a decimal point, you may have accidentally switched from mg/dL to mmol/L (the unit of measure used in Canada) while installing new batteries. The switch is located at the bottom of the battery compartment. (See *Measurement Conversion*.)

i. Use glucose control solution to check the system and confirm that you are following the correct procedure. (See *Checking the System*.)

Recalling tests from memory

Your ONE TOUCH™ Meter automatically stores up to 250 test results. When you have done more than 250 tests, the oldest tests are dropped from memory as new ones are added. The most recent test will always be displayed first.

To recall test results

> CODE 6

> INSERT

> STRIP

> AND

> RESTART

1. *Without* inserting test strip, push POWER to turn meter on. CODE (number) will appear, followed by INSERT STRIP AND RESTART.

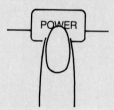

Procedure for using the One Touch Blood Glucose Meter—cont'd

2. Push MEMORY button.

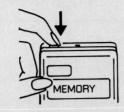

MEMORY appears on display for several seconds. Then, two numbers appear.*

The left one is the *number* of your most recent test.

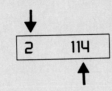

The right one is the *blood glucose result* of your most recent test.

3. To read results of tests before the most recent one, press MEMORY button again.

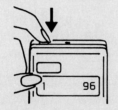

Continue pressing MEMORY to review previous results.

4. When you are finished with memory, push POWER to turn meter OFF.

*If no results are stored, NO DATA will appear on display.

5. If you want to perform another test, insert strip, close door, then push POWER to turn meter back ON and proceed as usual.

Each push of the MEMORY button calls up the test *before* the one just displayed, all the way back to test number 1. Then the meter starts over again with the most recent test.

If you want to return to a more recent test without going all the way back to the beginning, it may be faster to turn the meter off, then repeat the procedure from Step 1 above.

Your ONE TOUCH™ System Kit contains a logbook you can use to keep a permanent written record of your test results, together with information on diet and medication. Additional logbooks can be obtained from your Authorized Life-Scan Distributor or directly from LifeScan.

An optional LifeScan product called the DATA MANAGER™ unit is available for use with your meter. The DATA MANAGER lets you review the test results in the meter's memory with the date and time of each test. It also prints out your results in graphic format to help you and your health care professional better analyze your test results. For more information, ask your Authorized Life-Scan Distributor or call LIfeScan toll-free:

In the U.S.   1 800 227-8862
In Canada   1 800 663-5521

Complete Blood Count (CBC): Hematology Test

Since the complete blood count is the most common laboratory procedure ordered on blood, it will be discussed more fully than other tests. A CBC gives a fairly complete look at the components in blood, providing a wealth of information on a patient's condition. The tests performed in a CBC include red blood cell count (RBC), hemoglobin (Hgb), hematocrit (Hct), white blood cell count (WBC), differential (Diff) white cell count, and a stained red cell examination (red cell morphology). The first four tests are quantitative measurements, and the last two are qualitative. All these tests are performed on whole blood (Table 26.1).

Red cell count

The red cell count is the number of red blood cells found in each cubic millimeter of blood. *Manual counting in the past led to errors, thus was of questionable value. Presently with the automated counting equipment available, this determination is considered more reliable.* Elevated red cell counts indicate polycythemia or that the patient has moved to a location with a higher altitude at which the air contains less oxygen. In the latter case, the body requires more red cells to carry sufficient oxygen to meet its needs. Decreased numbers of red cells will be seen in patients with some form of anemia, after a hemorrhage, and also after the initial hemoconcentration of shock.

Hemoglobin

A hemoglobin determines the oxygen-carrying ability of the blood. It is a simple and most efficient method to detect any anemia (pernicious, iron deficiency, sickle cell) and the severity of the condition. It also helps the physician determine the effectiveness of treatments administered to the patient. A patient is considered anemic if the hemoglobin value is below 12 gm/100 ml. Low hemoglobin values will also be caused by hemorrhage. Elevated concentrations of hemoglobin may be seen in severely burned or dehydrated patients. This is because the body has lost considerable amounts of fluid; thus the red cells are suspended in less fluid, and more hemoglobin is present in each 100 ml of blood.

Hematocrit

The hematocrit, or packed cell volume, represents the percentage of red blood cells in the total blood volume. Elevated hematocrits will be seen in patients with polycythemia; a low hematocrit is seen

Table 26.1
Normal values for a complete blood count performed on whole blood

Test	Values
Red cell count	
Females	4,000,000-5,500,000/mm³ blood
Males	4,500,000-6,000,000/mm³ blood
Hemoglobin	
Females	12-16 g/100 ml blood
Males	14-18 g/100 ml blood
Hematocrit	
Females	37%-47%
Males	40%-54%
White cell count (females and males)	5,000-10,000/mm³ blood
Differential	
Polymorphonuclear neutrophils	60%-70%
Monocytes	2%-6%
Lymphocytes	20%-40%
Eosinophils	1%-4%
Basophils	0.5%-1%
Morphology (stained red cell examination)	Normal

in anemia and leukemia. Generally, the hematocrit and hemoglobin concentrations are related. Each 1% hematocrit contains .34 gm of hemoglobin; thus the hematocrit should equal three times the hemoglobin within 3%. Thus if a patient's hemoglobin is 14 gm/100 ml, the hematocrit should fall between 39% and 45% ($14 \times 3.0 = 42$, and plus or minus 3 = 39% to 45%). Deviations from this relationship usually indicate the presence of red cells of abnormal size or hemoglobin content.

White blood cell count

The white blood cell count is the number of WBCs found in each cubic millimeter of blood. As with the red cell count, automated equipment now provides us with a more reliable count. A person's white count will vary some during a day, because of exercise, emotional states, or digestion. Increases as great as 2,000 WBC/cu mm may be seen in these situations. Pathologically, the WBC count will increase in infections and leukemia. Decreased WBC count may be caused by radiation therapy, immunosuppressive therapy (chemotherapy) for cancer and transplant patients, toxic reactions, measles, typhoid fever, and infectious hepatitis. This is caused by a depression of the bone marrow's blood-forming centers.

Differential white cell count

The differential is a test that determines the percentage of each of the five different types of white blood cells in the blood. Each type of white cell has a specific function. Together, with the degree of increase or decrease in the total number of white cells and with the percentage of each type of white cell, the physician is able to make a more definite diagnosis. Characteristic abnormal numbers and types of white cells are seen in various diseases (Figure 26.12).

Neutrophils. The body's primary lines of defense against infection are the neutrophils. They seek and destroy any invading bacteria by the process of phagocytosis. Increased numbers of neutrophils are seen in conditions such as appendicitis, tonsillitis, pneumonia, abscesses, granulocytic leukemia, and meningitis. A decreased neutrophil count (neutropenia) is seen in mumps, hepatitis, measles, aplastic anemia, agranulocytosis, and in patients who are taking certain drugs, such as certain antibiotics, antihistamines, anticonvulsants, and sulfonamides. In these cases the decrease in the neutrophils causes an increase in one of the other white blood cells, especially in the lymphocytes. Thus one must know the actual value for each of the five types of WBCs to determine if this is the case.

Monocytes. The body's second line of defense against invasion by foreign substances is the monocytes. These are also phagocytes, as they ingest any foreign particles or bacteria that the neutrophils are unable to ingest. The monocytes will also clean up any cellular debris that remains after an infection or abscess subsides. Increased numbers of monocytes will be seen in patients who have tuberculosis, amebic dysentery, typhoid fever, Rocky Mountain spotted fever, subacute bacterial endocarditis, or monocytic leukemia, or in those patients who are recovering from a bacterial infection. Conditions with decreased numbers of monocytes are difficult to indicate, since the normal count of the cells is so low.

Lymphocytes. The lymphocytes circulate through the body to destroy the toxic products of protein metabolism and to identify and produce antibodies against foreign cells. Recent studies are identifying new roles of these cells, especially in the field of immunology. Increased numbers of lymphocytes (lymphocytosis) are seen in viral diseases such as influenza, German measles, mumps, whooping cough, and infectious mononucleosis, as well as in lymphocytic leukemia. Decreased numbers are seen in patients who are taking cortisone, ACTH, and epinephrine. Other types of leukemia and radiation also cause lymphopenia.

Eosinophils and basophils. Little is known about the eosinophils and basophils. It is thought that the eosinophils aid in detoxification by breaking down protein material and are associated with allergic reactions and production of antihistamine. Increased eosinophil counts are seen in patients who have hay fever, allergies, skin diseases, parasite infections, and asthma. Decreased counts are seen in patients who have increased levels of insulin, epinephrine, and ACTH. Stress following surgery may also cause eosinopenia.

Basophils are thought to produce heparin and histamine; thus some believe that they help prevent blood from clotting in inflamed tissues and play a role in clot breakdown. Increased basophil counts are seen in patients who have hemolytic anemias, chronic granulocytic leukemia, and have had their spleen removed (splenectomy) and exposure to radiation. Decreased conditions have not been identified.

Abnormal white cells

The five types of white cells just discussed are all normal cells found in peripheral blood. In some disorders and diseases immature neutrophils or atypical lymphocytes will be seen. The immature neutrophils are myeloblasts, promyelocytes, myelocytes, metamyelocytes, and band cells. You will see these terms on some laboratory reports included with a differential report.

Stained red cell examination

Using the same stained slide that was used for determining the differential, the laboratory technologist will then examine the red blood cells for any variation in size, shape, structure, color, or content. Anisocytosis, macrocytosis, microcytosis, and poikilocytosis are reported as slight, moderate, or marked.

Summary

As you can see, the significant findings obtained from a complete blood count are numerous. Evaluation of these findings, along with the total clinical picture of a patient's condition, provides the physician with valuable information for screening, diagnosing, treating, or evaluating and monitoring the progress of treatment for patient care.

Figure 26.12
For legend see opposite page.

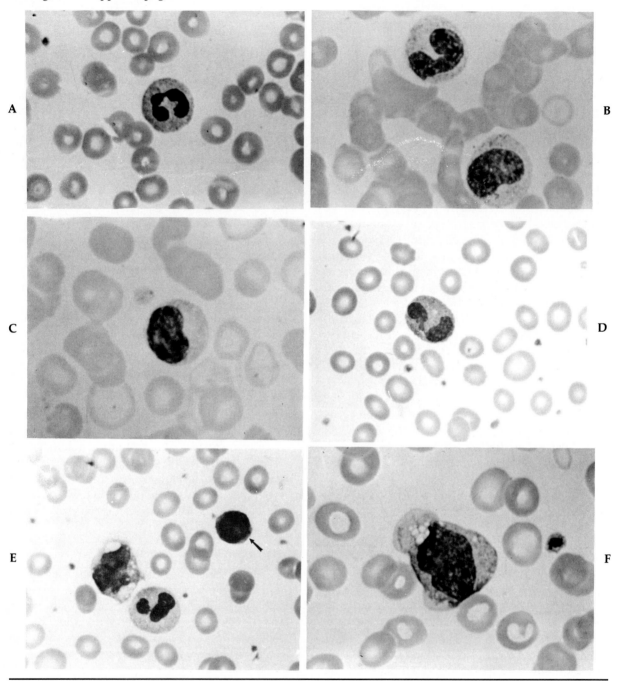

AUTOMATION IN THE CLINICAL LABORATORY

Within the past 15 to 20 years, clinical laboratories have been confronted with an ever-increasing workload. An answer to this problem has been sought in automated instrumentation. These specialized modular systems automate or semiauto-mate the time-consuming, step-by-step procedures formerly performed by manual analysis. With refinement of instrumentation, fast and accurate methods have been developed for reporting a wide variety of laboratory information on body fluids, which include whole blood, plasma, serum, urine, and cerebrospinal fluid. The human element of er-

Figure 26.12

Main types of leukocytes. **A,** *Granulocytes-neutrophils: Segmented neutrophils* are round or oval cells. The cytoplasm is a lavender or pink color, with pinkish or lavender granules. The nucleus is segmented, having from 2 to 12 segments, but usually 3 or 4, and it stains a purplish or lavender color. **B,** *Stab neutrophils* are round or oval, with a cytoplasm similar in color to that of the segmented neutrophils. It contains fine granules that are pinkish or reddish violet. The nucleus is one continuous piece that looks like a flexible rod. It commonly forms letter shapes, such as C, S, N, and U. The nucleus is colored a dark purple or lavender, and occupies about one fourth of the cell. **C,** *Juvenile neutrophils* are round or oval, and cytoplasm is usually a bluish pink, containing granules that may be definite or fine and of a purplish or reddish color. The nucleus is bean shaped, usually purplish in color and usually occupies about half the cell (juvenile neutrophil also appears at bottom of panel **B**). *Not shown, myelocyte neutrophils'* cytoplasm often takes an almost neutral stain, tinged with blue, and it, as well as the nucleus, is dotted with definite pinkish or purple granules. The nucleus is round or oval, ordinarily stains bluish purple, and takes up about two thirds of the cell. **D,** *Granulocytes-eosinophils.* Eosinophils' cytoplasm has light blue tinges and is covered with coarse, round, or oval bright pink or red granules. The nucleus is usually segmented and stains a deep lavender to light blue. **F,** *lymphocytes'* cytoplasm is usually a bright blue and at times may be almost negligible, as the purple or lavender nucleus may take up almost the entire cell. Immature lymphocytes are larger than mature cells, having much more cytoplasm, which generally stains a very pale, glasslike blue. Occasionally a few pink granules may appear in the cytoplasm. The nucleus is usually round or oval but may be indented as well. It stains a purple or lavender color. **F,** *Monocytes* are the largest of all the white cells. Often they are irregular in shape and usually take a pale stain. The cytoplasm is usually a smoky blue-gray, sometimes sprinkled with a fine pink dust. The nucleus generally is kidney shaped or round, often lobulated, staining a lavender color.

ror is virtually eliminated, assuring the absolute objectivity of measurement so important to accurate diagnosis and monitoring. Multiphasic tests, test panels, or profiles consist of a battery of automated tests performed on the same specimen at the same time. It has been found that it is more useful and economical to subject every specimen to a battery or panel of automated tests than to limit the examination to one or two tests. Through this system of routine total blood counts and biochemical profiling, additional disease screening tests may be routinely performed. Most hematology panels in laboratories that have any volume at all are done on the Coulter systems or other systems, such as the Technicon H-I system. There are several different machines; most of them automate or at least semiautomate the whole process, using only 1 ml of blood. Test results are obtained visually, on a digital display or video screen, or on a hematology printout card (Figure 26.13). The latest state-of-the-art systems use laser technology. Laser counters in hematology, such as the ELT-8, perform an automated CBC. The laser looks at the cells to determine the results. Traditionally the chemistry sections of laboratories are the most

heavily automated. Most laboratories will have at least some form of automation in chemistry if not in other departments. Frequently used biochemical panels are the SMA 12/60, SMA 18, SMA 20, SMAC 20 OR 24. SMA stands for sequential multiple analysis, the C indicates that it is computer-assisted, and the numbers indicate the number of tests that are performed. Another panel is simply called a Chemistry Screening Panel 12, 20, or 24. The numbers indicate how many tests are to be performed. These are general terms that are used, as the type of tests run in these panels will vary with the laboratory and how they have programmed the automated equipment for use. All of these panels are screening devices that allow the physician to focus on abnormal results for further study and investigation. Test results from the SMA systems are reported on an 8-½ × 11 inch sheet of precalibrated, vertical graph paper called an SCG (serum chemistry graph) or an SMA 12 or on a similar horizontal graph for the other systems (Figure 26.14). Rather than sending the physician this graph paper, many laboratories now have special computer printout forms that also record the results of the tests performed. The laboratory

Figure 26.13

A, The Coulter S-Plus for automated cell counting.

Courtesy Coulter Electronics, Inc, Hialeah, Fla.

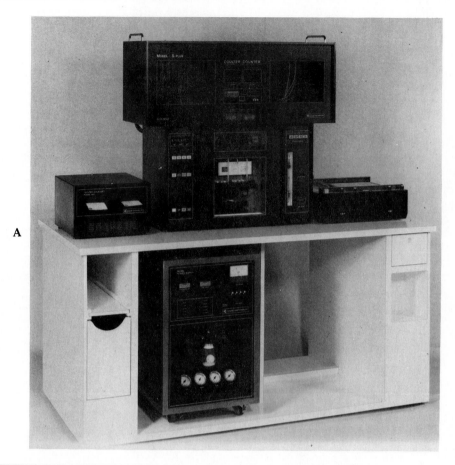

keeps the graph as its permanent record and sends the computer printout to the physician. One example of the computer forms used is a sheet divided into columns. In different columns the names of the tests, the normal values, and the results of the tests performed are recorded.

Many multiphasic tests, panels, or profiles are devised to provide information on particular body system disorders or suspected conditions and also for screening purposes, some of which include a hepatobiliary profile, diabetes profile, cardiac screening, renal function, thyroid function, and arthritis. The grouping of specific tests provides the physician with an overall view of the patient's sta-

tus that a single test could not provide. An example of a cardiac profile (panel) may include the following: an SGOT, SGPT, LDH, CPK, CBC, sedimentation rate, prothrombin time (PT), cholesterol, triglycerides, and potassium.

A kidney function profile may include the following: total protein, albumin, globulin, A/G ratio, creatinine, BUN, BUN/creatinine ratio, sodium, potassium, chloride, uric acid, and cholesterol. A liver function profile may include the following: alkaline phosphatase, LDH, SGOT, SGPT, total bilirubin, total protein, albumin, globulin, A/G ratio, and so on. See Table 26.2 for additional information on some of these tests and others.

Figure 26.13, cont'd
B, The Coulter diff3 System for automating the complete differential. **C,** The
Coulter Counter ZBI 6 System for semiautomated hematology profiles. It will
determine red blood cell count, white blood cell count, hemoglobin,
hematocrit, mean corpuscular volume, and platelet count. Test results are
obtained from digital readouts on equipment.

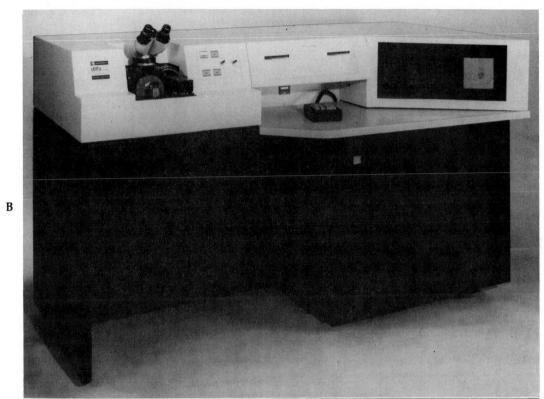

B

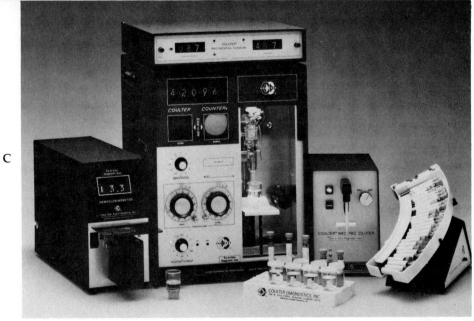

C

Continued.

Figure 26.13, cont'd
D, Hematology printout card that shows results of tests performed on Coulter S-Plus and on Coulter diff3 System.

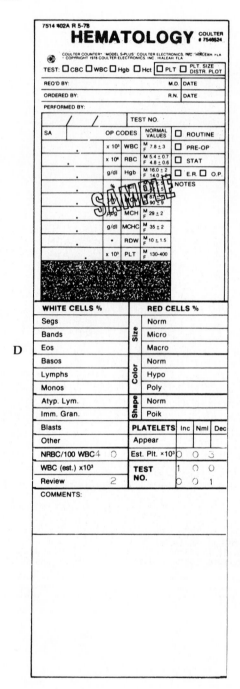

D

Figure 26.14
A, The SMA 12/60 for simultaneous performance of 12 biochemical tests on just
1.8 ml of untreated serum. **B,** Results are presented in concentration terms on a
precalibrated strip chart record, the Serum Chemistry Graph. Normal test ranges
for each parameter are printed as shaded areas; horizontal line crossing graph
represents the test results. Time from aspiration of given sample to finished chart
is only 8 minutes—less time than it takes to complete any one of these tests by
other methods.
Courtesy Technician Instruments Corp, Tarrytown, NY: TECHNICON, SMA, and SMAC are registered trademarks
of Technicon Instruments Corp.

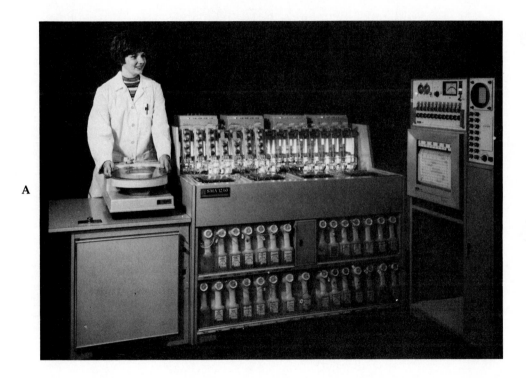

A

Continued.

Figure 26.14, cont'd
For legend see p. 551.

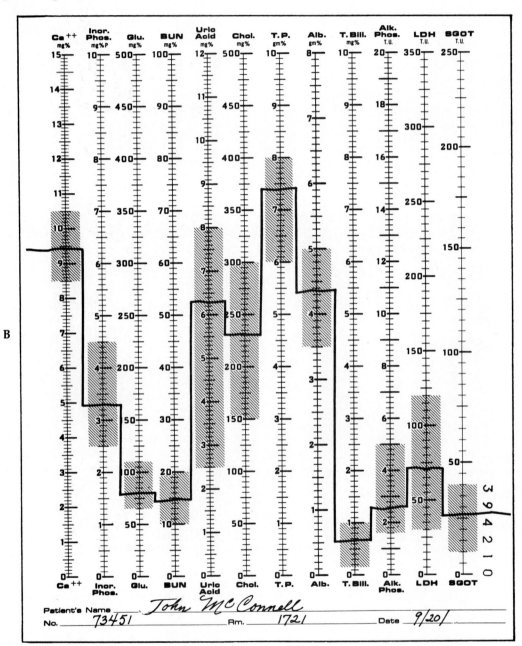

Table 26.2
Examinations made on blood

Test	Performed on	Normal values*	Significance
Hematology blood tests			
1. Sedimentation rate (sedate or ESR)	Whole blood	Wintrobe tubes: Female: 0-20 mm/hr Male: 0-9 mm/hr Wester: Female and male: 0-20 mm/hr	Increased in almost all infections, myocardial infarction, active rheumatoid arthritis, pulmonary infarction, shock, surgical operations, and pregnancy. Decreased in sickle cell anemia, polycythemia, cardiac decompensation, and newborn infants.
2. Microhematocrit (MCHC)	Whole blood	32%-36%	Same as for regular hematocrit.
3. Coagulation tests and platelets			
a. Coagulation or clotting time	Blood	Lee-White: 6-10 min Capillary tube: 3-7 min	Used as a measurement of the ability of blood to clot properly. May indicate that vitamin K or calcium levels are inadequate for clotting of blood.
b. Platelet count	Whole blood	200,000-400,000/cu mm blood	Decreased numbers may indicate disease of the spleen; also will cause bleeding.
4. Prothrombin time (PT or Pro-Time)	Blood serum	70%-110% of control value	Prolonged time may indicate vitamin K deficiency, liver disease, or an excessive use of dicumarol in treatment. When anticoagulation therapy used, PT kept at from 2 to 2½ times normal.
Blood chemistries			
1. Blood urea nitrogen (BUN)	Blood serum	10-20 mg/100 ml or 10-20 mg/dl	Increased in some kidney diseases.
2. Cholesterol	Blood serum	Up to 20 yrs.: 120-230 mg/100 ml or mg/dl 30 yrs.: 120-240 mg/100 ml or mg/dl 40 yrs.: 140-240 mg/100 ml or mg/dl 50 yrs.: 150-240 mg/100 ml or mg/dl 60 yrs.: 160-240 mg/100 ml or mg/dl 100 yrs.: 160-240 mg/100 ml or mg/dl	Increased in liver disease with obstructive jaundice, nephrosis, diabetes mellitus, hypothyroidism, and in diets too high in saturated fat or cholesterol. Decreased in anemia, malabsorption, hyperthyroidism, and hepatic failure.

Modified from Zakus SM: Clinical skills and assisting techniques for the medical assistant, ed 2, St Louis, 1988, The CV Mosby Co.
*NOTE: For many years laboratories have reported a number of their test results in milligrams (mg) percent, or milligrams (mg) per 100 milliliters (ml), or 100 cubic centimeters (cc). A newer method, used by many, is the use of a deciliter (dl); 1 dl = 0.10 L or 100 ml or 100 cc. Thus in a report, mg/dl is the same as mg% or mg/100 ml. Keep in mind that test values may differ, depending on the methods and procedures used by the laboratory.

Continued.

Table 26.2
Examinations made on blood—cont'd

Test	Performed on	Normal values*	Significance
Blood chemistries—cont'd			
3. Total protein (TP)	Blood serum	6.0-8.0 g/100 ml or 6.0-8.0 g/dl	Increased in dehydration, malignancy, hepatic disease, infection. Decreased levels in overhydration, hepatic insufficiency, burns, malnutrition, nephrosis.
4. Albumin (Alb)	Blood serum	3.5-5.5 g/100 ml or 3.5-5.5 g/dl	Increase seen in dehydration. Decreased in overhydration, hepatic insufficiency, malnutrition, burns, nephrosis.
5. Alkaline phosphatase (Alk phos)	Blood serum	2-4.5 Bodansky units 4-13 King Armstrong units 20-90 IU/L	Increased in children and in women in the third trimester of pregnancy; in hepatic disease, obstructive jaundice, bone growth, osteoblastic bone tumors, peptic ulcer, and colitis. Decreased in hypothyroidism, anemia, malnutrition, pernicious anemia.
6. LDH (Lactic dehydrogenase)	Blood serum	90-200 IU/L	Increased in myocardial infarction, muscle necrosis, hemolysis, kidney infarct, liver disease, and cerebral damage.
7. SGOT (Serum glutamic oxaloacetic transaminase)	Blood serum	10-40 units/L	Very high levels seen 24 hours after a myocardial infarction, in liver disease, complete biliary obstruction and jaundice with hepatic cirrhosis. Increased in skeletal trauma, hemolysis, cerebral damage. Lower levels seen in pregnancy, chronic dialysis, beri beri.
8. Triglycerides	Blood serum	40-140 mg/100 ml or 40-140 mg/dl	Increased in diets too high in saturated fat or cholesterol. High level is a risk factor for heart attack. Decreased in anemia.
9. CPK (Creatine phosphokinase)	Blood serum	1-10 units 0.2 to 1.42 units (two methods)	Increased in myocardial infarction, pulmonary edema, and pulmonary infarction, DTs, and muscular dystrophy.
10. Creatinine	Blood serum	0.7-1.7 mg/dl	Increased in nephritis and impaired kidney function.

Table 26.2
Examinations made on blood—cont'd

Test	Performed on	Normal values*	Significance
Other tests			
1. Glucose tolerance test (standard test)	Blood serum	(Results per 100 ml blood) *Fasting blood glucose:* 80 mg—120 mg *After ingesting test dose of glucose:* 30 min—150 mg 60 min—135 mg 2 hours—100 mg 2½ hours—80 mg	Used to detect abnormalities in carbohydrate metabolism such as occur in diabetes mellitus, hypoglycemia, and adrenocortical and liver dysfunction. In diabetes, fasting blood sugar (FBS) is around 120 mg/100 ml or higher. After 1 hour, level rises over 180 mg/100 ml, and does not return to normal in 2- and 3-hour specimens. Normally blood sugar will return to normal after 2 hours.
2. Blood typing	Whole blood or blood serum	*One of the following:* Type O—45% of the population (Universal donor) Type A—40% of the population Type B—10% of the population Type AB—5% of the population (Universal recipient) And either: Rh positive—85% of population Rh negative—15% of population	Must be done before a patient receives a blood transfusion to ensure a compatible transfusion; also important in pregnancy to help prevent erythroblastosis fetalis.
3. Radioimmunoassay for serum pregnancy *or* *HCG* Beta subunit for pregnancy	Serum	Quantitative results: 1st wk: 20-60 mIU/ml 2nd wk: 60-200 mIU/ml 3rd wk: 200-2000 mIU/ml 2nd or 3rd month: 20,000-200,000 mIU/ml 2nd trimester: 12,000-60,000 mIU/ml 3rd trimester: 10,000-30,000 mIU/ml	Results reported as either positive or negative for pregnancy. A result of 5-15 mIU/ml *may* indicate an ectopic pregnancy. A result of less than 5 mIU/ml would be considered negative for an ectopic pregnancy.
4. HIV III antibody for AIDS *NOTE:* In many states it is a state regulation that the patient must sign a consent form before this test is performed.	Serum or plasma	Negative	A negative result indicates that the antibody is not in the blood. A positive result indicates that the antibody is in the blood.

Conclusion

You have now completed the chapter on hematology. Practice the procedures, and when you feel that you know the equipment and steps of the procedures, arrange with your instructor to take a performance test. You will be expected to demonstrate accurately your ability to prepare for and perform all the procedures that have been presented.

Review Questions

1. Define *blood*.
2. List the white blood cells that are classified as granulocytes and those that are classified as agranulocytes.
3. When asked to obtain a blood sample for a battery of 12 blood chemistry tests, what method and body site would you use to obtain this sample?
4. You have obtained a skin puncture blood sample. What tests might you perform in the office on this sample?
5. The following blood report has been sent to your office. Indicate which test results are normal and which are abnormal.

   White blood cells—15,000/cu mm
   Red blood cells—5.6 million/cu mm
   Diff
     Lymphocytes—55%
     Eosinophils—8%
     Neutrophils—65%
   SGOT—65 units/ml
   Alkaline phosphatase—85 IU/L
   Prothrombin time—90% of control
   Hematocrit—45%
   BUN—18 mg/100 ml
   Cholesterol—160 mg/100 ml
6. The physician has ordered a CBC, an SMA-12, and a triglyceride test for a patient. Would you give this patient any special instructions before having a blood sample drawn? Could you collect one sample of blood in one tube? Would you use plain tube(s) or tube(s) with an anticoagulant additive? Explain the reasons for your answers.
7. What simplified test might you do in the office to determine the presence of sugar in the blood? Explain the method involved.
8. List the blood test(s) that a physician may order to help diagnose the following conditions or diseases:
   a. Liver disease
   b. Myocardial infarction
   c. A diet too high in fat content
   d. Kidney disease
   e. Leukemia
   f. Anemia
   g. Diabetes
9. Define the terms *multiphasic tests*, *test panel*, and *profile*.
10. List 3 blood tests that require a patient to fast before the blood sample is drawn.

SUGGESTED READINGS

Clarke WL and Pohl SL: New developments in blood glucose monitoring and insulin delivery, Occup Health Nurs 30:40, Dec 1982.

Leser DR: Synthetic blood: a future alternative, Am J Nurs 82:452, March 1982.

Stevens AD: Monitoring blood glucose at home—who should do it, Am J Nurs 81:2026, Nov 1981.

Thompson DA: Teaching the client about anticoagulants, Am J Nurs 82:78, Feb 1982.

Chapter 27

Diagnostic Radiology

- Radiological procedures
- X-rays
- Diagnostic radiology
- Position of patient for x-ray studies
- Radiological dangers, hazards, and safety precautions
- Medical assistant's responsibilities
- Storage and management in office

Objectives

On completion of Chapter 27 the medical assistant student should be able to:

1 Define and pronounce the terms listed in the vocabulary and text of this chapter.

2 Explain the medical specialty of diagnostic radiology, listing examples of procedures performed by this specialty; explain the nature and purpose of each procedure.

3 Define the term *contrast medium* as used in radiology; state the function of contrast media and list at least three examples of these.

4 List and explain the nature of at least 10 radiological procedures that use contrast media.

5 List and explain four basic positions used for proper exposure of the body part during radiography.

6 State and discuss the dangers, hazards, and safety precautions relevant to x-ray equipment and procedures.

7 List three body changes that may occur with overexposure to radiation.

8 Discuss the medical assistant's responsibilities relevant to radiological procedures.

9 Demonstrate proficiency in communicating proper preparation for x-rays to the patient.

10 Demonstrate the care and storage of the finished product when received in the physician's office.

11 Prepare and assist the patient for radiological procedures.

12 Position the patient correctly for different x-ray exposures (if licensed to do so).

Vocabulary

cassette (kah-set′) A light-proof aluminum or Bakelite container with front and back intensifying screens, between which x-ray film is placed when used for x-ray examinations.

detail The sharpness of the radiograph image.

density The quality of being dense or impenetrable.

fluoroscope (floo′or-o-skōp″) An instrument used during x-ray examinations for visual observation of the internal body structures by means of x-rays. The body part to be viewed is placed between the x-ray tube and a fluorescent screen. As x-rays pass through the body, shadowy images of the internal organs are projected on the screen.

fluoroscopy (floo″or-os′ko-pē) Visual examination by means of a fluoroscope.

ionizing (i″on-i′-zing) **radiation** Radiant energy given off by radioactive atoms and x-rays.

irradiate (ĭ-rā′dē-āt) To treat with radiant energy.

irradiation (i-rā″dē-ā′shun) Exposure to radiation; the passage of penetrating rays through a substance or object.

oscilloscope (ŏ-sil′ō-skōp) An instrument for visualizing the shape or wave form of sound waves, as in ultrasonography, or of electric currents, as when monitoring heart action and other body functions.

radiation (rā″dē-ā′shun) Electromagnetic waves of streams of atomic particles capable of penetrating and being absorbed into matter. Examples of electromagnetic waves are x-rays, gamma rays, ultraviolet rays, infrared rays, and rays of visible light. Atomic particles are alpha and beta particles.

radiogram (rā′dē-ō-gram″) A picture of internal body structures produced by the action of gamma rays or x-rays on a special film.

radiograph (rā′dē-ō-graf″) or **roentgenograph** (rent′gen-ō-graf) or **roentgenogram** (rent′gen-ō-gram″) The film or photographic record produced by radiography.

radiography (rā″dē-og′rah-fe) The taking of radiograms.

radioisotope (rā″dē-ō-ī′so-tōp) A radioactive form of an element consisting of unstable atoms that emit rays of energy or streams of atomic particles. Radioisotopes occur naturally, as in the case of radium, or can be created artificially, as in the case of cobalt.

radiolucent (rā″dē-ō-lū-sent) That which permits the partial or wholly passage of radiant energy, such as x-rays. Representative areas appear dark on the exposed x-ray film.

radionuclide (rā″dē-ō-nū′klīd) A radioactive substance.

radiopaque (rā-dē-ō-pāk′) Pertaining to that which is impenetrable by x-rays and other forms of radiant energy; matter that obstructs the passage of radiant energy. Representative areas appear light or white on the exposed film.

voltage (vōl-tij) The electromotive force measured in volts (the units of force for electricity to flow).

RADIOLOGICAL PROCEDURES

Radiology (rā″dē-ol′ō-jē) is the specialty of medical science that deals with the study, diagnosis, and treatment of disease by using x-rays, radioactive substances, and other forms of radiant energy such as gamma rays, ultraviolet rays, alpha and beta particles, sound, and magnetic waves.

The procedures involved in radiology can be divided into three specialties: diagnostic radiology, radiation therapy (radiation oncology), and nuclear medicine.

The equipment used for radiological procedures is very expensive and sophisticated; thus most physicians requisition these examinations or therapy from outside sources, such as from a major treatment center, local hospital, or private radiologist. However, some diagnostic radiology procedures, such as radiographs of the chest or skeletal fractures, may be performed in some larger offices or in physician's offices in rural areas. It takes special training and great skill to do radiological procedures properly and to accurately interpret the fluoroscopic, scanning, and x-ray images formed. Skilled radiology technologists called radiographers, prepare and position the patient and take the x-ray films. These individuals must be registered nationally to practice. In addition, those who practice in California, New York, and 20 other states must also be licensed or certified by the state. The radiologist, a licensed physician specially trained in radiological techniques, reads and interprets the films, scanning images, and fluoroscopic images.

For medical assistants to be well qualified and

able to contribute to total patient care, it is imperative that they know the varied techniques, the purposes, and the nature of the specialized and highly technical radiology procedures. *Medical assistants are not legally allowed to perform radiological procedures (unless licensed and registered to do so).* Descriptions of various x-ray and fluoroscopic studies follow (also see Chapter 24, Laboratory Orientation).

X-RAYS

X-rays are also called roentgen rays, after their discoverer, Wilhelm Konrad Roentgen (1845-1923), a physicist at the University of Würzburg, Germany, in 1895. They are a form of radiation that consists of energy waves of very short wavelength. It is this very short wavelength that gives x-rays the special power of penetration. Although not visible to the human eye, x-rays can be captured on film as visible images and can also be seen fluoroscopically by an image intensifier. The density of the matter at which x-rays are aimed and the voltage used determine the degree of penetration of x-rays.

X-rays, capable of penetrating the body completely or in varying degrees and also of changing the basic structure of cells of the body, are used beneficially in the diagnosis of conditions and in the treatment of tumors and other medical conditions, such as blood malignancies.

Various types of equipment are used for radiological procedures. The equipment used for diagnostic procedures is usually of lower voltage than that used for x-ray therapy.

DIAGNOSTIC RADIOLOGY

By exposing body parts to x-rays, diagnostic radiological procedures create images on films, views on the fluoroscope, and/or on videotape or videodisc that enable the physician to view the internal structures and functions of the body to pinpoint disease or anomalies. The observations made are then interpreted by the physician-radiologist, who then dictates the findings and radiological diagnosis. The findings interpreted from these procedures help the physician make a diagnosis or evaluate ongoing treatment; they are also used as a screening method to determine the patient's state of health and to determine the effectiveness of a treatment program after therapy has been completed. In addition to the routine chest or skeletal films, there are many special diagnostic procedures and techniques that reveal more specific information about the function and structure of an organ.

Fluoroscopy: Image Intensification

Fluoroscopy, an image-intensifier television system, is an x-ray examination using an instrument that permits visual observation of deep structures of the body. X-rays from the x-ray tube pass through the patient's body and project shadowy images of organs and bones through an image intensifier. This information is fed to television monitors so that images can be readily observed during the procedure. Videotape and/or videodisk systems can record these images. This allows for playback during the procedure or after it has been completed. A permanent recording of the fluoroscopic image can be made on 35 mm film. This is called *cinefluorography* and occurs simultaneously with television monitoring and/or image recording on a videotape and/or videodisk unit.

The major advantage of the fluoroscope over the usual type of x-ray film is that the action of organs, joints, or entire body systems can be observed in motion. The use of a contrast medium during fluoroscopy may be necessary in some procedures utilizing this system.

Contrast Medium Techniques

A contrast medium is a radiopaque substance that is used in diagnostic radiology to permit a more accurate visualization of internal body parts and tissues in contrast to their adjacent structures.

Contrast media include liquids, powders, gas, air, or pills that are administered orally, parenterally (by injection), or through an enema, each being specific for the examination of a particular organ or structure. The contrast medium opacifies the body part(s) under examination. Thus the structure and functions of the organ(s) can be observed and studied through x-ray films or fluoroscopy.

Artificial, positive contrast media include barium sulfate and iodine compounds. Because these media have more density, they absorb more of the radiation. They will appear white on x-ray images. Negative contrast media include air, gas, and carbon dioxide. They appear black on x-ray images.

Barium sulfate

Barium sulfate is a harmless chalky compound, now available commercially in a premixed flavored (such as cherry) liquid or paste. Often x-ray departments will buy the powder form and mix it with water to the desired consistency.

Barium sulfate is an opaque medium used for two main types of x-ray and fluoroscopic examinations of the gastrointestinal (GI) tract. A barium

Figure 27.1
Patient in position for a gastrointestinal study performed under fluoroscopic
control with VECTOR R/F table.
Courtesy Picker International, Cleveland, Ohio.

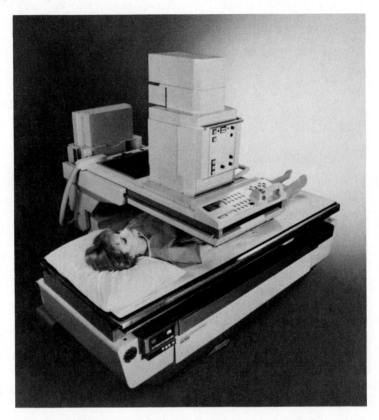

meal or upper GI series is the oral ingestion of the barium mixture to outline the esophagus, stomach, and if ordered, the small intestine, depending on the physician's request. A barium enema (BE), or lower GI series, outlines the colon for study after the instillation of the barium mixture through an enema. On occasion, a third examination, a barium swallow, is done to outline the esophagus (after the oral ingestion of the barium mixture) (Figure 27.1).

Iodine compounds

Containing up to 50% and more iodine, iodine radiopaque contrast media (dyes) are used for the following tests on various body systems. If the patient is allergic to iodine, these examinations should not be performed; other diagnostic techniques may then be employed. The iodinated contrast media used for these procedures will interfere with thyroid studies performed by the nuclear

medicine department; therefore these procedures should *not* be performed when the patient is having thyroid function tests.

angiogram X-ray record of blood vessels after injecting a contrast medium (dye) through a catheter inserted in the appropriate vessel (arteriogram, lymphangiogram, phlebogram) (Figure 27.2).
angiocardiogram X-ray record of the heart and great vessels after injecting a contrast medium into a large peripheral vein or into a chamber of the heart by direct heart catheterization.
arteriogram X-ray record of an artery or arterial system after injecting a contrast medium through a catheter inserted in an artery.
arthrogram X-ray record of a joint after injecting a contrast medium into the joint.
bronchogram X-ray record of the bronchial tree and lungs after instillation of a contrast medium into the bronchi via the trachea with a special instrument.
cerebral angiogram X-ray record of the cerebral vessels after injecting a contrast medium into the common ca-

Figure 27.2
Vascular procedures suite. Patient being prepared for bi-plane cerebral study with
an Angicon angiography system.
Courtesy Picker International, Cleveland, Ohio.

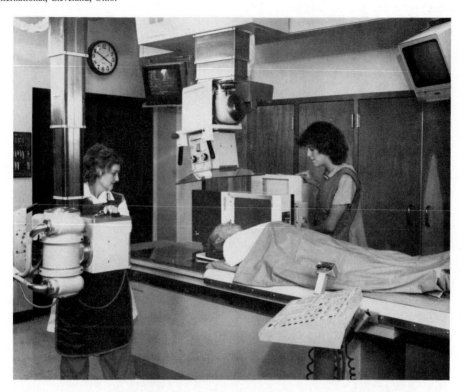

rotid artery; for x-ray records of the vessels in the posterior fossa or the occipital lobes, the medium is injected into the vertebral artery in the neck.

cholecystogram* X-ray record of the gallbladder after
oral ingestion of radiopaque granules or tablets taken
the evening before the examination.

diskogram X-ray record of the vertebral column after
injecting a contrast medium into an intervertebral
disk. This procedure is done very infrequently.

hysterosalpingogram X-ray record of the uterus and fallopian tubes after injecting a contrast medium through
the vagina into the uterus.

intravenous cholangiogram* X-ray record of the bile
ducts after injecting a contrast medium intravenously.
The dye is excreted by the liver into the bile ducts; x-
ray films are taken at intervals as the dye is excreted
through the hepatic, cystic, and common bile duct into
the duodenum

intravenous pyelogram (IVP) X-ray records taken at intervals after intravenous injection of a contrast medium at intervals to observe the excretion rate and the
concentration of the dye in the renal pelvis and the
outline of the ureters and urinary bladder.

lymphangiogram X-ray record of the lymphatic vessels
after the injection of a contrast medium into the lymphatic system.

myelogram X-ray record of the spinal cord after injection of a contrast medium into the subarachnoid space
through a lumbar puncture needle.

retrograde pyelogram X-ray record of the urinary tract
after introduction of a contrast medium through ure-
teral catheters.

urogram X-ray record of any part of the urinary tract
after intravenous injection of a contrast medium. See
also intravenous pyelogram.

retrograde urogram The contrast medium is injected
into the bladder through an urethral catheter.

Air, oxygen (O_2), and carbon dioxide (CO_2)

Since the introduction of computed tomography
and magnetic resonance imaging (see pp. 564 and

---

*In most facilities these procedures have been replaced by ultrasound ex-
aminations (sonography) of the gallbladder and bile ducts.

565), the frequency with which these negative contrast media have been used for cerebral pneumography (pneumoencephalography and pneumoventriculography) in radiology departments has essentially disappeared. Still at times these negative media can be used for examinations of the spinal cord, joints, and in combination with barium sulfate during a barium enema. Oxygen is rarely used. Carbon dioxide is used most frequently, as it is absorbed by the body faster than air or oxygen, thus limiting the duration of headaches that may follow a myelogram.

arthrogram   X-ray record of a joint after injecting air or other gas into the articular capsule. Air can be combined with an iodine compound for double contrast studies.

myelogram   X-ray record of the spinal cord after the injection of air or gas (carbon dioxide) into the subarachnoid space by means of a lumbar puncture.

Mammography

Mammography, an x-ray examination of the breast to identify breast lesions or tumors, involves detection of radiodense tissue or calcifications. Mammography is the most effective method for detecting early and curable breast cancer. The new dedicated mammographic units perform diagnostic x-ray examinations of the breast at radiation doses 5 to 10 times lower than the older units. Machines of this type provide enormous potential benefit for early cancer detection, and the minimal levels of

Figure 27.3
A, Technologist positioning patient for right craniocaudal view of breast for mammography.

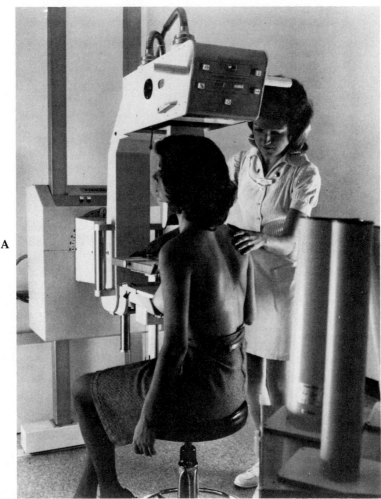

radiation exposure have essentially removed any meaningful risk. Radiation physicists have estimated that the radiation risk of a low-dose mammogram may be equivalent to the lung cancer risk of smoking one cigarette. In addition, this "state-of-the-art" machine obtains magnified and grid images that can more optimally evaluate the young, dense, and small breast. Two films are taken from different angles: (1) the sitting or standing axillary, and (2) the sitting or standing craniocaudal views (Figure 27.3).

To achieve diagnostic x-ray images of the breasts at extremely low radiation doses, the breast must be compressed firmly by a clear plastic plate. Many women find this uncomfortable but tolerable. Some women find breast compression intolerable. For women with painful, tender breasts, it is suggested that they (1) schedule the examination during the time in the menstrual cycle when the breasts are least tender. This corresponds to the first 10 days of the cycle for many women; (2) avoid caffeine-containing products such as coffee, tea, chocolate, coca, and soft drinks for 1 week before the examination; (3) verbally cooperate with the radiographer to mutually arrive at a degree of compression that is tolerable to them and consistent with the technical requirements of the examination. The patient should be asked not to wear any powder or deodorant on the day of the examination, as these products sometimes show up as artifacts on the x-ray images.

The American Cancer Society recommends that "women without symptoms of breast cancer, ages 35 to 39, should have one mammogram for the record; women age 40 to 49 should have a mammogram every 1 to 2 years, and women age 50 and over, once a year. All women are advised that monthly breast self-examination is an important health habit." (See Chapter 19, p. 334.)

Figure 27.3, cont'd
B, X-ray of female breast (mammography) showing the entire breast back to rib cage.

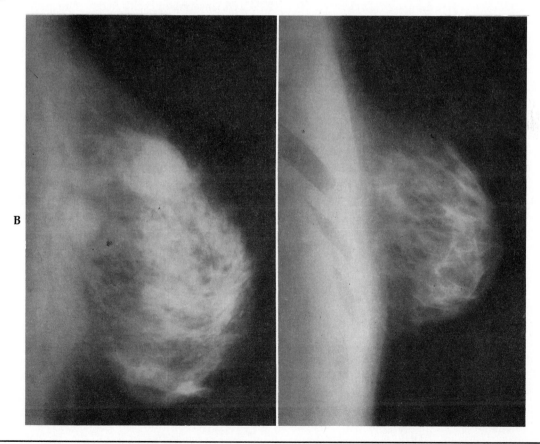

Xeroradiography

Xeroradiography uses a dry electrophotographic technique to produce images on specially treated photocopy paper. This system, used mostly for mammography, can also be used to obtain x-ray images in small areas in soft tissue and some bone. In general xeroradiography compares favorably with the radiation dose the patient receives from other film-screen recording systems. The major advantages over a conventional film-screen system is its ability to outline or enhance the edges of a density, for example, bone, tumors, or foreign bodies such as glass.

Thermography

Thermography is a heat-sensing technique used in the detection of breast tumors. Essentially, an apparatus makes a photographic image of the varying skin temperatures. Body areas that are warm appear light; cool areas appear dark; and medium temperature areas appear gray on the thermogram. Localized skin temperature elevations, such as occur over inflammatory or malignant lesions, are then sharply delineated against the temperatures of the surrounding tissues.

Though research continues, *the majority opinion is that thermography is not a sufficiently reliable procedure to use for screening or detecting breast cancer*. Thus it is *not recommended* and is *seldom used* now *except* in institutions continuing investigative work. X-ray mammography is the superior diagnostic tool for detecting breast cancer.

Tomography

Tomography, or sectional roentgenography, has a special ability to penetrate dense shadows. X-ray pictures are taken in sections at different depths in the patient's body, focusing on the plane of the structure to be studied. Structures in front of and behind the plane under examination are blurred out.

Because of this, tomography can be a valuable diagnostic procedure when a definitive diagnosis cannot be made from conventional radiographs. Used to demonstrate and evaluate a number of different disease processes, traumatic injuries, and congenital abnormalities, tomography can be used in any part of the body, but is most effective in areas of high contrast, such as in the lungs and bones. One of the most frequent uses is to demonstrate and evaluate benign and malignant processes in the lungs.

Although computed tomography (CT) and magnetic resonance imaging (MRI) (see p. 565) have replaced the use of tomography to a great extent, there are still times when tomography is the examination of choice. Many hospitals do not have the CT and MRI units because of the high cost. Also the cost to the patient is much higher for a CT or MRI examination. Tomography can often provide a satisfactory diagnosis or at least screen the patient for further evaluation by the other more sophisticated modalities.

Computed Tomography (CT Scan)

The CT scanner—the developers of which were awarded the Nobel Prize for medicine in October 1979—has been a most significant breakthrough in medical technology.

Computed tomography is an advanced radiological modality that provides valuable clinical information in the early detection, differentiation, and demarcation of diseases of the head and body. Quick and noninvasive, the CT scan is particularly helpful in solving problems in which there is conflicting information from other radiological or laboratory studies, and may be necessary for planning radiation therapy for certain tumor masses. Its use frequently does replace some examinations, such as echoencephalography (see "Diagnostic Ultrasound") and others, many of which carry greater risk and discomfort to the patient, such as the pneumoencephalogram and arteriogram. In addition, computed tomography does, in certain cases, replace procedures that would require the patient to be hospitalized. This technique is employed to detect cerebral abnormalities, for example, tumors, lesions, hematomas, and bleeding in the brains of newborn infants; to search for childhood cancer, to detect masses in the chest, abdominal, and pelvic cavities; and to examine the liver, spleen, pancreas, kidneys, adrenal glands, pituitary gland, optic nerve, and for a generalized survey for lymphoma or metastases (Figure 27.4).

Machines called scanners (such as ACTA, EMI, CT/T, Synerview, Delta, Syntex) beam x-rays to scan the body site in a series of x-rays. The scanner combines the capabilities of traditional x-ray with that of a computer, providing an image of soft tissue in three dimensions. The x-ray tube and detector source rotate 360 degrees around the patient's head or body part being studied, taking multiple "slices"—cross-sectional readings. Thus every tissue and organ is x-rayed from all sides. As they pass through the body, the absorption rates of the x-rays are detected, and the density of the tissue is relayed to the computer. From the calculations per-

Figure 27.4

A, Technolgist positioning patient for head scan with General Electric CT8800 Computed Tomography System. **B,** Control room for CT scanner. X-ray generation controls, scanning control console, and viewing monitors are found here. Main computer hardware is usually located in adjacent room.

Courtesy General Electric Co, Medical Systems Div, Milwaukee, Wis.

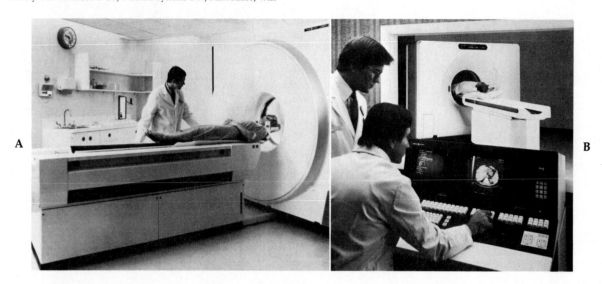

formed by the computer, densities are translated into a picture of the body as if it were neatly cut into slices, each a fraction of an inch thick. This picture is projected on a screen for the radiologist to study (Figure 27.5).

The conventional x-ray film reveals only certain organs and tissues, and requires multiple exposures to estimate the size and location of diseased areas. The CT scanner can distinguish nearly every type of tissue and has the ability to distinguish more minute differences in the various tissues. CT can determine the size and location of any pathologic condition with great accuracy. When first developed around the mid-1970s, the CT scans were slow, but now many machines in use can complete a scan in 4 to 5 seconds, and a more sophisticated machine can complete a scan in 1 second. Nevertheless, one of the limitations of CT is that it takes 15 to 30 minutes or longer to complete all the slices required for a complete examination. Thus most CT scanners can only be used for 15 to 20 examinations during an 8-hour work day.

Minimal patient preparation is required for CT scans. Some facilities require the patient to have nothing by mouth for 4 hours before the examination if a contrast medium is used. For abdominal and pelvic scans the patient preparation is usually the same as the one used for a barium enema (see p. 574). When a contrast medium is not used, no patient preparation is required. A contrast medium can be administered orally or intravenously.

Research is continuing for a scanner that can make clear x-ray images of the fast-beating human heart. Some researchers are presently testing it as a noninvasive method to determine whether vein grafts installed in a coronary bypass surgery are allowing blood to flow freely or have become closed and useless. The National Aeronautics and Space Administration (NASA) is also interested in this device, because it may be valuable in detecting the loss of calcium in bones, a serious consequence of weightlessness in space travel.

Although the use of the CT scan is superior in numerous situations, at times the findings obtained do indicate the need for additional and invasive procedures so that a conclusive diagnosis can be established.

Magnetic Resonance Imaging (MRI)

A newer and equally exciting form of imaging technique for examining the body is the MR. Mag-

Figure 27.5
Images from CT scan of head and
abdomen.
Courtesy General Electric Co, Medical Systems Div,
Milwaukee, Wis.

Head

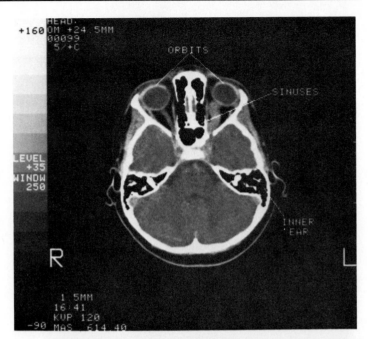

Abdomen

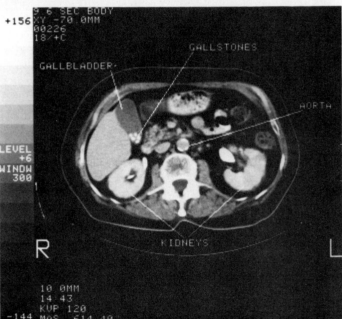

netic resonance is a computer-based, cross-sectional imaging modality that examines the interactions of magnetism and radio waves with tissue to obtain its images. Magnets, as the name suggests, are at the heart of this system. Many machines use superconducting magnets, as the more powerful the magnets, the clearer the images produced.

There are major advantages to the MR. It can examine properties of body tissue that have never before been visualized. Both anatomic and physiologic information can be obtained. No x-rays, that is no ionizing radiation of any kind, are used to obtain the MR image. It is a painless and noninvasive technique. There are no known harmful effects to the patient when exposed to the current levels of magnetic field strength and radiowave energy transmission.

Magnetic resonance is used to detect tumors in soft tissues because even in early stages malignant tissue responds to the magnetic pull differently from normal tissue. No other imaging technique can detect such subtle differences in soft tissues. It is also used to examine the brain (it can distinguish brain tumors from tiny blood clots and determine the chemical changes that cause dementia in the elderly); spinal cord tumors, cystic changes of the spine, and disc disease; the gastrointestinal tract; the heart muscle, septal defects and cardiac valve leaflets; the lungs; the extremities (but bone lesions and calcium within tumors are seen better with CT); tumors of the liver and spleen; pelvic structures, e.g., bladder tumors, neoplasms in the female genital tract, and may detect prostate tumors; and it can outline the kidneys, adrenal glands, and retroperitoneal structures such as lymph nodes (although there is limited evidence that MR is superior to CT in this area).

However, MRI has its limitations. It cannot see the hard part of the bones, so we still need x-rays, CT, or other techniques to diagnose fractures and malformations in bones. Also the strong magnetic field is potentially dangerous to patients with cardiac pacemakers and to those patients who have any type of metallic implants in them, such as aneurysm clips on blood vessels within the skull or clips tying off other blood vessels. The pull of the magnets could slip the clips out of place, and vessels could be torn. It is therefore important to check that the patient does not have a pacemaker or metallic implants before a MR is scheduled.

The image produced by the computer can be viewed on a television monitor. If desired, the images can be photographed for further study. These images can also be stored on a computer disk temporarily and then transferred to magnetic tape for permanent storage and retrieval.

The explosion of MR technology within the last decade still leaves questions on how far-reaching its applications will be and on the proof of its superior nature over other imaging modalities.

Diagnostic Ultrasound

Diagnostic ultrasound or ultrasonography, does *not* use ionizing radiation to diagnose or treat disease but uses very high frequency inaudible sound waves that bounce off the body to record information on the structure of internal organs.

In this examination, the patient's skin is covered with water, oil, or a special jelly that helps conduct the sound waves into the body. A special instrument emitting sound waves is placed and moved on or near the patient's skin. Sound waves pass through the skin, strike the body tissues, and pass an echo reflection back to the instrument. These ultrasonic echoes are then recorded on the oscilloscope as a picture of a series of dots. This record produced is called an echogram or sonogram. The method of image recording in which the data is stored on film, paper, or other recording material is called the hard copy.

Ultrasound can be used to detect abnormalities in the heart (echocardiography), major blood vessels, kidneys, abdominopelvic cavity, breast, scrotum, muscles, spine, and brain (echoencephalogram [EECG], although this has now been replaced by the CT scan, when available, because of the superiority of the CT images of the entire cranial vault versus very limited knowledge available from the EECG). It is also used to determine the presence of a pregnancy if other tests are unsuccessful, to differentiate between single and multiple pregnancies, or to view placental position, various stages, and fetal positions during pregnancy, and for neonate examinations (Figure 27.6). In some procedures body structures, such as the diaphragm, cardiac or fetal heart motion, or other organ structures that move with respiration, are visible as they change position in time.

Ultrasound has the advantages of being a painless, noninvasive procedure that does not expose the patient to ionizing radiation. After 30 years of use, physicians have found no evidence that diagnostic ultrasound causes any untoward biologic effect. Therefore it has generally been accepted as a safe technique.

Ultrasound is also used for treatment in physical medicine (by physical therapists) for deep muscle or tension pain. In this case a different machine with a different soundwave intensity is used. This is discussed in the physical therapy chapter.

Other Diagnostic Radiological Examinations
Abdomen

A survey film (flat plate) of the abdomen is ordered without the use of a contrast medium when abnormal conditions of the abdomen are suspected, such as tumors, abscesses, enlarged or perforated organs, or hematomas.

In the plain survey, three films are often taken. The patient may be placed in the erect, supine, prone, or lateral decubitus position, depending on

Figure 27.6
A, Sectorview ultrasound system for scanning abdominal organs. **B,** Ultrasound
system for scanning abdominal organs.
Courtesy Picker International, Cleveland, Ohio.

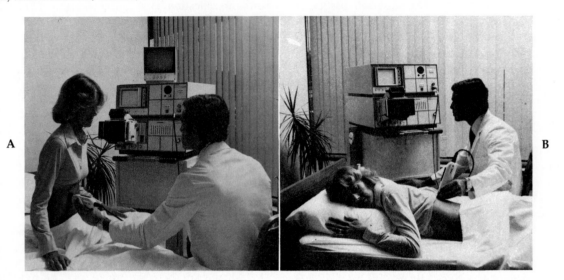

the suspected pathological condition to be studied
(Figure 27.7).

Routine chest x-ray film

An x-ray record of the chest is obtained with the
patient in the posteroanterior erect position. Generally, a lateral view is also taken.

Kidney, ureter, bladder (KUB) film

A flat plate of the abdomen is used to study the
kidneys, flank area, gas pattern, abdominal wall,
bones of the pelvis, and any unusual masses.

Skull series

A series of radiographs of the skull is used to determine cranial injuries or the effects of trauma to the
head and neck. Computed tomography has replaced the use of these films except in cases of severe trauma.

Paranasal sinuses films

X-ray records are made of the paired sinuses
within the frontal, ethmoid, sphenoid, and maxil-
lary bones of the face.

Bone x-ray films

X-ray records are made of bones suspected of disease or trauma, such as tumors and fractures or
displacement. X-ray studies of the vertebral column are common. Radiographs of the neck are referred to as cervical x-ray films; those of the middle back are referred to as thoracic x-ray films; and
those of the lower back are referred to as lumbo-
sacral x-ray films.

POSITION OF PATIENT FOR
X-RAY STUDIES

Radiograms are made by directing beams of x-rays
through the x-ray tube toward a specific body part.
The body part to be radiographed must be positioned correctly between the film-containing cassette and the x-ray source. The body part to be
filmed is positioned closest to the cassette.

When the physician orders x-ray film to be
taken, and when radiologists take and interpret the
film, they will use special terms to designate the
position or direction of the x-ray beam and the patient's position. Before the x-ray film is taken,
markers are placed on the film-containing cassette
to indicate the position used, the patient's identification, and the date (Figure 27.8).

Basic positions for proper exposure of body part

anteroposterior (AP) The x-ray beam is directed from
front to back. The patient may be in a supine or
standing position, having the back near the film and
the front facing the x-ray tube.

Figure 27.7
Radiologic technologist performing routine radiographic work (for example,
pelvis or abdomen) with ceiling tubemount.
Courtesy Picker International, Cleveland, Ohio.

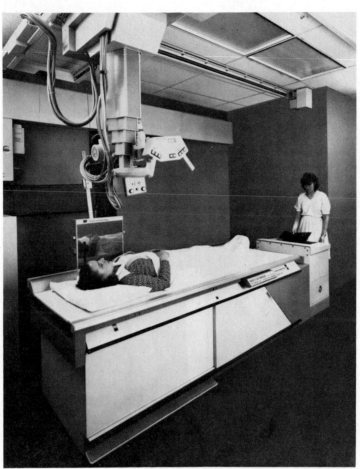

posteroanterior (PA) The x-ray beam is directed from
    back to front. The patient is usually in an upright po-
    sition, having the back facing the x-ray tube and the
    front near the film (Figure 27.9).
lateral The x-ray beam is directed from one side. In the
    right lateral (RL) view, the right side of the body is
    near the film, and the x-ray tube is pointed toward the
    left side (Figure 27.10). For the left lateral (LL) view,
    the left side of the body is nearest the film.
oblique The x-ray beam is directed at an angle. These
    views are often used to outline areas that would be
    hidden and superimposed in the AP and PA views.

Terms to describe patient's position

supine The patient is lying on the back, with face up
    (Figure 27.7).

prone The patient is lying on the abdomen, face down-
    ward.
recumbent The patient is lying down.

Other terms to describe direction of x-ray beam

axillary The x-ray beam is directed toward the axilla.
mediolateral The x-ray beam is directed from the mid-
    line toward the side of the part being filmed.
supine mediolateral The patient is in the supine posi-
    tion, and the x-ray beam is directed from the midline
    toward the side.
craniocaudal The x-ray beam is directed from the supe-
    rior to inferior levels (from head to toe).

Figure 27.8
A, Samples of various lead numbers and letters in different heights and thicknesses for radiographing directly onto x-ray film. **B,** X-ray cassettes showing placement of identification markers (lead) using Film Clip product.
Courtesy Picker International, Cleveland, Ohio.

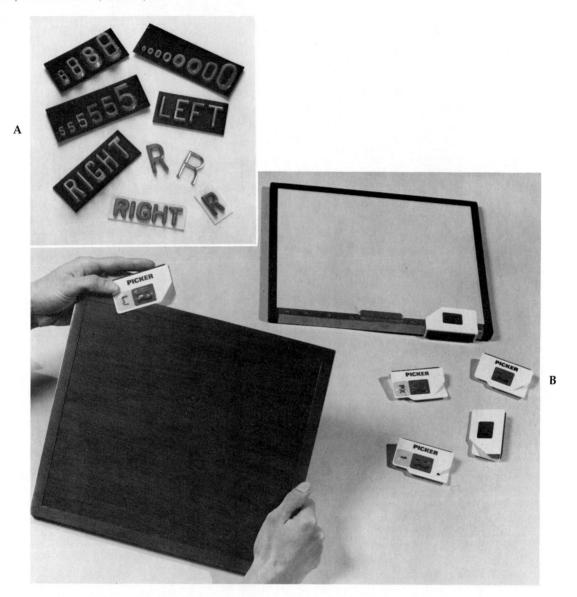

Figure 27.9
Patient in PA (posteroanterior) position for chest x-ray film.
Courtesy General Electric Co, Medical Systems Div, Milwaukee, Wisc.

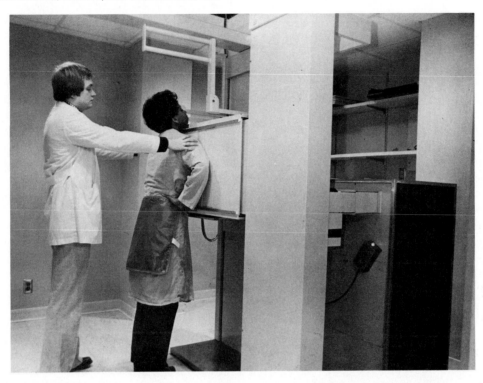

Figure 27.10
Patient positioned for right lateral view of chest (lung) on a Pickerchest system.
Courtesy Picker International, Cleveland, Ohio.

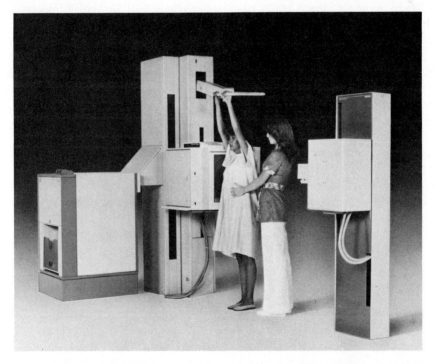

RADIOLOGICAL DANGERS, HAZARDS, AND SAFETY PRECAUTIONS

X-rays do constitute a potential danger both to patients and health personnel; therefore proper precautions must be taken at all times.

Dangers

Massive or excessive exposure to radiation can cause tissue damage and various ill side effects. Tissue destruction to diseased areas is aimed for in radiotherapy, but in diagnostic radiology exposure to radiation should be kept within safe limits, because radiation has a cumulative effect over a period of time. That is, the radiation a person receives today adds to the dose he will receive tomorrow, and these add to the dose he received yesterday to accumulate a total radiation dosage. (Doses of radiation are measured in rads or rems or roentgens: these units are all the same.) Thus everyone should avoid all unnecessary radiation exposure. On the other hand, patients must be helped to realize the importance of any radiological examination as an aid for the diagnosis and treatment of a disease process compared with the effects, if any, of the radiation dose that will be received. Newer machines and techniques currently used have significantly reduced the amounts of radiation exposure compared with the same examinations of 10 or more years ago.

When radiation goes beyond a safe limit, body tissues may begin to break down. Blood cells, skin, eyes, and reproductive cells are some of the tissues most sensitive to radiation. Overexposure to radiation can result in a lowered red blood cell and white blood cell count because of disturbances of bone marrow and other blood-forming organs; burns on the skin, and cancer; damage to the germinal cells in the ovaries and testes; and also damage to a fetus, especially in the first 3 months of pregnancy. Radiation also apparently predisposes individuals to the development of cataracts.

Studies have shown that massive and prolonged exposure to radiation can result in a higher incidence of cancer, especially of the lymph glands, and the various types of leukemia.

Hazards

Hazards of x-rays include the direct x-ray beam itself from the x-ray machine, which travels through an opening in the x-ray tube. Lead (which is able to stop x-rays from traveling) is in the x-ray tube housing to prevent the rays from escaping except through the opening.

A second hazard is scattered radiation of two types. *Leakage radiation* is radiation that may escape (leak) from the head of x-ray machines, and this is dangerous to the operator. Therefore, frequent inspection of all x-ray equipment is to be performed by a licensed radiation physicist. Once the primary beam of radiation strikes and reacts on the patient or anything else in its path, it is then called *secondary radiation,* which can be emitted in all directions. Secondary radiation is radiation that has deviated from its original path, being strongest close to the patient. Therefore distance is an important factor in radiation protection; that is, the further one is away from the patient, the better the protection one has from any form of radiation.

Lead screens or shields are used to separate x-ray personnel operating the controls of the machine from the patient receiving the radiation. These protect the personnel from secondary radiation. The walls of the x-ray room are also lined with lead, which absorbs secondary radiation when struck by it and thus prevents radiation from passing through the walls into adjacent areas, exposing others to the radiation. In most facilities, when x-ray machines are in use, a red light flashes on outside the room, indicating to others that radiation is being given and therefore they should not enter the room. In some facilities there are interlocking devices by which the door will not open when radiation is being used. Sometimes these devices interact with the x-ray equipment so that the machines will not work unless the door is locked.

Safety Precautions

X-ray personnel and medical assistants exposed to possible radiation can control the potential dangers by adhering to the following prescribed safety precautionary measures:

1. Have the equipment inspected frequently by a qualified person to assure that there is no leakage of radiation.
2. Stay behind the lead shield in a lead-lined room when the x-ray machine is being used.
3. Wear a lead apron and protective rubber-lead gloves if it is absolutely necessary to hold the patient or to remain in the room during any radiological procedure. On these occasions, always face the patient so that the lead apron is closest to the patient, or stay away from the patient. Never assume that you must hold or support the patient, and do not make this a routine. Certain techniques can be used to maintain the patient in the correct position.

4. Wear a film badge on outer clothing at all times when your job involves exposure to any type of radiation, including exposure to radionuclides. A film badge is a small device that contains x-ray film that is sensitive to radiation and thus records the level and intensity of radiation exposure, which is measured in rads, rems, or roentgens. These badges are to be submitted periodically (weekly in some facilities) to a film badge service for evaluation, thus providing a means for warning personnel when dangerous levels of radiation exposure are near.

5. Have a periodic blood count performed to determine if a blood dyscrasia is present. Blood counts do not measure the amount of radiation, but can indicate if there is any apparent radiation damage to blood cells. Generally, a yearly physical examination is required for all personnel working with radiological materials.

To protect the patient from unnecessary radiation exposure, adhere to the following:

1. Before making arrangements for a patient to have x-ray examinations, routinely ask the following:
   - If and when the patient has had other x-ray studies or therapy and the nature of these.
   - If the patient has been exposed to any radiation for other reasons, such as in employment or experimental situations.
   - If it is possible that a female patient is pregnant. These inquiries are important, as it may be that the patient has received excessive doses of radiation, and further exposure at that time may be detrimental to the patient's health status. When it appears that the patient has been exposed to a large amount of radiation recently, and when a woman suspects that she is pregnant, inform the physician of this, without alarming the patient and before making arrangements for the x-ray studies. Provided with this information, the physician may want to change the order for x-ray studies at that time. The physician will weigh the facts: that is, how urgent is the need for the x-ray examination versus what is the risk to the patient or fetus, who will receive the additional radiation exposure.

2. Position the patient correctly for the x-ray film when this is one of your assisting duties. Accuracy of the film requires that the patient assume and maintain the correct position without moving during the exposure time. If this is not attained, distortion on the film will result, thus requiring the patient to be exposed to additional radiation while a repeat film is taken.

3. Shield the patient's abdomen and reproductive organs with a lead apron or cover, especially patients who are pregnant or of childbearing age and children.

MEDICAL ASSISTANT'S RESPONSIBILITIES

The medical assistant's responsibilities relating to radiological procedures used in the physician's office or clinic are to prepare the patient, provide reassurance when needed, and employ the safety measures relevant to x-ray equipment. When the physician employs an x-ray technician, the assistant may not do any of these functions.

When outside sources are used, the assistant is responsible for calling the radiologist's office or hospital x-ray department to schedule the examination and for furnishing the patient's name, the referring physician's name, and the type of examination.

One of the most important communications between the medical assistant and radiology department involves the scheduling of multiple x-ray procedures that are ordered at one time for the patient. Consultation will be needed to sequence the procedures so that they will not interfere with each other and to decide how many procedures can be done on the same day. The medical assistant should give all the information to the radiology department so that they can schedule the examinations in proper sequence. The general rule is that examinations *not* using a contrast medium are done *before* examinations that do use a contrast medium; for example, a chest x-ray would be done before a barium enema. The patient is to take the physician's written requisition(s) to the x-ray department on the day of the examination.

In either situation, patients should be informed before the scheduled date of the approximate amount of time the examination will take so they can schedule other activities accordingly and not get unduly upset or surprised if the examination takes an hour or so. Also, certain x-ray examinations require special patient preparation the day before or the morning of the study or both. To prepare the patient, the medical assistant must know and go over the instructions orally with the patient to ensure that these are understood and provide written instructions to be taken home. Many physicians' offices and clinics have preprinted individual instructions to be followed before x-ray studies

Text continued on p. 576.

Table 27.1
X-ray examinations *requiring* special individual patient preparation

Examination	Time required	Sample preparation
Barium enema	30-60 min	Take 2 ounces (4 tablespoons) castor oil at 4 PM the day preceding x-ray examination (may be taken in grape juice or root beer). No solid foods on day preceding examination; just liquids such as fruit juice, clear soup, Jello, water, plain tea, or black coffee, but no milk products. NPO after midnight. No breakfast on day of examination. *or* Enemas till bowels are clear the evening before. NPO after midnight. Rectal suppository in the morning.
Barium meal (upper GI series)	30-60 min for stomach, but up to 90 min with small bowel examination. More films may be taken 6 hr or 24 hr later	Nothing to eat or drink after 10 PM the evening before examination. No breakfast, no fluids, and no cigarettes in the morning. Stomach must be empty. *or* Nothing to eat or drink after 8 PM. Do not eat breakfast. No water. Report to x-ray office.
Angiogram	1-3 hr	No breakfast when any of these examinations are done in the early morning; or no lunch if they are done in the afternoon.
Arteriogram	1-3 hr	
Angiocardiogram	2 hr	
Cerebral angiogram	2-3 hr	
Bronchogram	1 hr	NPO
Myelogram	1 hr	NPO
Computed Tomography	1 to 2 hr	NPO for 4 hr before if a contrast medium is used
Cholecystogram (gallbladder series)	1-2 hr	Evening before x-ray examination, eat a light supper, consisting of nonfatty foods such as lean meat (small portion) and fresh vegetables cooked without butter and no eggs, mayonnaise, French dressing, or fried or fatty foods. After supper swallow gallbladder tablets with water, taking one at a time. Eat nothing after evening meal. Water, however, may be taken in moderate amounts until bedtime. Do not take a laxative. Do not eat breakfast. Report to x-ray department. *or* Low-fat evening meal. Iapanoic acid (Telepaque) tablets the evening before. NPO after midnight.
Intravenous cholangiogram	3 hr	NPO

From Zakus SM: Clinical skills and assisting techniques for the medical assistant, ed 2, St Louis, 1988, The CV Mosby Co.

Examination	Time required	Sample preparation
Intravenous pyelogram (IVP)	1½ hr	Take 2 ounces (4 tablespoons) of castor oil or 3 tablets bisacodyl (Dulcolax) at 4 PM the day before x-ray examination. Eat a light supper. Do not drink anything, even water, after midnight. Eat no breakfast, no fluids. *or* Laxatives or enemas night before examination. NPO for 8 hours before examination.
Retrograde pyelogram	1-1 ½ hr; usually done in operating room	NPO
Pneumoencephalogram	2-4 hr	NPO
Pneumoencephalomyelogram	2-4 hr	NPO
Ultrasonography	25-45 min up to 2 hr	
Pelvic ultrasound		Afternoon before the examination, take 3 bisacodyl tablets and 3 glasses of water to clear the bowel. On the day of examination, use a bisacodyl rectal suppository 3 hours before examination. Then take 3 to 4 glasses of water 45 minutes before the exam and do not urinate. *A full urinary bladder is essential for this examination!* *or* A full urinary bladder is essential. Please do not empty your bladder for 1-2 hr before examination. Drink 4-6 glasses of any liquid 45 min before examination. Use one bisacodyl suppository 3 hr before examination.
Abdominal ultrasound		Take 1 simethicone (Mylicon) tablet 4 times daily for 2 days before examination. *Do not eat* solid food after 8 AM on day of examination. You may take fluids as desired. *or* Take 10 ounces of citrate of magnesia and 3 glasses of water at noon the day before examination. Take 3 bisacodyl tablets at 6 PM with an additional 3 glasses of water. The evening meal should consist of clear fluids but no milk products. Have nothing other than liquids after midnight. Do not eat breakfast the day of examination.
Renal ultrasound		Drink 2 glasses of water 1 hr before examination.
Thyroid ultrasound		No preparation needed. Nothing in mouth 3 hr before examination.
Obstetrical ultrasound		A full urinary bladder is essential. Do not empty your bladder for at least 1 hr before examination. Drink 4-6 glasses of any liquid 45 minutes before examination.

or they may use product literature provided by pharmaceutical companies for patient use. Written instructions are essential, as oral instructions can easily be forgotten. Repeat examinations required because of poorly given or misunderstood instructions are unnecessary radiation exposures and expenses for the patient.

For the x-ray studies discussed in this chapter,

Table 27.1 lists the studies that require individual patient preparation (listed as individual, because the specific preparation may vary among different radiology departments). The approximate amount of time required for each examination is also listed. Samples of individual patient preparations are given for common examinations. Similar reference sheets should be made available for the medical as-

---

Preparation of Patient and Assisting with Radiographs in Physician's Office

Procedure	*Rationale*
1. Identify the patient, check if the special preparation was followed (when applicable), and explain the following: • The value of the examination • How the machine operates • Whether it will hurt • What clothing and other articles must be removed • How to put on the patient gown, that is, with the opening in the front or back • What position will be required • The importance of remaining still during the examination	X-ray procedures performed in the office are used for diagnostic or screening purposes. If a required special preparation was not followed, the examination must be cancelled and rescheduled. The patient can be told that x-ray examinations are painless, with the exception of those requiring the instillation of a contrast medium. Then, on these occasions an uncomfortable feeling can be expected, rather than pain. The patient is to remove clothes, watches, all metal, dentures, jewelry, and hairpins, which may interfere with the accuracy of the x-ray film. These objects will produce shadows on the film and may obscure details that should be observed. The patient gown is usually to be put on with the opening in the back. For films of the breast, all clothing from the waist up is removed. The physician will determine the position to be maintained by the patient; you will explain to the patient what it will be. Movement of the body during the examination will cause distortion on the film. It is then necessary to repeat the examination, which provides additional radiation exposure for the patient.
2. Drape the patient as necessary. Shield the abdominal regions with a lead apron, especially for patients who are pregnant, of childbearing age, or children.	Drapes may be used to provide warmth and to protect the patient's modesty, but are *not* to interfere with the body part being filmed.
3. Reassure the patient as required. Radiographs are taken on either very sick patients or those who come in for diagnostic purposes, but they all must be given support and attention.	Careful and complete explanations to the patient help provide reassurance and reduce fears and confusion. Offer assistance to the patient when getting on and off the x-ray table. Remain calm and quietly cheerful. Any reassurance to a nervous patient is helpful.
4. Be empathetic and courteous; remain calm.	The patient will be lying on or standing against a cold, hard plate. In an empathetic and courteous manner, emphasize the importance of remaining still in the proper position. Distortion on the film will occur unless the required position is maintained.
5. When the examination has been completed by the physician or x-ray technician or technologist, ask the patient to wait in the dressing room while the films are developed.	The patient remains while films are developed to ensure that clear films have been obtained for study. This is much more convenient for everyone than to have the patient return later for retakes if the preliminary films are not clear.
6. If it is necessary to obtain another film, explain to the patient that the physician requires another film for study.	Careful communication is important, as you must avoid creating fears in the patient that unnecessary exposure to radiation will result or that the individual taking the x-ray was incompetent, thus the need for another film.
7. Dismiss the patient after it has been determined that the films are satisfactory. If the x-ray film showed the presence of a fracture, make arrangements for immediate treatment.	The physician will read the films later, then the patient is to be notified; OR schedule a future appointment for a time at which the physician can review the results with the patient.
8. Record the procedure on the patient's chart.	Charting example: August 1, 19_____. PA and lateral chest x-rays taken by Dr. Mouer. Results—negative. Detailed report to follow. Film No. 8179. Cassandra Quinn, CMA

sistant in the physician's office or clinic.

After the x-ray examination has been completed, the medical assistant must check to ensure that a written report is received and then filed in the patient's chart after being reviewed by the physician and that the x-ray films, when sent to or when taken in the physician's office, are stored and handled correctly.

STORAGE AND MANAGEMENT IN OFFICE
X-ray Materials

When x-ray materials are used in the office, they require special storage attention. These supplies must be protected from damage caused by exposure to moisture, heat, and light. Film must be kept in a dry, cool place, preferably in a lead-lined box. The lead-lined box protects the film from any x-rays that may escape during filming.

When unexposed film is to be placed into a cassette for use, the film packets are to be opened only in the darkroom with only the darkroom light on. Before development, the exposed film obtained after the radiological procedure is completed must also be stored in a lead-lined box to protect it from secondary radiation, which would spoil the radiograph recorded on the film.

X-ray developer solutions must also be stored in a moisture-free, cool location, because they are of extreme importance in the processing of quality radiographs.

X-ray Films, Reports, and Records

Frequently there is much controversy over the ownership of medical records, reports, and x-ray films. The important thing to remember is that this type of property legally belongs to the medical facility at which it is made or recorded. It does not belong to the patient. All x-ray films obtained on a patient are the sole property of the physician's office or hospital that performed the radiological examination. Written x-ray reports from the radiologist are to be sent to the referring physician, but the actual films usually remain in the files of the office or hospital that did the filming. At times these films can be loaned out to the referring physician for further study, reference, or review as needed to confirm a diagnosis or to compare old films with current ones. At other times the radiologist's office routinely sends the films to the referring physician so that they may be kept as part of the patient's permanent medical record in the office, but they still remain as the legal property of the radiologist. Presently in a few states patients can request, pay for, and obtain copies of the original x-ray film.

Radiological films are permanent records for current or future reference (as opposed to fluoroscopy, which can be viewed only at the time of the examination). Special file envelopes are available to keep exposed film in. These envelopes must be labeled with the patient's name, the date, and the number, if and when used. (Some agencies file film by number rather than by the patient's name. In this case, the number *must* be recorded on the patient's medical record for a cross reference.)

X-ray films placed in filing envelopes should be filed in a dry, cool storage area, preferably in a metal cabinet; ones no longer needed for current reference should be filed in a permanent storage file so that they are available for future reference.

Conclusion

This chapter has given you an exposure to various diagnostic procedures used in the field of radiology. In addition, the medical assistant's responsibilities in these fields, though limited, have been discussed. Numerous additional studies may be performed in these specialty areas of medicine for the diagnosis and treatment of disease processes. It is not within the scope of this book to discuss all of them in detail. There are various sources to which you may refer to expand your knowledge on these procedures. Check with your instructor for additional enrichment assignments and references in areas of your own particular need and interest. A tour through the radiology and nuclear medicine departments of a modern hospital, especially a large teaching hospital, would make you aware of the dramatic progress that has been made in these fields of medicine.

When you feel that you know the information presented in this chapter, arrange with your instructor to take a performance test.

Review Questions

1. Mrs. G.B. Emerson, a 46-year-old, 164-pound woman, has been scheduled for a barium enema and a cholecystogram. Mrs. Emerson does not understand why she must have these tests. Explain the nature and purpose of these tests to her and the special directions that she must follow before having these tests performed.

2. The physician has ordered a PA and lateral chest x-ray film to be taken on Mr. T. Rankin. Explain how the patient will be positioned when these films are taken.

3. Ms. B. Milius has discovered several lumps in her breast while doing a breast self-examination and has now come to the physician for a checkup. List three studies that the physician may order for this patient to help diagnose the condition.

4. Mrs. Gwen Boyd is scheduled for ultrasonography to determine if she is pregnant, because other tests have proved unsuccessful. She feels very apprehensive about having this test done and is fearful of the pain she expects to have during this test. Explain the nature and purpose of this test, indicating if pain is to be expected.

5. Explain the nature and purpose of computed tomography (CT). State the advantages of this technique and equipment over other types of radiological examinations.

6. List three ways to protect the patient from unnecessary radiation exposure when having x-ray examinations.

7. Discuss the medical assistant's responsibilities relevant to x-ray procedures performed in the physician's office and at an outside facility.

8. Describe how an x-ray film should be stored in the office.

9. Mr. B. Wingate had a myelogram performed last month and now is in your office stating that he wants the x-ray films to take home. Define *myelogram*. Explain to Mr. Wingate why he cannot have the films to take home. Does Mr. Wingate have an option?

SUGGESTED READINGS

Ehrlich RA and Givens EM: Patient care in radiography, St Louis, 1981, The CV Mosby Co.

Phelps J: Radiation protection and the medical assistant, Prof Med Assist 10:32, July/Aug 1977.

Chapter 28

Electrocardiography

- The cardiac cycle and ECG cycle
- ECGs
- Phone-A-Gram—the computerized ECG

Objectives

On completion of Chapter 28 the medical assistant student should be able to:

1 Define and pronounce the terms in the vocabulary and text of this chapter.

2 Explain the cardiac cycle and conduction system of the heart.

3 List eight components recorded on the ECG cycle and relate these to the electrical activity of the heart.

4 Describe electrocardiograph paper and indicate the significance of each small block and each large block.

5 List four factors that are interpreted from an ECG.

6 Describe how to monitor an ECG for abnormal and erratic tracings.

7 List three types of common artifacts that may be seen on an ECG and the causes for each.

8 Describe electrodes and electrolytes and state the purpose of each.

9 List the 12 leads recorded on a standard ECG, state the electrical activity that each records, and recognize each recorded lead by interpreting the identification code used.

10 Discuss the phrase, *standardizing the electrocardiograph,* indicating the importance of this. Illustrate and explain the universal standard of electrocardiograph measurement.

11 Discuss the concepts of the Phone-A-Gram, the computerized electrocardiograph.

12 Discuss the automatic electrocardiograph. State the advantages of this electrocardiograph.

13 Demonstrate proficiency in communicating proper preparation of the patient for electrocardiography and in preparing the room and equipment.

14 Demonstrate the proper procedures for applying the electrodes and lead wires to the patient, recording the ECG with a standard electrocardiograph and the Phone-A-Gram system, mounting the finished product, and caring for the equipment after use.

Vocabulary

amplify (am′plĭ-fī) To enlarge, to extend.

arrhythmia (ah-rith′mē-ah) A variation from the normal or an irregular rhythm of the heartbeat.

atrium (ā′trē-um) One of the upper chambers of the heart. The right atrium receives deoxygenated blood from the body, whereas the left atrium receives oxygenated blood from the lungs. (The plural is *atria*).

cardiac (kar′dē-ak) **arrest** Sudden and often unexpected cessation of the heartbeat. Permanent damage of vital organs and death are probable if treatment is not given immediately.

defibrillation (dē-fĭ″brĭ-lā′shun) The application of electrical impulses to the heart to stop heart fibrillation.

electrocardiograph (ē-lek″trō-kar′dē-ō-graf″) The instrument used in electrocardiography.

fibrillation (fĭ″brĭ-lā′shun) A cardiac arrhythmia characterized by rapid, irregular, and ineffective electrical activity in the heart. Ventricular fibrillation is a common cause of cardiac arrest.

myocardial infarction (MI) (mi″ō-kar′dē-al in-fark′shun) The formation of ischemic necrosis in the heart muscle caused by an interference of blood supply to the area.

myocardium (mī″ō-kar′dē-um) The heart muscle.

oscilloscope (ŏ-sil′o-skōp) An instrument used to display the shape or waveform of the electrical activity of the heart and other body organs (comparable to a television screen).

pacemaker (pās′māk-er) The pacemaker of the heart is the sinoatrial node located in the right atrium.

pericarditis (per″ĭ-kar-di′tis) Inflammation of the pericardium, the fibroserous sac enveloping the heart.

rhythm strip A rhythm strip is an ECG recording of a single lead that is used to determine the *rhythm* of the heartbeat, such as a fast, slow, regular, or irregular rhythm, and certain types of ventricular fibrillation. It is also used to determine if the patient is in any type of heart block, such as third-degree heart block. The rhythm strip gives a one-dimensional picture of the beating of the heart, which determines *only* the rhythm of the heartbeat in contrast to the 12-lead ECG, which can show damage to the heart and other conditions as listed on p. 583.

Data from the rhythm strip can be a useful "screening" tool because frequent runs of arrhythmias can be more easily observed. The rhythm strip can also be used to confirm the basic assessment made on the 12-lead ECG.

Currently for the rhythm strip most practitioners will record lead V_1, and possibly leads V_2 and V_5, although one could record any lead that is desired. Rhythm strips are frequently recorded from a continuous cardiac monitor in intensive care units in the hospital and by paramedics out in the field in emergency situations.

ventricle (ven′trĭ-kl) One of the lower chambers of the heart. The right ventricle receives deoxygenated blood from the right atrium and pumps this blood through the pulmonary arteries to the lungs; the left ventricle receives oxygenated blood from the left atrium and pumps this blood out through the aorta to all body tissues. Additional terms are defined in the text of this chapter.

The science and art of electrocardiography combine advanced electromedical technology with the science and art of medical practice. Present-day electrocardiographs present physicians with precise information by amplifying the minute electrical currents produced by the heart on a graphic record or tracing. This record or tracing is called an electrocardiogram, abbreviated ECG or EKG, defined simply as a graphic representation of the electrical activity (currents) produced by the heart during the processes of contraction and relaxation. More precisely, the ECG records the amount of electrical activity, the time required for this activity to travel through the heart during each complete heartbeat, and the rate and rhythm of the heartbeat. Many physicians now include an ECG as part of a complete physical examination, especially for patients 40 years of age and older. It is also advisable to have an ECG or a treadmill stress ECG before any serious jogging or other exercise program is started.

The *treadmill stress test* is used for noninvasive cardiac evaluation to aid physicians in patient diagnosis and prognosis with ECGs taken under controlled exercise stress conditions. During this test of increased stress and work, abnormal electrocardiographic tracings (that do not appear during an ECG taken when the patient is resting) may appear. The test is done in the presence of a physician, and the patient is constantly monitored. Systems used record and monitor the patient's ECG while it is being monitored by the physician.

Frequently physicians will have medical assistants take ECGs. To be valuable members of the health team, those who take ECGs must acquire related knowledge and develop skills; that is, they must know what they are doing, why and how to do it, and then do it well.

The following pages are designed to help medical assistants acquire this knowledge and skill by discussing the nature and purpose of the ECG, the equipment and materials needed, preparation of the patient and equipment, ways to monitor the record for abnormal and erratic tracings, procedure for taking the ECG, and mounting the record obtained.

Before going further, it is suggested that you review the anatomy of the heart to maximize your understanding of electrocardiography (Figure 28.1).

THE CARDIAC CYCLE AND ECG CYCLE

The term *cardiac cycle* refers to one complete heartbeat, which consists of contraction (systole) and relaxation (diastole) of both atria and both ventricles. The many cells of the heart are arranged so that they act together as one network or system. Throughout this network, two types of electrical processes, called depolarization and repolarization, are transmitted. When depolarization occurs, the cells are stimulated, and the myocardium (the heart muscle) contracts; as repolarization occurs, the myocardium relaxes. To understand the electrical activity of the heart, think of the heart as consisting of two separate cell networks—one being the atria and the other the ventricles. The two atria contract simultaneously. Then as they relax, the two ventricles contract and relax; the entire heart does not contract as a unit. Any disturbance in the processes of the cardiac cycle will cause a change in the electrical forces needed to maintain normal, rhythmic heartbeats and may produce an arrhythmia. Depending on the degree of the disturbance, it could be a minor disruption of rhythm or a major life-threatening arrhythmia.

Each of these cell networks (the atria and the ventricles) is considered separately on the ECG, the graphic recording of these electrical forces produced by the heart. That is, the waves or deflections recorded on the electrocardiograph paper represent the sequence of events that occurs during the cardiac cycle. The normal ECG cycle consists of waves that have been arbitrarily labeled P, QRS, and T waves. Each wave corresponds to a particular part of the cardiac cycle (Figure 28.2). The *P wave* reflects contraction (depolarization) of the atria. The *QRS wave* (QRS complex) reflects the contraction (depolarization) of the ventricles. This wave follows the P wave. The *T wave* reflects ventricular recovery (repolarization of the ventricles). A T wave reflecting the repolarization of the atria is not visible, because it is obscured by the QRS wave. A T wave follows every QRS wave. Occasionally another wave, the *U wave*, appears after the T wave. It is a small wave and usually shows up on ECGs of patients who have a low serum potassium level. In some animal laboratory studies, U waves have been produced during the repolarization stages of the Purkinje fibers.

Because the ventricles are much larger than the atria, the QRS and T waves are normally much larger than the P wave.

The *P-R interval* reflects the time it takes from the beginning of the atrial contraction to the beginning of ventricular contraction. The P-R interval is measured from the beginning of the P wave to the beginning of the QRS complex (Figure 28.3).

The *ST segment* reflects the time interval from the end of the ventricular contraction (depolarization) to the beginning of ventricular recovery (repolarization). It is normally a flat (isoelectric) line that is measured from the end of the S wave (of the QRS complex) to the beginning of the T wave.

The *Q-T interval* reflects the time it takes from the beginning of ventricular depolarization to the end of ventricular repolarization. This interval gives a better picture of the total ventricular activity. It is measured from the beginning of the QRS complex to the end of the T wave.

The *baseline*, a flat horizontal line that separates the waves, may be seen to run the length of the ECG tracing. This is known as the isoelectric line. The waves of the ECG cycle will deflect either upward (positive deflection) or downward (negative deflection) from the baseline (isoelectric line). This line is present when there is no current flowing in the heart, that is, after depolarization or after repolarization of the heart. The baseline (isoelectric line) present after the T wave reflects the period in which the entire heart is resting or in its polarized state.

Observing and measuring the configuration and location of each wave in relation to the other waves and baseline, the intervals and the segments in each cycle, and then between each ECG cycle al-

Figure 28.1
Your heart and how it works.
© Reproduced with permission. American Heart Association.

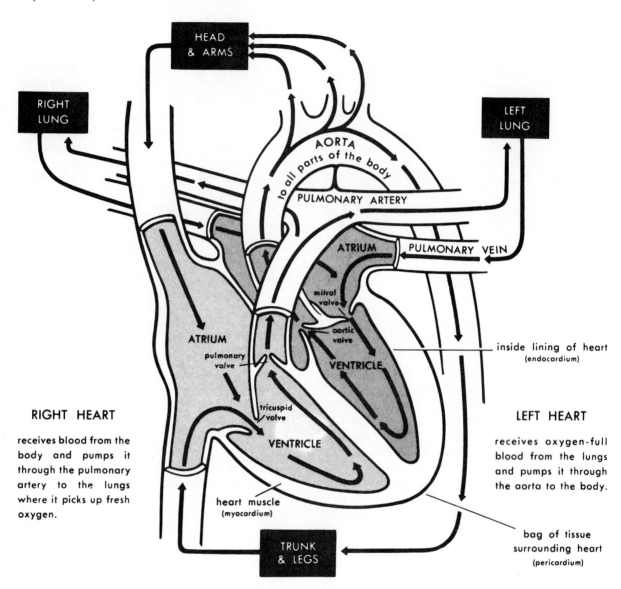

RIGHT HEART

receives blood from the body and pumps it through the pulmonary artery to the lungs where it picks up fresh oxygen.

LEFT HEART

receives oxygen-full blood from the lungs and pumps it through the aorta to the body.

Your heart weighs well under a pound and is only a little larger than your fist, but it is a powerful, long working, hard working organ. Its job is to pump blood to the lungs and to all the body tissues.

The heart is a hollow organ. Its tough, muscular wall (myocardium) is surrounded by a fiberlike bag (pericardium) and is lined by a thin, strong membrane (endocardium). A wall (septum) divides the heart cavity down the middle into a "right heart" and a "left heart". Each side of the heart is divided again into an upper chamber (called an atrium or auricle) and a lower chamber (ventricle). Valves regulate the flow of blood through the heart and to the pulmonary artery and the aorta.

The heart is really a double pump. One pump (the right heart) receives blood which has just come from the body after delivering nutrients and oxygen to the body tissues. It pumps this dark, bluish red blood to the lungs where the blood gets rid of a waste gas (carbon dioxide) and picks up a fresh supply of oxygen which turns it a bright red again. The second pump (the left heart) receives this "reconditioned" blood from the lungs and pumps it out through the great trunk-artery (aorta) to be distributed by smaller arteries to all parts of the body.

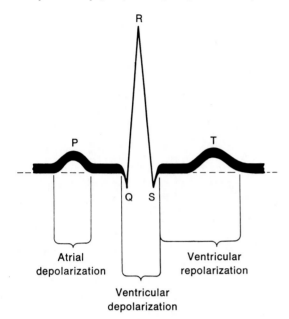

Figure 28.2
Normal ECG deflections.
From Conover MB: Understanding electrocardiography: physiological and interpretive concepts, ed 3, St. Louis, 1980, The CV Mosby Co.

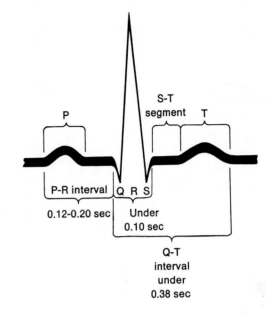

Figure 28.3
ECG intervals.
From Conover MB: Understanding electrocardiography: physiological and interpretive concepts, ed 3, St Louis, 1980, The CV Mosby Co.

low the physician to interpret and analyze the rate, rhythm, and conduction of the heart. Abnormalities detected in the ECG cycles help diagnose cardiac problems, for example, myocardial infarction (MI), pericarditis, myocarditis, left ventricular hypertrophy, atrial and ventricular arrhythmias, nodal block, atrial and ventricular fibrillation, and a variety of other conditions such as acid-base imbalance, effects of various drugs, metabolic diseases, autonomic hyperactivity, and hyperventilation.

Control of the Heartbeat—Conduction System of the Heart

To understand the interpretation of an ECG, one must know the mechanism by which the heartbeat originates. Stimulation of the heartbeat originates in the sympathetic (acting to increase the heart rate) and parasympathetic (the vagus nerve, acting to slow the heart rate) branches of the autonomic nervous system. Although the heart is under the control of the nervous system, the myocardium (heart muscle) itself is capable of contracting rhythmically independently of this outside control. Despite this property of automaticity, impulses from the autonomic nervous system are required to produce a rapid enough beat to maintain circula-

tion and life effectively. Without the nerve connection, the heart rate may be less than 40 beats per minute instead of the usual 70 to 90 per minute (average 80 beats per minute).

Specialized masses of tissue in the heart form the conduction system, regulating the sequence of events of the cardiac cycle. These include the sinoatrial node (SA node), the "pacemaker" of the heart, located in the upper right-hand corner of the right atrium adjacent to the opening of the superior vena cava; the atrioventricular node (AV node), located near the intraventricular septum in the inferior wall of the right atrium and near the tricuspid valve; the bundle of His (or atrioventricular bundle), located in the interventricular septum, which then divides into the left and right bundles; and the Purkinje fibers, which terminate in the ventricles.

The electrical impulse of the cardiac cycle travels first to the sinoatrial node, from which wavelike impulses are sent through the atria, stimulating first the right and then the left atrium, and eventually sweep over the heart. In a comparable manner, if one drops a pebble in water it will generate waves that travel outward from the point of origin.

When the atria have been stimulated, the impulse slows as it passes through the atrioventricular node. Slowing of the impulse at the AV node allows the resting ventricles (in diastole) to fill with blood from the atria. This wave of excitation (stimulation) then spreads down to the bundle of His, then to the right and left bundle branches, which then relay the impulse to the Purkinje fibers, an interlacing network terminating in the ventricle's musculature. The Purkinje fibers distribute the impulse in the right and left ventricles, causing them to contract. Stimulation of the muscle of the ventricle begins in the intraventricular septum and moves downward, causing ventricular depolarization and contraction. Mechanically, the ventricles empty blood into the pulmonary (or lesser) circulation by way of the pulmonary artery and the right and left pulmonary branches, and into the systemic (or greater) circulation by way of the aorta. This stimulation or impulse must spread through the muscle of both atria and both ventricles before mechanical contraction can occur. To complete the cardiac cycle, the entire heart now relaxes momentarily, and then a new impulse is initiated by the SA node to repeat the whole cycle.

The electrical wave front that originates in the SA node and spreads throughout the heart then spreads through the body. From the body surface it is possible to pick up these electrical impulses and record them on specialized paper (the electrocardiograph) or display them on an oscilloscope (comparable to a television screen).

Time Required for Cardiac Cycle

Each cardiac cycle takes approximately 0.8 second. With this time limit, there are 75 heartbeats per minute. When the heart beats more than 75 times per minute, the cycle requires less time. Conversely, when the heart beats fewer than 75 beats per minute, the cardiac cycle requires more than 0.8 second.

Heart Sounds During Cardiac Cycle

Typical sounds are elicited from the heart during each cardiac cycle. These sounds are described as *lubb dupp*, as they are heard through a stethoscope. The first sound, *lubb* or systolic sound, is a longer and lower-pitched sound and is believed to be from the contraction of the ventricles and vibrations from the closing of the cuspid valves. The second sound, *dupp* (the diastolic sound), is shorter and sharper and occurs during the beginning of ventricular relaxation. It is thought to be caused by the vibrations of the closure of the semilunar valves (pulmonic and aortic valves). Since these sounds provide information about the

valves of the heart, they have clinical significance. Variations from normal in these sounds indicate imperfect functioning of the valves. Heart murmurs are one type of abnormal sound heard and may indicate stenosis or incomplete closing of the valves (valvular insufficiency). It is important to remember that the electrocardiograph does not record these sounds. They can be heard when a stethoscope is put on the chest wall over the apex region of the heart.

ECGS
Electrocardiograph Paper

To understand the significance of each wave and interval of various heights and widths recorded by an electrocardiograph, the medical assistant needs to know the significance of the small and large blocks on the electrocardiograph paper (Figure 28.4, *A*). On the horizontal line, one small block represents 0.04 seconds (Figure 28.4, *B*). On the vertical axis, one small block represents 1 mm. Since a large block is five small blocks wide and five deep, each of them represents 0.2 second (horizontal) and 5 mm (vertical).

Notice all the lines. Every fifth line (horizontal and vertical) is usually printed darker than other lines, producing blocks (squares) that are 5 mm × 5 mm. Thus two of the larger blocks equal 10 mm or 1 cm.

These measurements, accepted internationally, allow physicians to interpret cardiac time (rate) on the horizontal line and cardiac voltage on the vertical axis, and thus determine if the electrical activity of the heart is within normal limits.

Electrocardiograph paper is heat-sensitive and pressure-sensitive. When the machine is on and running, a heated stylus moves over the paper to record the cardiac cycles. Being pressure-sensitive, electrocardiograph paper must be handled carefully to avoid markings that would blemish the actual tracing.

Interpretation

When the physician interprets an ECG, the following factors are usually determined:

rate How many beats per minute; determined are the atrial rate and the ventricular rate.
rhythm Whether the heart rhythm is regular or irregular; determined are the atrial rhythm and the ventricular rhythm.
conduction time How long it takes for the impulse originating at the SA node to simulate ventricular contrac-

Figure 28.4
ECG paper with a section enlarged. **A,** Number of large squares between recorded R waves will indicate rate of heartbeat per minute. **B,** One large square enlarged.

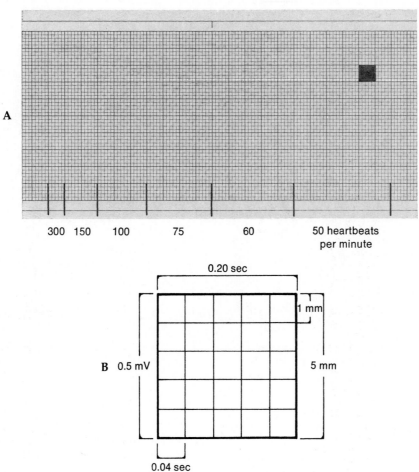

tion (review the conduction system); determined are the P-R interval and the QRS duration.

configuration and location Of each wave, the ST segment, the P-R interval, and sometimes the Q-T interval.

These findings are then recorded and reviewed by the physician to help establish a diagnosis or evaluate current treatment.

Since many physicians expect the medical assistant who takes a patient's ECG to monitor the graph for abnormal or erratic tracings, you should be aware of the following.

Heart rate and rhythm

In a normal ECG, all heartbeats consist of three major units, the P wave, the QRS complex, and the T wave, and appear as a similar pattern, equally spaced.

Briefly, the rate of a particular rhythm may be determined from the ECG simply by noting the distance between two R waves. As seen in Figure 28.4,*A*, two large squares between R waves means that the rate is 150 beats per minute; three large squares between R waves means that the rate is 100 beats per minute. Similarly, four large squares between R waves indicates a heart rate of 75 beats per minute. To get this rate per minute, divide the number of large squares between the R waves into 300. NOTE: If the rhythm is irregular, counting the squares in a single R-R interval will give an approximate rate rather than the precise rate that would be obtained with a perfectly regular rhythm.

To determine if heart rhythm is regular or irregular, the distance between each P wave and then between each R wave is measured. If the distance between all P waves is the same, atrial rhythm is regular; if the distance varies, it is irregular. Similarly, if the distance between R waves is the same,

Figure 28.5

ECG artifacts. **A,** Somatic tremor artifact. **B,** Wandering baseline. **C,** Alternating
current artifact.

From Conover MB: Understanding electrocardiography: physiological
and interpretive concepts, ed 3, St Louis, 1980, The CV Mosby Co.

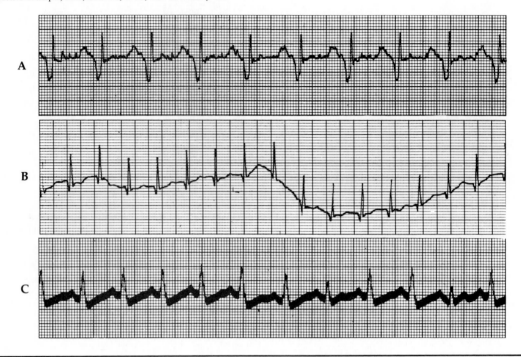

ventricular rhythm is regular, and if not, it is irregular.

Artifacts

Artifacts are defects (unwanted activity) on the
electrocardiograph *not* caused by the electrical activity produced during the cardiac cycle. Since the
electrocardiograph will pick up and record every
kind of electrical activity it can find, artifacts may
appear, making the recording difficult to interpret.
To remedy this situation, the medical assistant
should understand what causes artifacts and how
they can be eliminated or greatly minimized and
use the correct recording technique.

There are several types of artifacts, the most
common being somatic tremor (muscle movement),
wandering baseline (baseline shift), and alternating
current (AC) interference.

Somatic tremor. Somatic tremor artifacts can
be identified by the unnatural baseline deflections,
ranging from irregular vibrations in amplitude and
frequency (jagged peaks of irregular height and
spacing) to large shifting of the baseline (Figure
28.5,*A*). Muscle movement, either voluntary or involuntary, produces artifacts caused mainly when
the patient does the following:

- Is tense and/or apprehensive;
- Moves or talks;
- Is in an uncomfortable position; or
- Suffers from a nervous disorder that causes
constant tremors, such as Parkinson's disease.

The best way to avoid these patient-produced artifacts is to prepare the patient well, both emotionally and physically, preferably in a pleasant and relaxing atmosphere. The following will aid in patient preparation:

- Gain the full cooperation of the patient;
- Explain the procedure and what you will be
doing;
- Position the patient comfortably, with limbs
well supported;
- Offer assistance and reassurance as needed;
and
- Have patients suffering from a nervous disorder put their hands, palms down, under their
buttocks or take a deep breath. This will help
reduce artifacts. (See also "Patient Preparation," p. 590)

Wandering baseline (baseline shift) (Figure 28.5, B)

Causes of wandering baseline include the following:

- Electrodes that are applied too tightly or too loosely;
- Tension on an electrode as a result of an unsupported lead wire that is pulling the electrode away from the patient's skin;
- Too little or poor quality electrolyte gel or paste on an electrode;
- Corroded or dirty electrodes; or
- Skin creams or lotions present on the area to which the electrode is applied.

To prevent artifacts, correct and attentive technique when applying the electrodes with the electrolyte gel or paste is a must. Wash the electrodes after each use and occasionally with kitchen cleanser, but *never* use steel wool. Electrolyte gels or pastes that are left on the electrode can cause corrosion, which makes the electrode a poor conductor of cardiac electrical currents. The tips of the lead wires must also be kept clean.

Ensure that the patient's skin where the electrodes will be applied is clean; if necessary wash the area briskly with alcohol or the presaturated electrolyte pads before applying the electrode.

Alternating current (AC) interference

AC artifacts appear as a series of small regular peaks (or spiked lines) on the ECG (Figure 28.5, C).

Alternating current is our standard source for electrical power. AC present in electrical equipment or wires can radiate or leak a small amount of energy into the immediate area. When a patient is present in this area, some of the AC may be picked up by the body, which in turn is detected by the electrocardiograph. Thus an ECG with AC artifacts results. Common causes of AC interference artifacts include the following:

- Improper grounding of the electrocardiograph;
- Presence of other electrical equipment in the room;
- Electrical wiring in walls or ceilings;
- X-ray or other large electrical equipment being used in adjacent rooms;
- Lead wires crossed and not following the contour of the patient's body;
- Corroded or dirty electrodes; and
- Faulty technique of the operator.

To minimize or eliminate AC interference, correct technique is required. The electrocardiograph must be properly grounded. Check the instructions in the operator's manual supplied with each unit by the manufacturer. Newer units have three-prong plugs that are inserted into a properly grounded three-receptacle outlet. Older units may have a two-prong plug. In this case a ground wire from the unit is connected to a suitable ground, such as a cold water pipe.

Unplug other electrical equipment in the room. When x-ray equipment is being used in adjacent rooms, it may be necessary for you to wait until that procedure is completed or move to another room to record the ECG. Moving the patient table away from the wall may help minimize interference caused from electrical wiring. Lead wires must be straight and positioned to follow body contour; the line cord is to be away from the patient, and the unit should be near the feet of the patient, not the head. Electrodes must be cleaned after each use and occasionally should be scrubbed with a kitchen cleanser.

Additional problems

When recording on ECG, you may encounter a few additional erratic tracings, which may appear as follows:

- An indistinct tracing usually caused by (1) the stylus heat being too low, (2) a bent stylus, (3) incorrect stylus pressure, or (4) a broken stylus heating element, which results in no tracing;
- A straight line but no tracing, caused by the patient cable not being plugged in correctly; or
- A break between complexes, caused by a loose or broken lead wire.

When you cannot correct the cause of an artifact, inform the physician and call the manufacturer's or other repair service, according to office policy.

Electrocardiograph Electrodes and Electrolytes

Electrodes (also called sensors) are small metal plates placed on the patient to pick up the electrical activity of the heart and conduct it to the electrocardiograph. The standard 12-lead electrocardiograph has five electrodes—two to be attached to the fleshy part of the arms, two to the fleshy part of the legs, and one floating electrode that will be placed in six different positions on the chest when recording the chest leads.

In the machine, this electrical current is changed into mechanical action, which is recorded on the electrocardiograph paper by a heated stylus. To help conduct this electric current, an electrolyte is applied to each electrode. Electrolytes are available in the form of gels, pastes, or flannel materials presaturated with an electrolyte solution.

Once the electrodes are correctly secured to the

Figure 28.6
A, Lead triangle showing position of standard limb leads. **B,** Lead triangle showing position of augmented leads.

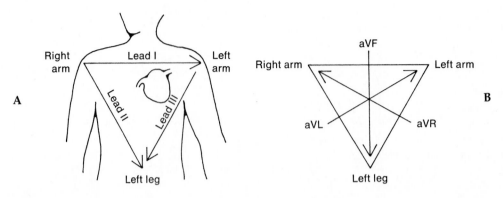

patient with rubber straps, lead wires are fastened to them. These lead wires extend off the patient cable, which is attached to the electrocardiograph.

Electrocardiograph Leads

The standard 12-lead electrocardiograph system records electrical activity from the frontal and horizontal planes of the body by using 12 leads as follows.

Standard limb or bipolar leads

The first three leads to be recorded on a standard ECG are known as Lead I, Lead II, and Lead III. These are called bipolar leads, because each of them uses two limb electrodes that record simultaneously the electrical forces of the heart from the frontal plane, that is, Lead I records electrical activity between the right arm and left arm; Lead II records activity between the right arm and left leg; Lead III records activity between the left arm and left leg (Figure 28.6, *A*).

Upright (positive) deflections on the ECG indicate current flowing toward a positive pole; inverted (negative) wave deflections indicate current flowing toward a negative pole. For example, in Lead I, the flow of current will be from a negative to a positive pole; thus the wave deflections on the recording will be upright.

Augmented leads

The next three leads are the augmented leads, designated as a V_R, a V_L, and a V_F. The *aV* stands for augmented voltage; the *R*, *L*, and *F* stand for right, left, and foot (leg). Augmented leads are unipolar and also record frontal plane activity.

- *Lead aV_R* records electrical activity from the midpoint between the left arm and left leg to the right arm.
- *Lead aV_L* records electrical activity from the midpoint between the right arm and left leg to the left arm.
- *Lead aV_F* records electrical activity from the midpoint between the right arm and left arm to the left leg (Figure 28.6, *B*).

Chest or precordial leads

The last six leads of the standard 12-lead electrocardiograph are the chest or precordial leads. These leads are also unipolar and are designated as V_1, V_2, V_3, V_4, V_5, and V_6.

This third set of leads records electrical activity between six points on the chest wall and a point within the heart. To obtain these recordings, the chest electrode is to be moved to six predesignated positions on the chest. Figure 28.7 shows the location of these positions. It is imperative that the correct position be used for each lead recording.

All 12 leads discussed can be interpreted separately or in combination. Each lead presents a picture of a different anatomical part of the heart, thus allowing the physician to determine areas of damage or problem areas.

When doing an ECG, the machine automatically

Figure 28.7

Leads of routine electrocardiogram.
Courtesy The Burdick Corporation, Milton, Wis.

Standard or bipolar limb leads	Electrodes connected	Marking code	Recommended positions for multiple chest leads (Line art illustration of chest positions)
Lead I	LA & RA	— 1 dot	
Lead II	LL & RA	— 2 dots	
Lead III	LL & LA	— 3 dots	
Augmented unipolar limb leads			
aVR	RA & (LA-LL)	1 dash	V₁ Fourth intercostal space at right margin of sternum
aVL	LA & (RA-LL)	2 dashes	V₂ Fourth intercostal space at left margin of sternum
aVF	LL & (RA-LA)	3 dashes	V₃ Midway between position 2 and position 4
Chest or precordial leads			V₄ Fifth intercostal space at junction of left midclavicular line
			V₅ At horizontal level of position 4 at left anterior axillary line
V	C & (LA-RA-LL)	(See data on right)	V₆ At horizontal level of position 4 at left midaxillary line

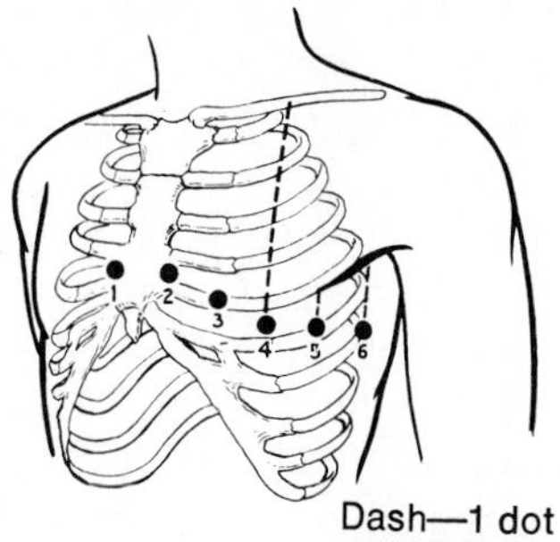

Dash—1 dot

connects the proper electrode potentials for Leads I, II, III, aV_R, aV_L, and aV_F. To record the chest leads, the chest electrode must be moved manually to each of the assigned chest positions.

Suggested codes for marking leads

Certain codes are used to identify each lead recorded. Without these codes it would be difficult to determine which lead one was interpreting, and it would be impossible to mount the recording with proper lead identification. An example of codes used is seen in Figure 28.7. On older machines the leads are coded (marked) by depressing the lead marker button. New machines will automatically code for each lead as it is being recorded.

Standardizing the Electrocardiograph

The diagnostic value of an ECG depends on an accurate recording. Standard techniques have been adapted to provide a recording that can be interpreted anywhere in the world, assuming the electrocardiograph used has been calibrated according to universal measurements.

The universal standard of electrocardiographic measurement is: 1 millivolt of cardiac electrical activity will deflect the stylus precisely 10 mm (1 cm) high. This is equal to 10 small blocks on the electrocardiograph paper (see also the section on electrocardiograph paper).

Before any ECG is recorded, the machine must be standardized; that is, it must be checked to determine if it is set to record according to the universal measurement.

To standardize the machine, turn the main power switch on. The stylus should be positioned to run along on one of the dark horizontal lines. Set the lead selector switch to STD and the record switch to RUN. Quickly depress and release the standardization button. The standardization mark should go 10 mm high and 2 mm wide. It will appear as an open-ended rectangle (the open end being along the baseline). A slight slant may be seen in the top right corner, which is normal, but any other deviation from this is not and must be corrected. To correct any deviation, turn the standardization adjustment knob and repeat the procedure until the correct standardization mark is obtained.

It is important to consult the instruction manual provided by the manufacturer of each electrocardiograph, as this procedure may vary slightly among the various machines on the market.

The universal standard for recording an ECG is at a speed of 25 mm/second. This can be increased on the machine to run the paper at 50 mm/second when segments of the ECG are close together or when heart rate is rapid. A notation of this *must* be made to alert the physician of this change to allow an accurate interpretation of the record.

Preparation and Procedure for Obtaining ECGs
Equipment

- Bed or examining table (preferably without any metal attachments)
- Linen sheet or blanket
- Electrocardiograph with patient cable lead wires
- Electrolyte gel *or* paste *or* presaturated electrolyte pads
- Electrodes and rubber straps
- Gauze squares
- Patient gown

Preparation of electrocardiograph room

1. The room should be as far away as possible from all x-ray and other electrical equipment that may cause artifacts on the electrocardiogram.
2. The room should be comfortably warm, quiet, pleasant, and not crowded with medical instruments, which may make the patient apprehensive.
3. The electrocardiograph (and patient) should be positioned away from wires, cords, and any other source of AC interference.
4. The bed or examining table must be wide enough that the patient may rest comfortably with the extremities well supported; otherwise muscle tension or tremors may cause artifacts.

Preparation of patient

The quality of the record obtained is influenced by scrupulous attention to fundamental rules regarding the preparation of the patient. The medical assistant who is confident, but empathetic, will make it easier for the patient to relax, both mentally and physically.

1. Explain the nature and purpose of the electrocardiograph to the patient. Tactfully help the patient realize that full cooperation (that is, relaxing and not talking, moving, or chewing gum) will help produce a recording that will help the physician diagnose and treat the patient's condition (when applicable).
2. Assure the patient that no shock or other sensation will be felt.
3. Have the patient remove any jewelry that would interfere with electrode placement or come in contact with the electrolyte.
4. Have the patient remove shoes and clothing from the waist up; women are to remove nylons. A patient gown should be put on with the opening in the front.
5. Help the patient assume a recumbent position on the table with arms at the sides and legs not touching. The extremities must be well supported on the table.
6. Place a cover over the patient with arms and lower legs exposed. Protecting the patient from cold or any other discomfort is very important. A small pillow can be placed under the head.
7. Locate and mark the six chest locations on the patient. (You can use a felt tip pen or such and wash the markings off afterwards with an alcohol sponge.) The patient gown over a woman's chest can be adjusted so as not to expose the breasts and cause possible embarrassment and apprehension and still allow you to adequately locate and record the chest lead positions.
8. Inquire if the patient has any questions before you begin the recording.

Application of electrodes and connection of lead wires

1. Expose the patient's arms and legs.
2. Attach one end of each rubber strap to each electrode (Figure 28.8, *A*).
3. Place a small amount of electrolyte gel or paste, about the size of a pea, on the electrode (Figure 28.8, *B*).
4. Using the side of the electrode, rub the electrolyte into the skin on the fleshy part of the right arm. The area rubbed should not be much larger than the size of the electrode and should be slightly reddened by the rubbing. (If there is

Figure 28.8
A, Attaching rubber strap to electrode. **B,** Place small amount of electrolyte gel
on electrode. **C,** Presaturated electrolyte pad and electrode applied to arm. **D,**
Electrolyte pad, electrode, and rubber strap applied to arm.
Courtesy The Burdick Corporation, Milton, Wis.

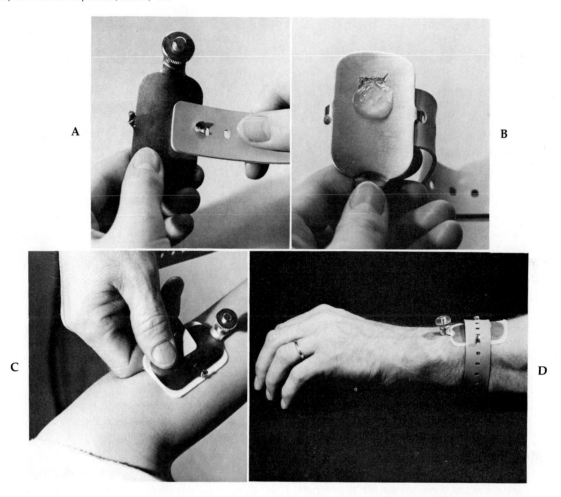

lotion or cream on the skin, it must be removed with an alcohol sponge before the electrolyte and electrode are applied.)

5. Place the electrode on this skin area, pull the rubber strap around, and fasten it to the electrode. The electrode must not be pressing against the table or other body parts. The electrode must not be fastened too loosely or too tightly. Try to move the electrode about once secured in place. If it slips or slides on the limb, it is too loose and must be tightened; if the skin is pinched on either side of the electrode, the strap is too tight and must be loosened.

6. Using a gauze square, wipe any excess gel or paste from around the electrode.

7. Follow this same procedure to apply the electrodes to the left arm and to the right and left legs over the fleshy part of the lower leg, not over the bone. By applying the electrodes to the fleshy areas on the limbs, the chance of undesirable muscle artifacts is minimized. Also use equal amounts of gel or paste on each electrode.

8. When using presaturated electrolyte pads rather than a gel or paste, rub the skin with the pad, then place it on the skin. The electrode is to be placed directly on top of the pad (Figure 28.8, *C* and *D*).

9. *If taking an ECG on a patient who has a cast, amputation, or prosthesis, place the electrode above the affected area. The electrode for the other extremity must then be placed in the same location opposite the first. For example,*

Figure 28.9
A, Portable automatic three-channel electrocardiograph records all 12 leads simultaneously on a single 10-second record. **B,** Single-channel electrocardiographs record 12 leads individually on strip of ECG paper as it is run through the machine.
Photo courtesy Hewlett-Packard, Palo Alto, Calif.

A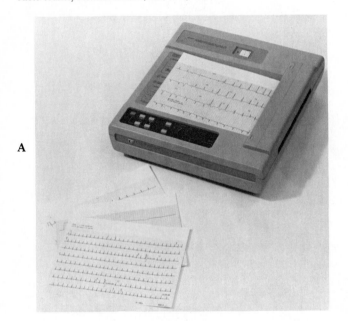

B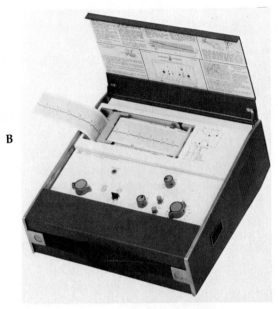

if the patient has a cast extending from the knee to the ankle on the right leg, place the electrode on the inside of the upper right leg. The electrode for the left leg must then be placed on the inside of the upper left leg. If the electrodes are not placed in this manner, that is, if one electrode is placed on the upper part of the right limb above the cast and the other electrode is placed on the fleshy part of the lower left leg, the electric vector would be changed, and abnormal results would occur on the ECG.

10. Leave the chest electrode unattached but not touching a direct surface, *or* position it on the first chest position using the electrolyte of choice.

11. Firmly connect the patient cable lead wires to the proper electrodes so that the lead wire connector faces the patient's feet. Each wire is alphabetically coded: RA—right arm, LA—left arm, RL—right leg, LL—left leg, and C—Chest. In addition, each lead wire is color coded to provide additional identification for the operator. It is very important that the lead wires are connected and arranged to follow the contour of the body without any strain

placed on the electrodes so that the possibility of AC artifacts is minimized.

12. Plug the patient cable into the patient cable jack on the machine. Make sure that it is pushed all the way in.

13. Before beginning the recording, routinely check that all connections are secure, that the patient cable is supported on the table or over the patient's abdomen to prevent pulling of the cable, and to see if the patient has any questions.

Recording the ECG (Figure 28.9)

Limb leads

1. Set the lead selector switch to STD (standard).

2. Turn recorder switch to ON. (Some machines will require a warm-up period before recording. Check the instruction manual to determine if this is the case for the equipment that you are using.)

3. Turn recorder switch to RUN.

4. Center the baseline by turning the centering dial or position control knob.

5. Check the standardization: quickly depress and release the standardization button sev-

eral times while the lead selector is on STD and the recorder switch is on RUN. The height of the standardization measurement should be 10 mm or two large squares from the baseline.

6. Turn the lead selector switch to Lead I.

7. Mark the identification code for the lead immediately after it is selected, unless the machine does this automatically.

8. Run for a few heartbeats; depress the standardization button quickly if the physician requires proof of standardization for each lead. This standardization mark should be inserted between the T wave (or U wave when present) of one complex and the P wave of the next complex.

9. Record at least 8 to 10 inches. This provides ample tracing of the lead.

10. Turn lead selector to Lead II.

11. Repeat steps 7, 8, and 9.

12. Turn the lead selector to Lead III and repeat steps 7, 8, and 9.

Augmented levels—aV_R, aV_L, aV_F

13. Turn the lead selector to lead aV_R, mark the identification code, insert a standardization mark if required, and record 5 to 6 inches (see steps 7 and 8).

14. Turn the lead selector to lead aV_L, and repeat step 13.

15. Turn the lead selector to lead aV_F, and repeat step 13.

16. Turn the machine off.

Chest leads

17. Leave the limb electrodes and patient cable wires in place.

18. Position the chest electrode over the first chest position, V_1, applying the electrode with gel *or* paste *or* presaturated electrolyte pad in the same manner used on the limbs.

19. Turn the lead selector to STD, the recorder switch to RUN, and depress the standardization button.

20. Turn the recorder switch to OFF to prevent excessive movement of the stylus.

21. Turn the lead selector switch to V.

22. Turn the record switch to ON.

23. Mark the identification code for the lead, and insert standardization marks as described in step 8, when required.

24. Record 5 to 6 inches.

25. Turn the recorder switch to OFF.

26. Move the chest electrode to the next position. Start again with step 21; repeat until all the chest leads have been recorded, that is, lead V_1 through lead V_6.

27. When all the leads have been recorded satisfactorily, turn the lead selector to STD, the recorder switch to OFF, and unplug the power cord.

28. Disconnect the lead wires, unfasten the rubber straps, and remove the electrodes from the patient.

29. Wipe any electrolyte from the patient's skin.

30. Assist the patient as needed. Provide further instructions as indicated.

31. Label the recording with patient's name, date, and your initials.

32. Clean all equipment, and return it to the proper storage area.

33. Wash your hands.

34. Record the procedure.

35. Mount the recording, using the preferred mount as indicated by the physician; record the required information on the mount. Sign your name to the mounted ECG.

36. Give the mounted ECG to the physician for review and interpretation.

Throughout the recording of the ECG, make sure that the stylus stays on the same baseline (Figure 28.10). Use the position control knob if any adjustment is necessary. Constantly watch for the appearance of any artifact. If they do occur, determine the cause and correct the problem.

Mounting an ECG

Mounting the ECG is important so that the recording can be protected, easily seen by the physician, and inserted into the patient's medical record after the physician has it reviewed and interpreted. There are a variety of commercially prepared mounts available for use, or the recording can be mounted on a plain piece of paper. Regardless of the method chosen to mount the ECG, each lead must be correctly identified. In addition, the patient's name, address, age, sex, and the date of the recording must be documented. Other information may be included varying with the physician's request, such as drugs the patient is taking, especially cardiac drugs such as digitalis and quinidine, height, weight, blood pressure, and occupation. See Figure 28.11 for sample mounts and specific directions for mounting the ECG.

PHONE-A-GRAM— THE COMPUTERIZED ECG

For over 2,000 years, physicians from Hippocrates to Laënnec and Einthoven and many others have

Figure 28.10
Electrocardiograph paper and recording.
Courtesy Sanborn Company, Boston, Mass.

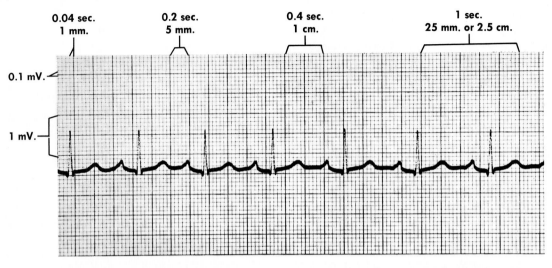

sought to improve diagnostic accuracy. Phone-A-Gram joined this distinguished group in 1971 by providing a computerized ECG system to help physicians diagnose heart disease. In the late 1950s the U.S. Public Health Service started investigating the use of computers in the analysis of ECGs. By 1969, following the expenditure of millions of dollars, the Health Care Technology Division, National Center for Health Service Research and Development, had approved a computer-assisted ECG analysis program. In 1971 Phone-A-Gram System received the Public Health Service certificate, ensuring faithful reproduction of an ECG analysis program.

Today Phone-A-Gram provides a complete ECG *service* and all the necessary equipment to over 2,400 physicians, hospitals, and clinics throughout the United States. The unmatched speed and accuracy of the computer now provide physicians everywhere with a second opinion for the diagnosis of a patient's condition and save much time and money.

Phone-A-Gram's ECG system includes a portable automatic ECG transmitter (a standard model, a scout model, or the stripchart recorder model), all the auxiliary equipment, and a personal hookup into the national network (Data Center), which receives, converts, processes, analyzes, and prints out all ECG information for ready reference.

All ECG transmitting units are single-channel units with the features of automatic lead switching and standardization across all 12 leads. The units are compact, portable, and extremely reliable. The *standard model unit* is the simplest to operate and *does not* produce a stripchart. This eliminates the need for and cost of graph paper. It is battery powered and can be easily transported from one location to another. The *scout model* is the same as the standard unit but can be used in conjunction with a conventional electrocardiograph to produce an on-site tracing as the ECG is being transmitted. When using this model to get an on-site tracing, an audiocable is attached to the standard electrocardiograph. The *stripchart recorder* (Figure 28.12) is a compact, single-channel, automatic lead-switching electrocardiograph with a built-in transmitter. It can run a preview tracing and then produce single-channel tracings simultaneously as the ECG is transmitted.

The patient is prepared for the ECG by attaching the electrodes to the chest, arms, and legs in the usual manner, although when using the Phone-A-Gram system, all six chest lead electrodes are applied to the patient's chest before you begin to record the ECG.

A standard telephone is used to dial the Data Center (Figure 28.13). The telephone handset is placed on the Phone-A-Gram unit, and the ECG is transmitted at the push of a button (Figure 28.12). The unit picks up signals from the patient and transmits them over the telephone to the Data Center.

Text continued on p. 599.

Figure 28.11
A, Sample ECG mount for mounting a three-channel electrocardiogram strip.
Directions are given on mount.
Photo courtesy Hewlett-Packard, Palo Alto, Calif.

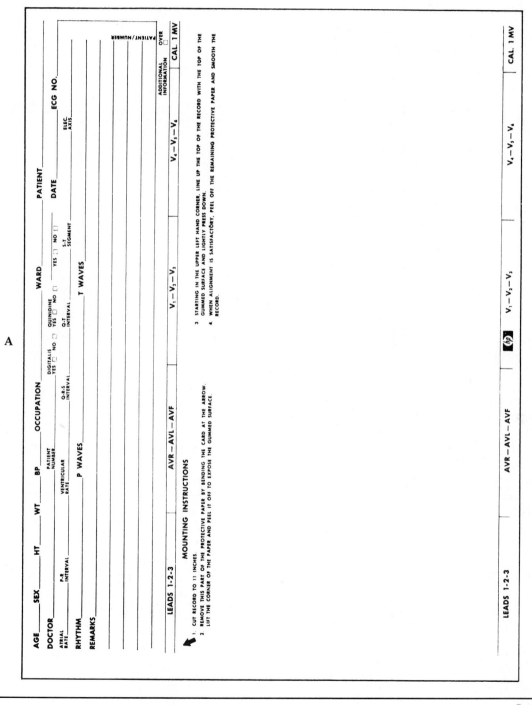

Figure 28.11, cont'd
For legend see opposite page.

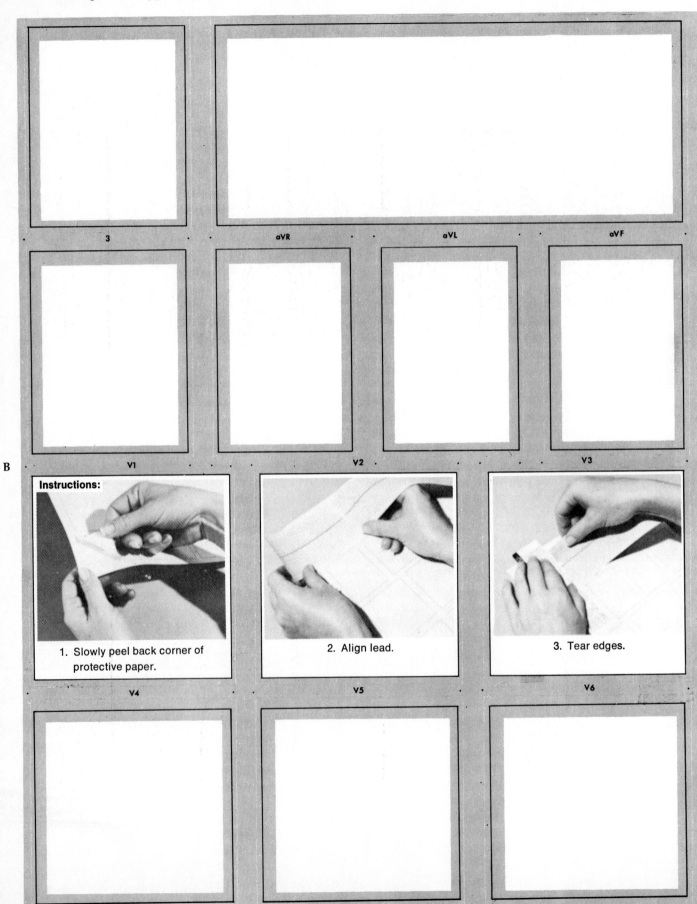

3   aVR   aVL   aVF

V1   V2   V3

Instructions:

1. Slowly peel back corner of protective paper.

2. Align lead.

3. Tear edges.

V4   V5   V6

B

Figure 28.11, cont'd
B, Sample ECG mount with instructions for use with single-strip
electrocardiograms. **C,** Information to be recorded on back of single-strip ECG
mount.

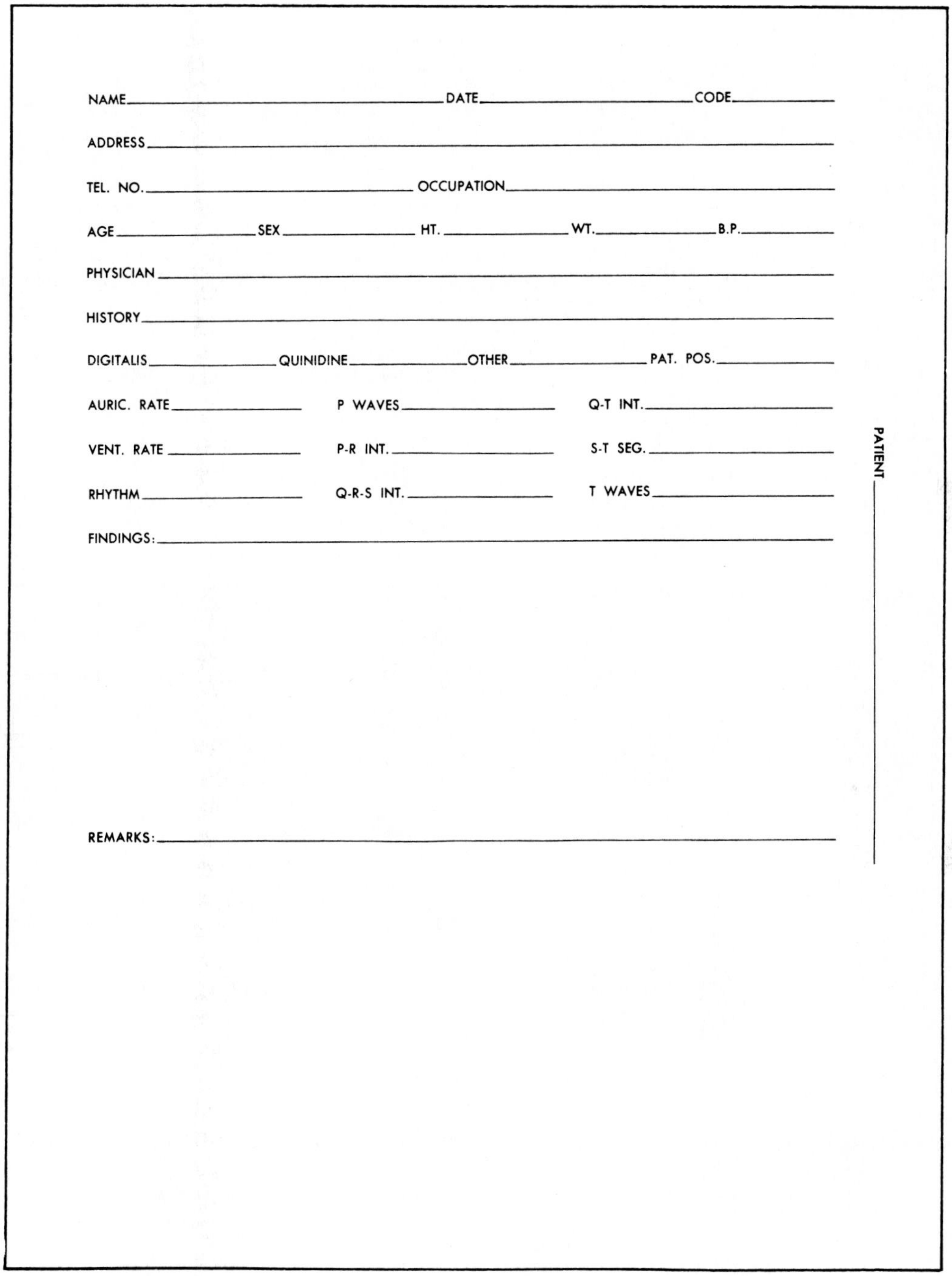

NAME_____ DATE_____ CODE_____

ADDRESS_____

TEL. NO._____ OCCUPATION_____

AGE_____ SEX_____ HT._____ WT._____ B.P._____

PHYSICIAN_____

HISTORY_____

DIGITALIS_____ QUINIDINE_____ OTHER_____ PAT. POS._____

AURIC. RATE_____   P WAVES_____   Q-T INT._____

VENT. RATE _____   P-R INT._____   S-T SEG._____

RHYTHM_____   Q-R-S INT._____   T WAVES_____

FINDINGS:_____

REMARKS:_____

PATIENT_____

C

Figure 28.12
Phone-A-Gram stripchart model.
Courtesy Phone-A-Gram System, San Francisco, Calif.

1. Start/reset switch: Used to start the instrument. Instrument will automatically stop at the end of test. If the instrument stops in the middle of a test, this is because an electrode has either fallen off or is not making proper contact with the patient's skin.

2. Recorder chart switch: This three-position switch allows the user the option of either producing or not producing a tracing at the time the ECG is being transmitted to Phone-A-Gram system. When a tracing is not desired the switch should be set on STOP position. When a tracing is desired it should be set on AUTO position. The FEED position is only used at the end of a test to feed the tracing out of the recorder so it can be torn off.

3. Gain switch: This switch is normally left in the *1* position. If the patient's heart waves are large enough to go off the graph the switch should be moved to the ½ position. If the patient's heart waves are too small to measure the switch should be moved to the *2* position.

4. Strip chart recorder: Produces a 12-lead tracing automatically. Use only ECG paper provided by Phone-A-Gram system. Other types may damage recorder. When your supply of paper is low you may reorder by calling our customer service department.

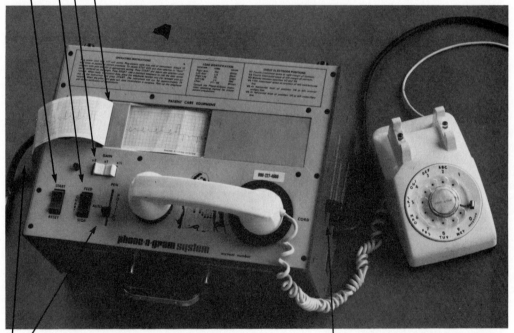

5. Stylus/pen position knob: Allows user to center the baseline in the middle of the tracing before the test begins.

6. Patient cable socket: Patient cable plugs in here.

7. Fuse access: If fuse blows replace with your spare ½ amp slo-blow type fuse only.

Figure 28.13
Phone-A-Gram Data Center, equipped with most technically advanced telephone
system. Phone-A-Gram unit picks up signals from patient and transmits these
signals over telephone to Data Center, where ECG is processed.
Courtesy Phone-A-Gram System, San Francisco, Calif.

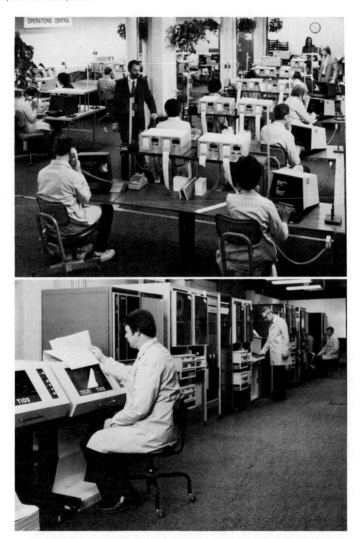

Phone-A-Gram Data Centers are staffed 24 hours a day, 7 days a week, by technicians fully trained to receive and process computer-interpreted ECGs. They monitor transmissions, evaluate the quality of ECG tracings, and identify and solve common technical problems. Phone-A-Gram's computer prints out the 12 lead measurements and interpretations. The complete printout, stripchart, and analysis are mailed to the physician the same day (Figure 28.14). In an emergency or when requested, the technician calls the reports back to the physician within minutes. Phone-A-Gram's staff cardiologists will automatically review ECGs when necessary and will also provide special optional services as required, such as telephone consultations. In addition, other special services such as serial comparison of ECGs and pediatric ECG interpretations can be obtained on request.

The accuracy of a computer-analyzed ECG, like the manually read ECG, depends on the current state of the art and science of electrocardiography. The criteria for diagnosis incorporated into the Phone-A-Gram computer software analysis program represent the most recent in the state of the science. Phone-A-Gram ECG interpretations are a

Figure 28.14

Latest, most technologically advanced computer system in combination with revolutionary device called Printer Plotter produce unique Phone-A-Gram report format. Printer Plotter format *eliminates hand mounting* of tracing, because it is produced on one sheet of paper. *File storage convenience* is afforded, because report can be folded to an 8½ × 11 size before being placed on the patient's chart.
Courtesy Phone-A-Gram System, San Francisco, Calif.

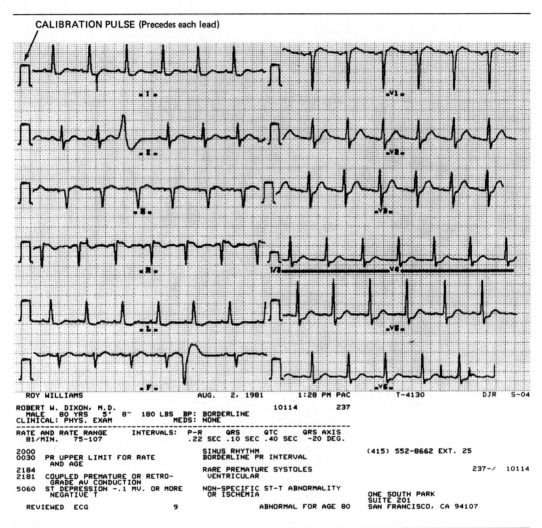

combination of computers and cardiologists. Expert cardiologists agree that this method represents the optimum in ECG analysis and provides the most clinically relevant and accurate interpretations available.

The physician receiving a Phone-A-Gram computer or cardiologist's report should relate the interpretive statements to the clinical circumstances, symptomatological findings, and other diagnostic test results in determining the appropriate plan of treatment for the patient.

Procedure for Using the Phone-A-Gram System for ECGs*

1. Prepare the electrocardiograph room.
2. Obtain the pertinent patient data: name, sex, age, height, weight, blood pressure, medication, and the clinical reason for the ECG. This information is needed when you call the Data Center before transmitting the ECG recording.

*Modified from Phone-A-Gram System Operating Handbook, San Francisco, Phone-A-Gram System.

Phone-A-Gram Codes for Blood Pressure, Medication, and Clinical Reason Information

The listed *Blood Pressure, Medication Class,* and *Clinical Reason* codes are the ones the Phone-A-Gram computer program takes into account in producing the analysis. You should use the appropriate codes whenever possible, particularly for medications, since Phone-A-Gram is not familiar with all brand name drugs.

Code   Blood pressure

B0   Normotension—Systolic pressure 100 to 139 mm and diastolic pressure 89 mm or below
B1   Borderline hypertension—Systolic pressure 140-159 mm or diastolic pressure 90-94 mm
B2   Hypertension—Systolic pressure 160 or above or diastolic pressure 95 mm or above
B3   Hypotension—Systolic pressure 99 mm or below
B4   Unknown

Code and medication class

D0	None	D8	Antihypertensive
D1	Digitalis	D9	Alpha-adrenergic
D2	Quinidine/procaine/lidocaine	D10	Beta-adrenergic
D3	Antiarrhythmic	D11	Parasympathomimetic
D4	Diuretic	D12	Phenothiazine
D5	Potassium	D13	Tranquilizer
D6	Nitroglycerin	D14	Thyroid
D7	Beta-blocking	D15	Unknown/other

Code and clinical reason

R0	None given	R8	Arrhythmia
R1	Physical exam	R9	Pacer, demand rate
R2	Pre-op	R10	Pacer, fixed rate
R3	Chest pain	R11	Lung disease
R4	Acute myocardial infarct	R12	Cardiac surgery
R5	Prior myocardial infarct	R13	Rheumatic heart disease
R6	Congestive heart disease	R14	Congenital heart disease
R7	High blood pressure	R15	Pericarditis

Courtesy and with permission of Phone-A-Gram System, San Francisco, Calif.

It is recommended that you convert the last three items to the appropriate codes listed above to expedite the telephone procedure.

3. Prepare the patient (see p. 590).
4. Insert the patient cable into the side of the instrument. Push it straight in all the way. *Do not* attempt to screw it in or twist it in any way, since this could cause damage to the unit and/or cable.
5. Attach the 10 suction cup electrodes to patient cable tips and check to see that each electrode fits snugly onto the tip of each lead wire. If any are loose, gently expand the metal tip of the lead wire with a small screw driver until a secure fit is achieved. The tips of the lead wires are color-coded and lettered for ease of identification (Figure 28.15).
6. When all electrodes are attached to the patient cable, anchor the cable under one of the patient's legs or right arm and rest the cable on the patient's lap while you apply the electrode gel to the skin.
7. Rub the skin area for each electrode position vigorously with gauze saturated in alcohol (particularly during cold, dry weather) to remove dead skin and oils from the body surface. Next apply a drop of electrode gel to the appropriate areas and work it into the skin in a circular pattern about the size of a nickel, being careful that gel from one electrode position does not overlap onto that for another position. Since the gel forms a seal around the rim of the suction cup, a sufficient amount should always be used to ensure good contact. If the patient has an extremely hairy chest, use additional gel, spread the hair, and if necessary shave the area before attaching the electrodes. Figure 28.15 illustrates the correct positions for the V_1 through V_6 electrodes to obtain accurate results. It is important that actual counting and feeling for rib (intercostal) spaces is done routinely, since patient anatomies may differ. NOTE: *Spacing should appear equidis-*

Figure 28.15
Phone-A-Gram System's lead wire color codes, alphabetical codes, and six chest electrode positions.
Courtesy Phone-A-Gram System, San Francisco, Calif.

LEAD WIRE COLOR CODES AND ALPHABETICAL CODES

Electrode location	Alphabetical code	Color code
Right arm	RA	White
Left arm	LA	Black
Right leg	RL	Green
Left leg	LL	Red
Chest	V1-V2-V3-V4-V5-V6	Brown

ELECTRODE POSITIONS

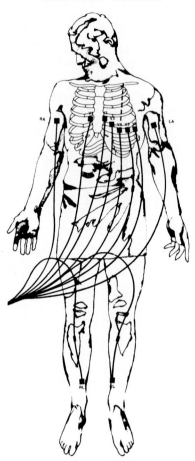

The four limb electrodes should be adhered to the following areas shown

Left arm/Right arm/
Left leg/Right leg

SIX CHEST ELECTRODE (PRECORDIAL) POSITIONS

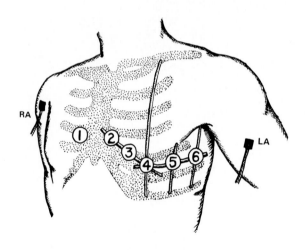

V1	Fourth intercostal space, right margin of sternum
V2	Fourth intercostal space, left margin of sternum
V3	Midway between position V2 and V4
V4	Fifth intercostal space at junction of left mid-clavicular line
V5	Fifth intercostal space at anterior axillary line
V6	Fifth intercostal space at left midaxillary line

tant from one electrode to the next with no crowding or gaps.

8. Properly applying the six chest electrodes and two arm electrodes is a quick and easy procedure. To achieve maximum suction and contact, grasp the electrodes in a syringe-type manner, depress the rubber bulb with your thumb, and push down firmly on the patient's skin before releasing.

9. Attach the leg electrode to a meaty area of the calf. Arrange excess lead wires on the patient's

lap so that there is no strain or pull on any of the electrodes. If strain exists or any electrode is leaning to one side, hold the electrode in place by the rubber bulb and swivel the lead wire (where it is labeled, for example, LA) clockwise or counterclockwise so that the electrode cup ultimately lies flat on the patient's skin.

10. *Standard model only*—After all electrodes are attached to the patient, press the START button and allow the unit to run for at least 15

Figure 28.16
Phone-A-Gram ECG being recorded on site and transmitted to Data Center.
Courtesy Phone-A-Gram System, San Francisco, Calif.

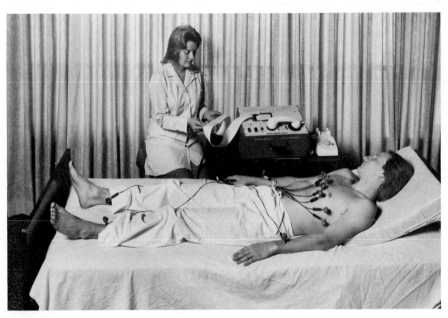

seconds to test that all connections are properly made. If the red light comes on, this indicates that one or more of the electrodes is not making proper contact, a lead has actually fallen off, or the patient cable is not inserted properly into the unit. Recheck the patient and test the instrument again. When the red light stays out, press the RESET button to stop the unit (see Figure 28.12 for operation if you have the stripchart model equipment). Instruct the patient to lie still, relax, and breathe normally without expanding the chest excessively and not to talk or move. Do not touch the patient, the cable, or the Phone-A-Gram instrument during transmission.

11. Now you are ready to make the telephone call to the Data Center, using the Data Center number that is affixed to the transmitting unit.

12. Telephone procedure—Proceed as follows when the Data Center operator takes your call:
    • This is account number #_____
    • Dr. _____ office (or _____ Hospital)
    • The patient's name is _____
    • Sex _____
    • Age _____

• Height _____
• Weight _____
• Blood pressure*_____
• Medication*_____
• Clinical reason*_____

If you desire any special service(s), such as an immediate callback report, it should be requested at this time.

13. The Phone-A-Gram operator will then advise you when to start the transmission process. The patient should again be reminded to lie still, breathe normally, and not talk.

14. To transmit, simply place the mouthpiece of the telephone snugly in the black cup and then press the START button. The instrument will then automatically calibrate itself, switch from one lead to the next, and shut itself off at the end of the test. It takes a total of 75 seconds to transmit the ECG (Figure 28.16).

15. When the white light goes off and the tone stops, pick up the telephone and the Data Center operator will inform you within seconds if the ECG was of good quality. If the tracing was of poor quality, the Data Center operator

---

*It is recommended that a code be used to expedite the telephone procedure. Please see the list of codes on p. 601.

will ask you to rerun the test after the problem is corrected. If for any reason you get cut off before getting confirmation on the quality of the tracing from the operator, call the Data Center back immediately before disconnecting the patient and inform the operator that you were cut off.

16. The tracing and complete computer printout will be mailed to you on the same day. If you requested an immediate callback on the ECG, the results will be called back before being mailed. Approximately 5 seconds of heartbeat is automatically recorded at the Phone-A-Gram Data Center for each of the 12 leads (Figure 28.14).

17. Disconnect the patient cable tips from the electrodes and remove the electrodes from the patient.

18. Wipe any electrode gel from the patient's skin.

19. Assist the patient as needed. Provide further instructions as indicated.

20. Clean all equipment and return it to the proper storage area.

21. Wash your hands.

22. Record the procedure on the patient's chart.

Cleaning Electrodes

All 10 of the suction cup–type electrodes must be wiped clean immediately after each ECG is completed to prevent residual buildup and subsequent contact problems. Use only alcohol or soap and water to clean electrode surfaces, since polishes, commercial cleaners and other such items if used can cause artifacts in the ECG tracing. Also, never use a scrub brush to clean the electrode surfaces, because the metal plating is very thin and can be scraped away, thus rendering the electrodes useless.

The Role of the Computer in ECG Analysis

The computer is used to obtain a large number of precise measurements from the ECG waveforms. These measurements coupled with the pertinent patient data—sex, age, height, weight, blood pressure, medications, and clinical reason for the ECG—are then compared against range criteria for normal and abnormal cardiac conditions. The results of these comparisons are printed out along with the patient and account data and a set of routinely used ECG interval measurements (P-R, QRS, QTC, QRS axis) in an easy-to-read, understandable report. The computer-generated report repre-

sents, in the majority of cases, what would be reported by a cardiologist reading the same ECG.

The Effect of Combining Computer Analysis and Cardiologist Review

Inherent to the computer analysis program are two automatic flagging systems. One identifies possible and actual acute conditions (for example, acute myocardial infarction), which are automatically reviewed by a cardiologist. An immediate callback report is then given to the physician. The other flagging system represents an array of preselected cardiac conditions (for example, complex arrhythmias) that are routinely reviewed by a staff cardiologist before being sent back to the physician.

Reports that have been reviewed by a staff cardiologist will contain the statement *Phone-A-Gram reviewed ECG* at the bottom of the left-hand corner of the printout, in addition to the signature of the reviewing cardiologist.

Optimal Use of the Phone-A-Gram ECG Report

The unique Phone-A-Gram ECG report format includes the *interpretive statements* (descriptive) on the right-hand column and the *diagnostic criteria statements* (objective ECG findings) on the left-hand column. Simply stated, the criteria reflect the objective ECG data that were used to arrive at each interpretation. This criteria–interpretive statement format allows the physician to apply the diagnostic criteria to the actual tracing to verify the reported interpretation(s). Directly above this data is the rate and rate range, interval measurements, and pertinent patient information that was used in arriving at the interpretation(s). In the lower right-hand corner is an overall severity classification of the ECG, which summarizes the interpretive statements and suggests clinical significance (for example, *within normal limits for age* or *abnormal for age*) (Figure 28.14).

NEWEST TECHNOLOGY: AUTOMATIC ELECTROCARDIOGRAPHS

The newer electrocardiographs have fewer operating controls, and are much easier to use. With these new machines controls such as position, sensitivity, heat, paper speed, run, and lead markers *do not* need to be adjusted. Set one switch to select the format which is to be recorded. Different *positions* on the electrocardiograph set it at different speeds and sensitivities. On Hewlett-Packard's

4700 models many different formats can be selected. The 10 preset ECG format selections are on a pull-out card under the machine. Directions for use are on top of the electrocardiograph. Thus there is no need to memorize the format selection available.

There are different operating modes of the electrocardiograph that will produce three different ECG reports. These modes include the following:

- Auto Mode: By pushing this button to select a format position when turning the format switch, the electrocardiograph is instructed to automatically record the routine diagnostic 3-channel 12-lead ECG. Multiple leads are recorded simultaneously. If desired, a rhythm strip recording can also be added. The final single-page report will have 10 seconds of continuous 12-lead information plus the rhythm strip.
- Manual Mode: By pushing this button to select a format position when turning the format switch, the electrocardiograph is instructed to record three leads for detailed waveform examinations. A choice of which leads will be recorded can be made from one of the preset formats.
- Rhythm Mode: By pushing this button to select a format position when turning the format switch, the electrocardiograph is instructed to record a single-lead rhythm strip. Format selection determines which and for how long the rhythm strip will be recorded.

These electrocardiographs allow an exact copy of the ECG which was just taken to be made simply by pushing the *copy* button. Lead identification marks, lead switching marks, and frequency changes are printed on every record. A one-page ECG on standard 8½ × 11-inch heavy-weight paper is produced. The page is easy to read, handle, store, and interpret, and does not require mounting.

Some electrocardiographs have a complete alphanumeric keyboard through which a wide range of patient data can be entered including the patient's name, the requesting physician, name of the facility, and the operator's initials on the ECG record. Other 3-channel electrocardiographs can be operated manually or automatically by the push of a touch pad. The ECG record is produced on standard size paper that can be mounted on card or folder-format mounts (Figure 28.17). When operating these new electrocardiographs, which is relatively easy, first attach all 10 electrodes (one on each arm, one on each leg, and six on the chest) to

Figure 28.17
The high-volume, easy-to-operate, three-channel ECG that makes its own copies. Can be operated manually or automatically.
(Courtesy The Burdick Corp, Milton, Wisc.)

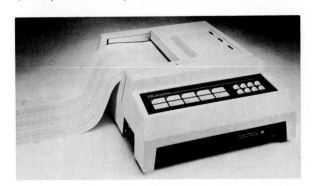

Figure 28.18
Portable Burdick E500 interpretive ECG.
(Courtesy The Burdick Corp, Milton, Wisc.)

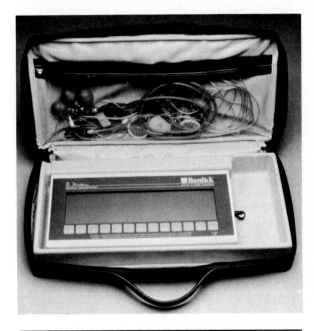

the patient and then select the type of report that needs to be recorded.

There are also single-channel electrocardiographs that can be operated manually or automatically.

Another new machine, the *portable interpretive* electrocardiograph, is also available (Figure 28.18).

Using a clinically proven computerized program, the Burdick E500 analyzes 10 seconds of data from all 12 leads simultaneously in just 3 seconds and also provides the reason for its interpretation. Up to 60 ECGs can be stored in memory for review and printout at a later time. Wherever there is a phone line, the E500 can transmit data from the patient's location to other units for overread so that the physician can take it along if visiting the patient at home or in a care facility. The unique LCD display shows actual waveforms for each lead, permitting continuous monitoring while the ECG is being taken. The display also indicates if leads are improperly connected, thereby eliminating paper waste caused by false starts. A comprehensive report of all pertinent information is provided on one compact $8\frac{1}{2} \times 11$-inch, easy-to-file sheet. Demographic information on the patient in addition to medications that the patient may be taking, heart rate interval measurements, date, and time is included on every printout.

Conclusion

Having completed the chapter on electrocardiography, you should have acquired a basic understanding of the technique for taking ECGs and the importance of this vital diagnostic procedure.

After you have practiced the procedures and are ready to demonstrate your skills and knowledge attained, arrange with your instructor to take a performance test.

Review Questions

1. Mr. Perry Bloom is having an ECG done and wants to know if the record will pick up his heart sounds and what each of the little squares on the electrocardiograph paper mean. State and explain the answers that you would give to this patient.
2. The physician expects you to monitor the recording of Mr. Bloom's ECG. List three items that you will look for.
3. During the recording of Max Sugar's ECG, he continually coughs and moves his hand to cover his mouth. What type of artifact would you expect to see on the record?
4. Explain to Ms. Maurine McArthur how and why the physician in your office can read her ECG taken on another machine by a different physician in another city.
5. Mrs. D. Bernstrom wants to know why you have to put that "gooey paste" on her body when you are applying the electrodes. State your reply to this patient.
6. Mrs. Sara Pace wants to know how you can tell if your electrocardiograph is working properly and what all those "funny little" waves on the electrocardiograph paper mean. What would you tell her?
7. State what the following items on the electrocardiograph are used for:
   a. The STD button
   b. The position control knob
   c. The lead selector knob
   d. The recorder switch
8. Illustrate identification codes for each of the 12 leads on a standard ECG.

SUGGESTED READINGS

Conover MB: Understanding electrocardiography: physiological and interpretive concepts, ed 3, St Louis, 1980, The CV Mosby Co.

Hammond C: ECG's made easier than ever—when the natural pacemakers fail, RN 11:30, Nov 1979.

Phibbs B: The cardiac arrhythmias, ed 3, St Louis, 1978, The CV Mosby Co.

Chapter 29

Physical Therapy

- Ultraviolet light
- Diathermy
- Ultrasound
- Local applications of heat (thermotherapy) and cold (cryotherapy)
- Electrotherapy using galvanic and faradic currents
- Electrodiagnostic examinations

Objectives

On completion of Chapter 29 the medical assistant should be able to*:

1 Define and pronounce the terms listed in the vocabulary.

2 Differentiate between physical medicine and physical therapy; a physiatrist and a physical therapist.

3 List six modalities and/or techniques employed for treatments in physical therapy, indicating the nature and purpose or use of each.

4 Describe the differences between ultraviolet radiation, diathermy, ultrasound, and local applications of heat and cold.

5 State the physiological reactions that occur with applications of heat and with applications of cold.

6 List examples of dry and moist applications of heat and cold, and apply these to a patient using safety precautions to avoid injury to the patient or the medical assistant.

7 Differentiate between electrotherapy and electrodiagnostic techniques, explaining the nature and purpose of each.

8 Identify the medical assistant's responsibilities relevant to physical therapy procedures.

9 Demonstrate proficiency in communicating proper preparation of the patient for physical therapy treatments.

10 Design his or her own step-by-step procedures for each procedure discussed in this chapter.

*It is suggested that the student review "Diagnostic and Therapeutic Procedures," p. 486, before proceeding with this chapter.

Vocabulary

arthritis (ar-thrī'tis) Inflammation of a joint.

bursitis bur-sī'tis) Inflammation of a bursa. The most commonly affected is the bursa of the shoulder.

conduction (kon-duk'shun) The passage or conveyance of energy, as of electricity, heat or sound.

debridement (da-brēd-ment') The process of removing foreign material and devitalized tissue.

hypothermia (hī˝pō-ther'mē-ah) Low body temperature.

modality (mō-dal'ĭ-tē) Therapeutic agents used in physical medicine and physical therapy.

light therapy or **phototherapy (fō'tō--ther'ah-pē)** The use of light rays in the treatment of disease processes. By custom, this includes the use of ultraviolet and infrared or heat rays (radiation).

psoriasis (so-rī'ah-sis) A chronic inflammatory recurrent skin disease characterized by scaly red patches on the body surfaces. The lesions are seen most commonly on knees, elbows, scalp, and fingernails. Other areas frequently affected are the chest, abdomen, palms of the hands, soles of the feet, and backs of the arms and legs. The cause is unknown, although a hereditary factor is suggested.

sprain (sprān) A joint injury in which some fibers of a supporting ligament are ruptured but continuity of the ligament remains intact. There may also be damage to the associated muscles, tendons, nerves, and blood vessels.

strain (strān) An overexertion or overstretching of some part of a muscle.

tendinitis (ten'dĭ-nī'tĭs) Inflammation of a tendon; one of the most common causes of acute pain in the shoulder.

Physical medicine or physiatrics (fiz'ē-ah'triks) is the medical discipline that uses physical and mechanical agents in the diagnosis, treatment, and prevention of disease processes and bodily ailments. The therapeutic use of these agents in conjunction with patient education and rehabilitation programs (rather than by medicinal or surgical means) is called physical therapy (PT). Physicians who specialize in this field are physiatrists (fiz˝ē-ah'trist). Specially trained licensed individuals skilled in the techniques of physical therapy (physiotherapy) and qualified to administer treatments and tests prescribed by a physician are physical therapists (physiotherapists).

A great variety of modalities and techniques using the properties of heat, cold, electricity, water, light, mechanical manuevers, and exercise are used in physical therapy. The *purpose* and *aim* of physical therapy is to relieve pain, increase circulation, restore and improve muscular function, build strength, and increase the range of motion or mobility of a joint. Aside from treating patients with neuromuscular conditions, physical therapy is involved with a significant number of physical conditioning programs, particularly for patients with cardiac and pulmonary conditions. Chest therapy is also given to patients with pulmonary conditions to help clear secretions and keep the air passageways open and clear. Patient education is a major area in physical therapy—that is, physical therapists teach and train patients how to perform essential activities that they can do themselves for their condition and how to avoid recurrences of certain problems.

Generally speaking, physical therapy treatments are given by physical therapists or the physician; therefore the duties of the medical assistant may be limited. However, the medical assistant in the physician's office is often required to administer some types of physical therapy treatments under the direction and supervision of the physician. In addition, at the physician's request, the medical assistant should be able to explain the nature and purpose of the treatment or test to the patient or provide adequate instructions to be followed by the patient at home. It is too often assumed that patients who are to use heat or cold applications at home know how to do so without assistance. The medical assistant will wish to ensure that these patients understand the dangers of using heat or cold to excess and the importance of using the correct solution at the proper temperature.

Some acquaintance with the various modalities used in physical therapy is therefore a requirement for the well-trained medical assistant. The following pages are devoted to briefing the medical assistant on various physical therapy modalities and techniques employed and their uses and purposes. Additional materials that may be studied or demonstrations for using the equipment are provided by the manufacturers of the modalities.

For any of the subsequent treatments that may fall within the scope of the medical assistant's duties on the job, the basic steps as stated in previous chapters for all procedures must be implemented. The medical assistant should now be able to organize the information that will be presented on various treatments into the following briefly stated procedural steps. These steps can also be used as a guideline for a performance test checklist.

1. Check the physician's order.
2. Wash your hands.
3. Assemble the equipment and supplies needed.
4. Identify the patient and explain the nature and purpose of the treatment.
5. Prepare the patient: position correctly and comfortably and drape as necessary.
6. Prepare supplies for use.
7. Proceed with the treatment and time it accurately.
8. Observe the area to which the treatment has been applied frequently for desired or adverse reactions.
9. Remove the application used for the treatment.
10. Attend to the patient's safety and comfort; provide further instructions as indicated.
11. Properly care for the used equipment and supplies.
12. Wash your hands.
13. Record the treatment and the results obtained.
    Charting example:
    September 9, 19_____, 9 AM
    Hot moist compress applied to a wound on the inner aspect of the right forearm at 110° F for 1 hour. On completion of the treatment, the skin appeared pink, and the wound appeared clean; no evidence of suppuration present. Dry dressing was applied. Patient stated that most of the pain was relieved and that the compress provided much comfort.

Kim Worth, CMA

ULTRAVIOLET LIGHT

Ultraviolet rays are rays beyond the violet end of the visible spectrum. They are produced by the sun and by sun lamps. Although ultraviolet rays produce very little heat, they can cause tanning on the skin or a sunburn (redness, erythema) and are capable of killing bacteria and other microorganisms and activating the formation of vitamin D.

Ultraviolet rays (light) are used therapeutically in the treatment of acne, psoriasis, pressure sores, and wound infections. The purposes of this treatment are to stimulate growing epithelial cells and cause capillary hyperemia and to increase cellular metabolism and vascular engorgement, which increases the skin's defenses against bacterial infections.

Various forms of apparatus provide ultraviolet rays. Before receiving ultraviolet treatment, the patient's sensitivity must be determined. This is done by exposing different areas of the patient's skin to different dosages of the rays for different time periods. The following day the patient returns so that the response can be determined. A little redness on the skin area is wanted, but not a real burn. For example, if 20 seconds of exposure gives the maximum coloration to the skin that is wanted without giving any more, the treatment is started with a 20-second exposure period to the ultraviolet light; then, depending on the light used, the exposure time is usually increased by 10-second intervals. The number of treatments to be given depends on how well the patient is responding.

When this treatment is given, the light must be placed at least 30 inches away from the patient and directed *only* on the area(s) to be treated.

Timing of the exposure period *must be exact*, as excessive exposure can cause severe sunburn up to second- and third-degree burns. Dark goggles should be worn by both the patient and the operator of the light to protect their eyes.

The patient *must never* be left unattended while being exposed to this light. If you are timing the exposure period and for some reason have to leave the room, you must disconnect the light and resume the treatment when you return. Some lights will turn off automatically, but it is still important for the operator to be present in the room when the patient is receiving this treatment to ensure that burns do not result.

DIATHERMY

Diathermy is a heat-inducing wavelength that is part of the electromagnetic spectrum. It is the therapeutic use of a high frequency current, the purpose being to generate heat within a part of the body. Diathermy works by inducing an electrical field, a conduction field in the tissues, and thereby heating the tissues and increasing the circulation.

Diathermy is used in the treatment of muscular problems and sometimes for the treatment of arthritis, bursitis and tendinitis.

The term *diathermy* is also applied to the many different machines available for this purpose.

Depending on the machine used, the applicator is generally placed at least 1 inch away from the patient's skin. The heating element of some machines has a spacer built into it—that is, there is a space between the outside cover on the unit and the actual heating element. With these machines the element is placed directly against the skin, because it is the outside cover of the unit and not the actual heating element that is in contact with the skin. The built-in spacer of these machines provides the required distance between the skin and the heating element.

Other machines have pads on the applicators. When these machines are used, towels (1-inch thickness) are placed between the pad and the patient's skin.

When giving diathermy treatments, you must watch for desensitized skin areas, because patients have to be able to feel the heat; otherwise they can get burned without realizing that they are getting burned. Areas of skin breakdown and other reactive areas such as inflamed areas must be avoided.

The electrical field of diathermy is attracted by metal. Therefore patients who have metal implants, such as joint implants, cannot receive diathermy treatments. Also patients cannot be wearing jewelry or other metal objects such as buckles and hairpins, and cannot be positioned on a metal table or chair, but must be on wooden furniture. If these practices are not followed, the patient may receive severe burns, because metal will become hot once the diathermy unit is turned on. Duration of the treatment is usually 15 to 20 minutes and should be timed carefully. It must be explained to the patient that a warm comfortable feeling should be experienced, and if it becomes uncomfortable, to inform the operator of the unit. If the patient complains that the treatment is becoming too hot, it must be stopped to avoid burning the patient. To operate any of the diathermy units available, you must carefully follow the instructions for use supplied by the manufacturers of each unit. Currently, diathermy is no longer used very much in many facilities. It has been replaced by ultrasound.

ULTRASOUND

Ultrasound is also part of the electromagnetic spectrum. Therapeutic ultrasound is a very specific part of the sound spectrum that provides acoustic vibration with frequencies beyond human ear perception. This form of treatment uses high frequency sound waves to penetrate deep tissue layers. (Ultrasound is also used for diagnostic purposes. Review p. 567 in Chapter 27.)

Ultrasound vibrates a molecular level. The two effects obtained from ultrasound are a mechanical effect and a heating effect. The mechanical effect, the vibration that causes the heating, is most noticeable on connective tissues, such as tendons and ligaments. A heating effect is produced on almost all tissues with the exception of bone, because ultrasound is reflected from bone.

Ultrasound is of value for the treatment of pain syndromes, to relax muscle spasm, and to provide deep penetration of heat and stimulate circulation in small areas, as when used to increase blood supply to tissues in patients with vascular disorders. It is also used in breaking up calcium deposits and in loosening scars.

Ultrasound is applied by means of an applicator with a sound head, approximately 2 inches in diameter, that extends off from the special machine. Since ultrasound is not conducted through the air, a conducting medium must be spread on the patient's skin over the area to be treated. Special gels are available for this; mineral oil can also be used, but it is not as effective. After the gel is applied to the skin, the operator of the machine holds the sound head and moves it in a steady up-and-down and rotary motion over the skin. The applicator must be in motion when used to prevent internal burns or tissue damage. Special care must also be taken when the treatment is used on patients with implants, such as joint implants, as ultrasound will tend to vibrate and loosen the implant. Also heat will build up in the metal (Figure 29.1).

Ultrasound can also be applied underwater for treatment of the hands and feet. The water then acts as the conducting medium for the ultrasound. The length of any treatment will depend on the size of the area being treated, but is usually under 10 minutes. For example: ultrasound treatment to the lower back is applied for 6 to 7 minutes on one side. The minimal number of ultrasound treatments to be given to be effective varies from 5 to 12.

After use, the sound head should be cleansed with alcohol. Instructions for use of the ultrasound machines are supplied by the manufacturers and must be followed very carefully.

LOCAL APPLICATIONS OF HEAT (THERMOTHERAPY) AND COLD (CRYOTHERAPY)

Dry and moist applications of heat and cold have been employed universally as an effective means of treatment by individuals in the home and by physicians, nurses, medical assistants, and physical ther-

Figure 29.1
Ultrasound equipment being used on a patient's leg in physical therapy. A special agent, such as a gel, is first applied to the clean, dry skin of the area to be treated to aid in the conduction of ultrasonic energy. Note proximal electrode pad, which is used to give electrical stimulation to relieve muscle spasm.

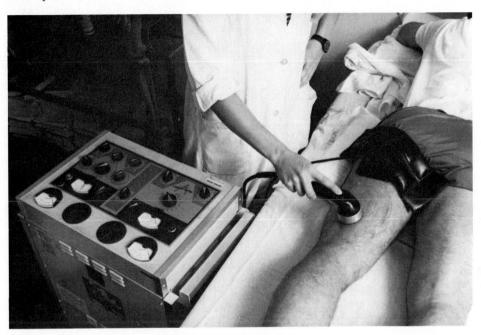

Table 29.1
Physiological reactions produced by heat and cold applications

Body function	Heat	Cold
Blood vessels in area	Dilated (increasing circulation)	Constricted (decreasing circulation)
Heat production	Decreased	Increased (by shivering)
Blood pressure	Lowered	Elevated
Respiratory rate	Increased	Increased
Tissue metabolism	Increased	Decreased

apists, either in an office or hospital setting. Tolerance for the temperature changes that occur when heat or cold is applied to the body varies with the individual and also varies in different parts of the body. Generally, the more sensitive skin areas to these changes are those that are not usually exposed; the less sensitive areas are those that are exposed, usually having thicker and tougher layers of skin, such as areas on the soles of the feet or the palms of the hands.

Once heat or cold is applied to the skin, certain physiological reactions occur in the body. Heat has the opposite effect to that of cold, except for respiratory rate changes (Table 29.1).

Heat or cold modalities are to be placed on a bare body surface for only *short durations*. An important fact to remember is that the prolonged use of heat (more than 1 hour) produces reverse secondary effects; that is, blood vessels will then constrict, thus decreasing blood supply to the area. The prolonged use of cold (more than 1 hour) also has a reverse secondary effect; that is, blood vessels will dilate, thus increasing circulation and tissue metabolism, in other words, the immediate effect of heat applications is vasodilation; whereas the prolonged effect is vasoconstriction. Likewise, the immediate effect of cold applications is vasconstriction; whereas the prolonged effect is vasodilation. Therefore heat applications should not be left in place for long periods of time. Cold applications can be used for longer periods than heat, depending on the desired effects. The physician will usually indicate the temperature (that is, warm or hot, tepid, cool, cold, or very cold) and the time period to be used for the following applications of dry and moist hot and cold applications.

Principles for Preparation and Patient Care

Because applications of heat and cold are common treatments, the medical assistant should keep in mind the following principles regarding preparation and patient care:

1. Learn exactly where and for how long the application is to be placed on the patient's body.
2. Position the patient comfortably so that the treatment can be maintained for the designated period.
3. Avoid accidents—be sure that the patient is positioned safely and will not fall. Place solutions in a convenient location and so that they will not spill.
4. Test the solution (with a bath thermometer) or the device you are using to be sure that it is at the exact temperature that the physician ordered or the recommended temperature for the method used.
5. Remove any dressings covering the area to be treated. (Review the procedure for a dressing change in Chapter 21). Apply a clean dressing, if ordered, when the treatment is completed.
6. Keep the application at the ordered temperature. Generally, compresses and packs cool off within 15 or 20 minutes and then will have to be reheated and reapplied. If the temperature of the device or the solution changes, it will not accomplish its purpose and may even harm the patient.
7. Keep the patient warm during the application of heat; drape sheets or blankets can be used to cover the patient. When blood vessels dilate (as with the application of heat), more blood comes to the surface of the body and the body is cooled by the surrounding air. Thus the patient can easily become chilled unless protected with coverings.
8. Check the patient's skin frequently during the application to observe for any skin changes, as well as any signs of burns or frostbite. Report any signs of burns or frostbite *immediately*.

9. Provide further instruction to the patient, as indicated, on completion of the treatment.

Thermotherapy

Superficial heat treatments can be administered with dry or moist heat applications. These local heat applications are used to relieve pain, to promote muscle relaxation and reduce spasm, to increase circulation to an area to relieve congestion and swelling by dilating the blood vessels, and to speed up the inflammatory process to promote suppuration (pus formation) and drainage from an infected area. In addition, dry heat applications are used to dry and heal surgical incisions and sutures, perineal lacerations, and skin ulcers.

Dry heat

Dry heat applications commonly used include the following:

- Infrared radiation (heat lamps);
- Electric light bulbs;
- Electric heating pads; and
- Hot water bottles.

Infrared radiation is dry heat application by means of a heat lamp. The term *infrared* usually refers to the heat lamp. Infrared rays from these lamps provide surface heat and penetrate the skin to a depth of about 5 to 10 mm. At times, a plain gooseneck lamp is used, because the *incandescent light bulb* is a source of infrared rays. Heat lamps must be kept at least 2 to 4 feet away from the skin, varying with the type and intensity of the lamp used. The skin must be clean and free of any ointment or medicinal substances. The duration of the treatment is *usually 15 to 20 minutes,* because prolonged or intense application can lead to burning and blistering of the skin.

Electric heating pads are to be placed in a protective covering, such as a towel or pillow case, and then applied to a dry area (Figure 29.2). They must never be used over moist or wet areas or dressings where moisture could come in contact with the electricity. Patients must be instructed not to lie on the pad, because burns could result. The heat selector switch is usually set on low or medium setting and left for an accurately timed period. (The amount of heat and period of time to be applied are to be designated by the physician).

A *hot water bottle* is to be filled only about half full and have the air expelled before it is sealed. This allows the hot water bottle to be lighter and more pliable so that it can be molded to the area where it is to be applied. It is essential to test the temperature of the water accurately with a ther-

Figure 29.2
Place an electric heating pad in a protective cover before applying to skin area that is dry.

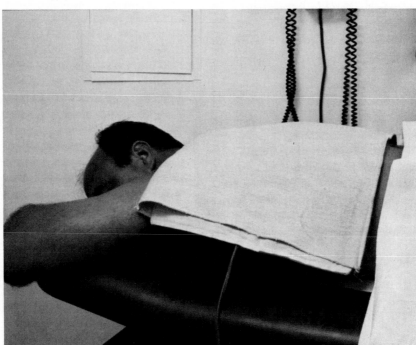

mometer before it is poured into the hot water bottle. Water not exceeding 125° F (32° C) is to be used. The accepted temperature ranges are from 115° to 125° F (46° to 52° C) for patients 2 years and older, and from 105° to 115° F (41° to 46° C) for children under 2 years and elderly patients. (The very young and the very old tend to be more sensitive to applications of heat and to cold.) Hot tap water is placed into a pitcher so that the temperature can be tested with a bath thermometer. The outside of the hot water bottle must be dry and then placed into a protective covering, such as a pillow-case or towel, before it is applied to the patient. This protective covering should remain dry unless the hot water bottle is placed over moist dressings to keep them warm (Figure 29.3).

The patient should experience a feeling of warmth but not be uncomfortable; burns must be avoided. When the hot water bottle is left on for any length of time, it will need to be refilled with hot water so that the desired temperature is maintained. After use, the hot water bottle must be washed thoroughly with warm water and detergent, rinsed, and allowed to dry before being stored. The bottle should be stored with the stopper in place and air inside to prevent the sides from sticking.

Moist heat applications

Moist heat applications commonly used include the following:

- Hot soaks;
- Hot compresses; and
- Hot packs.

For a *hot soak*, the body part to be treated is immersed gradually (to allow the patient to become accustomed to the heat change) in tap water or a medicated solution of 105° to 110° F (41° to 44° C). *Unless otherwise ordered, the body part is kept immersed for 15 to 20 minutes.* This form of treatment can be used for heat applications to the hands, arms, feet, or legs. The process of having the body from the neck down immersed in water in a special tank called the Hubbard tank or the body or a limb immersed in a whirlpool tank, is more commonly referred to as *hydrotherapy*. Soaks applied to open wounds require the use of sterile (aseptic) technique, a sterile container, and a sterile solution. The water or solution temperature should be maintained as much as possible throughout the

Figure 29.3
A, Testing temperature of hot water before placing it into hot water bottle. **B,** Expel air from half-filled hot water bottle before using. **C,** Cover the hot water bottle before applying to the patient.

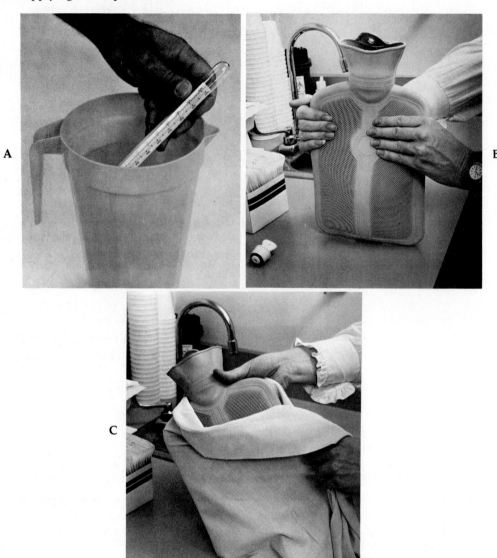

treatment. This can be accomplished by removing some of the solution every 5 minutes or so and adding more hot solution. Care to avoid burning the patient must be taken when the hot solution is added. The hot solution should be added to the container at the point farthest away from the patient's skin and stirred quickly into the cooler solution (Figure 29.4).

The patient should be positioned comfortably to prevent strain or pressure on the area treated and to prevent fatigue. The patient's skin is to be ob-

served during the treatment for excessive redness, at which time the limb is to be removed until the solution has cooled. Remember that the observations made during the treatment must be recorded on the patient's record. On completion of the treatment, the limb should be dried with a towel by patting, *not* rubbing. For an open wound, only the surrounding area should be patted dry. The towel used should not touch the open wound. Observation of the area is necessary after the treatment, because this information is to be recorded on the pa-

Figure 29.4
During a hot soak, add more hot solution to container at point farthest away
from patient's skin and stir quickly into cooler solution.

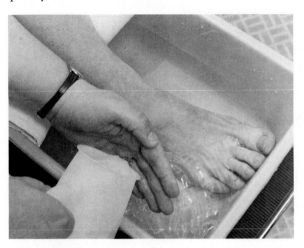

tient's record. Soaks *differ* from compresses and packs in that soaks are used for shorter periods of time and usually at lower temperatures.

There are two basic differences between hot moist compresses and packs: (1) different materials are used for each, and (2) a pack is usually applied to a more extensive body area than a compress is.

A *compress* used for the application of moist heat is prepared by taking a soft square of gauze or similar absorbent material (a clean washcloth can also be used), soaking it in hot water, then wringing it out manually or with the use of forceps to avoid excessive wetness. This material is then applied to a limited body area, such as the finger or a small area on the arm, for a designated period of time (Figure 29.5). (*Dry compresses* are used to apply pressure or medications to specific restricted areas.)

A *pack* used for the application of moist heat is prepared in the same manner as a compress except that flannel or similar materials are used. Commercially prepared hot packs filled with a silica gel (for example, Hydrocollator* packs) are also used (Figure 29.6). Packs are usually applied to a more extensive body area.

Both compresses and packs are to be applied to the skin area slowly so that the patient can gradually adjust to the heat. The recommended water temperature for soaking gauze, flannel, or similar

*Chattanooga Corp., Chattanooga, Tenn.

materials is 105° to 110° F (41° to 44° C). Commercially prepared packs are kept in a hot water bath at 140° to 160° F (60° to 71° C) until used and then wrapped in towels before being applied to the patient's skin. Both compresses and packs should be as hot as the patient can comfortably tolerate. A plastic covering can be placed over or wrapped around the compress or pack to concentrate and hold the heat over the area treated for as long a time as possible.

During these treatments, the patient's skin should be checked frequently to ensure that it is not burning and to observe for signs of increased redness or swelling. All observations must be recorded on completion of the treatment. If the patient experiences pain or is uncomfortable, the plastic covering should be removed or unwrapped to release some of the confined heat. If the area remains painful, the pack or compress is to be removed and cooled some before being reapplied. This is done to prevent burning the skin.

Additional compresses or packs should be made ready for use when the applied one cools. The length of these treatments will vary according to the physician's order. *Generally they will be prescribed for 15 to 20 minutes,* but at times may be applied for 1 hour. On completion of the treatment, the compress or pack is removed and the skin patted dry. When these treatments have been applied to an open wound, *only* the surrounding area is to be patted dry. The open wound is *not* to be touched. A clean sterile dressing is applied to an

Figure 29.5
A, Wring out hot compress to avoid excessive wetness before it is applied. **B,** Applying hot compress to body area.

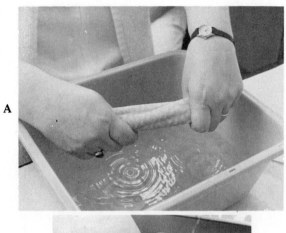

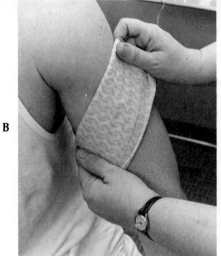

Figure 29.6
Commercially prepared hot pack.

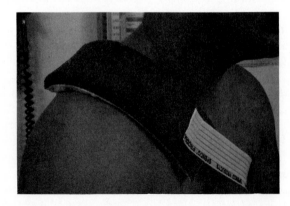

open wound when ordered by the physician. Used equipment and supplies are to be cared for properly. The treatment and all observations are to be recorded on the patient's record.

Cryotherapy

Cryotherapy, the therapeutic use of cold, is applied with dry or moist cold applications. Cold applications are used to do the following:

- Prevent edema or swelling;
- Relieve pain or tenderness (cold produces a topical anesthetic effect);
- Reduce inflammation and pus formation (cold inhibits microbial activity in the early stages of the infectious process);
- Control bleeding (the peripheral vessels constrict with the application of cold, thus resulting in a decreased blood flow); or
- Reduce body temperature.

Cold is commonly used following strains, sprains, bruises, and for muscle spasm and tenderness. Any type of acute injury responds fairly well to cold applications. During the acute phase of an injury, in which there may be bleeding in the area, do not use heat. The old rule of thumb for treating such injuries was to apply cold applications for the first 24 hours, then apply heat applications. Currently, many health care practitioners commonly wait longer than 24 hours before using heat applications on patients, and often use cold applications continually when good results are being obtained.

The physician should indicate the temperature to be used for cold applications. The temperatures of the water are described as follows:

- Tepid: 80° to 93° F (26.7° to 33.9° C);
- Cool: 65° to 80° F (18.3° to 26.7° C);
- Cold: 55° to 65° F (12.3° to 18.3° C); and
- Very cold: Below 55° F (below 12.5° C).

The selection of the temperature to use will depend on the following:

- Condition of the patient;
- Sensitivity of the patient's skin;
- Area to be covered; and
- Method to be used.

The duration of the application depends on the temperature; for example, an ice massage will be given for a shorter time period (5 minutes) than a cold compress or pack (20 to 30 minutes). Colder temperatures can be tolerated best on small areas for short periods of time. It is usually considered dangerous to keep skin temperatures below 40° F (4.4° C) for long periods except when ice is used for anesthesia.

Dry cold

Dry cold applications commonly used include the following:

- Ice bags; and
- Ice collars.

An *ice bag* is filled one half to two thirds full with *small* pieces of ice; air is expelled from the bag by twisting the top and then capped (Figure 29.7). At this time the bag should be checked for leaks. Small ice pieces reduce the amount of air spaces in the bag, which results in better conduction of cold and also allows the bag to mold better to the contour of the body part. Once sealed, the ice bag is dried and placed in a protective covering, which provides comfort for the patient and absorbs moisture that condenses on the outside. To be effective, the ice bag is placed on the skin for 30 to 60 minutes, as designated by the physician. If the treatment is to be continuous, the ice bag is applied for 30 to 60 minutes and then removed for 1 hour. By doing the procedure in this manner, the tissues are allowed to react to the immediate effects of the cold.

The patient's skin must be checked periodically for signs of decreased swelling or redness. Signs of excessive coldness, which include mottled and pale skin and excessive numbness in the body part, must be noted when present. When or if this occurs, the ice bag must be removed and the physician notified.

Ice collars are rubber or plastic devices that are smaller than ice bags and look like a medium-sized rectangle. They are used on the neck or on small areas or wrapped around a body part (Figure 29.8).

Moist cold

Moist cold applications commonly used include the following:

- Cold compresses;
- Cold packs; and
- Ice massage.

Moist cold compresses are generally applied to small areas, and *cold packs* are used on larger body areas, as are hot applications. Compresses may be used for treating a headache, a tooth extraction, or an eye injury. The area to which the compress is to be applied will determine the type of material used. For example, a clean washcloth can be used on the head or face; surgical gauze dressings with a small amount of cotton filling can be used for eye compresses. The material used for the compress is immersed in a clean basin containing

Figure 29.7
Expel air from ice bag by twisting the top and then replacing cap.

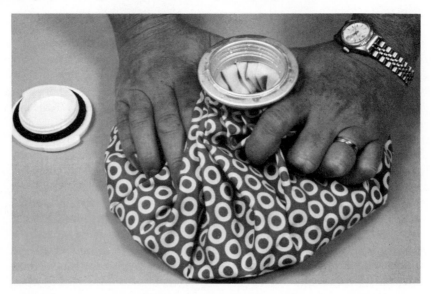

Figure 29.8
Ice collar applied to patient's neck.

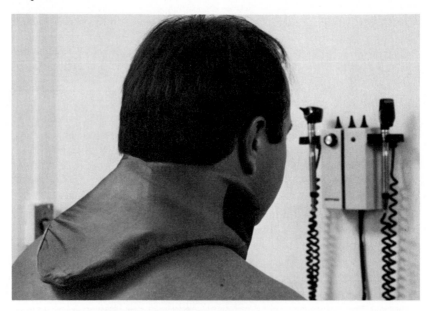

ice chips or small pieces of ice and a small amount of cold water. To avoid dripping, the material is wrung out manually or with the use of forceps and then placed on the skin for the time period designated by the physician *(usually 20 to 30 minutes and then repeated every 2 hours)*. Compresses should be changed frequently to maintain a cold application. Most patients will tell you when the compress no longer feels cold. Placing an ice bag over the compress helps keep the compress cold and reduces the number of times that it must be changed. The patient must be checked periodically during this treatment for any changes, such as a decrease or increase in swelling or redness on the area or a decrease or increase of pain. On completion of the treatment, the skin should be patted dry if necessary. The treatment and observations made are to be recorded on the patient's record.

Cold packs (ice packs) may be applied to a small area, but are generally used on larger areas, such as an arm or leg. At times they can be applied to the whole body to lower the temperature. In this case, hypothermia pads or blankets may be used, rather than ice packs. These are used in hospitals with the patient under close observation for temperature and skin changes. Manufacturers of hypothermia units provide complete instructions for use, which must be followed precisely.

To apply a cold or ice pack, first wrap the extremity in wet toweling and then pack ice chips around it; place an additional towel over the ice to reduce the melting rate. Generally, these are applied for 20 to 30 minutes. Commercial cold packs are also available. These are kept in a freezer until used. They do not freeze stiff, thus are pliable and can be molded to fit the contour of the body part.

Ice massage is simply massaging the area with ice. This can be as simple as freezing water in a paper cup and then rubbing it over the affected area for approximately 5 minutes (Figure 29.9).

ELECTROTHERAPY USING GALVANIC AND FARADIC CURRENTS

Galvanic current is a steady direct current (DC); faradic current is alternating current (AC) produced by induction. Both are currents of low voltage that are used for many therapeutic purposes. The basic use for galvanic and faradic currents is for muscle stimulation, used to retrain patients who have had nerve injuries. For example, as the injured nerve regenerates, the body may have forgotten how to contract a muscle, so commonly these treatments are given to somewhat remind them and get them functioning once again.

Galvanic stimulation (or faradic if it works) can be used just to maintain the contractility of the muscle while waiting for the nerve to regenerate. Once the nerve is cut or degenerates, or if the nerve itself does not conduct stimuli, galvanic current (direct current) is the only thing that can be used. Direct current will work directly on muscle tissue even when there is no intact nerve. Faradic current (alternating current) cannot be used, as it will not work on muscle tissue in this case. Galvanic current is also used for **iontophoresis** (ī-on″to-fo-rē′sis). Iontophoresis or ionotherapy is the introduction of ions

Figure 29.9
Ice massage is one form of cryotherapy that can be used to decrease pain. Freeze water in paper cup and then rub it over affected area.

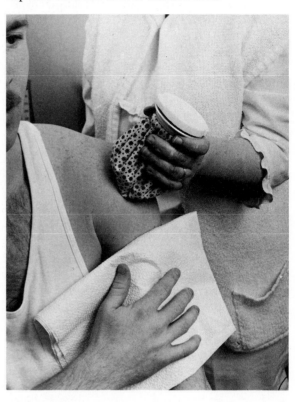

into the body through the skin by means of an electric current for therapeutic purposes.

Faradic current is used mainly for the stimulation of weak muscles that have a normal nerve supply. This current causes contractions, which in turn increase blood supply to the muscle and thus help the muscle gain strength.

These treatments can be applied in various ways. To stimulate muscles, the current must be interrupted. This is accomplished by a hand interrupter or an interrupter that is built into the equipment. Basically, to apply these currents, two electrodes padded with cotton that has been soaked in salt water are placed over the area to be treated. The soaked pads prevent the occurrence of severe wounds. When small muscles are worked on, a very small applicator can be used. This has a push button on it so that specific jolts of current can be given. This apparatus can also be used when using what is called a surged current or a ramped current. These are currents that start out with nothing, then begin and increase up to a designated point, and then decrease. With these a smooth contraction and then a smooth relaxation is obtained. In addition to muscle stimulation, these currents can also be used on muscle spasms and on areas around hematomas, bruises, and so on. Electrostimulation therapy is also used with biofeedback for muscle reeducation. The biofeedback machine allows the patient to hear the muscle contract and relax. This is especially helpful postoperatively and for controlling chronic pain.

ELECTRODIAGNOSTIC EXAMINATIONS

Electrodiagnostic examinations used by physical therapists and physiatrists are performed by means of electrical stimulation applied to muscles and nerves. Various types of examinations are available, all having clinical value in the diagnosis and prognosis of some neuromuscular disorders. Two additional major electrodiagnostic examinations used for different clinical purposes are the electroencephalogram (EEG), which records the electrical impulses of the brain, and the electrocardiogram (ECG), which records the electrical action of the heart. The ECG is discussed in Chapter 28.

Electromyographic examinations measure very specifically the electrical activity in a muscle as a result of nerve conduction. A needle electrode is introduced into a muscle belly to study muscle action potentials. It will also measure just the general electrical excitability of the muscle cells. The recording obtained (the electromyogram) can be very specific diagnostically, because it not only tells you that something is wrong but points out exactly what is wrong. It helps distinguish any weakness from neuropathy from that of other causes.

Other examinations available test the reaction time of a muscle to a shot of electricity; the threshold is tested, that is, how much electricity it takes to get a reaction from the muscle. The results obtained are compared with normal levels. Any deviation or fluctuation from the established norm helps diagnose certain problems, such as damaged nerve and muscle tissues.

Nerve conduction studies are performed to test the speed with which the nerve is conducting; again, this helps the physician diagnose.

Special electrodiagnostic equipment is used for each of these tests, which are generally performed by a physical therapist or a physician. The medical assistant will not operate this equipment but may be expected to keep it clean and ready for use. The medical assistant may also be expected to explain the nature and purpose of the examination to the patient.

Conclusion

You have now completed the chapter on physical therapy. After you have practiced the procedures and are ready to demonstrate your skills and knowledge attained, arrange with your instructor to take a performance test.

There are various types of patient conditions and disabilities that benefit from physical therapy.

Numerous other procedures, tests, and modalities are used in a physical therapy department. It is not within the scope of this book to discuss all of them in detail. A clinical experience or a field trip to a physical therapy facility would be most valuable to you; here you could see firsthand the use of the various modalities and techniques.

Review Questions

1. Define and state the purposes and time duration of application for each of the following:
   a. Ultraviolet light treatments
   b. Diathermy treatments
   c. Ultrasound treatments
   d. Applications of moist and dry heat
   e. Application of moist and dry cold
2. How full should a hot water bottle be filled when applied to a patient? Why?
3. State the temperature of the water you would use when applying a hot water bottle to a 70-year-old man and to a 2-year-old child.
4. Outline the instructions that you would give to a patient who is to soak her foot in hot water four times a day at home.

5. Why should the patient's skin be checked frequently during any form of hot or cold application?
6. List five situations in which cold applications may be used for treatment.
7. List five situations in which hot applications may be used for treatment.
8. State two types of electrodiagnostic examinations and explain each briefly.

SUGGESTED READINGS

Ciuca R, Bradish J, and Trombly S: Passive range-of-motion exercises: a handbook, Pt 1, Nursing 78 8:59, July 1978.

Krusen FH: Handbook of physical medicine and rehabilitation, ed 2, Philadelphia, 1971, WB Saunders Co.

Yates DA: The electrodiagnosis of muscle disorders, Proc R Soc Med 65:617, July 1972.

Chapter 30

Common Emergencies and First Aid

- Cardiopulmonary resuscitation in basic life support for cardiac arrest
- Heart attack—signals and actions for survival
- Cardiopulmonary resuscitation (CPR)
- Choking
- Emergency management of the obstructed airway
- Emergency Medical Services System (EMSS)
- Shock
- Abdominal pain
- Allergic reaction to drugs
- Asphyxia
- Severe bleeding (hemorrhage)
- Burns
- Cerebral vascular accident
- Chest pain
- Convulsions
- Epistaxis (nosebleed)
- Fainting (syncope)
- Foreign bodies in the ear, eye, and nose
- Head injuries
- Hyperventilation
- Insulin reactions and diabetic coma
- Open wounds
- Poisoning
- Poison Control Centers
- First aid kit

Objectives

On completion of Chapter 30 the medical assistant student should be able to:

1   Define *first aid* and the related terminology presented in this chapter.

2   State what factors constitute a medical emergency.

3   List four fundamental rules and general procedures to follow in a medical emergency.

4   List six common warning signals of a heart attack.

5   List five types of shock, the usual causes of each, and at least 10 signs and symptoms.

6   Differentiate between arterial, venous, and capillary bleeding.

7   List and demonstrate four methods used to control severe bleeding.

8   Differentiate between a first, second, and third degree burn.

9   Explain what is meant by the *rule of nine* in reference to burns.

10   Differentiate between insulin reaction and diabetic coma by stating the signs, symptoms, and causes of each.

11   List at least 15 items that should be included in a first aid kit.

12 Discuss the 911 emergency telephone system.

13 State the purpose of a poison control center.

14 Define and list eight signs and symptoms of a cerebral vascular accident (CVA).

15 Demonstrate and describe the proper first aid care to be used for all the medical emergencies presented in this chapter.

Vocabulary

antidote (an′tĭ-dōt) An agent used to counteract a poison.

biological death The condition that results when the brain has been deprived of oxygenated blood for a period of 6 minutes or more and irreversible damage has probably occurred.

clinical death The state that results when breathing and circulation have stopped.

concussion (kon-kush′un) The injury that results from a violent blow or shock.

concussion of the brain A violent disturbance of the brain caused by a blow or fall.

contusion (kon-too′zhun) A bruise, indicating injury to tissues without breakage in the skin. Discoloration appears because of

blood seepage under the surface of the skin.

epinephrine (ep″ĭ-nef′rin) A hormone produced by the adrenal glands. Epinephrine can be administered parenterally, topically, or by inhalation. It is used as an emergency heart stimulant, to relieve symptoms in allergic conditions, and to counteract the lethal effects of anaphylactic shock.

tourniquet (toor′nĭ-ket) A constricting device used to compress an artery or vein to stop excessive bleeding or to prevent the spread of snake venom.

Additional terms will be defined under their respective topics in this chapter.

When someone is injured or suddenly becomes ill, there is a critical period—before medical help is obtained—that is of the utmost importance to the victim. What you do, or what you do not do, in that interval can mean the difference between life and death. For serious conditions, the victim *must* receive medical attention; first aid is not meant to resolve serious problems.

First aid is defined as the immediate and temporary care given the victim of an accident or sudden illness until the services of a physician can be obtained. It is the help that *you* can provide in emergencies until trained medical emergency personnel or a physician takes over. You owe it to yourself, the patients under the care of your physician-employer, your family, and the general public to know and understand the simple procedures that can be rendered quickly and intelligently in an emergency.

First aid is more than a dressing or a cold compress. The victim suddenly has new problems and needs. Both emotional and physical needs of the victim must be cared for. Your contributions include offering well-chosen words of encouragement, a willingness to help, the uplifting effect of your evident capabilities and calmness, and the performance of temporary physical care to alleviate pain or a life-threatening situation.

It is commonly a responsibility of the medical assistant to deal with an emergency before the physician or other emergency teams arrive. The medical assistant who can exercise good judgment, remain calm, avoid panicking others, and, being familiar with the procedures for emergency care, administer care in an orderly manner, renders great service to the patient and the physician. Whether in the physician's office, at home, or on the street, *prompt action must be taken*.

Each year more than 1 million Americans die from sudden death. In many cases of sudden death, especially death from heart attacks, the victim could have been saved if the early warning signs of heart attack were known, if someone close by could have performed cardiopulmonary resuscitation, or if the victim had been transported quickly to a hospital or received first aid or medical attention at the scene of sudden illness or injury. *Time* is of essence in any medical emergency in which breathing and heartbeat have ceased. Within 4 to 6 minutes after the heart stops, brain damage begins. Thus the importance of the medical assistant knowing what to do and acting quickly in a medical emergency cannot be overemphasized. *Know what constitutes an emergency, whom to call for help, and what to do.* An emergency exists when life is threatened, when situations develop that endanger a person's physical and/or psychological well-being, or when pain and suffering occur.

When an emergency occurs in the physician's office, the medical assistant should notify the physician. If the physician is *not* in the office and is not expected momentarily, the assistant should call for a nearby physician; if none can be reached for immediate help, call the local emergency medical service system, or an ambulance, or the fire and rescue squad, or the police department. The medical assistant is not to assume the responsibility for making a diagnosis and providing medical treatment, but *is* expected to make a reasonable judgment (that may require medical knowledge) of the situation and to provide immediate first aid care.

Medical assistants should perform *only* those procedures that they have been trained to do, and when in the office or health care agency, only with the prior consent of the physician-employer. An office policy should be established between the physician and assistant as to what should be done in the case of office emergencies, and in the case of emergency telephone calls received from patients (see Chapter 10).

The fundamental rules and general procedures to follow in an emergency are few but very important.

1. Remain calm, reassure the patient, be empathetic, and do not panic. Act in an orderly, organized manner.
2. Survey the situation to determine the nature of the emergency. A primary survey includes the ABCs for all emergencies; that is, check the patient for an open *a*irway, for *b*reathing, and for *c*irculation. A secondary survey is to examine the total body to determine what is wrong.
3. Take immediate steps to remedy the situation. Your responsibilities for the type of care to provide will vary in each situation and depend on the nearness of medical help, the seriousness of the injury or illness, and the immediate environment.
4. Seek medical help if needed and be able to describe the nature of the patient's condition. Think of yourself as a reporter who must obtain concise and relevant information to act on and then report. Seek answers to questions that begin with who, what, when, where, why, and how.

Provided in this chapter is important information in concise and convenient form on common emergencies and the first aid treatment to be administered. Cardiopulmonary resuscitation (CPR) and care for choking victims and then care for patients in shock are presented first. Other common emergencies are then discussed in alphabetical order. Read and study the contents of this chapter carefully and keep this or other first aid references in a convenient place where they will be on hand for quick reference when needed.

The purpose of this chapter is to provide a review and reference source for first aid treatment to use for common emergencies. It is not intended to be used as a substitute for a certified first aid program of study. Currently it is a requirement of all accredited medical assistant programs of study for the students to complete a recognized certified first aid and CPR course. Medical assistants who completed their training and studies before this requirement was made should enroll in a certified first aid and CPR course if they have not already done so. Courses are offered by the American Red Cross and at many community colleges. Cardiopulmonary resuscitation courses for basic life support are also provided by the American Heart Association in numerous communities. All medical assistants should then take a refresher course in first aid every few years, and in CPR every year.

CARDIOPULMONARY RESUSCITATION IN BASIC LIFE SUPPORT FOR CARDIAC ARREST

Cardiopulmonary resuscitation, commonly known as CPR, is a combination of artificial respiration and artificial circulation. CPR should be started immediately by individuals properly trained to do so in emergency situations in which cardiac arrest occurs. To repeat, CPR must be performed by those properly trained in the skill. The performance of CPR is *not recommended unless one has had proper training and practice in the procedure*, because serious adverse consequences may result because of faulty technique. Therefore the following information is to serve as a review and reference source *after* you have completed a training course and before you take your next refresher course.

The *goal* of CPR is life support. When trained in CPR techniques, you must start life support techniques as quickly as possible and continue them until one of the following has occurred:

- An effective respiration and pulse are restored to the victim;
- You are completely exhausted and cannot continue CPR;

- Care of the victim is turned over to medical or other properly trained personnel; or
- The victim is pronounced dead.

Basic and Advanced Life Support

Life support is divided into two systems: basic and advanced life support. Basic life support can be carried out by trained lay and medical persons and includes the following (Figure 30.1):

Basic ABC steps

    A—airway opened

    B—breathing restored

    C—circulation restored

Supplementary techniques

    Proper positioning of the victim, that is, in the supine position

    Jaw thrust maneuver, may be required when the head tilt alone is unsuccessful for opening the airway

    Opening the mouth, at times it may be necessary to force the mouth open for ventilation or to remove foreign bodies or to allow drainage of vomitus or blood

    Mouth-to-stoma resuscitation, when the victim has had a laryngectomy, a stoma will be present in the neck through which the person breathes; in this case, mouth-to-stoma resuscitation must be performed

    Adjunctive equipment, to be used only by those trained in its use

Advanced life support is to be performed *only* by trained medical personnel and includes the following:

    Definitive therapy

        Diagnosis

        Drugs

        Defibrillation

    Cardiac monitoring and stabilization

    Transportation

    Communication

HEART ATTACK—SIGNALS AND ACTIONS FOR SURVIVAL*

There are many causes of sudden death: poisoning, drowning, suffocation, choking, electrocution, and smoke inhalation. But the most common cause is heart attack. Everyone should know the usual early signals of heart attack and have an emergency plan of action.

---

*©Reproduced with permission. American Heart Association, Inc.

The most *common signal* of a heart attack is:

- Uncomfortable pressure, squeezing, fullness or pain in the center of the chest behind the breastbone, which may spread to the shoulder, neck, jaw, or arms (the pain may not be severe)

Other signals may be:

- Sweating
- Nausea, and maybe vomiting
- Shortness of breath *or*
- A feeling of weakness
- Apprehension

Sometimes these signals subside and return.

1. *Action:*
1. Recognize the "signals"
2. Stop activity and sit or lie down
3. *Act at once if pain lasts for 2 minutes or more*—call the emergency rescue service or go to the nearest hospital emergency room with 24-hour service.

CARDIOPULMONARY RESUSCITATION (CPR)

Basic CPR is a simple procedure, as simple as A-B-C, Airway, Breathing, and Circulation. *The following brief review is based on the 1986 standards for CPR. This is to be used only for review purposes. It is not to be used for learning the procedure for performing CPR. Mouthpieces, resuscitation masks, resuscitation bags, or other ventilation devices should be available for use in clinics and physicians' offices. Use these devices on all patients instead of mouth-to-mouth resuscitation.*

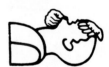

Airway. If you find a collapsed person, determine if the victim is conscious by shaking the shoulder and shouting "Are you all right?" If no response, shout for help. Then open the airway. If the victim is not lying flat on the back, roll the victim over, moving the entire body at one time as a total unit.

To open the victim's airway use the head-tilt/chin-lift maneuver. Lift up the chin gently with one hand while pushing down on the forehead with the other to tilt head back. Once the airway is open, place your ear close to the victim's mouth:

- Look at the chest and stomach for movement,
- Listen for sounds of breathing, and
- Feel for breath on your cheek.

Figure 30.1
CPR in basic life support. **B,** First aid for choking.
Reproduced with permission, American Heart Association.

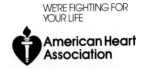

WE'RE FIGHTING FOR
YOUR LIFE

Cardiopulmonary Resuscitation (CPR)

Place victim flat on his/her back on a hard surface.

1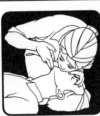

If unconscious, open airway.

Head-tilt/chin-lift.

2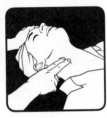

A

If not breathing, begin rescue breathing.

Give 2 full breaths. If airway is blocked,
reposition head and try again to give breaths.
If still blocked,
perform abdominal thrusts (Heimlich maneuver).

3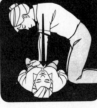

Check carotid pulse.

4

If there is no pulse, begin chest compressions.

Depress sternum 1½ to 2 inches.
Perform 15 compressions (rate: 80–100 per minute)
to every 2 full breaths.

Continue uninterrupted until advanced life support is available.

©1986, American Heart Association
77-0153 (CP)

Figure 30.1, cont'd

FIRST AID FOR CHOKING

CALL-FOR-HELP NUMBER:

_____

WE'RE FIGHTING FOR YOUR LIFE

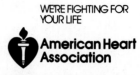 American Heart Association

CONSCIOUS VICTIM

1 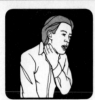 Ask the victim: "Are you choking?"
If the victim can speak, cough, or breathe, do not interfere.

2 If the victim cannot speak, cough, or breathe,
apply subdiaphragmatic abdominal thrusts (the Heimlich maneuver)
until the foreign body is expelled or the victim becomes unconscious.

B ## IF VICTIM BECOMES UNCONSCIOUS

1 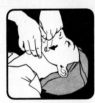 Open mouth and perform finger sweep.

2 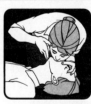 Open airway and try to ventilate.

3 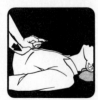 If unsuccessful, apply 6-10 subdiaphragmatic abdominal thrusts.

BE PERSISTENT

Activate the EMS system as soon as possible.
Repeat sequence: thrusts, finger sweep, attempt to ventilate.
Continue uninterrupted until advanced life support is available.

If none of these signs are present, the victim is not breathing.

If opening the airway does not cause the victim to begin to breathe spontaneously, you must provide rescue breathing.

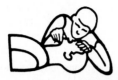

Breathing. The best way to provide rescue breathing is by using the mouth-to-mouth technique. Take your hand that is on the victim's forehead and turn it so that you can pinch the victim's nose shut while keeping the heel of the hand in place to maintain head tilt. Your index and middle fingers of your other hand should remain under the victim's chin, lifting up.

Immediately give two full breaths (1 to 1.5 seconds per breath) using the mouth-to-mouth method.

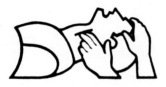

Check pulse. After giving the two breaths, locate the victim's carotid pulse to see if the heart is beating. To find the carotid artery, take your hand that you are using on the victim's chin and locate the voice box. Slide the tips of your index and middle fingers into the groove beside the voice box. Feel for the carotid pulse. Cardiac arrest can be recognized by absent breathing and an absent pulse in the carotid artery in the neck.

If you cannot find the pulse, you must provide artificial circulation in addition to rescue breathing.

Activate the Emergency Medical Services System (EMSS). Send someone to call 911 or your local emergency number if this has not already been done. If you are alone, perform CPR for 1 minute, then call the EMSS if possible. If it is not feasible to summon the EMSS, continue with CPR.

Cardiac Compression

Artificial circulation is provided by external cardiac compression. In effect, when you apply rhythmic pressure on the lower half of the victim's breastbone, you are forcing the heart to pump blood. To perform external cardiac compression

properly, kneel at the victim's side near the chest at the level of the victim's shoulders. Locate the notch at the lowest portion of the sternum with your hand that was on the victim's chin. Put your middle finger on this notch and your index finger next to it. Using your hand that was on the victim's forehead, place the heel of this hand on the lower half of the sternum, close to the index finger of your other hand. Place your other hand on top and parallel to the one that is in position. Be sure to keep your fingers off the chest wall. You may find it easier to do this if you interlock your fingers.

Bring your shoulders directly over the victim's sternum as you compress downward, keeping your arms straight. Depress the sternum about 1½ to 2 inches for an adult victim. Then relax pressure on the sternum completely. However, *do not* remove your hands from the victim's sternum, but *do* allow the chest to return to its normal position between compressions. Relaxation and compression should be of equal duration.

If you are the only rescuer, you must provide both rescue breathing and cardiac compression. The proper ratio is 15 chest compressions to 2 full, slow breaths. You must compress at the rate of 80 to 100 times per minute when you are working alone since you will stop compressions when you take time to breathe.

When there is another rescuer to help you, position yourselves on opposite sides of the victim if possible. One of you should be responsible for interposing a breath (1 to 1.5 seconds) after each fifth compression, maintaining an open airway, and monitoring the carotid pulse for adequate chest compressions. The other rescuer, who compresses the chest, should use a rate of 80 to 100 compressions per minute.

Rescuers	Ratio of Compressions to Breaths	Rate of Compressions
1	15:2	80 to 100 times/min
2	5:1	80 to 100 times/min

CPR FOR INFANTS AND SMALL CHILDREN

Basic life support for infants and small children is similar to that for adults. A few important differences to remember are given below.

Airway. Be careful when handling an infant that you do not exaggerate the backward position of the head tilt. An infant's neck is so pliable that forceful backward tilting might *block* breathing passages instead of opening them.

Breathing. Do not try to pinch off the nose. Cover both the mouth and nose of an infant or *small* child who is not breathing. Use small breaths with less volume to inflate the lungs. Give one small breath every 3 seconds for an infant (0 to 1 year) and one small breath every 4 seconds for a child (1 to 8 years). (For a child, a mouth-to-mouth seal should be made with the nose pinched tightly, as is done for adults.)

Check pulse. The absence of a pulse may be more easily determined by feeling for the brachial pulse for infants (0 to 1 years). (Locate the carotid pulse for children 1 to 8 years, as you would for an adult.)

Circulation. The technique for cardiac compression is different for infants and small children. In both cases, only one hand is used for compression. The other hand may be slipped under the child to provide a firm support for the back.

For infants, use only the *tips* of two or three fingers to compress the chest. Place the index finger of the hand nearest the infant's legs just under an imaginary line between the nipples where it intersects with the sternum. Compress the chest one fingerbreadth below this intersection, at the location of the middle and ring fingers. Depress the sternum between ½ to 1 inch at a fast rate of 100 times a minute.

For children 1 to 8 years, use only the *heel* of one hand to compress the chest. Depress the sternum between 1 and 1½ inches, depending upon the size of the child. The rate should be 80 to 100 times per minute.

In the case of both infants and small children, breaths should be administered during the relaxation after every fifth chest compression.

	Part of Hand	Depress Sternum	Rate of Compression
Infants	Tips of 2 or 3 fingers	½ to 1 inch	100 per minute
Children	Heel of hand	1 to 1½ inches	80 to 100 per minute

Neck injury. If you suspect the victim has suffered a neck injury, you must not open the airway in the usual manner. If the victim is injured in a diving or automobile accident, you should consider the possibility of such a neck injury. In these cases, the airway should be opened by using a jaw thrust, keeping the victim's head in a fixed, neutral position.

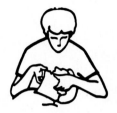

CHOKING

The urgency of choking cannot be overemphasized. Immediate recognition and proper action are essential. If the victim has good air exchange, or only partial obstruction, and is still able to speak or cough effectively, *do not interfere with his or her attempts to expel a foreign body.* The distress signal for choking is the gesture of clutching the neck between the thumb and index finger. *Prompt action is urgent in every case of choking.*

When you recognize complete airway obstruction by observing the conscious victim's inability to speak, breathe, or cough, the following sequence should be performed quickly on the victim in the sitting, standing, or lying position:

1. Manual thrusts (abdominal or chest) until effective, or the person becomes unconscious.
2. Finger sweep if the victim is unconscious.
3. If the victim becomes unconscious, shout for help. Place the victim on the back, face up. Open the airway and attempt to ventilate. If unsuccessful, deliver 6 to 10 manual thrusts, probe the mouth with the finger, and attempt to ventilate. It may be necessary to repeat these steps. *Be persistent.*

EMERGENCY MANAGEMENT OF THE OBSTRUCTED AIRWAY
Heimlich Maneuver

The Heimlich maneuver (subdiaphragmatic abdominal thrusts or abdominal thrusts) is the technique recommended for relieving foreign-body air-

Figure 30.2
For legend see opposite page.

A person choking on food will die in 4 minutes – you can save a life using the HEIMLICH MANEUVER®

Food-choking is caused by a piece of food lodging in the throat creating a blockage of the airway, making it impossible for the victim to breathe or speak. The victim will die of strangulation in four minutes if you do not act to save him.

Using the Heimlich Maneuver (described in the accompanying diagrams), you exert pressure that forces the diaphragm upward, compresses the air in the lungs, and expels the object blocking the breathing passage.

The victim should see a physician immediately after the rescue. Performing the maneuver could result in injury to the victim. However, he will survive only if his airway is quickly cleared.

If no help is at hand, victims should attempt to perform the Heimlich Maneuver on themselves by pressing their own fist upward into the abdomen as described.

WHAT TO LOOK FOR

The victim of food-choking:

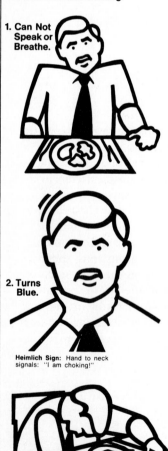

1. Can Not Speak or Breathe.

2. Turns Blue.

Heimlich Sign: Hand to neck signals: "I am choking!"

3. Collapses.

HEIMLICH MANEUVER®
RESCUER STANDING
Victim standing or sitting

☐ Stand behind the victim and wrap your arms around his waist.
☐ Place your fist thumb side against the victim's abdomen, slightly above the navel and below the rib cage.
☐ Grasp your fist with your other hand and press into the victim's abdomen with a **quick upward thrust.**
☐ Repeat several times if necessary.

When the victim is sitting, the rescuer stands behind the victim's chair and performs the maneuver in the same manner.

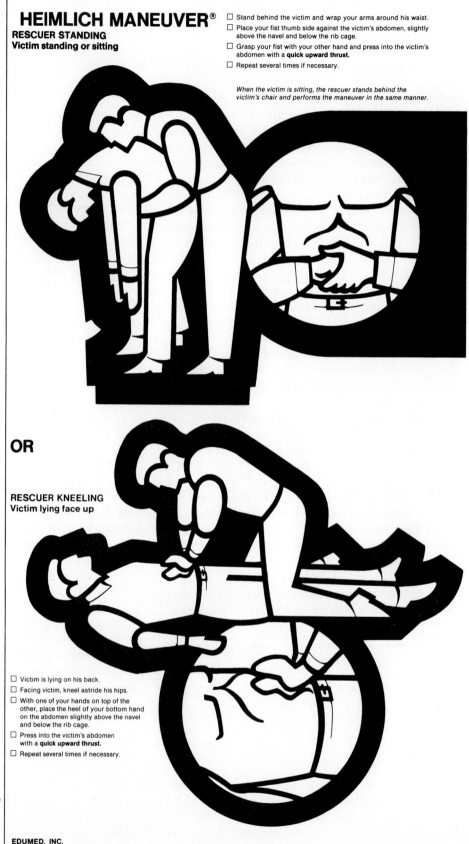

OR

RESCUER KNEELING
Victim lying face up

☐ Victim is lying on his back.
☐ Facing victim, kneel astride his hips.
☐ With one of your hands on top of the other, place the heel of your bottom hand on the abdomen slightly above the navel and below the rib cage.
☐ Press into the victim's abdomen with a **quick upward thrust.**
☐ Repeat several times if necessary.

EDUMED, INC.
BOX 52, CINCINNATI, OHIO 45201

Figure 30.2
Heimlich Maneuver. Heimlich Maneuver is a registered service mark of EDUMED, INC, which reserves all rights to its use. Posters, flyers, wallet cards, teaching slide/cassette program narrated by Dr. Heimlich, inventor of the Heimlich Maneuver, with study guide and T-shirts are available. Material is available in Spanish, and other languages are in work. EDUMED, INC., P.O. Box 52, Cincinnati, Ohio 45239
Courtesy EDUMED, INC, Cincinnati, Ohio.

way obstruction. It may be necessary to repeat the thrust 6 to 10 times to clear the victim's airway. Never have your hands on the victim's xiphoid process of the sternum or on the lower margins of the victim's rib cage when performing this maneuver (Figure 30.2).

Manual thrusts are a rapid series of thrusts to the upper abdomen or chest that force air from the lungs.

Heimlich maneuver (abdominal thrusts) with victim sitting or standing

1. Stand behind the victim; wrap your arms around the waist.
2. Place the thumb side of your fist against the victim's abdomen in the midline slightly below the rib cage well below the tip of the xiphoid process and slightly above the umbilicus.
3. Grasp your fist with your other hand and press it into the victim's abdomen with a *quick upward thrust.*
4. Repeat if necessary.

Heimlich maneuver (abdominal thrust) with victim lying

1. Place the victim in a supine position; kneel astride the victim's hips/thighs.
2. Place the heel of your hand in the middle of the abdomen, slightly below the rib cage well below the tip of the xiphoid process and slightly above the umbilicus. Place your other hand on top of your bottom hand.
3. Rock forward, having your shoulders directly over the victim's abdomen and press into the abdomen and toward the diaphragm with a *quick upward thrust. Do not* press to either side.
4. Repeat if necessary.

Chest Thrusts

Chest thrusts are to be used *only* when the victim is markedly obese or in the later stages of pregnancy. The downward thrusts will generate effective airway pressures.

Chest thrust with the victim standing or sitting

1. Standing behind the victim, place your arms under the victim's armpits, and encircle the victim's chest.
2. Place the thumb side of your fist on the victim's sternum (breastbone), but not on the xiphoid process.
3. Grasp this fist with your other hand, and press on the victim's sternum with a quick backward thrust.

Chest thrust with the victim in a lying position

1. Place your hands in the same position used for closed chest compression.
2. Exert quick downward thrusts.

Infants and Children

For infants up to 1 year of age, the combination of back blows and chest thrusts continues to be recommended. *Back blows* are a rapid series of sharp whacks delivered with the hand over the spine and between the shoulder blades. The blows should be applied quickly, forcefully, and in rapid succession. For a child 1 to 8 years of age, the Heimlich maneuver is recommended.

Other Causes of Airway Obstruction

An adequate open airway must be maintained at all times in all unconscious patients.

Other conditions that may cause unconsciousness and airway obstruction include stroke, epilepsy, head injury, alcoholic intoxication, drug overdose, and diabetes.

Remember:
1. Is the victim unconscious?
2. If so, shout for help, open the airway, and check for breathing
3. If no breathing, give two breaths
4. Check carotid pulse
5. Activate the EMSS: Send someone to call 911 or your local emergency number
6. If no pulse, begin external cardiac compres-

sion by depressing the lower half of the sternum 1½ to 2 inches (for adults)

7. Continue uninterrupted CPR until advanced life support is available

CPR for one rescuer:

15:2 compressions to breaths at a rate of 80 to 100 compressions a minute (four cycles per minute)

CPR for two rescuers:

5:1 compressions to breaths at a rate of 80 to 100 compressions a minute

Periodic practice in CPR is essential to ensure a satisfactory level of proficiency. A life may depend on how well you have remembered the proper steps of CPR and how to apply them. You should be sure to have both your skill and knowledge of CPR tested at least once a year. It could mean someone's life. (See also Chapter 20 for AIDS infection precautions and CPR.)

EMERGENCY MEDICAL SERVICES SYSTEM (EMSS)

Any victim on whom you begin resuscitation must be considered to need advanced life support. He or she will have the best chance of surviving if your community has a total emergency medical services system. This includes an efficient communications alert system, such as 911, with public awareness of how or where to call; well-trained rescue personnel who can respond rapidly; vehicles that are properly equipped; an emergency facility that is open 24 hours a day to provide advanced life support; and an intensive care section in the hospital for the victims. You should work with all interested agencies to achieve such a system.

911: Emergency Telephone System

Many communities participate in the nationwide 911 emergency telephone system. To find out if it is in effect in your community, call information in your area.

The 911 telephone system *must be used only in emergency situations when you need help quickly.* Dial 911 only when you or someone nearby needs emergency medical help or an ambulance, when you see a fire or a crime in progress, and even when you suspect that a stranger may be in your home or you see him/her trying to enter or leave. Since 911 is a local service in each area, it is not necessary to dial any special access codes before the number. You only need to use three telephone digits—911. You can dial 911 from any type of telephone, including coin-operated public telephones, without any charge (you don't have to put coins into a coin-operated telephone to dial 911). If you are calling for help for someone who does not live in your area, you should call the "O" operator instead of 911. This is because 911 is a *local* service and cannot be used to obtain help outside of your immediate area.

When you dial 911 you will reach a specially trained emergency operator. This operator will ask you a few important questions so that the type of help you need will be obtained without delay. Information that you will be asked includes the following:

- What is the emergency?
- Where is the emergency? (Include cross-reference streets when applicable.)
- What is your name and address?

Even if you can't talk, stay on the line. In many communities, the special nature of the 911 system allows the emergency operator to know exactly where you are so that help can come quickly. The emergency operator immediately assesses the problem and by pressing a button, notifies the appropriate public emergency agency. The operator stays on the line to be sure that your problem is handled properly to get the fastest emergency service and to see if other emergency services are necessary. The emergency operator also serves to keep the caller calm while waiting for help to arrive. Callers who are disconnected after dialing 911 can be called right back and in even greater emergencies, the operator can trace the location of the phone.

Remember to stay calm and don't hang up. The emergency operator should hang up before you do. Often people panic in an emergency situation. They may give the operator information in a hurried fashion and hang up to go back to the emergency scene before the operator has obtained adequate and correct information. When this happens, the proper help may not be able to reach you in an adequate time to meet the needs of the situation. In some communities your line can be left open until the proper type of emergency help arrives. This would allow special instructions to be given for the emergency while you wait for help to arrive, and if necessary, to determine your address if you are unable to give it.

Remember, 911 must be used only to report "real" emergencies. It must not be used for every call that you may have to make to the police department, the fire department, or an ambulance service.

SHOCK

Shock, a state of collapse or a depressed condition of the circulatory system, occurs when the vital organs of the body are deprived of circulating blood flow necessary to sustain their normal cellular activity. It is a physiological reaction of the body to severe injury or insult. Circulatory collapse may occur following hemorrhage, severe trauma, dehydration, massive infection, severe burns, surgery, increased peripheral resistance, decreased cardiac output, drug toxicity, pain, fear, or emotional distress.

Shock may be immediate or delayed, slight or severe, or even fatal. Every injury is accompanied by some degree of shock and so should be treated promptly.

Types of Shock

Shock may be divided into five basic types, as the exact cause of shock is not always the same for every patient.

Traumatic shock

Traumatic shock is the direct result of extracellular fluid loss, as in extensive contusions or loss of plasma from large burned areas.

Hemorrhagic or hypovolemic shock

Hemorrhagic or hypovolemic shock is produced by a decrease in the circulating blood volume. The blood loss may be external or internal (into a body cavity from which it is no longer accessible to the circulatory system).

Cardiogenic shock

Cardiogenic shock is the result of conditions that interfere with the heart's function as a pump. This may be a result of cardiac failure or secondary to myocardial infarction, coronary thrombosis, or certain disorders of the rate and rhythm of the heart.

Septic shock

Septic shock results from bacterial infection. It may occur when there is massive infection of traumatized tissue or when toxic tissue products are absorbed. Gram-negative shock is a form of septic shock caused by infection with gram-negative bacteria (see Chapter 22).

Neurogenic shock

Neurogenic shock is the result of loss of peripheral vascular tone with subsequent dilation of the blood vessels, decreased heart rate, and a drop in the blood pressure to the point at which the supply of oxygen carried to the brain by the blood is insufficient. The patient then faints; thus this type of shock is commonly called fainting.

Signs and Symptoms of Shock

Five Ps denote the outstanding signs and symptoms of shock.
- Prostration;
- Pallor;
- Perspiration;
- Pulselessness; and
- Pulmonary deficiency.

These will all vary in intensity depending on the patient's condition and the injury or cause.

The most outstanding signs and symptoms of severe shock or the later stages of shock include the following:

1. The pulse is weak, rapid, and irregular.
2. Respirations increase in rate and are shallow.
3. Blood pressure is lowered—less than 90 mm Hg systolic.
4. The skin is markedly pale and may feel cold to the touch and moist with perspiration.
5. The lips, nailbeds, tips of the fingers, and lobes of the ears may be bluish (cyanosis).
6. The face may appear pinched and without expression.
7. There may be a staring of the eyes, which often lose their characteristic luster.
8. The pupils may be dilated, especially in the late stages.
9. Occasionally, the patient may be unusually anxious, restless, or excited.
10. When conscious, the patient appears quite disinterested in the surroundings and complains little of pain, although he may be groaning.
11. Later the patient may become apathetic and unresponsive. Eyes are sunken with a vacant expression.
12. If untreated, the patient will eventually lose consciousness. Vital signs drop, and death may occur.

First Aid Care

In any emergency situation a routine procedure is to evaluate the situation for the possibility of shock and take measures to prevent it. The following objectives for preventing or treating shock should be met:

- Improve circulation of blood; control bleeding when necessary;
- Ensure an open airway and an adequate supply of oxygen;
- Maintain normal body temperature and keep the patient at rest; and
- Obtain medical assistance as and when required.

When treating a patient in shock:

1. Do a quick primary survey of the situation. Ensure the ABCs of all emergencies; that is, maintain an open airway and check for breathing and circulation. Be prepared to give cardiopulmonary resuscitation if necessary.

2. Control severe bleeding if present.

3. Position the patient in a supine (lying) position with the lower extremities elevated 8 to 12 inches, *except* when there is a head injury, or if breathing difficulty is thereby increased, or if the patient complains of pain when this is attempted, or if the patient is vomiting. A patient with a head injury should be kept flat, or the head and shoulders may be propped up slightly.

4. Keep the patient warm but do not overheat.

5. Loosen tight clothing.

6. Do not move the patient unnecessarily.

7. Avoid disturbing the patient with noise and questions.

8. Fluids may be given *only* when there are no contraindications and when medical help cannot be obtained for an hour or more. Fluids are not given to patients who are unconscious, have head injuries, are vomiting, are convulsing, have abdominal injuries, or are likely to require surgery. The recommended fluid to give is water, preferably water with 1 teaspoon of salt and ½ teaspoon of baking soda to each quart of water. Give this at 15-minute intervals as follows:
   • 4 ounces for adults;
   • 2 ounces for children ages 1 to 12 years; and
   • 1 ounce for infants under 1 year of age.

9. When necessary, administer oxygen, but only with the consent and directions of the physician.

10. Provide constant, kindly, tactful encouragement and extreme gentleness when caring for the patient.

11. Call the physician or hospital promptly when the patient is going into or is in the state of shock.

12. Arrange for ambulance transport as indicated. Do not attempt to move the patient alone without explicit instructions from the physician, unless the immediate surroundings would cause further harm to the patient.

ABDOMINAL PAIN

All abdominal pain should be investigated, especially unusual pain that occurs rather suddenly and is accompanied by fever. Treatment varies with the cause of pain. For pain caused by trauma, keep the patient lying flat if possible, in case of internal bleeding. For pain caused from metabolic or pathologic causes, keep the patient in a comfortable position until medical help arrives or the patient is transported to the hospital. For any abdominal pain, do the following:

• Keep the patient quiet and warm. Keep activity to a minimum.
• Do not apply heat.
• Do not give foods, liquids, or laxatives.
• Place an emesis basin nearby in case the patient vomits.
• Check the patient frequently.
• Be empathetic.

Pathologic processes causing acute abdominal emergencies are inflammation, hemorrhage, perforation, obstruction, and ischemia (lack of adequate blood supply). These medical emergencies require immediate care by a physician, because most often they require surgical intervention, although at times some may be treated medically.

ALLERGIC REACTION TO DRUGS

Usually in an anaphylactic reaction or in any type of drug overdose reaction, the airway, breathing, and circulation will become impaired because of the effects of drugs on the central nervous system. Thus a primary survey (the ABCs) must be done.

A = airway
  Ensure that the airway is open.
B = breathing
  After you ensure that the airway is open, make sure that the breathing is spontaneous; in other words, make sure that the patient is breathing on his or her own.
C = circulation
  Check for a pulse beat. The best place to check the pulse rate is at the carotid artery.

When any of these areas require stabilization, do nothing else except stabilize the ABCs and call or send for medical help. A secondary survey should also be made to ensure that additional injury is not done to the patient. This is a quick head-to-toe check to observe for any obvious bleeding or injury that may require immediate attention. Oxygen and epinephrine should be available for administration on the physician's order. Usually 4 to 8 liters of oxygen is administered by mask or nasal cannula, and 1 to 3 ml epinephrine 1:1,000 IU is administered subcutaneously. It is necessary to stay with the patient until medical help arrives to ensure the ABCs.

Constantly monitor the level of consciousness and vital signs and maintain an adequate airway and ventilation.

Positioning the patient is also very important. Commonly when a patient goes into anaphylaxis, a lying position cannot be tolerated. Usually the patient must be in a sitting or a semi-Fowler position to expand the lungs and breathe more easily. Monitor the vital signs carefully, approximately every 2 or 3 minutes, note the skin color, and again monitor the airway. An oropharyngeal airway may be used at times to allow more air to get into the air passageways. When there is not a reversal within a reasonable time, rapid transport to the hospital is necessary.

Encourage patients with known allergies to wear a Medic-Alert bracelet or necklace.

ASPHYXIA

Asphyxia may occur whenever there is an interference with the normal exchange of oxygen and carbon dioxide between the lungs and outside air. Common causes include obstruction of the airway caused by foreign bodies or the tongue or by edema of the tissues, as seen in burns or inflammatory processes of the air passages. Drowning, electric shock, inhalation of smoke and poisonous gases, trauma to or disease of the lungs, bronchi, and trachea, or allergic reactions can all cause asphyxia. Basically the patient is apneic (not breathing). Treatment must be an immediate remedy of the situation. Follow the ABCs—check for an open airway, breathing, and circulation. Open the airway if necessary and give artificial ventilation. Remove the underlying cause whenever possible. When there is absence of both breathing and heartbeat, cardiopulmonary resuscitation must be given immediately. Have oxygen available; it may be given when the patient is having difficulty breathing, and also is frequently administered after breathing resumes to treat the resultant hypoxia. Send for medical help or call the physician.

SEVERE BLEEDING (HEMORRHAGE)

Three types of bleeding can be observed from open wounds. Spurting of bright red blood from a wound indicates arterial bleeding; continuous flow of dark red blood indicates venous bleeding; and oozing of blood indicates capillary bleeding. Arterial bleeding is the most serious, requiring immediate control and medical intervention after the initial control to prevent severe shock or death. Generally, venous bleeding is easier to control than arterial bleeding, because there is less pressure on the blood flow in the veins than in the arteries. However, venous bleeding may also be life-threatening, especially if several large veins are involved. Capillary bleeding is easily controlled by first aid measures and the body's own clotting mechanisms.

Immediate action is imperative for any wound accompanied by severe bleeding, because shock, loss of consciousness, and even death may occur from a rapid loss of blood in a very short time.

Objectives of Wound Care

- To control the bleeding immediately;
- To protect the wound from contamination and infection (as is feasible; in emergency situations where sterile dressings are not available, you must use materials on hand, even if they are not sterile. It is more important to save the person's life by controlling the bleeding than it is to worry about preventing infection);
- To treat for shock; and
- To obtain medical attention.

Methods to Control Severe Bleeding (In Order of Preference)
Direct pressure

Place a sterile dressing (or the cleanest cloth item on hand) over the wound site and apply hard, firm, direct pressure. This will usually be effective in controlling severe bleeding. In the absence of dressing or cloth materials, apply direct pressure with the hand or fingers, but only until a compress is obtained. If a dressing becomes saturated with blood, do not remove it, but place additional dressings directly over the saturated one and continue firm, direct pressure.

Maintain direct pressure by applying a pressure bandage over the dressings on the wound site until medical help is obtained. If bleeding resumes once pressure is released, reapply it, and get the person to the physician immediately.

Elevation

Elevate a limb above the person's heart level in conjunction with direct pressure, unless there is evidence of a fracture. Elevation helps reduce blood

Figure 30.3
Location of pressure points.
From Parcel GS: First aid in emergency care, St Louis, 1977, The CV Mosby Co.

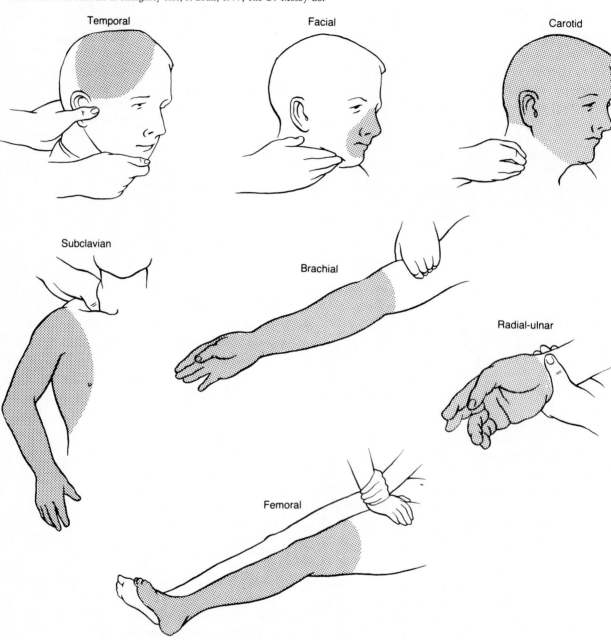

pressure within the limb, thus slowing down blood loss from the wound.

Pressure points

When severe bleeding is not controlled with direct pressure and elevation of an affected limb, the pressure point method can be applied in conjunction with the first two methods. The pressure point method compresses the blood vessel supplying blood to the wound against an underlying bone or muscle tissue in an effort to close it off and reduce the amount of blood flowing through the vessel to the wound site. This method will control bleeding in all but a few circumstances. The exact position of the pressure point must be known and located quickly; otherwise significant blood loss will result. The seven pressure points follow (really fourteen, because there is one on the right and one on the left) (Figure 30.3).

Temporal artery. Compression on the temporal artery may be used to control superficial wounds of the forehead or the frontal part of the scalp.

Facial artery. Upward and outward compression of the facial artery against the jawbone with two or more fingers may be used to control bleeding in the facial region.

Carotid artery. Compression of the carotid artery in the neck against underlying muscle tissue may be used to control *only* serious hemorrhaging in the head. When this pressure point is used, extreme care must be taken to avoid obstructing the person's airway. *Do not* apply pressure dressings around the neck.

Subclavian artery. Downward compression with the fingers of the subclavian artery just behind the collar bone (the clavicle) may be used to control bleeding in the arm and upper shoulder regions.

Brachial artery. Compression of the brachial artery against the bone with the fingers applied midway between the shoulder and elbow on the inside of the arm may be used to control bleeding from the arm, hand, and fingers.

Femoral artery. Compression of the femoral artery (in the center of the groin area) against the pelvic bone with the heel of the hand may be used to control bleeding from the leg.

Radial artery. Compression of the radial artery on the anterior side of the wrist on the thumb side may be used to control severe bleeding from the hand or fingers.

Compression of the ulnar artery (on the little finger, anterior side of the wrist) should be used in conjunction with compression of the radial artery when there is profuse hemorrhaging from the hand. If bleeding does not stop with compression on the radial and ulnar arteries, apply pressure to the brachial artery to control the bleeding.

Tourniquet

The use of a tourniquet is dangerous and should be used *only as a last resort* to control severe, life-threatening hemorrhage when direct pressure, elevation, and pressure point methods fail to control the bleeding. The dangers of nerve damage, blood vessel damage, and tissue damage exist when a tourniquet is applied; thus a tourniquet must be avoided unless a life could be lost. In essence, the decision to apply a tourniquet is a decision to risk the loss of the person's limb to save life. After the application of a tourniquet, it is imperative that the person be attended to by a physician. The following directions *must* be observed when a tourniquet is applied (Figure 30.4):

Figure 30.4
Procedure for application of a tourniquet.
From Parcel GS: First aid in emergency care, St Louis, 1977, The CV Mosby Co.

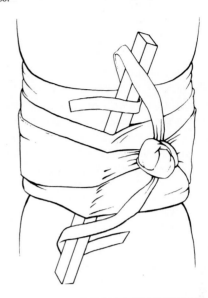

1. Use appropriate materials at least 2 inches wide, such as a stocking, a cloth, a folded triangular bandage, or a blood pressure cuff, if available.
2. Apply the tourniquet just above the wound, or just above the joint when the wound is in or below a joint area.
3. Wrap the tourniquet material around the limb twice, and secure it with a knot.
4. Insert a strong stick or similar object between the two loops and twist this object to tighten the tourniquet until bleeding stops. Tourniquets must be applied tightly enough to stop the bleeding; if applied too loosely, bleeding will increase.
5. Wrap the ends of the tourniquet material around the stick or similar object, and tie it in place.
6. Make a written note of the time of application and the location of the tourniquet, and attach this to the person's clothing, or mark this information on the person. Commonly people will mark a large *TK* (for tourniquet) on the injured person's forehead with lipstick when at the scene of the accident.
7. *Never* release a tourniquet once it has been applied. A tourniquet must be removed only by a physician, who can provide supportive treatment for shock.

8. Elevate the limb slightly if this will not cause further injury.
9. Treat for shock and give first aid for other injuries as required.
10. Transport the person immediately to receive medical attention.

Amputation

In cases of amputation, the amputated part should be kept cool and moist if possible and taken with the victim to the physician. With the advent of microsurgery, amputated limbs can frequently be reattached successfully, provided there is minimal tissue damage to the surrounding tissues.

Further Wound Care

For capillary bleeding, direct pressure and the application of ice wrapped in a towel or plastic bag are useful. Remember that ice is not effective in controlling *severe* bleeding.

In all cases when caring for bleeding wounds, provide reassurance and emotional support to the victim and remain calm. If possible, estimate how much blood was lost, because this will help the physician treat the person and determine if fluid replacement is necessary. However, remember that even an ounce of blood can discolor large numbers of dressings; and a cup of blood poured on the floor or ground covers a fairly large area, because when blood first comes from the vessels it is thin, and a small amount looks like a lot. Also observe the actual bleeding—is it a minimal, moderate, or heavy flow? This information will aid the physician, in addition to guiding your decision for the use of a tourniquet.

When bleeding stops, bandage the dressings firmly in place. Do not remove the initial dressings, because blood clots may be disturbed and bleeding resumed. Leave the cleaning and treatment of the wound to the physician.

Prevention of Contamination and Infection

To prevent infection, avoid, if possible, touching the wound with an unsterilized dressing or your unscrubbed hands. Do not disturb or remove the initial dressing placed over the wound.

BURNS

Burns are wounds caused by body contact with fire (dry heat), steam and scalding water (moist heat), electricity, chemicals, radiation (sun or nuclear rays), or lightning. Each year thousands of burns occur, many of which could have been prevented, and many of which are fatal in both the young and old. Burns involving over one third to one half of the body are often fatal, especially in children. Theories on the treatment for burns have undergone many changes over the years; many remedies were advocated and later rejected. Current thought on the matter can best be summed up by following the three Bs and the three Cs.

B = *burn*
   Stop the burning
B = *breathing*
   Check the breathing
B = *body examination*
   Examine where and how extensively the body has been burned, and assess any associated injuries
C = *cool*
   Cool the burn
C = *cover*
   Cover the burn
C = *carry*
   Carry the burn patient to the nearest medical treatment facility

In addition, current treatment practices *condemn* the application of greasy substances, ointments, powders, or antiseptics to a burned area.

Classification of Burns

Burns are classified as first, second, and third degree, depending on the depth of the wound; they are also classified according to the percentage of body surface involved (Figures 30.5 and 30.6).

Depth of wound

First-degree burns involve only the outer layers of the skin. The skin is reddened without blister formation and is painful. The best example is a sunburn. *Second-degree burns* involve deeper layers of the epidermis, are painful, and usually form blisters. *Third-degree burns* are the most serious, destroying all layers of the skin including the hair follicles, and the sebaceous and sweat glands. Nerves are destroyed, thus the wound is painless. Muscles, blood supply, and bones may also be destroyed in third-degree burns.

Body surface

The percentage of total body surface involved usually determines the severity of the burn. The body surface is divided into areas by the rule of nine. Each arm is 9%, each leg is 18%, the front or back

Figure 30.5
A, Cross-section showing structures of skin. **B,** Classification of burns by degree.
From Parcel GS: First aid in emergency care, St Louis, 1977, The CV Mosby Co.

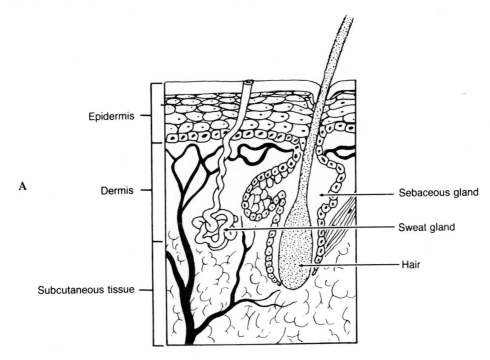

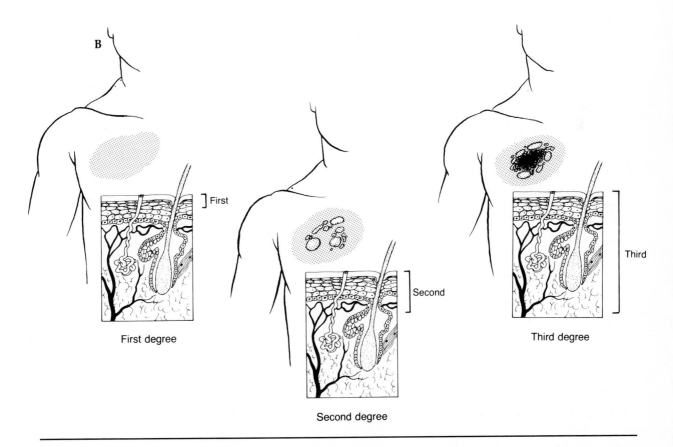

Figure 30.6
Classification of burns by body surface area.
From Parcel GS: First aid in emergency care, St Louis, 1977,
The CV Mosby Co.

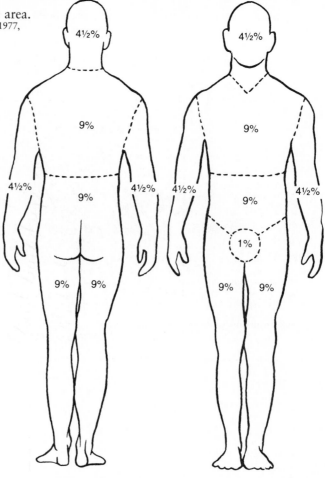

of the trunk is 18%, and the head and neck are 9% of the total body surface.

A first-degree burn involving more than 20% of total body surface, or involving the face and airway, or impairing the person when walking or wearing clothes should receive medical attention. Any second- or third-degree burn involving more than 20% of the total body surface, or the feet, hands, or genitalia is considered a serious burn in need of medical attention. When more than 40% of total body surface is burned, it is considered a *severe burn*.

First Aid Treatment for Burns
Objectives for care of first-degree burns

- To relieve pain.
- To prevent the formation of blisters.

Treatment

1. Immediately submerge the burned part in ice water or place cold compresses directly on the burn.

2. Continue this treatment until pain has subsided when the cold is discontinued.
3. Apply a dry sterile dressing if the burn is in an area that will be irritated by clothing.
4. When running water is available, it is best to place the burned part under cold running water for 20 minutes. The reason for this is that, even though the top layers of the skin are cooled within a few minutes, the underlying tissue is still very heated, and the burn continues to cause tissue damage up to periods of 20 minutes after the initial burn.

Objectives for treating second- and third-degree burns

- Treat the person for shock;
- Prevent infection; and
- Relieve pain.

Second-degree burn care

1. Immediately submerge the burned part in cold water for 1 to 2 hours, *or* place under running water for 20 minutes.

Figure 30.7
For chemical burns, wash immediately with copious amounts of cool running water for at least 5 minutes.

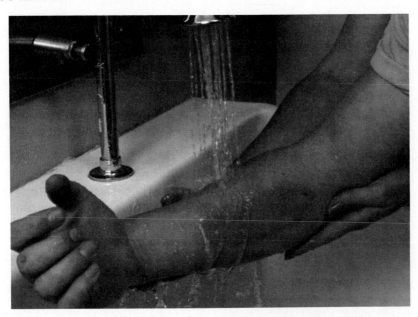

2. *Do not* break blisters or remove tissue.
3. Cover with a dressing or clean cloth that has been wrung out in ice water.
4. Apply a dry dressing as a protective bandage.

Third-degree burn care

1. Stop the burning; check for breathing; remove the burning agent. Remove any smoldering clothing; certain synthetics retain heat. Remove any jewelry on the burned area. Clothing and jewelry retain heat and also can become constricting as edema develops. Do a quick body assessment to determine the extent and severity of the burn.
2. Keep the person lying down with the head a little lower than the legs and hips, unless there is a chest or head injury or if the person has difficulty breathing in this position.
3. Cool and cover the wound. Cover the burned areas with sterile dressings if available, or a cloth or sheet. Pour copious amounts of cool water, or saline, if available, onto the material covering the wound. Continue pouring cool water onto the material every so often, because the burn continues to heat the water up to the level of the material. If clean material is not available, water may be poured directly onto the wound. When the wound is cooled, wrap the person for transport to a medical fa-

cility. *Never open any blisters.* Covering the wound prevents moving air from reaching the wound, lessens pain, and reduces contamination.
4. If adjoining surfaces of skin are burned, separate them with gauze or cloth to keep them from sticking together (such as between the toes or fingers, ears and head, arms and chest).
5. If the victim is conscious, is not nauseated or vomiting, and medical help cannot be obtained for an hour or more, make a solution of ½ teaspoon baking soda and 1 teaspoon salt in a quart of water. Allow the adult patient to sip a half glass every 15 minutes to replace lost body fluids; a child 1 to 12 years, 2 ounces, and an infant about 1 ounce. Discontinue fluid if vomiting occurs.
6. For *chemical burns,* wash immediately with *copious* amounts of cool running water for at least 5 minutes (Figure 30.7). Remove any clothing that was in contact with the chemical. If the chemical got on the face or eyes, flush the face and eyes with a gentle flow of cool water for at least 15 minutes (Figure 30.8). Remove contact lenses if the victim is wearing them. Try to find out what chemical caused the burn so that you can tell the personnel at the emergency department where the victim will be taken. Also see the above steps.

Figure 30.8
If chemical gets on face, flush face and eyes with a gentle flow of cool water.

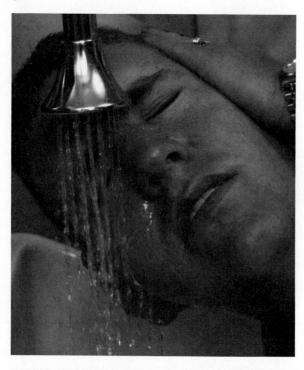

NOTE: *Never* flush a phosphorus burn with any type of solution, including water, as this could cause tissue sloughing. Instead, *soak* the affected area in water.

7. If possible while awaiting transport for the person, take the pulse, respiration, and blood pressure to assess impending shock.

8. Keep the patient resting quietly and warm. Chilling must be avoided to prevent additional discomfort and loss of energy.

9. Constantly provide emotional support for the patient.

10. Inform the patient before transfer is undertaken.

What *not* to do about burns

• *Do not* pull clothing over the burned area—cut it away if necessary.

• *Do not* try to remove any pieces of cloth or bits of debris or dirt that are stuck to the burn.

• *Do not* try to clean the burn; do not use iodine or other antiseptics on it; and do not open any blisters that may form on the burn.

• *Do not* use grease, butter, ointment, salve, petro-

leum jelly, or any type of medication on *any* burn.

• *Do not* breathe on the burn and do not touch it with anything except a sterile or clean dressing.

• *Do not* change the dressings that were initially applied to the burn until directed to do so by a physician.

CEREBRAL VASCULAR ACCIDENT (STROKE)

A cerebral vascular accident (CVA), also called a stroke, is a disorder of the blood vessels of the brain. It results in a lack of blood supply to parts of the brain. Main causes of a CVA include a cerebral thrombus or a cerebral embolus, cerebral hemorrhage, compression of cerebral arteries (as from edema or tumors), and arterial spasms. The symptoms and effects of a CVA vary greatly. They can be slight or severe, temporary or permanent, depending on the cause, location, and extent of the damage in the brain. Signs and symptoms of a CVA may include the following:

• Dizziness, mental confusion, headache, and poor coordination;
• Difficulty in speaking or loss of speech;
• Loss of bladder and bowel control;
• Paralysis or weakness on one or both sides of the body;
• Loss of vision, especially in one eye;
• Difficulty in breathing and in swallowing;
• Unequal size of the pupils; and/or
• Loss of consciousness.

First aid measures for a cerebral vascular accident include the following:

1. Loosen all constricting clothing, especially around the neck. This may help to improve breathing and circulation to the head.

2. Maintain an open airway.

3. Position the victim on the affected side so that secretions will drain from the mouth and thus prevent aspiration of saliva and mucus.

4. Keep the victim calm and provide reassurance that care is being provided.

5. If conscious, the victim may sit up or have the head elevated. This will help to lessen blood pressure in the head.

6. Do not give fluids unless the victim is able to swallow and is fully conscious. Discontinue all fluids if the victim vomits.

7. Seek medical attention as soon as possible. The victim will usually need to be hospitalized.

8. Be prepared to administer cardiopulmonary resuscitation if required.

CHEST PAIN

Chest pain can be associated with heart disease, lung disease, pain in the muscle fibers of the chest wall, and a few other conditions. It can be serious. It is advisable to treat all patients with chest pain as if they are heart patients. First aid measures include the following:

1. Observe the symptoms.
2. Keep the patient quiet and warm. Allow the patient to rest. Commonly the patient will find it easier to breathe when in a semisitting or upright position. Do not have the patient walk any distance.
3. Loosen all tight clothing.
4. Administer 4 to 6 liters of oxygen (if you are in the office and have prior directions and permission from the physician).
5. Contact the physician. When the physician cannot be reached, call the emergency medical system in your community, or an ambulance, or the fire department.
6. Stay with the patient until medical help arrives.
7. If the patient is conscious, inquire if she or he has any medication with her or him that is used for attacks of chest pain. The medication will usually be nitroglycerin tablets, which are taken sublingually. You may give them to the patient with the patient's consent.
8. When feasible, obtain pertinent information from the patient. Use the PQRST method:
   P = provoking
   What provoked the pain, what was the patient doing or experiencing when the pain started, such as any physical activity, emotional upset or excitement, or was the patient just sitting quietly reading or such?
   Q = quality of pain
   Is it a sharp pain, prolonged oppressive pain, or unusual discomfort?
   R = radiation of pain
   Where, if at all, does the pain radiate to? Is it in the center of the chest? Is it in the chest wall? Does it radiate to the abdomen or to the neck or to the left arm?
   S = severity
   How severe is the pain—mild, moderate, or severe?
   T = time

When did the pain start? How long does it last? How frequently does it recur?
9. Keep an emesis basin handy in case the patient vomits.
10. At times it may be necessary to start artificial respiration or cardiopulmonary resuscitation if breathing and heartbeat have ceased.
11. If in the physician's office, you may connect the patient to the electrocardiograph and record a few tracings for the physician to interpret. Lead II and Lead V_1 are considered the monitoring leads.
12. Remain calm; offer emotional support and reassurance to the patient, because most patients will be anxious and frightened.

CONVULSIONS

Convulsions are the involuntary spasms or contractions of muscles caused by an abnormal stimulus to the brain or by changes in the chemical balance in the body. The primary effort in first aid for convulsions is to protect the patient from causing harm to the body during the convulsion.

1. Move items near the patient that may cause harm. Ask curious onlookers to remove themselves from the immediate area.
2. Loosen clothing around the neck and in any other area where it is constricting.
3. Place a padded bite block between the teeth to protect against biting of the tongue. *Do not* insert a bite block if force is required to get it in place. If an appropriate bite block is not available, one can be made by wrapping and taping a couple pieces of gauze around two tongue blades.
4. Do not restrain the patient's movements except to prevent injury. Protect the head at all times.
5. When movement has ceased, keep the patient lying down and allow to rest.
6. Ensure an open airway.
7. If bleeding from a bitten tongue, or excessive saliva, or vomit is present, turn the patient's head to one side to prevent aspiration of these excretions.
8. After all seizure activity has ceased, allow the patient to rest or sleep in a quiet, comfortable place until sufficiently oriented to time and place and capable of moving without weakness.

Anyone who has experienced a seizure (convulsion) should be seen by a physician, although the occurrence of one seizure is not considered an emergency. If convulsive activity is repeated or occurs frequently, medical attention must be sought.

If reporting the convulsion to the physician, it is very important that you describe the convulsive activity; that is, was the convulsion generalized or localized, how and where did it start, how many convulsions were there, and how long did they last.

EPISTAXIS (NOSEBLEED)

Most nosebleeds are not serious and can be easily controlled. However, excessive bleeding requires medical attention and may require electrocauterization of the ruptured vessels causing the bleeding.

First aid for nosebleeds is relatively simple. Have the patient in a sitting position, and pinch the lower portion of the nose between the thumb and index finger for 5 to 10 minutes. When this does not control the bleeding, apply ice packs to the nasal and facial areas. Place a moistened gauze pad gently into the bleeding nostril, leaving one end of the gauze outside so that it can be removed easily, then pinch the nose between the thumb and index finger for 10 minutes. If this does not control the bleeding, medical attention should be obtained.

FAINTING (SYNCOPE)

Fainting is a partial or complete loss of consciousness of limited duration caused by a decreased amount of blood to the brain. A person may feel weak and dizzy, cold, nauseated, appear pale, perspire, and have numbness or tingling in the hands and feet before fainting; or one may faint suddenly. First aid management for patients who faint is as follows:

1. Lay the person flat with the head lowered slightly.
2. Ensure an open airway.
3. Loosen tight clothing.
4. Apply cold cloths to the face. These are beneficial because of their stimulating effect.
5. Pass aromatic spirits of ammonia back and forth in front of the person's nose to allow inhalation. Avoid holding them too close to the person's nose.
6. Observe the person carefully, looking for anything unusual.
7. Observe for local weakness of the arms and legs and locate and count the pulse. These observations may be of great importance if the condition turns out to be something other than a fainting episode.

8. Keep the person resting quietly for at least 10 minutes after full consciousness has been regained.
9. Lower the head between the legs when the person is in a sitting position and begins to feel faint. Stay with the person and protect against falling should fainting occur.
10. When fainting lasts more than a minute or two, keep the person warm and resting quietly and summon the physician or transport to the hospital, because the condition may not be a simple episode of fainting. It may, in fact, be a symptom of diabetes, heart disease, epilepsy, stroke, or any one of many diseases.

FOREIGN BODIES IN THE EAR, EYE, AND NOSE
Ear

Foreign bodies lodged in the ear canal are commonly seen in children. *Do not* attempt to remove them. They must be removed by the physician, because of the possibility of injury to the eardrum (tympanic membrane) and ear canal tissue.

If the foreign body in the ear is a live bug or insect, instill a few drops of sterile oil into the ear canal. This will asphyxiate and stop the movement of the intruder.

Eye

Foreign bodies in the eye are very irritating and can be harmful because of the possibility of their scratching the eye surface or becoming embedded in the eye tissue.

Instruct the patient not to rub the affected eye.

Wash your hands and examine the eye by pulling the lower lid down and turning the upper lid back. If the object is on either lid, take a moistened corner of a clean cloth and touch it lightly to try to remove it. Avoid applying any pressure on the eye. If the object is on the eye itself, do not attempt to remove it this way. At times when the object is located under the upper eyelid or on the eye, it may be dislodged by pulling the upper eyelid forward and down over the lower lid; tears may dislodge the object. The eye then may be flushed with clean water.

When the previous methods do not remove the object, it may be embedded. Cover the closed eye with a dressing, and summon the physician.

Nose

When an object in the nose cannot be removed easily, a physician must be consulted. Instruct the patient to avoid violent nose blowing and probing the nose, because these acts may only push the object deeper or injure the tissues of the nose.

HEAD INJURIES

The severity of head injuries can vary greatly. The patient may appear normal, experience a headache, have a momentary loss of consciousness or lack of memory, be dazed, or be unconscious. Bleeding from the mouth, nose, ears, or scalp may be present; pulse may be rapid and weak; pupils of the eyes may be unequal in size; and pallor, vomiting, or double vision may be present. *In all cases medical attention is imperative.* When the initial symptoms are minor, it must be remembered that even after a period of time, hours or days, the injured person may become drowsy or confused or unconscious as a result of a head injury. A prompt recovery from a state of minor signs and symptoms may not be an indication of the seriousness of the injury. The following steps and precautions should be taken:

1. Assess the patient's physical and mental status. For physical assessment, check for signs as just stated, and take the blood pressure if equipment is available. For mental assessment when the patient is conscious, check for orientation as to time, place, name, and alertness, and ask the patient to repeat a simple phrase. Talking with the patient is a good way to check the level of consciousness and alertness.
2. Keep the patient at rest in a supine position if the face is ashen and gray, or raise the head and shoulders (together) if the face is flushed. *Never position the patient with the head lower than the rest of the body.*
3. Always ensure an open airway. Be prepared to give artificial respiration when necessary.
4. Control hemorrhage if present.
5. Do not give fluids by mouth.
6. Apply a dressing to a scalp wound and bandage it in place with a head bandage.
7. Take note of any period of unconsciousness and record it.
8. Observe and record any changes in the pupils of the eyes.
9. Take and record the blood pressure and the time of any changes (if the equipment is available). When the blood pressure begins to rise and if the pupils begin to dilate, or the state of consciousness begins to decrease, this usually indicates an elevation of intracranial pressure.
10. If the patient is unconscious, gently turn the head to one side to prevent aspiration of any blood or mucus that may be present.
11. Keep the patient resting quietly until medical help arrives or the patient is transported to the hospital.

HYPERVENTILATION

Hyperventilation is a common complication of emotional upsets or hysterical situations. It usually affects persons who are anxious and high-strung and have a history of job or home stress, anxiety from lack of sleep, sudden stoppage of prescribed drugs such as diazepam (Valium), or a history of drug use that increases sensitivity of the respiratory centers, such as high concentrations of salicylate. These individuals usually unknowingly breathe too rapidly, which disturbs the normal balance of carbon dioxide in the blood.

At the outset, individuals may feel a tightness in the chest and have a feeling of air hunger; they feel that they cannot fill the lungs because they cannot get enough air. Commonly these individuals will become very apprehensive, which only leads to increased hyperventilation and at times to syncope (fainting). Palpitation of the heart, abdominal pain, and a feeling of fullness in the throat may also occur.

Immediate first aid treatment is to have the individual breathe into a paper bag held tightly over the mouth and nose for 10 minutes or more to replace the carbon dioxide that has been given off during hyperventilation. Removing the victim from the surroundings is helpful, because commonly people who are trying to help the victim become very excited and anxious and unknowingly only promote the victim's anxiety and subsequent hyperventilation. In all cases, the first aider or medical assistant should be the calming influence and provide reassurance to the victim.

When frequent attacks of hyperventilation occur, it is recommended that the victim seek medical attention for treatment of the underlying cause(s).

INSULIN REACTIONS AND DIABETIC COMA

Diabetes mellitus is a disorder of carbohydrate metabolism in which the ability to oxidize and use carbohydrates is lost and a subsequent derangement of protein and fat metabolism occurs. This results from disturbances in the normal insulin mechanism, a hormone secreted by the islands of Langerhans in the pancreas.

Table 30.1

Signs and symptoms of insulin reactions and diabetic coma

	Insulin reaction	Diabetic coma
Onset	Gradual	Sudden
Skin	Perspiration, pallor, cold and damp skin	Flushed and dry skin, dry tongue
Behavior	Tremors, restlessness, fatigue, faint feeling, headache, confusion or strange behavior	Weakness, drowsiness, lethargy
Gastrointestinal tract	Extreme hunger, nausea	Thirst, nausea, and vomiting
Vision	Double vision	Eyeball tension low
Respiration	Shallow	Difficulty in breathing or air hunger
Pulse	Rapid or normal	Rapid, weak
Speech	Slurred	
Breath	No acetone smell	Sweet or fruity odor; smell of acetone
Level of consciousness	May have loss of consciousness	Coma if unattended
Blood glucose	Low (40-70 mg/100 ml)	High (over 200 mg/100 ml)
Urine test	Sugar—absent, or a trace at most Acetone—negative	Sugar—positive in high amounts Acetone—positive

From Zakus SM: Clinical skills and assisting techniques for the medical assistant, ed 2, St Louis, 1988, The CV Mosby Co.

Adverse conditions can occur when a diabetic is undiagnosed or does not follow the therapy prescribed or when there is a disturbance in the normal functions of the body. All persons with diabetes, their immediate families, and persons in the health care professions should know the signs and symptoms and the treatment or immediate first aid for an insulin reaction (too much insulin or presence of insulin without food) and diabetic coma (a condition that may develop when there is lack of insulin in the diabetic patient's system) (Table 30.1). Diabetics should carry a card stating the fact that they are diabetic, their daily insulin or oral hypoglycemic drug dosage, their address, and the name and address of their physician. Many diabetics wear Medic-Alert bracelets or necklaces, which indicate their condition in case of emergency situations requiring treatment.

First Aid
Insulin reaction

1. If the patient is conscious, give some form of simple sugar, such as hard candy, sugar, or sweetened orange juice.
2. Seek medical attention if the patient does not respond readily to these measures.
3. If the patient is unconscious, do not force fluids or food. Call the physician, or get the patient to the hospital immediately.

Diabetic coma

There is *no adequate first aid* treatment for hyperglycemia or diabetic coma. *Immediate medical treatment is necessary.*

OPEN WOUNDS

Types of wounds include abrasions, avulsions, incisions, lacerations, and puncture wounds. See pp. 394 and 395 and Figure 21.22.

First Aid Care for Minor Wounds

1. Wash your hands thoroughly before treating any wound to minimize the possibility of infection.
2. Observe the wound to check for foreign objects, such as pieces of glass, wood, and dirt.
3. Control bleeding (see pp. 635-638).
4. Gently wash the skin around the wound with soap and water. Wash away from the wound, not toward it.
5. For minor cuts, scratches, and abrasions, wash the wound well with soap and water to remove foreign matter.
   - Lacerations and incisions may be irrigated with large amounts of water or normal saline. Do not apply an antiseptic unless instructed to do so by the physician.
   - For puncture wounds, gently squeeze the

wound to encourage a small amount of bleeding to help wash out microorganisms. Then wash the wound with soap and water.
- Wounds with severe bleeding should not be cleansed.

6. Cover the wound with a sterile dressing, and bandage it in place. Use the cleanest material on hand when sterile dressings are not available.

7. Refer the person to the physician for follow-up care. Tetanus immunization may be required. Lacerations, incisions, and avulsions will require medical attention, because they may have to be sutured.

8. Advise the person to be alert for signs of infection, and if present, to seek medical attention. Signs to watch for are as follows:
   - Redness and swelling;
   - Heat and increasing tenderness;
   - Drainage;
   - Red streaks away from the wound;
   - Fever; and
   - Excessive pain.

POISONING

The symptoms of poisoning vary greatly and depend on the type and amount of substance taken. All types of poisonings are considered emergencies that require immediate attention. Points that should be considered when poisoning is suspected follow:

- Look for any physical changes, such as an abrupt onset of pain or illness; burns or stains around the mouth or on the face, which would indicate poisoning with a caustic substance; breath odor, which may indicate the type of poison ingested; or depressed consciousness and an irregular heartbeat.
- Observe the surroundings for empty containers, spilled fluids, or containers of substances that would be poisonous if ingested.
- Obtain information from the person or an observer when possible.

Objectives of First Aid Measures

- To dilute or neutralize the poison.
- To induce vomiting, *except* when the person has swallowed corrosive or petroleum products, when the person is unconscious, or when the person is convulsing.
- To prevent absorption of the poison.
- To maintain an open airway, breathing, and vital functions.
- To obtain medical attention without delay.

First Aid

Speed is essential to stop absorption of a poison. First aid for poisoning depends on the type of poison ingested. It is not possible for the first aider or medical assistant to know exactly what to do for all cases, but general guidelines must be followed.

1. In all cases, monitor the person's vital signs, maintain an open airway, and be prepared to administer cardiopulmonary resuscitation if necessary.

2. Make every effort to determine what, when, and how much was ingested.

3. Obtain specific information to follow when this is possible. Call the physician, or the poison control center that is in the nearest city, or the hospital emergency physician. Antidote labels may be on the product ingested, but *caution* must be taken, because the label may be out of date and incorrect. Poison control centers are open 24 hours a day and maintain antidote information on several thousand available commercial products. Most states have a poison control center in the major cities. Keep this number on hand with other important telephone numbers.

4. Carry out the specific first aid instructions obtained.

5. When specific directions cannot be obtained, the following may be performed:

- If the person is awake and able to swallow, milk or water may be given to dilute the poison.
- *Do not induce vomiting* if the person (1) is unconscious or in a coma; (2) is having a convulsion; (3) has ingested a petroleum product, such as kerosene, lighter fluid, gasoline; (4) has ingested a corrosive substance, for example, strong acids or alkalis. In these situations, if the person can swallow, give the following:
  - (a) For acids: milk, water, or milk of magnesia (1 tablespoon to 1 cup of water).
  - (b) For alkalis: milk, water, any fruit juice, or vinegar; for persons 1 to 5 years old—1 to 2 cups, for persons 5 years and older—up to 1 quart.
- If the person has ingested a *noncorrosive* substance and is *not* unconscious or convulsing:
  - (a) Give 1 tablespoon of syrup of ipecac, followed by 1 cup of water. Keep children active. Repeat the same dose in 15 minutes if vomiting has not occurred. *Repeat only once.*
  - (b) If ipecac is not available, attempt to induce vomiting by giving milk or water and then placing the blunt end of a

spoon or your finger at the back of the person's throat. Mild soapy water may also induce vomiting if ipecac is not available.

(c) When retching and vomiting begin, place the person's head down with the head lower than the hips. This prevents vomitus from entering the lungs, causing further injury.

(d) When the poison is unknown, save the vomitus, and take it to the physician or hospital for analysis.

NOTE: The universal antidote of 2 parts burned toast, 1 part milk of magnesia, and 1 part strong tea that was formerly recommended is now believed to be *useless*. Therefore, *do not* waste time preparing this mixture for administration.

6. Arrange for transportation of the person to the physician or the hospital. *All cases of poisoning must receive medical attention.*

7. Remain calm at all times. Stay with the person, and provide reassurance.

POISON CONTROL CENTERS

Poison control centers have been established in many cities across the nation to provide quick and reliable information on possible poisonings or drug-related problems. They provide information on the appropriate first aid and clinical management to use for cases of suspected or known poisoning. Some centers also offer specialized poisoning treatment and consultant services, professional training, and poisoning prevention education for consumers. Many centers are staffed by clinical pharmacists 24 hours a day, every day of the year.

Not all states have poison control centers, but rely on centers in nearby cities. Some states have state designated centers that are located in two or three major cities in that state. Other states have poison control centers that are regional centers established by a particular city. These centers are normally financed locally and are usually located at major hospitals or major medical universities. The telephone number of the nearest poison control center should be posted at a nearby telephone at work and at home so that information can be obtained as quickly as possible when the need arises.

For a list of poison control centers in the United States write to: Publication Office of Veterinary and Human Toxicology, Comparative Toxicology Laboratories, Kansas State University, Manhattan, KS 66506; telephone: (916) 532-5679.

FIRST AID KIT

The best time to provide the office, home, or automobile first aid kit is *before* it is needed. Check the first aid kit kept in the office, home, and family automobile *now*. A properly equipped kit, with fresh supplies that are kept replenished after use, is a practical aid in relieving many minor injuries and ailments. It may even be lifesaving before medical help arrives. The following first aid supplies are suggested:

- Sterile gauze pads;
- Sterile gauze roller bandages;
- Adhesive tape;
- Adhesive dressings;
- Sterile absorbent cotton;
- Triangular bandage;
- Elastic bandage;
- A mild antiseptic;
- Syrup of ipecac;
- Analgesic, such as aspirin and/or acetaminophen;
- Petroleum jelly;
- Calamine lotion;
- Aromatic spirits of ammonia;
- Tweezers;
- A scissors with rounded ends;
- Clinical thermometer;
- Flashlight;
- Safety pins;
- Sugar for diabetics; and a
- First aid book.

For automobiles, the American National Red Cross suggests a specially designed compact unit with standardized first aid materials fitted into a case, like blocks. The packet is readily stored, and the supplies do not become easily disarranged. Each packet is clearly labeled, and instructions for use are included. These kits can be obtained at automobile supply stores and department stores with contents selected to meet the purchaser's particular needs. Ask your physician regarding other medications for such things as car sickness, upset stomach, and allergies. Take some road flares for car safety.

Regardless of how well equipped the first aid kit is, its effective use depends on individuals knowing how to give aid properly. A course in first aid, as well as training in cardiopulmonary resuscitation (CPR), can be an invaluable investment.

For additional drugs and supplies that may be kept in the physician's office or clinic for emergency situations, see "Emergency Tray" in Chapter 23.

Conclusion

In the event of a sudden illness or an accident that causes trauma to a person, the trained, competent medical assistant should be prepared to properly administer the appropriate first aid treatment and obtain medical assistance as needed. In time of emergencies, prompt action must be taken. It is important that the medical assistant remain calm in all cases and provide care in a competent, orderly, and organized manner. Do not perform procedures that you have not been trained to do. To maintain your skills and knowledge in first aid and cardiopulmonary resuscitation, it is suggested that you enroll in a refresher course every few years.

Review Questions

1. Define cardiopulmonary resuscitation. State the goal of CPR, and discuss the ABCs of basic life support.
2. List three factors that determine if a situation is an emergency.
3. As a medical assistant you are responsible for rendering first aid when the need arises. Define first aid, and state the contributions you can make for the physical and psychological care of the victim in an emergency situation.
4. List four fundamental rules and procedures to follow in a medical emergency.
5. Mr. Bill Bailey has been experiencing uncomfortable pressure and pain in the center of the chest, shortness of breath, and slight nausea for the past 3 minutes. What medical condition would you suspect him to have? What type of action should be taken for this condition?
6. Define shock. List and explain the five types of shock. List eight outstanding symptoms of shock.
7. Dave Rubin has just had minor surgery in the physician's office. As you are assisting him after the procedure, you observe that he is very pale and his skin quite cold to the touch. You immediately take his vital signs and find that the pulse is weak and rapid, the blood pressure 92/70, and respirations 34 and shallow. What condition would you suspect that he is experiencing? What must be your immediate actions?
8. Ray Wood is cleaning the windows in your office. By accident, he breaks a window. He comes running to you at the desk. You observe that he is clutching his wrist and that there is bright red blood spurting from his wrist as well as from his hand and fingers. State the type of bleeding this would indicate, the vessel that may be cut, and the first aid treatment that you would administer.
9. Ann O'Brien, a diabetic patient, is displaying the signs and symptoms of an insulin reaction. List six signs and symptoms of insulin reaction. State the immediate care that you could provide for Ann.
10. List at least 15 items that you would include when compiling supplies for a first aid kit.

SUGGESTED READINGS

Daleske EE and others: The who, what, and when of tetanus prophylaxis, Patient Care 10:144, Aug 1976.

National Safety Council: Accident facts, Chicago, 1981, The Council.

Renshaw D: Psychiatric first aid in an emergency, Am J Nurs 72:497, 1972.

Appendix A

Common Medical Terminology Combining Word Parts

In this appendix the basic elements of medical word-making are presented. A scientific vocabulary that conveys complex ideas and descriptions is needed. Our medical traditions and word sources have been commonly taken from Greek and Latin writings.

Learning a medical vocabulary becomes a matter of memorizing a few score Greek and Latin prefixes, suffixes, and word roots and combining them systematically to make thousands of precise terms.

When studying, the student should have at hand a good medical dictionary. Spelling, pronunciation, word structure, and usage need to be verified constantly if one is to build a medical vocabulary.

The base word we call the *root;* the combining modifier (or affix) we call the *prefix* when it is placed *before* the root, or the *suffix* when we place it *after* the root. Thus in the foregoing sentence, *pre-* and *suf-* are prefixes to *-fix. Ophthalmo-* (eye) and *-scope* (instrument for viewing) become *ophthalmoscope,* an instrument for examining the eye. *Oto-* (ear) and *-scope* become *otoscope,* an instrument for examining the ear. Combining the suffix *-itis,* meaning inflammation, with the base words *tonsilla, peritoneum, otos,* and *osteon,* we get *tonsillitis, peritonitis, otitis,* and *osteitis.*

Prefixes and suffixes give special meaning to the ideas the roots express. In English we have, for example, *before*hand, handi*ness* and handi*craft.* Memorize the following commonly used prefixes, world elements, and suffixes. Get the feel of their usage in medical-word construction.

Prefixes and word elements	Common usage	Examples*
a-, an-	without, absent,	*a*plasia
ab-	away from	*ab*duct
ad-	to, at	*ad*hesive
aden/o	gland	*aden*osis
alb/o	white	*alb*icans
album-	white, albumin	*album*inuria
alveolo-	alveoli	*alveolo*tomy
ana-,/an-	up, too much, backward	*ana*phylaxis
angi/o	blood vessel	*angi*ogram
ankyl/osis	bent, crooked, adhesion	*ankyl*osis
ante-	before	*ante*febrile
antero-	in front of, before	*antero*grade
anti-	against, opposed to	*anti*biotic, *anti*body
aort/o	aorta	*aort*itis
appendic/o	appendix	*appendic*itis
arteri/o	artery	*arteri*osclerosis
arthr/o	joint	*arthr*opathy
audi/o	hearing	*audi*ogram
auto-	self	*auto*graft
bacteri/o	bacteria	*bacteri*uria
bi-	two	*bi*lateral
blast-	germ cell	*blast*oma
blenno: see muco-		
blephar/o	eyelid	*blephar*oplasty
brady-	slow	*brady*cardia
bronch/o	bronchus	*bronch*itis
bucc/o	cheek	*bucc*al
burs/o	bursa	*burs*itis
cardi/o	heart	electro*cardi*ogram
cephal/o	head	*cephal*ogram
cerebr/o	cerebrum	*cerebr*opathy
cervic/o	neck, cervix	*cervic*al; *cervic*itis
cheil/o	lip	*cheil*oplasty
cholecyst-	gallbladder	*cholecyst*ectomy
chondr/o	cartilage	*chondr*itis
coccus	coccus (bacterium)	strepto*coccus*
col/o	colon	*col*ostomy
colp/o	vagina	*colp*ostenosis
cost/o	rib	*cost*overtebral
crani/o	cranium	*crani*otomy
cyan/o	blue	*cyan*osis
cyst/o	bladder	*cyst*ocele
cyto-	cell	*cyto*plasm
dacry/o	tears	*dacry*agogic
dacryocyst/o	lacrimal sac	*dacryocyst*itis
dent/o	tooth	*dent*algia
derm-	skin	*derm*al
dermat/o	skin	*dermat*ology
dextr/o	to the right side	*dextr*ocardia
dia-	through	*dia*phragm

*As you study, find these words in the medical dictionary and include them in your vocabulary. Also note that the terminal vowel of some prefixes, usually *o* but often *i* or even *a*, is dropped when the word root begins with a vowel, such as *hyp*esthesia, *kal*emia, and *lamin*ectomy.

Continued.

Prefixes and word elements	Common usage	Examples*
diplo-	double	*diplo*pia
dis-	to separate	*dis*articulate
doch/o	duct	chole*doch*ectomy
duoden/o	duodenum	*duoden*oscopy
dys-	difficult, painful	*dys*pnea
ec-, ex-	out of, away from	*ec*topy, *ex*crete
ecto-	outside	*ecto*pic
electro-	electric in nature	*electro*cardiogram
emesis	vomit	hemat*emesis*
emesis	vomit	hemat*emesis*
encephal/o	brain, or enclosed within the head	*encephal*ogram
endo-	within, inside of	*endo*cardium
enter/o	intestine	*entero*colitis
epi-	on, over	*epi*dermis, *epi*dural
erythr/o	red	*erythr*ocyte
esophag/o	esophagus	*esophag*itis
esthesia	sensation	an*esthesia*
eti-	causation	*eti*ology
ex/o	outside	*exo*cardia
extra-	outside of	*extra*dural, *extra*peritoneal
gastro-	stomach	*gastro*enteritis
gen/o	producing	*gen*esis
gingiv/o	gums	*gingiv*itis
gloss/o	tongue	*gloss*itis
glyc/o	sugar	*glyc*ogen
gyne-, gyneco-	women	*gyne*cology
hemat/o	blood	*hemat*emesis
hemi-	one half	*hemi*plegia
hem/o	blood	*hem*atoma
hepat/o	liver	*hepat*itis
hidr/o	sweat	*hidr*osis
hist/o	tissue	*hist*ology
hydr/o	water	*hydr*otherapy
hyper-	over, excessive, increased	*hyper*alimentation, *hyper*esthesia, *hyper*trophy
hyp/o	under, below, less	*hypo*tension, *hypo*dermic, *hypo*gastric,
hyster/o	uterus	*hyster*ectomy
iatro	physician, medicine	*iatro*genic
im- (replaces *in-* before *b, m,* or *p*)	negative prefix, not	*im*balance
in-	negative prefix, not	*in*operable
in-	in, into	*in*clusion
infra-	below	*infra*patellar
inter- (contrast *intra-*)	between, among	*in*ercostal
intra-	within, inside of (separate the double *a* with a hyphen)	*intra*-articular, *intra*muscular, *intra*venous,
intro-	into, within	*intro*spection
intus-	in, into	*intus*susception
ipsi-	self, the same	*ipsi*lateral
ir-	not	*ir*regular, *ir*reversible
ir-	in, into	*ir*radiate

Prefixes and word elements	Common usage	Examples*
ir/o, irid/o	iris	*irid*ocele
isch- (pronounced *isk*)	to suppress	*isch*emia
ischi/o (pronounced *iskee [o]*)	ischium	*ischi*ectomy, *eischio*dynia
iso-	equal, alike	*iso*tonic
juxta-	near	*juxta*-articular, *juxta*position
kal-, kali-	potassium (K⁺)	*kal*emia
karyo-	nucleus	*karyo*cyte
kerat/o	horny tissue, cornea	*kerat*osis, *kerat*itis
keto-	carbonyl group (through German from Latin *acetum*, vinegar)	*keto*genic, *keto*sis
kilo-	one thousand	*kilo*gram, *kilo*meter, *kilo*volt
kine-, kinesi/o	movement	*kinesi*ology
labio-	lip (compare *labium*, lip, and *labrum*, edge of lip)	*labio*plasty
lacrima, lacrimo-	tears	*lacrima*tory
lact/o	milk	*lact*igenous
lalo-	speech; babbling	*lalo*gnosis, *lalo*plegia, *lal*orrhea,
lamell/a	thin leaf or plate (a little lamina)	*lamell*iform
lamin/a	thin plate or layer	*lamin*ectomy
lapar/o	abdomen	*lapar*otomy
laryng/o	larynx	*laryng*itis
lepto-	delicate, slender, thin	*lepto*cyte, *lepto*meninges
leuko-, leuco-	white (*leuko-* is preferred)	*leuko*cyte, *leuk*emia (o omitted before another vowel)
levo-	to the left side	*levo*cardia, *levo*rotation
lip/o	fat, lipid	*lip*ase, *lipo*tropic
litho-	stone, calculus	*litho*nephritis
lob/o	lobe	*lob*ectomy
lymphaden/o	lymph gland	*lymphaden*opathy
lympho-	lymph	*lympho*blast, *lympho*sarcoma
macro-	large, abnormally long	*macro*scopic, *macro*cyte
malacia	softening	cerebro*malacia*
mamm/o	breast	*mammo*gram
mast/o	breast	*mast*ectomy
melan/o	black	*melan*oma
mening/o	meninges	*mening*eal
meso-	middle, intermediate, mesentery	*meso*derm, *meso*appendix
metr/o	uterus	*metr*optosis
micro-	small (in Greek originally *short*)	*micro*scopic, *micro*cyte
mito-	thread, threadlike, mitosis	*mito*chondria, *mito*genesis
mon/o	one, single	*mono*blast, *mono*cular
mortem	death	post*mortem*

Continued.

Prefixes and word elements	Common usage	Examples*
muco- (Latin); *myxo-* and *blenno-* (Greek)	mucus	*muco*sa, *muco*purulent, *myxo*ma, *myxo*rrhea or *blenno*rrhea
multi-	many, much	*multi*factorial, *multi*form
my-; see *myo-*		
mycet-, *myc/o*	fungus	*myco*logy, *myco*bacterial
myelo-	marrow, often specifically spinal cord	*myelo*blastoma, *myelo*cele, *myelo*cyte
my/o	muscle	*my*atrophy or *myo*atrophy, *myo*cardial, *myo*tonia
myring/o	eardrum	*myringo*plasty
nas/o	nose	*naso*pharyngitis
natal	birth	*natal*ity
natr/i	sodium (Na⁺)	*natr*emia
necr/o	death	*necr*osis
neo-	new	*neo*natal, *neo*plastic
nephr/o	kidney	*nephr*itis, *nephr*ostomy
neur/o	nerve or nervous system	*neur*ectomy, *neuro*dermatitis, *neuro*fibroma
non-	without; not	*non*union
normo-	normal, usual	*normo*blast, *normo*calcemia
nos/o	disease	*noso*comial, *noso*logy
oculo-	eye	*oculo*facial, *oculo*motor
odont/o	teeth	*odont*algia, *odonto*blast
olig/o	few, scanty	*olig*uria
onc/o	mass, bulk, tumor	*onco*logy
onych/o	nails	*onycho*dystrophy, *onycho*gryphosis, *onycho*mycosis
oo- (Greek); *ov/i*, *ov/o* (Latin)	egg, ovum	*oo*genesis, *ovi*parous, *ov*iod
oophor/o	ovary	*oophor*ectomy
ophthalm/o	eye	*ophthalmo*scope
orchi/o	testes	*orchio*plasty
orchid/o	testes	*orchid*ectomy
orth/o	straight, normal, correct	*ortho*pedic
ost-, *osteo-*	bone	*ost*ectomy, *osteo*malacia
ot/o	ear	*oto*scope
ox/o, *oxy*	oxygen	*oxy*genation
pan-	all	*pan*carditis, *pan*hysterosalpingo-oophorectomy
para-	beyond, beside, apart, accessory to	*para*-appendicitis, *para*colitis
partum	birth	post*partum*
ped-	child; foot	*ped*iatrics; *ped*al
peri-	around	*peri*anal, *peri*osteum
phagia	swallowing	dys*phagia*
pharyng/o	pharynx	*pharyng*itis
phasia	speech	dys*phasia*
phleb/o	vein	*phleb*itis

Prefixes and word elements	Common usage	Examples*
phobia	fear	acro*phobia*
phon/o	sound	*phono*cardiogram, *phono*-myogram
phot/o	light (the radiation)	*phot*ometer
phren-, phrenic-	diaphragm, mind, of the phrenic nerve	*phren*ectomy or *phrenic*ectomy
phys-, physio-	nature, physiology, or physical things	*phys*iatry, *physio*therapy
pilo-	hair	*pilo*nidal
plegia	paralysis	para*plegia*
pneumato-, pneumo-, pneumon-	lungs, air in lungs, breath	*pneumo*encephalogram, *pneumon*ia
post-	after	*post*partum
pre-	before	*pre*natal
proct/o	rectum	*prot*oscope
prostat/o	prostate gland	*prostat*ectomy
pseud/o	false	*pseud*oankylosis
pulm/o	lung; air or gas	*pulm*onary
py/o	pus	*py*ocyst
pyel/o	kidney pelvis	*pyel*ogram
quadri-, quadru-	four	*quadri*ceps, *quadri*plegia
radi/o	x radiation, radius bone, short-wave radiation	*radio*active, *radio*carpal, *radio*thermy
recto-	rectum	*recto*cele, *recto*sigmoid
ren/o	kidney	*ren*al
retin/o	retina	*retin*itis
retro-	backward, behind	*retro*cecal, *retro*bulbar
rhin/o	nose, noselike	*rhin*itis
sacr/o	sacrum	*sacro*coccygeal, *sacr*oiliac
salping/o	tube (uterine or auditory)	*salping*ectomy, *salpin*gopharyngeal
sangui-	blood	*sangui*nous
sarc/o	flesh	*sarc*oidosis, *sarc*oma
scler/o	hard	*scler*edema, *sclero*derma
semi-	half, partly	*semi*coma, *semi*flexion
sinistr/o	left side; left	*sinistr*aural, *sinistro*manual
spleno- (lien/o)	spleen	*spleno*megaly, *lien*ectomy
spondyl/o	vertebra, vertebrae, spinal column	*spondyl*itis, *spondyl*olysis
staped/o	stapes	*staped*ectomy
staphyl/o	resembling a bunch grapes	*staphyl*ococcus
sten/o	narrow, contracting	*sten*osis
stere/o	solid, three dimensional	*stere*ognosis, *stere*ogram
stomatlo	mouth	*stoma*titis
sub-	under, near, almost	*sub*acute, *sub*clinical, *sub*ungual
supra-	above	*supra*renal
sym-, syn-, sys-, sy-	together; union or association	*sym*physis, *syn*apse, *syn*drome
synov/io	synovial	*synov*itis
tachy-	swift, rapid	*tachy*cardia

Continued.

Prefixes and word elements	Common usage	Examples*
teno- (less used: tendo-, tendino-, tenonto-)	tendon	tenoplasty (tendinoplasty, tendoplasty), tenodesis, tenotomy
tetra-	four	tetrabasic, tetralogy
therm/o	heat	thermal, thermometer
thorac/o thoracico-	chest	thoracalgia, thoracocentesis
thromb/o	clot, thrombus	thrombectomy; thromboembolism
thyr/o	thyroid	thyrotomy
tomo-	a cutting, a section	tomography
trachel/o	trachea	tracheostomy
trans-	through, across	transfusion
tri-	three	triceps
tympan/o	tympanic membrane or eardrum	tympanitis
ungu/o	nail	unguinal
uni	one	unilateral
ureter/o	ureter	ureteritis
urethr/o	urethra	urethritis
urin/o, ur/o	urine	urinalysis, urinometer
vas/o	vessel, a duct	vasoconstriction, vasectomy
ven/o	vein	venogram
xanth/o	yellow	xanthelasma, santhochromia
xer/o	dry; dryness	xeroderma, xerography
xiph-, xiphi-, xipho-	xiphoid process (swordlike)	xiphisternal, xiphocostal
zoo- (pronounced zō-ō, not zū)	animal	zoonosis
zyg/o	yoked, joined	zygapophysis, zygote

Suffixes	Common usage	Examples*
-ac	pertaining to	cardiac
-al	pertaining to	oral
-algia	pain	arthralgia
-ase	an enzyme	amylase
-centesis	puncture and aspiration of	paracentesis, amniocentesis, anthrocentesis
-cele	hernia, cavity, tumor	hydrocele, rectocele
-clasis	breaking	osteoclasis
-clysis	to wash out	hypodermoclysis
-desis	binding	arthrodesis
-dynia	pain	cephalodynia
-ectasis	dilatation, distention	colpectasis
-ectomy	excision of an organ or part	appendectomy, gastretomy
-emia	blood condition	hypervolemia, septicemia
-gnosis	knowledge	diagnosis
-gram	recorded; written	electrocardiogram

Suffixes	Common usage	Examples*
-graphy	making a graphic tracing or recording	electrodardio*graphy*
-ia	state; condition; disease	card*ia*
-iac	pertaining to	card*iac*
-iasis	condition of; process or its result	cholelith*iasis*
-itis	inflammation	gingiv*itis*, gloss*itis*
-logy	word, reason, science, study of	patho*logy*, etio*logy*, embryo*logy*
-lysis	dissolution, releasing, freeing	hemo*lysis*
-megaly	enlarged	hepato*megaly*
-meter	measure	sphygmomano*meter*
-odynia	pain condition	ophthalm*odynia* (same as ophthalm*algia*)
-oid	resembling, like	lip*oid*
-ologist	specialist; expert in the study of	cardi*ologist*
-ology	study or science	cardi*ology*
-oma	tumor	aden*oma*
-opia, opsia	vision	dipl*opia*, hemian*opsia*
-ose	carbohydrate (sugars, starches, and cellu-loses)	glu*cose* cellul*ose*
-osis	process, disease, abnormal increase	hepat*osis*
-para	bring forth (woman who has born viable young)	multi*para*, nulli*para*, primi*para*
-pathy	disease	neuro*pathy*, myo*pathy*, osteo*pathy*
-penia	abnormal reduction in number	erythro*penia*, leuko*penia*, neutro*penia*
-pexy, -pexia	surgical fixation of an organ, suspension	nephro*pexy*
-plasty	shaping or surgical formation of	arthro*plasty*, mamma*plasty* or mammo-*plasty*, rhino*plasty*
-pnea	breathing	dys*pnea*
-ptosis	drooping; sagging	nephro*ptosis*
-ptysis	cough up	hemo*ptysis*
-rrhage, -rrhagia	a bursting forth, excessive flow	hemo*rrhage*, meno*rrhagia*, metro*rrhagia*
-rrhaphy	surgical repair by suture	hernio*rrhaphy*, teno*rrhaphy*
-rrhea	flow, discharge	dysmeno*rrhea*
-scope	instrument for observing	oto*scope*, ophthalmo*scope*, broncho*scope*, arthro*scope*, sigmoido*scope*, laryngo-*scope*
-scopy	examination of	gastro*scopy*
-sect	act of cutting, sectioning	dis*sect*
-stomy	(mouth) surgical creation of an opening of a viscus for drainage or for communica-tion from one viscus to another	colo*stomy*, tracheo*stomy*, gastrojejunos-*tomy*
-tome	instrument for cutting	myringo*tome*, osteo*tome*
-tomy	act of cutting, incising	tracheo*tomy*, gastro*tomy*
-trophy	nutrition, as it has to do with vitality and growth	a*trophy*, hyper*trophy*
-uria	urine condition	dys*uria*, an*uria*, olig*uria*

Appendix B

Medical Abbreviations

In a patient's medical case history, physical examination report, and notes on the chart, you will encounter a variety of abbreviations. The following list includes some of the more common abbrevations. They are grouped together according to general usage. You should recall some of these, while others are new. Pay special attention to when capital letters are used and when not used. Prescription abbreviations are given in Chapter 23. Others were given in the appropriate chapters.*

    Body systems
        HEENT—head, eyes, ears, nose, and throat
        ENT—ear, nose, and throat
        CR—cardiorespiratory
        CVS—cardiovascular system
        GI—gastrointestinal
        GU—genitourinary
        CNS—central nervous system
        MS—musculoskeletal
        NM—neuromuscular
    Patient's history
        CC—chief complaint
        PI *or* HIP—present illness or history of present illness
        PH—past history
        LMD—local medical doctor
        UCHD *or* UCD—usual childhood diseases
        FH—family history
        a & w *or* A & W—alive and well
        ROS—review of systems
        PTA—prior to admission
        c/o—complains of
    Physical examination (PE)
        wd—well-developed

        wn—well-nourished
        IPPA—inspection, percussion, palpation, and auscultation
        P & A—percussion and auscultation
        BP—blood pressure
        TPR—temperature, pulse, and respirations
        WNL—within normal limits
        wt—weight
        ht—height
    Diagnosis
        Diag *or* Dx—diagnosis
        R/O—rule out
        POS—problem-oriented system
    Ears
        TM—tympanic membrane(s)
    Eyes
        REM—rapid eye movements
        L & A—light and accommodation
        PERLA—pupils equal and reacting to light and accommodation
        EOM—extraocular movements
        RRE—round, regular, and equal
        OS—left eye
        OD—right eye
        OU—both eyes
    Chest (heart and lungs)
        P & A—percussion and auscultation
        PND—paroxysmal nocturnal dyspnea
        SOB—shortness of breath
        PMI—point of maximal intensity (or impulse)
        MCL—midclavicular line
        ICS—intercostal space
        NSR—normal sinus rhythm
        RSR—regular sinus rhythm
        ASHD—arteriosclerotic heart disease
        MI—myocardial infarction
        EKG *or* ECG—electrocardiogram
        AV—arteriovenous, atrioventricular
        CHF—congestive heart failure

*According to the style of the American Medical Association, medical and pharmaceutical abbreviations are to be written *without* the use of periods. That is, rather than writing a.c. as was done in the past, you will now write ac, and so on.

RHD—rheumatic heart disease
URI—upper respiratory infection
COPD—chronic obstructive pulmonary disease
CHD—coronary heart disease
Abdomen and GI
LKS—liver, kidney, spleen *or* LKKS—liver, kidneys, and spleen
GB—gallbladder
BM—bowel movement
Female reproductive system
BUS—Bartholin, urethral, and Skene glands
LMP—last menstrual period
OB—obstetrics
PID—pelvic inflammatory disease
GYN—gynecology
EDC—expected date of confinement
FHT—fetal heart tones
L & D—labor and delivery
PP—postpartum
IUD—intrauterine device
SAB—spontaneous abortion (miscarriage)
Musculoskeletal system
EMG—electromyogram
MS—multiple sclerosis
LOM—loss of movement or motion
cva—costovertebral angle
DTR—deep tendon reflexes
Fx—fracture
ROM—range of motion
Central nervous system
CSF—cerebrospinal fluid
CVA—cerebrovascular accident
EEG—electroencephalogram
DTR—deep tendon reflexes
Laboratory
CBC—complete blood count
UA—urinalysis
O_2—oxygen
CO_2—carbon dioxide
CSF—cerebrospinal fluid
SMA—sequential multiple analysis
HGB *or* HG *or* HB—hemoglobin
Hct—hematocrit
WBC—white blood count
RBC—red blood count
Diff—differential (blood count)
Protime *or* PT—prothrombin time
pH—hydrogen ion concentration, referring to the degree of acidity or alkalinity of a solution
BUN—blood urea nitrogen
Sedrate—sedimentation rate
Rh—Rhesus blood factor

PKU—phenylketonuria
FBS—fasting blood sugar
PBI—protein-bound iodine
PCV—packed cell volume
RhA—rheumatoid arthritis
STS—serologic test for syphilis
VDRL—Venereal Disease Research Laboratory
C & S—culture and sensitivity
CPK—creatine phosphokinase
LDH—lactic dehydrogenase
X-ray studies
A-P and Lat—anterior, posterior, and lateral
IVP—intravenous pyelogram
GBS—gallbladder series
CT—computed tomography
MRI—magnetic resonance imaging
BE—barium enema
KUB—kidneys, ureter, bladder
UGI—upper gastrointestinal series
Surgical terms
T & A—tonsillectomy and adenoidectomy
D & C—dilation and curettage
I & D—incision and drainage
TUR—transurethral resection
TURP—transurethral resection of the prostate
Hospital departments
ICU—intensive care unit
CCU—coronary care unit
ER—emergency room
OR—operating room
RR *or* PAR—recovery room or postanesthetic room
Lab—laboratory
Path—pathology
OPD—outpatient department
Peds—pediatrics
RT—respiratory therapy
General
Ca *or* CA—cancer or carcinoma
d/c *or* D/C—discontinue
DOA—dead on arrival
OD—overdose
cm—centimeter
lb—pounds
kg or kilos—kilograms
ac—before meals
pc—after meals
stat—immediately
prn—whenever necessary
ad lib—as desired
ASAP—as soon as possible
BR—bed rest

BP—blood pressure
I & O—intake and output
IM—intramuscular
IV—intravenous
sc or SubQ—subcutaneous
LP—lumbar puncture
NPO—nothing by mouth
D/W—dextrose in water
S/W—saline in water
DOB—date of birth
FUO—fever of unknown (or undetermined)
  origin
GC—gonococcus or gonorrhea
K—potassium
LE—lupus erythematosus
NYD—not yet diagnosed
PM—postmortem
TB—tuberculosis
O_2—oxygen
CO_2—carbon dioxide
pt—patient
TLC—tender loving care

Symbols
>—greater than
<—less than
♂—male
♀—female
↑—above, increase
↓—below, decrease
×—times (multiply by)
%—percentage
#—number
=—equals
+—plus
−—minus
ō—none
c̄—with
s̄—without
ā—before
p̄—after

Appendix C

Special Vocabulary and Sample Reports

SPECIAL VOCABULARY
Part 1—Vocabulary Used to Decrease Pain
Types of pain

In performing the complete history and physical examination, the examiner must deal with a variety of terms relating to pain. The following are some of these particular terms, along with an explanation of each term.

- Superficial or cutaneous;
- Deep pain—from muscles, tendons, joints;
- Visceral pain—from the viscera; any large interior organ in any great body cavity, especially those in the abdomen.

Adaptation does not exist in the sense of pain. This is especially important, because pain may be a warning signal of danger, and if one became used to pain and ignored it, damage to the body would follow.

Terms relating to pain

radiating Pain diverging from a common central point; for example, gallbladder pain begins in the right upper quadrant of the abdomen, and it is diverted from that central point to the right flank and right scapular area.

stabbing Deep, sharp intermittent pain.

intractable Unmanageable, not controllable with conventional means, that is, rest, heat, medication.

colicky Acute intermittent abdominal pain usually caused by spasmodic contractions.

excruciating Torturing, extreme pain, often intractable.

exquisite Intense pain to which an individual is extremely sensitive.

transient Fleeting, brief, passing, coming and going.

threshold The level that must be exceeded for an effect to be produced; the level of pain that an individual can tolerate without external inter-

vention. Threshold is unique to each individual, and the overall physiopsychological makeup of an individual must be considered when evaluating pain.

guarding A reflex usually related to abdominal pain; the action of muscles tensing, knees drawn up and/or hand placed over a part to prevent examination and/or protect against increasing pain.

rebound tenderness A sensation of pain felt when pressure applied on a body part is released.

Part 2—Vocabulary Used when Recording Information Obtained from the Review of Systems

The following vocabulary lists *some* of the terms that an examiner may use when recording the *subjective* findings of the review of systems (ROS) of a patient. Terms are presented in the order in which they appear in the patient's ROS and under the body part or system for which they are used in describing ROS findings (see also Chapter 18).

Eyes

photophobia (fo"to-fo′be-ah) An abnormal visual intolerance to light.

Ears

tinnitus (tĭ-nī′tus) A ringing or buzzing noise in the ears.

Nose

coryza (ko-rī′zah) A head cold; an acute inflammation of the nasal mucous membrane with a profuse discharge

epistaxis (ep″ĭ-stak′sis) A nosebleed; hemorrhage from the nose. Many episodes of epistaxis are caused by the rupture of the small vessels over the anterior part of the cartilaginous nasal septum.

Respiratory

asthma (az'mah) Recurrent attacks of difficulty in breathing (dyspnea) with wheezing that is caused by spasms in the bronchial tubes.

expectoration (ek-spek"to-ra'shun) The coughing up, expulsion, or spitting out of material (mucus, sputum, or phlegm) from the throat, trachea, bronchi, or lungs.

hemoptysis (he-mop'tĭ-sis) The spitting and/or coughing up of blood from the respiratory tract caused by bleeding in any part of the respiratory tract. In true hemoptysis sputum is frothy with air bubbles and bright red. (Hemoptysis must not be confused with *hematemesis,* in which a dark red- or black-colored substance is ejected from the gastrointestinal tract.)

hyperventilation (hi"per-ven"tĭ-lā'shun) Abnormal deep and prolonged breathing; increase in the inspirations and expirations of air resulting from an increase in the depth or rate of respirations or both. This results especially with depletion of carbon dioxide. This condition is often associated with emotional tension or acute anxiety situations.

Cardiovascular (CV)

palpitation (pal"pĭ-tā'shun) An unusually strong, rapid, or irregular heartbeat, usually over 120 beats per minute (normal heart rate varies between 60 to 100 beats per minute). Palpitation is often the result of strong exertion, nervousness, excitement, or the taking of certain medications. Palpitations may also result from a variety of heart disorders.

peripheral edema
(pĕ-rif'er-al) Pertaining to the periphery, which means   the surface or outward structures.
(e-de'mah) An abnormal accumulation of fluid in the   intercellular spaces of the body.

varicosity (var"ĭ-kos'ĭ-te) Pertaining to a varicose condition; distended, swollen veins.

Gastrointestinal (GI)

anorexia (an"o-rek'se-ah) Loss of appetite. Anorexia can be caused by illness, emotional upsets, or unattractive food.

colic (kol'ik) Pertaining to the colon; abdominal pain caused by spasmodic contractions of the intestinal tract.

constipation (kon"stĭ-pa-shun) Difficult elimination of fecal material from the intestinal tract; often the infrequent passage of waste material that is hard to eliminate easily results in the passage of unduly dry and hard fecal material.

diarrhea (di"ah-re'ah) The rapid movement of fecal material through the intestine, the feces having more or less fluid consistency; primarily a result of increased peristalsis in the intestinal tract.

distention (dis-ten'shun) The state of being stretched out, or distended.

dysphagia (dis-fā'jē-ah) Difficulty in swallowing.

flatus (fla'tus) Air or gas in the gastrointestinal tract.

hemorrhoid (hem'ŏ-roid); also called *piles* A dilated blood vessel in the anus that may bleed, cause discomfort or pain, and itch.

jaundice (jawn'dis); also called *icterus* (ik'ter-us) A symptom of different disorders of the gallbladder, liver, and blood characterized by yellowness of the skin, mucous membranes, and whites of the eyes caused by excessive bilirubin in the blood and deposition of bile pigments.

melena (mĕ-lē'nah) Black fecal material; blood pigments darken the feces.

Genitourinary (GU)

enuresis (en"u-re'sis) The involuntary excretion of urine, especially at night during sleep; bedwetting; most commonly seen in children with physical or emotional problems.

frequency (fre'kwen-se) The need to urinate frequently.

hesitancy Dysuria caused by nervous inhibition or obstruction in the vesical outlet.

incontinence (in-kon ti-nens) The inability to refrain from the urge to urinate. This may occur in times of stress, anxiety, or anger; or because of obstructions that prevent the normal emptying of the urinary bladder, spasms of the bladder, irritation caused by injury or inflammation of the urinary tract, damage to the spinal cord or brain, or the development of a fistula (an abnormal tubelike passage) between the bladder and the vagina or urethra. The word also may refer to fecal incontinence caused by nervous disorders or weakening of the anal sphincter.

nocturia (nok-tu're-ah) Excessive urination at night.

potency (po'ten-se) The ability of a male to have sexual intercourse.

renal colic (re'nal kol'ik) Spasms accompanied by pain that radiates from the kidney region around to the abdomen and into the groin. Renal colic is experienced during movement of a stone in the ureter.

retention (rē-ten'shun) The process of urine accumulating the bladder because of the individual's inability to urinate.

urgency The immediate need to urinate.

urination (u"rĭ-na'shun); also called *micturition* (mik"tu-rish'un) Voiding; the act of passing urine from the body.

venereal (vĕ-ne're-al) *disease* A disease that is transmitted by sexual contact and intercourse. Venereal disease is now more commonly referred to as a *sexually transmitted disease*. Abbreviations used are VD and STD.

Female reproductive

abortion (ah-bor'shun) The termination of a pregnancy before the fetus is capable of surviving outside of the uterus. In lay terminology, *abortion* refers to a deliberate interruption of pregnancy by various methods, and *miscarriage* refers to the natural loss of the fetus *(spontaneous abortion)*.

dyspareunia (dis'pah-ru'ne-ah) Difficult or painful genital sexual intercourse in women.

gravida (grav'ĭ-dah) A pregnant woman. During the first pregnancy the woman would be referred to as Gravida I *(primigravida)*, and so on with each succeeding pregnancy.

leukorrhea (loo"ko-re'ah) An abnormal yellow or white mucus discharge from the cervix or vaginal canal. Leukorrhea may be a symptom of pathological changes in the vagina and endocervix.

menarche (mĕ-nar'ke) The beginning of the menstrual functions in a woman.

menopause (men'o-pawz) The period in a woman's life at which the menstrual cycles decrease and gradually stop; the period when menstruation and the ability to have a child cease because the ovaries stop functioning. Menopause is often referred to as *the change of life* and also called the *climacteric*.

parous (pa'rus) Having borne at least one child. For example, if a woman has one live child and is now pregnant for the second time, she would be referred to as Gravida II, Para I (see *gravida*).

Endocrine

goiter (goi'ter) An enlargement of the thyroid gland.

Skin

allergy (al'er-je) An abnormal condition of individual hypersensitivity to substances *(allergens)* that are usually harmless. Allergens, substances capable of inducing hypersensitivity, can be almost any substance in the environment. Examples of allergens to which people become sensitive include dust, animal hairs, plant and tree pollens, mold spores, soaps, detergents, cosmetics, dyes, foods, feathers, plastics, and even some valuable medicines. When the allergen is in contact with or enters the body, it sets off a chain of events that brings about the allergic reaction. The allergen itself is not directly responsible for the allergic reaction. An allergy does not develop on the first contact with the allergen, but can develop on the second contact or even years later, after repeated contact with the allergen. Signs and symptoms of the allergies include sneezing, stuffed up and running nose, watery eyes, itching, coughing, shortness of breath, wheezing, rashes, skin eruptions, slight local edema, and also mild to severe anaphylactic shock, which can be fatal unless treated.

mole (mōl) A discolored blemish or growth on the skin; also called a *nevus*.

ulcer (ul'ser) An open sore or lesion on the surface of the skin or mucous membranes of the body, produced by the sloughing of dead inflammatory tissues.

Musculoskeletal

atrophy (at'ro-fe) A wasting away and decrease in size of a normal tissue or organ.

dislocation (dis'lo-ka'shun) The displacement of a bone from its normal position in a joint.

fracture (frak'chŭr) A break in the continuity of a bone. Broad classification of fractures are *open fracture*, in which the bone penetrates the skin, producing an open wound; and *closed fracture*, in which there is no break in the skin.

spasm (spazm) An involuntary sudden movement or contraction of a muscle or group of muscles, commonly accompanied by pain, and varying from mild twitches to severe convulsions. Spasms may be *clonic*, in which muscles alternate between contracting and relaxing; or *tonic*, in which the contraction of the muscle is sustained. Tonic spasms are the more severe type, because they are caused by diseases that affect the brain or central nervous system, such as rabies or tetanus.

tetany (tet'ah-ne) A continuous tonic spasm of a muscle without distinct twitching. The spasms are usually sudden, periodic, or they involve the extremities.

Neurologic

convulsion (kun-vul′shun) Involuntary spasms or contractions of muscles caused by an abnormal stimulus to the brain or by changes in the chemical balance of the body.

paralysis (pah-ral′ĭ sis) A state caused by damage to parts of the nervous system resulting in impairment or loss of motor function in a part or parts of the body.

paresthesia (par″es-the′ze-ah) An abnormal sensation experienced without an objective cause. Examples include a burning, tingling, or numb feeling.

tremor (trem′or) An involuntary quivering or trembling movement of the body or limbs caused by alternate contractions of opposing muscles. Tremors may have a psychological or a physical cause or both.

vertigo (ver′tĭ-go) A sensation of dizziness, rotation of oneself or of external objects in one's surroundings.

Part 3— Vocabulary Used in Recording Physical Findings

The following vocabulary lists *some* of the terms that an examiner may use in recording the *objective* findings of the physical examination of a patient. Each term is presented under the body part or system for which it is used when describing the findings of the physical examination. The order in which the body part or system is presented follows the usual sequence that examiners follow in performing a physical examination.

Skin

abrasion (ah-bra′zhun) A scrape on the surface of the skin or on a mucous membrane, for example, a skinned knee.

avulsion (a-vul′shun) A piece of soft tissue that is torn loose or left hanging as a flap.

contusion (kon-too′zhun) A bruise; an injury to the tissues without skin breakage. In a contusion blood seeps into the surrounding tissues from the injured and broken blood vessels, causing pain, tenderness, swelling, and discoloration of the surface skin.

cyanosis (si″ah-no′sis) A bluish discoloration of mucous membranes and skin.

ecchymosis (ek″ĭ-mo′sis) A round or irregular nonelevated hemorrhagic spot on mucous membranes or skin. The appearance is that of a blue-black or purplish patch changing to yellow or greenish brown. An ecchymosis is *larger* than a petechia.

erythema (er″ĭ-the′mah) A redness of the skin caused by capillary congestion in the lower layers of the skin. Erythema will be present in any inflammatory process, infection, or injury of the skin.

jaundice (jawn′dis) See in ROS vocabulary

laceration (las″ĭ-rā′shun) A tear or jagged-edged wound of body tissue.

petechia (pe-te′ke-ah) A tiny, round, nonraised, purplish red spot caused by submucous or intradermal hemorrhage. Later a petechia will turn blue or yellow. Small red patches.

purpura (per′pu-rah) Purpura is a hemorrhagic disease of obscure cause. It is characterized by the escape or discharge of blood from vessels into tissues under the skin and through mucous membranes, producing small red patches and bruises on the skin.

turgor (tur′gor) The condition of normal tension or fullness in a cell.

ulcer (ul′ser) See under ROS vocabulary.

urticaria (ur″tĭ-ka′re-ah) Also called *hives*. An inflammatory reaction of the skin characterized by the appearance of slightly elevated red or pale patches that are often itchy.

Eyes

acuity (ah-ku′ĭ-te) Clearness, sharpness, or acuteness of vision.

adnexa (ad-nek′sah) Accessory organs of the eye.

arcus senilis (ar′kus seni′lis) An opaque white ring partially surrounding the margin of the cornea, usually seen in people 50 years old or older. This condition often occurs bilaterally and is a result of fat granules depositing in the cornea or lipoid degeneration.

fundus (fun′dus) (of the eye) The back portion of the interior of the eye. The physician can observe this part of the eye by looking into or through the pupil of the eye with an ophthalmoscope.

nystagmus (nĭs-tag′mus) The constant, involuntary, rhythmic movement of the eyeball in any direction.

papilledema (pap″il-ĕ-de′mah) Edema and inflammation of the optic nerve, usually caused by intracranial pressure as a result of a brain tumor pressing on the optic nerve.

ptosis (to′sis) A drooping of the upper eyelids caused by paralysis.

Ears

cerumen (sĕ-roo′men) Earwax.

tympanic (tim-pan′ik) *membrane; also called eardrum*   A thin membrane that separates the middle ear from the outer ear.

Nose

nares (na′rēz)   The external openings into the nasal cavity; the nostrils.

nasal septal defect   A deviation of the bone and cartilage that divides the nasal cavity so that one part of the nasal cavity is larger than the other. On occasion this may produce difficulty in normal breathing, prevent normal drainage from infected sinuses, and interfere with the normal flow of mucus from the sinuses when one has a cold.

Neck

supple (sup′l)   Easily movable.

Respiratory system

fremitus (frem′ĭ-tus)   A vibration or tremor felt through the chest wall, usually during palpation.
  tactile fremitus   A vibration felt when a person speaks.
  tussive fremitus   A vibration felt when a person coughs.
  vocal fremitus   A vibration heard during auscultation of the chest wall when a person speaks.

friction rub; also called *rub*   A sound heard during auscultation that is produced when two serous membrane surfaces rub together.

rale (rahl)   An abnormal respiratory sound heard when the physician auscultates the chest. A rale indicates a pathological condition. There are many types of rales. Examples include a *dry rale*, which is a whistling or squeaky sound as heard in a person who has bronchitis or asthma; a *moist rale*, which is produced by fluid in the bronchial tubes; and a *crepitant rale*, which is a dry, crackling sound heard in the early stages of pneumonia when the person completes an inspiration.

resonance (rez′o-nans)   The quality of sound heard when the physician is examining the chest wall by percussion.

rhonchus (rong′kus) (pl. *rhonchi*)   A dry rale in the bronchus or a rattling in the throat.

rub   See under friction rub, above.

sputum (spu′tum)   The mucus secretion that comes from the lungs, bronchi, and trachea and that is ejected from the mouth. *Saliva* is not the same as sputum; saliva is secreted from the salivary glands in the mouth.

stridor (stri′dor)   A harsh shrill respiratory sound heard during inspirations in individuals who have laryngeal obstruction.

Cardiovascular system (CVS)

bruit (brū′ē)   A blowing sound heard over an aneurysm during auscultation of the cardiovascular system.

congestion (kon-jes′chun)   An abnormal accumulation of blood in a body part.

ecchymosis   See under Skin, p. 664.

engorgement (en-gorj′ment)   A distention of a body part with blood.

erythema   See under Skin, p. 664.

gallop (gal′op)   A disordered rhythm of the heart heard during auscultation. In a gallop rhythm three or four extra sounds are heard during the diastolic phase; the sounds are related to atrial contraction.

infarction (in-fark′shun)   A localized area of deficiency of blood in a part causing death to the cells. This is caused by blockage of arterial blood supply to the area. With reference to the heart, the term *myocardial infarction* is used. This pertains to the death of the cells in the myocardial layer of the heart caused by the lack of blood supply to the area.

ischemia (is-ke′me-ah)   The deficiency of blood in a body part. Ischemia may be caused by an obstruction in a blood vessel, such as from a clot or cholesterol deposits, or by a functional constriction.

murmur (mer′mer)   A sound heard during ausultation that is cardiac or vascular in origin, especially a periodic sound of short duration. This sound may be heard over the aortic valve, over the apex of the heart, or over an artery; all of these indicate possible disease in the particular area.

petechia   See under Skin, p. 664.

purpura   See under Skin, p. 664.

resuscitation (rĕ-sus″ĭ-ta′shun)   The act of restoring life or consciousness to a person whose respirations have stopped and who is thought to be dead.

rub; also called *friction rub*   See under Respiratory System.
  pericardial rub   A rub associated with inflammation of the pericardium. When this condition is present during auscultation the physician will hear a grating or scraping sound with the heartbeat.

thrill (thril)   A vibration that is felt by the physician when palpating the area over the heart, either during diastole or systole.

Abdomen

ascites (ah-si'tēz) An abnormal excessive accumulation of serous fluid in the peritoneal cavity that may cause abdominal distention. Ascites can be caused by a variety of conditions, some of which are tumors, kidney and heart disease, inflammation of the abdominal cavity, and cirrhosis of the liver.

contour (kon'toor) The outline or shape, as of the abdomen.

distention See under ROS vocabulary.

flaccid See under Musculoskeletal System.

hernia (her'ne-ah) An abnormal projection or protrusion of an organ or tissue or part of an organ through the wall of the cavity in which it is normally contained.

protuberant (pro-tu'ber-ant) With reference to the abdomen, an area that projects out or is prominent beyond the usual surface abdominal area.

scaphoid (skaf'oid) In reference to the abdomen, appearing as having a hollowed anterior wall; boat-shaped.

rigidity See under Muscloskeletal System.

Gastrointestinal system (GI)

caries (ka're-ēz, kăr'ēz) The decay of teeth or bone.

distention (dis-ten'shun) See under ROS vocabulary.

fissure (fish'er) A slit or cracklike sore. For example, an anal fissure is a lineal ulcer at the border of the anus.

fistula (fis'tu-lah) An abnormal tubelike passage from a tube, organ, or cavity to another cavity or organ or from an internal organ to a free body surface.

hemorrhoid (hem'o-roid) A varicose (enlarged) vein in the mucous membrane just outside (external hemorrhoid) or inside (internal hemorrhoid) the rectum. Also called piles, these enlarge veins may be painful and itchy and may bleed.

peristalsis (per"ĭ-stal'sis) A wavelike movement by which tubular organs and the alimentary canal propel their contents. Peristalsis is an involuntary movement seen in tubes that have both circular and longitudinal layers of smooth muscle fibers.

Reproductive system

adnexa (ad-nek'sah) Accessory organs of the uterus (ovaries, uterine tubes, and ligaments).

atrophy (at'ro-fe) A decrease in size of organs or tissues after having reached full functional development. Atrophy is seen in the female reproductive organs after menopause.

gravida See under ROS vocabulary.

introitus (in-tro'ĭ-tus) The opening into a body cavity or canal, as the opening into the vagina.

involution (in"vol-lu'shun) The retrogressive change in the size and the vital processes of organs and tissues after they have fulfilled their functions, such as is seen after menopause or in the reduction in size of the uterus after birth.

parous See under ROS vocabulary.

Musculoskeletal system (MS)

crepitation (krep"ĭ-tā'shun) A crackling, grating sound produced by movement of the ends of a fractured bone.

exostosis (ek"sos-to'sis) A new bony growth arising and projecting from the surface of a bone, characteristically capped by cartilage.

flaccid (flak'sid) Relaxed, soft, weak, flabby; applied especially to muscles that lack muscular tone.

gait (gāt) The style or manner in which a person walks.

kyphosis (ki-fo'sis); also called *hunchback* When viewing a person from the side, the examiner sees an abnormal convexity in the curvature of the thoracic spine.

lordosis (lor-do'sis) An abnormal forward curvature of the lumbar spine.

protuberance (pro-tu'ber-ans) A part that projects or is prominent beyond the usual surface area.

rigidity (rĭ-jid'ĭ-te) A state of being stiff or inflexible.

scoliosis (sko"le-o'sis) A lateral curvature of the vertebral column that usually consists of two curves, one in the opposite direction from the first.

supple (sup'l) Flexible, limber, or easily bent.

Extremities

claudication (klaw"dĭ-kā'shun) Limping, lameness.
  intermittent claudication A severe pain, tension, and weakness in the calf muscles that occurs after walking is begun and that subsides when walking stops and the limb has been resting. This condition is seen in patients with occlusive arterial disease in the limbs.

clubbing (klub'ing) A process or result of rapid reproduction of the soft tissue on the ends of the fingers and toes, as seen in adults with long-standing pulmonary disease.

edema (ĕ-de'mah) An abnormal accumulation of fluid in the body's intercellular spaces. It can be local or general.

passive congestion (kon-jes'chun) An abnormal accumulation of blood in an area on the body.

ulcer (ul'ser) See under ROS vocabulary.

varicosity (var″ĭ-kos′ĭ-te) (pl. *varicosities)* The condition of being varicose; a swollen, distended, enlarged, and twisted vein.

General

cachexia (kah-kek′se-ah) A general state of ill health, wasting away, and malnutrition, as seen in many chronic diseases.

diaphoresis (di″ah-fo-re′sis) Perspiration.

dehydration (de″hi-dra′shun) The condition that results when water output exceeds water intake; the excessive loss of water from the tissues or body.

emaciation (e-ma″se-a′shun) A condition in which the body is extremely thin and wasting away. Emaciation is generally caused by extreme malnutrition or diseases of the gastrointestinal tract.

fingerbreadth (fing′ger-bredth) The width of the finger from side to side, used when measuring the width of something, such as a lesion, or when measuring the distance between two areas, for example, "two fingerbreaths from the umbilicus."

lethargic (leth′ar′gic) The state of being indifferent, drowsy, or sluggish.

patulous (pat′u-lus) The state of being open, spread apart widely, or distended.

tenderness (ten′der-nes) A sensitivity to touch or pressure.

Part 4—Sample Reports

The following are samples of medical reports as dictated by a physician. Terms that have been defined for you in this appendix are italicized in the first report. You should be able to discuss the contents of each report and define the medical terms used. See pp. 668-670.

Patient #1—physical examination

General

Blood pressure 140/96 lying, with a pulse of 92, going to 140/100 standing up, with a pulse of 116. Respirations were 20, temperature was 37°. Generally a well-developed male appearing in no acute distress.

Skin

The skin had a midline abdominal scar and a healing *laceration* on the left medial buttock area. There was no *diaphoresis* or *jaundice*. *Turgor* was good; was not *dehyrated*.

Head, eyes, ears, nose, and throat

Atraumatic; extraocular movements were positive; pupils were equal, round and reactive to light, without *nystagmus*. The *fundi* were remarkable for increased tortuosity of vessels, with hemorrhages and exudates present in both retinae; his discs were flat. *Tympanic membranes* showed old scarring, but normal light reflexes. Moderate amount of *cerumen* in both ears. Oropharynx was clear and edentulous. Slight *rhinitis* present.

Neck

Supple, without increase, decrease, or asymmetrical thyroid enlargement. There were no *bruits.*

Nodes

No cervical, supraclavicular, or axillary nodes. He did have positive occipital and inguinal nodes, old.

Lungs

Decreased respiratory movements; there was a slight increase in his AP diameter; positive end-inspiratory wheezing, with inspiration; expiration ratio of 1:1.2. The patients was without *rales;* he did have scattered *rhonchi*. There was no increased or decreased vocal or tactile *femitus.*

Cardiovascular examination

Examination of the heart showed a point of maximal impulse in the fifth intercostal space, midclavicular line; no heave, *thrill,* or thrust; no S-3, S-4, or *murmur*. Pulses were 2+ and equal throughout, without *bruits.* The carotids were good and up bilaterally without bruits.

Abdomen

The liver was 12 cm by *percussion;* no spleen, kidney, or bladder palpable; bowel sounds were active, without *distention*. *Hernia* repair scar in right inguinal region.

Rectal examination

The rectal examination was guaiac-negative. Prostate was symmetrically enlarged, without nodularity or mass.

Extremities

There was full range of motion, without *cyanosis, clubbing,* or *edema.*

Neurologic examination

Oriented times three. Abstract thought and short- and long-term memory were intact. There was no sensory, motor, or cerebellar abnormality in his lower or upper extremities. His cranial nerves II through XII were within normal limits. His reflexes were 1+ and equal throughout except for absent ankle jerks, with downgoing toes. Negative straight leg raising. No root, grasp, or suck reflexes were noted. *Gait* was normal.

Patient #2—admission history and physical

CARDIUM, Mr. Perry
#35-28-27
Room 385

Date of admission

September 3, 1991

Physician

Hardnose, Christopher, MD

Chief complaint

Swelling of the feet.

Present illness

This patient is seen by me for the first time for Dr. Richards. He is a 62-year-old man who complains of swelling of the feet, painless, of some days duration. The history is not clear. The patient is somewhat confused. He had alcoholic breath at the time of entry. He denies having any pains in his chest or shortness of breath and cannot tell me if he has gained or lost weight. Medications taken, to the best of my knowledge, are Pro-Banthine, 15 mg, four times a day, which the patient had with him, and he says that he has taken "water pills."

Past history

He appears to have been under the care of a number of doctors in the preceding years. He denies ever being icteric, except that he was told by a doctor some months ago that he had a yellow color to his eyes. The patient says he is allergic to penicillin. He tells me that he was assaulted and robbed approximately 18 months ago, knocked unconscious, and that the left side of his jaw was fractured at the time. The patient is unable to give me any additional history, except that he says that he had an operation on his left knee many years ago.

Family history

Unobtainable at this time.

Social history

The patient denies the consumption of alcohol. He is a cigarette smoker. He used to be in the Navy and subsequently he was a merchant seaman.

Review of systems
HEENT

The patient had bilateral cataract removal sometime in the past. So far as his hearing, smell, taste, voice, swallowing, etc. there is no difficulty.

Cardiorespiratory

There is no complaint of palpitation, weight gain, chest pain, cough, or wheezing.

Extremities

The patient states that his feet have been swollen.

Gastrointestinal

He denies indigestion, melena, nausea, or vomiting.

Genitourinary

He states that of recent date he has burning on urination.

Neuromuscular

Noncontributory.

Physical examination

Large, well-developed man, confused, with a pleasant personality, tending to joke. He is quite agreeable for all the things being done to him. He appears to be cooperative. There is an alcoholic odor to his breath. There is no dyspnea, or cervical venous stasis, or cough, or pallor, but his sclerae are deeply icteric. There is no wheezing present.

HEENT

Previous surgery on the eyes for the removal of cataracts.

Skin

Extremely dry. The tongue is in the midline, coated, or good color, and well papillated. The buccal lining appears to be unremarkable.

Lymph nodes

No adenopathy.

Neck

The thyroid is clinically normal.

Chest

Clear.

Heart

Heart tones are of faint quality. There are no murmurs, enlargement, thrills, rubs, or decompensations made out at the moment, except for the fact that on the basis of percussion there may be enlargement of his heart to the left.

Breasts

There is some gynecomastia.

Abdomen

Shows no distention or ascites, muscle spasm, or masses. No areas of tenderness are present. His liver is enlarged 7 fingerbreadths below the xiphoid and extremely tender. Nodules cannot be made out. The gallbladder, spleen, and kidneys are not palpable or tender.

Extremities

The tip of his left index finger is absent. The skin is very dry. The patient has considerable pitting edema of his feet, extending just above the ankles. Both calf muscles are quite tender. There is no phlebitis or varicosity present. The temporal, carotid, subclavian, radial, and femoral arteries are normal and equal. I do not feel the dorsalis pedis or posterior tibial pulses.

Cardiac

ECG taken on entry showed some ischemic changes. I suspect that there is a prolongation of the Q-T interval. U waves are not identified at this reading.

Genitourinary

Voided urine specimen at the time of his entry is extremely dark. External genitalia are unremarkable.

Rectal

Anus and digital exploration of the rectum and prostate are unremarkable. Rectal sphincter tone is practically absent. The stool is medium brown color on the glove and shows a trace of occult blood.

Impression

An inflammatory involvement of the liver at present, quite possibly as a result of alcohol. A secondary consideration is cardiovascular decompensation, but this is much less likely.

HC: bkr
D: 9-3-91
T: 9-7-91

Hardnose, Christopher, MD

Appendix D

Two-Letter State Abbreviations

Alabama	AL	Montana	MT
Alaska	AK	Nebraska	NE
Arizona	AZ	Nevada	NV
Arkansas	AR	New Hampshire	NH
California	CA	New Jersey	NJ
Canal Zone	CZ	New Mexico	NM
Colorado	CO	New York	NY
Connecticut	CT	North Carolina	NC
Delaware	DE	North Dakota	ND
District of Columbia	DC	Ohio	OH
Florida	FL	Oklahoma	OK
Georgia	GA	Oregon	OR
Guam	GU	Pennsylvania	PA
Hawaii	HI	Puerto Rico	PR
Idaho	ID	Rhode Island	RI
Illinois	IL	South Carolina	SC
Indiana	IN	South Dakota	SD
Iowa	IA	Tennessee	TN
Kansas	KS	Texas	TX
Kentucky	KY	Utah	UT
Louisiana	LA	Vermont	VT
Maine	ME	Virginia	VA
Maryland	MD	Virgin Islands	VI
Massachusetts	MA	Washington	WA
Michigan	MI	West Virginia	WV
Minnesota	MN	Wisconsin	WI
Mississippi	MS	Wyoming	WY
Missouri	MO		

Appendix E

English Words Commonly Misspelled or Misused

absence
accessible
achieve
alignment
analyses (pl.)
analysis (sing.)
analyze
argument
auxiliary
believe
brochure
changeable
clientele
concede
conscientious
conscious
corroborate
definitely
desirable
development
dilemma
discreet
discrete
dissatisfaction
dissipate
drunkenness
ecstasy
eligible
embarrass

exceed
exhilaration
independent
indispensable
inevitable
inoculate
insistent
irregular
irrelevant
irresistible
irreversible
irritable
judgment
labeled
license
liquefy
maintenance
maneuver
miscellaneous
noticeable
occasion
occurrence
pamphlet
parallel
pastime
perseverance
persistent
personal
personnel

precede
precedent
predominant
prerogative
prevalent
principal
principle
questionnaire
rearrange
receive
recommend
recurrence
refer
referring
separate
sizable
stationary
stationery
subpoena
succeed
suddenness
superintendent
supersede
thorough
tranquility
transferred
unnecessary
vacuum
warrant

Appendix F

Medical Words Commonly Misspelled

abscess
adhesion
aerosol
anastomosis
anesthetic
aneurysm
arrhythmia
asthma
bruit
bulbous
cachexia
callus
capillary
catarrh
cholecystectomy
cirrhosis
coccyx
concussion
convalescence
coryza
curettage
cyanosis
diaphoresis
diarrhea
dissect
distention
dyspareunia
dyspnea
ecchymosis
eczema
epididymis
erythema
fascia
fibrillation
fissure
flatulence
gait
gonorrhea
graafian
hemoptysis
hemorrhage
hemorrhoid
idiosyncrasy
immunology
infarct

inflammation
inpatient
introitus
ischemia
keloid
laryngitis
larynx
malaise
malleolus
melena
menarche
menstruation
metastasis
metastasize
mucous
mucus
occlusion
ophthalmology
ophthalmoscope
orchitis
outpatient
palliative
paralyze
parietal
parous
paroxysm
paroxysmal
penicillin
perineal
peripheral
pernicious
phalanx
pharynx
phlebitis
phlegm
pneumococcus
pneumonia
pneumothorax
polyp
postoperative
presbyopia
prophylaxis
prostate
pruritus

pseudarthrosis
psoriasis
psychiatric
psychoanalysis
ptosis
pupillary
purulent
pyelitis
pyorrhea
pyrexia
rale
recurrence
rheumatism
rhinitis
rhythm
roentgenogram
salicylates
saphenous
schizoid
schizophrenia
sciatica
sclerosis
seizure
semiconscious
spherical
sphincter
sphygmomanometer
spondylosis
stimulant
subconscious
supple
suppuration
susceptible
staphylococcus
symmetrical
syphilis
thrombophlebitis
tinnitus
tonsil
tonsillectomy
urinalysis
varicose
venous
xiphoid

Suggested Readings

American Association of Medical Assistants: American Association of Medical Assistants bylaws, Chicago, 1979, The Association.

American Medical Association: Current opinions of the Judicial Council, Chicago, 1982, The Association.

American Medical Association: Professional liability and the physician, Chicago, 1963, The Association.

American Medical Association: The wonderful human machine, Chicago, 1976, The Association.

American Medical Association: Winning ways with patients, Chicago, 1979, The Association.

American National Red Cross: Advanced first aid and emergency care, ed 2, Garden City, NY, 1979, Doubleday & Co, Inc.

American Sterilizer Co: Sterilization aids, Erie, Pa, 1975.

Ames Co: Modern urine chemistry, a guide to the diagnosis of urinary tract diseases and metabolic disorders, rev reprint, Elkhart, Ind, 1982.

Ames Co: Urodynamics: concepts relating to routine urine chemistry, Elkhart, Ind, 1978.

Anderson RA, Kumpf W, and Kendirck RE: Business Law, principles and cases, ed 5, Cincinnati, 1971, South-Western Publishing Co.

Anthony CP and Thibodeau GA: Textbook of anatomy and physiology, ed 11, St Louis, 1983, The CV Mosby Co.

Artz C: Trauma can be conquered, Emerg Med Today pp 1-6, July 1974.

Asperheim M: Pharmacology for practical nurses, ed 5, Philadelphia, 1981, WB Saunders Co.

Austrin M: Young's learning medical terminology step by step, ed 5, St Louis, 1983, The CV Mosby Co.

Bauer JD, Ackermann PG, and Toro G: Clinical laboratory methods, ed 9, St Louis, 1982, The CV Mosby Co.

Beaumont E: Blood pressure equipment, Nursing 75 5:56, Jan 1975.

Beaumont E: Diagnostic kits, Nursing 75 5:28, April 1975.

Bergeron JD: First responder, ed 2, Bowie Md, 1987, Robert J Brady Co.

Bergersen B: Pharmacology in nursing, ed 14, St Louis, 1979, The CV Mosby Co.

Bird B: Talking with patients, ed 2, Philadelphia, 1973, JB Lippincott Co.

Black HC: Black's law dictionary, ed 6, 1983.

Blainey C: Site selection in taking body temperature, Am J Nurs 74:1859, Oct 1974.

Bolles, RN: What color is your parachute? Rev ed, Berkeley, Calif, 1987, Ten Speed Press.

Bredow M and Cooper M: The medical assistant, ed 4, New York, 1978, McGraw-Hill Book Co.

Brunner LS and others: The Lippincott manual of nursing practice, ed 4, Philadelphia, 1986, JB Lippincott Co.

Buckner J: Interpersonal skills: necessary conditions for professional helpers, Prof Med Assist 9:17, March/April 1976.

Burdick Corp: Electrocardiography: a better way, Milton, Wis, 1976.

California Medical Association: Arbitration for physicians in private practice, San Francisco, 1971, The Association.

California Medical Association: Professional liability, San Francisco, 1971, The Association.

Chabner DE: The language of medicine, ed 2, Philadelphia, 1981, WB Saunders Co.

Clarke WL and Pohl SL: New developments in blood glucose monitoring and insulin delivery, Occupational Health Nursing 30:40, Dec 1982.

Conover MH: Understanding electrocardiography: physiological and interpretive concepts, ed 4, St Louis, 1984, The CV Mosby Co.

Cope Z: Cope's early diagnosis of acute abdomen, ed 15, New York, 1979, Oxford University Press, Inc.

DeWeese DD and Saunders WH: Textbook of otolaryngology, ed 6, St Louis, 1982, The CV Mosby Co.

Dison N: Clinical nursing techniques, ed 4, St Louis, 1979, The CV Mosby Co.

Dison N: Simplified drugs and solutions for nurses, including arithmetic, ed 8, St Louis, 1984, The CV Mosby Co.

Dubay EC and Grubb RD: Infection: prevention and control, ed 2, St Louis, 1978, The CV Mosby Co.

DuGas B: Introduction to patient care, ed 4, Philadelphia, 1983, WB Saunders Co.

Ehrlich RA and Givens EMC: Patient care in radiography, ed 2, St Louis, 1985, The CV Mosby Co.

Fischer P and others: The office laboratory, Norwalk, Ct, 1983, Appleton-Century-Crofts.

Fowler NO: Inspection and palpation of venous and arterial pulses, New York, 1970, American Heart Association, Inc.

Frederick P and Kinn M: The medical office assistant: administrative and clinical, ed 5, Philadelphia, 1981, WB Saunders Co.

French RM: Guide to diagnostic procedures, ed 5, New York, 1981, McGraw Hill Book Co.

Frew MA and Frew DR: Medical office administrative procedures, Philadelphia, 1982, FA Davis Co.

Garb S: Laboratory tests in common use, ed 6, New York, 1976, Springer Publishing Co.

Garfield SR and others: Evaluation of new ambulatory medical care delivery system, N Engl J Med **294:**426, 1976.

Geolot D and McKinney N: Administering parenteral drugs, Am J Nurs **75:**788, May 1975.

Gordon M: Initial care of burn victim often a matter of life or death, Occupational Health and Safety, p 34, Jan 1984.

Gould JA and Davies GJ, eds: Orthopaedic and sports physical therapy, St Louis, 1985, The CV Mosby Co.

Govoni L and Hayes J: Drugs and nursing implications, ed 4, New York, 1985, Appleton-Century-Crofts.

Guthrie HA: Introductory nutrition, ed 5, St Louis, 1983, The CV Mosby Co.

Hahn RL, Burgess A, and Oestreich SJK: Pharmacology in nursing, ed 15, St Louis, 1982, The CV Mosby Co.

Hammond C: ECG's made easier than ever, RN **10:**42. Oct 1979.

Hammond C: ECG's made easier than ever—when the natural pacemakers fail, RN **11:**30, Nov 1979.

Hanna JM, Popham EL, and Tilton RS: Secretarial procedures and administration, ed 6, Cincinnati, 1973, South-Western Publishing Co.

Heidrich G and Perry S: Helping the patient in pain, Am J Nurs **82:**1828-1833, 1982.

Hemelt MD and Mackert ME: Dynamics of law in nursing and health care, Reston, Va, 1978, Reston Publishing Co, Inc.

Hicks DJ, Innes BS, and Shores WL: Patient care techniques, Indianapolis, 1975, The Bobbs-Merrill Co, Inc.

Hill G: Outpatient surgery, ed 2, Philadelphia, 1980, WB Saunders Co.

Hirsch CS, Moritz, AR, and Morris, RC: Handbook of legal medicine, ed 5, St Louis, 1979, The CV Mosby Co.

Hobson L: Examination of the patient, New York, 1975, McGraw-Hill Book Co.

Holvey DN and others: The Merck manual of diagnosis and therapy, ed 12, Rahway, NJ, 1972, Merck, Sharp and Dohme Research Laboratories.

Horsley JE: Don't close your practice until you read this, Med Econ, p 187, June 14, 1976.

Hughes EC, ed: Obstetric-gynecologic terminology, Philadelphia, 1972, FA Davis Co.

Insel PM and Roth WT: Core concepts in health, ed 4, Palo Alto, Calif, 1985, Mayfield Publishing Co.

Iorio J: Childbirth: family-centered nursing, ed 3, St Louis, 1975, The CV Mosby Co.

Jennings LM: Secretarial and administrative procedures, ed 2, Englewood Cliffs, NJ, 1983, Prentice-Hall, Inc.

Johnson MM and Kallaus NF: Records management, ed 2, Cincinnati, 1974, South-Western Publishing Co.

Kent TH, Hart MN, and Shires TK: Introduction to human disease, ed 2, New York, 1986, Appleton-Century-Crofts.

Kirkindall WM and others: Recommendations for human blood pressure determination by sphygmomanometers, New York, 1979, American Heart Association.

Krause MV and Mahan LK: Food, nutrition and diet therapy, ed 7, Philadelphia, 1984, WB Saunders Co.

Lewis L: Fundamental skills in patient care, ed 3, Philadelphia, 1984, JB Lippincott Co.

Littmann D: The electrocardiogram, New York, 1973, American Heart Association, Inc.

Loebl S, Spratto G, and Wit A: The nurse's drug handbook, ed 3, New York, 1983, John Wiley & Sons, Inc.

Long BC and Phipps WJ: Essentials of medical-surgical nursing, St Louis, 1985, The CV Mosby Co.

Malasanos L: Health assessment, ed 2, St Louis, 1981, The CV Mosby Co.

McCormick J, Rushing RL, and Davis WG: The Management of medical practice, Cambridge, Mass, 1978, Ballinger Publishing Co.

Mechner F: Examination of the eye. I. Am J Nurs **74:**2039, Nov 1974.

Memmler RL and Wood DL: The human body in health and disease, ed 6, Philadelphia, 1986, JB Lippincott Co.

Menard RH: Introduction to arrhythmia recognition, San Francisco, 1968, California Heart Association.

Meschan I: Radiographic positioning and related anatomy, ed 2, Philadelphia, 1978 WB Saunders Co.

Meshelany CM: Post-op wound dressing, RN **42:**22, May 1979.

Miller B and Keane C: Encyclopedia and dictionary of medicine, nursing, and allied health, ed 3, Philadelphia, 1983, WB Saunders Co.

Mueller C: Perfecting physical assessment. I. Nursing 77 **7:**28, May 1977.

Mueller C: Perfecting physical assessment. II. Nursing 77 **7:**38, June 1977.

Mueller C: Perfecting physical assessment. III. Nursing 77 **7:**44, July 1977.

Nealon T: Fundamental skills in surgery, ed 3, Philadelphia, 1979, WB Saunders Co.

Newton D and Newton M: Needles, syringes and sites for injectable medications, Am Pharmaceut Assoc J, **NS17:**685-687, Nov 1977.

Nichols GA and Kucha DH: Taking adult temperatures: oral measurement, Am J Nurs **72:**1090, 1972.

Oppenheim I: Textbook for laboratory assistants, ed 3, St Louis, 1981, The CV Mosby Co.

Parcel GS: First aid in emergency care, ed 3, St Louis, 1985, The CV Mosby Co.

Perkins J: Principles and methods of sterilization in health sciences, ed 2, Springfield Ill, 1982, Charles C Thomas, Publisher.

Pfizer Laboratories: How to give an intramuscular injection, New York, 1976.

Phelps J: Radiation protection and the medical assistant, Prof Med Assist 10:32, July/August 1977.

Phipps WJ, Long BC, and Woods NF: Medical-surgical nursing: concepts and clinical practice, ed 2, St Louis, 1983, The CV Mosby Co.

Pitel M: The subcutaneous injection, Am J Nurs 71:76-79 Jan 1971.

Pomerleau OF and Brady JP, eds: Behavioral medicine: theory and practice, Baltimore, 1984, The Williams & Wilkins Co.

Potts AM, ed: The assessment of visual function, St Louis, 1972, The CV Mosby Co.

Poulos J: Diagnostic tests: a guide to patient instruction, Prof Med Assist 8:15, May/June 1975.

Raphael S: Lynch's medical laboratory technology, ed 4, Philadelphia, 1983, WB Saunders Co.

Raus E and Raus M: Manual of history taking, physical examination and record keeping, Philadelphia, 1974, JB Lippincott Co.

Resler MM and Tumulty G: Glaucoma update, Am J Nurs 83:752-756, 1983.

Saver GC: Manual of skin diseases, ed 3, Philadelphia, 1973, JB Lippincott Co.

Scherer J: Introductory clinical pharmacology, ed 2, Philadelphia, 1982, JB Lippincott Co.

Shanas E: Health status of older people, Am J Public Health 64:261, 1974.

Sloboda S: Understanding patient behavior, Nursing 77 7:74, Sept 1977.

Smith AL: Microbiology and pathology, ed 12, St Louis, 1980, The CV Mosby Co.

Soukhanov AH and Haverty JR, eds: Webster's medical office handbook, Springfield, Mass, 1979, G & C Merriam Co, Publishers.

Stein E: The electrocardiogram: a self-study course in clinical electrocardiography, Philadelphia, 1976, WB Saunders Co.

Stephenson HE Jr, ed: Immediate care of the acutely ill and injured, ed 2, St Louis, 1978, The CV Mosby Co.

Stevens AD: Monitoring blood glucose at home—who should do it, Am J Nurs 81:2026, Nov 1981.

Strand MM and Elmer LA: Clinical laboratory tests, ed 3, St Louis, 1983, The CV Mosby Co.

Superintendent of Documents, US Government Printing Office: The postal manual, Washington, D.C.

Thomas V: Life sciences for nursing and health technologies, Long Beach, Calif, 1974, Technicourse Inc.

Thompson JM and Bowers AC: Health assessment—a pocket guide, St Louis, 1984, The CV Mosby Co.

Tilkian SM, Conover MB, and Tilkian AG: Clinical implications of laboratory tests, ed 3, St Louis, 1983, The CV Mosby Co.

US Department of Health, Education, and Welfare: Collection handling and shipment of microbiological specimens, Atlanta, 1973, Center for Disease Control.

US Department of Health, Education, and Welfare: Criteria and techniques for the diagnosis of gonorrhea, Atlanta, 1974, U.S. Public Health Service.

Van Meter M: What every nurse should know about EKGs, Nurs 75 5:19, April 1975.

Vaughan-Wrobel BC and Henderson B: The problem-oriented system in nursing—a workbook, ed 2, St Louis, 1982, The CV Mosby Co.

Walter JB: An introduction to the principles of disease, ed 2, Philadelphia, 1983, WB Saunders Co.

Warner CG: Emergency care: assessment and intervention, ed 3, St Louis, 1982, The CV Mosby Co.

Weed LL: Medical records, medical education, and patient care, Cleveland, 1971, The Press of Case Western Reserve University.

Westfall E: Electrical and mechanical events in the cardiac cycle, Am J Nurs 76:23, Feb 1976.

Williams RB Jr and Gentry WD, eds: Behavioral approaches to medical treatment, Cambridge, Mass, 1977, Ballinger Publishing Co.

Williams SR: Nutrition and diet therapy, ed 4, St Louis, 1982, The CV Mosby Co.

Wood L and Rambo B: Nursing skills for allied health services, ed 3, Philadelphia, 1982, WB Saunders Co.

Woolley F and others: Problem-oriented nursing, New York, 1974, Springer Publishing Co, Inc.

Wu R: Behavior and illness, Englewood Cliffs, NJ, 1973, Prentice-Hall, Inc.

Wyeth Laboratories: Intramuscular injections, Philadelphia, 1984.

Young CG and Barger JD: Introduction to medical science, ed 3, St Louis, 1977, The CV Mosby Co.

Zakus SM: Clinical skills and assisting techniques for the medical assistant, ed 2, St Louis, 1988, The CV Mosby Co.

Zimmer MJ: Quality assurance for outcomes of patient care, Nurs Clin North Am 9:305-315, June 1974.

Index